CARDIOVASCULAR/ RESPIRATORY PHYSIOTHERAPY

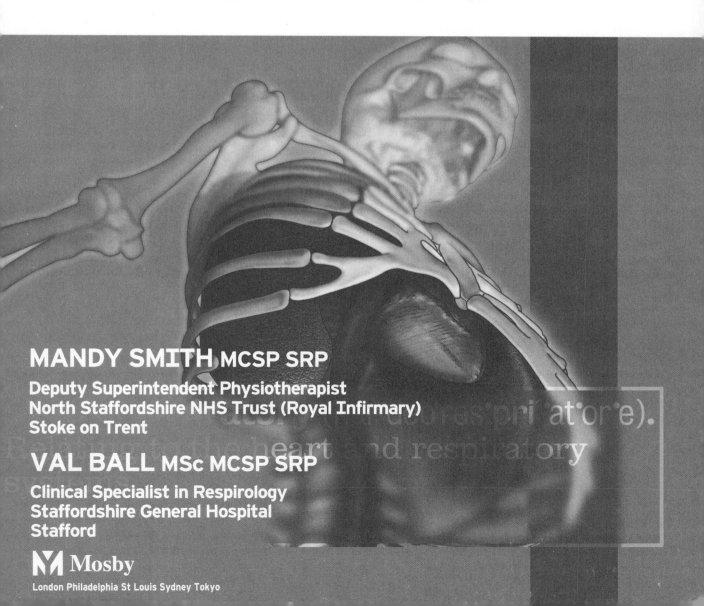

MANDY SMITH MCSP SRP

Deputy Superintendent Physiotherapist
North Staffordshire NHS Trust (Royal Infirmary)
Stoke on Trent

VAL BALL MSc MCSP SRP

Clinical Specialist in Respirology
Staffordshire General Hospital
Stafford

Mosby

London Philadelphia St Louis Sydney Tokyo

Publisher	**Jill Northcott**
Development Editor	**Gillian Harris**
Project Manager	**Adèle Collins**
Production	**Hamish Adamson**
Design	**Greg Smith**
Layout	**Gisli Thor**
Index	**Nina Boyd**
Cover Design	**Greg Smith**
Cover Illustration	**Mike Saiz**
Illustration Manager	**Danny Pyne**
Illustrators	**Deborah Gyan**
	Matthew McClements
	Marion Tasker
	Lynda Payne

Published in 1998 by Mosby, an imprint of Mosby International Limited

ISBN 0 7234 2595 7

Printed by Printer Trento s.r.l., Trento, Italy

Set in: Scala: Fontworks. Interstate: Font Bureau. (Supplied by Fontworks UK)

For full details of all Mosby titles, please write to Mosby International Publishers Limited, Lynton House, 7–12 Tavistock Square, London WC1H 9LB, UK.

A CIP catalogue record for this book is available from the British Library.

Library of Congress Cataloging-in-Publication Data has been applied for.

The aim of this textbook is to provide a compact, precise reference for undergraduate and immediate postgraduate physiotherapy staff dealing with respiratory and cardiovascular patients. The book also caters for physiotherapists re-entering or up-dating their respiratory skills.

With the changing structure of the National Health Service, physiotherapy has advanced to meet the demands of the developments and the needs of the patients around whom the service revolves. This requires closer management of resources both human and financial and is achieved by evidence-based practice, audit mechanisms and research to facilitate and justify appropriate use of our skills and therefore better time spent treating the patients who will benefit from our expertise.

The book acknowledges the role of enhanced nursing practice and demonstrates the move forward for physiotherapists from routine physiotherapy that is catered for by specialist nurses, to the advisory and preventative role, problem solving and the increase importance of early exercise.

The book highlights conditions, pathologies, treatment methods, team-players and the physiotherapy in common scenarios met in the general hospital.

The book emphasises the holistic approach to treating patients and the importance of the team and collaborative care. This enhances improved communication and ensures a high standard and quality of treatment.

We acknowledge that the diagnosis is often not the reason for a patient to benefit from physiotherapy but it is the reason for his signs and symptoms and hence our intervention.

SECTION 1: PHYSIOLOGY AND ASSESSMENT

These chapters cover aspects such as exercise physiology, control of ventilation, gaseous exchange and acid–base balance, and also assessment, including lung function, chest assessment, chest radiology and electrocardiography. Basic anatomy can be catered for by a reputable anatomy book.

SECTION 2: ADULT MANAGEMENT

This section includes adult management in hospital from the intensive care patient to the cancer victim.

SECTION 3: ON-CALL

The on-call service is an area of physiotherapy that causes much controversy in the shape of inappropriate use of the service. This section aims to support the physiotherapist in dealing with the on-call situation.

SECTION 4: PAEDIATRIC MANAGEMENT

This section encompasses all aspects of paediatric care from physiology to surgery and the physiotherapy management of common conditions. Clearly, major paediatric surgery is seen in specialist centres but the reader is presented with typical scenarios.

SECTION 5: RESEARCH AND AUDIT

Finally, Chapter 21 introduces the reader to research and clinical audit.

As experienced clinical educators, the design and content of the book results from the many questions and diversity of comments received from physiotherapy students and postgraduates.

The theme through the book is for easy, enjoyable reading and the content can be applied to any acute scenario. We acknowledge the lack of reference to the community physiotherapy service but feel this topic should be dealt with in a separate book.

We would like to thank all the contributors whose compliance and hard work allowed us to produce the work and extend special thanks to Mr CJ Smallpiece for his recommendations for the contributors and for his support. We also thank Janice Martin and Liz Murray for their critique and constructive advice. Please note that because many chapters are written by multi-authors, their names appear in alphabetical order.

Mrs Angela Adams RGN
Clinical Nursing Specialist, Intensive Care, North Staffordshire NHS Trust (City General), Newcastle Road, Stoke on Trent, Staffordshire ST4 6QG

Dr Martin B Allen MB FRCP
Consultant Physician, Department of Respiratory Medicine, North Staffordshire NHS Trust, Newcastle Road, Stoke on Trent, Staffordshire ST4 6QG

Mrs Val Ball MSc MCSP SRP
Clinical Specialist in Respirology, Staffordshire General Hospital, Weston Road, Stafford ST16 3SA

Mrs Samantha Brean MCSP SRP
Senior Physiotherapist, Cardiac Rehabilitation, Wythenshaw Hospital, South Moor Road, Wythenshaw, Manchester M23 9CT

Mr Graham Brett MCSP SRP
Senior Physiotherapist, Intensive Care and Surgery, North Staffordshire NHS Trust (City General), Newcastle Road, Stoke on Trent, Staffordshire ST4 6QG

Mr Gary Buchanan RGN BA ONC
Director of Training, Emergency Care Training Centre, HCI International Medical Centre, Beardmore Street, Clyde Bank, Glasgow G81 4HX

Dr Richard Carroll MB ChB MRCP
Specialist Registrar in Cardiology and British Heart Foundation Clinical Research Fellow, University College Hospital, Gower Street, London WC1E 6AU

Mrs Jane Chapman MA MCSP SRP
Acting Physiotherapy Manager, North Staffordshire Hospital NHS Trust, Physiotherapy Department (City General), Newcastle Road, Stoke on Trent, Staffordshire ST4 6QG

Dr Steve J Connellan DM FRCP
Consultant Physician, New Cross Hospital, Wolverhampton WV10 0QF

Mrs Maureen Conway MCSP SRP
Senior Douglas Macmillan Physiotherapist, Weston Infirmary, Glasgow G11 6NT

Mr Mark Danton FRCS
Specialist Registrar to Mr McGuigan, Northern Ireland Regional Thoracic-Surgical Department, Royal Victoria Infirmary, Grosvenor Road, Belfast BT12 6BA

Mrs Sarah Davey MCSP SRP
Senior Intensive Care Physiotherapist, Sheffield Children's Hospital, NHS Trust, Weston Bank, Sheffield S10 2TH

Mr Abdul K Deiraniya MB ChB FRCS
Consultant Cardiothoracic Surgeon, Wythenshaw Hospital, South Moor Road, Wythenshaw, Manchester M23 9CT

Dr Jane M Eddleston FRCS anaes
Clinical Director of Critical Care, Critical Care Unit, Manchester Royal Infirmary, Oxford Road, Manchester M13 9WL

Mr Ahmed El Gamel MB BCh FRCS
Specialist Registrar in Cardiothoracic Surgery, Wythenshaw Hospital, South Moor Road, Wythenshaw, Manchester M23 9CT

Mrs Denise Glover BSc MCSP SRP
Senior Physiotherapist, Blackfriars School, Priory Road, Newcastle under Lyme, Staffordshire ST5 2TS

Dr Melanie Greaves FRCR
Consultant Radiologist, North Staffordshire NHS Trust (Central Outpatients), Hartshill Road, Stoke on Trent ST4 7PA

Mr Kumarasingham Jeyansingham ChM FRCS
Consultant Thoracic Surgeon, Department of Thoracic Surgery, Frenchay Hospital, Bristol BS16 1LE

Mr Robin Kanagasabay BSc MRCS FRCS
Specialist Registrar in Cardiothoracics, St. George's Health Care, Blackshaw Road, London SW17 0QT

Mr Adrian Kendrick BA PhD
Clinical Scientist in Respiratory Physiology and Medicine, Sleep Unit, Bristol Royal Infirmary, Maulin Street, Bristol BS2 8HW

Mr Fergus MacBeth MA DM FRCP FRCR
Consultant Oncologist, Llandough Hospital, Penylan Road, Penarth CF6 2XX

Dr Andrew R Magnay MA MB Bchir MRCP (UK) FRCPCh
Consultant in Paediatric Intensive Care, North Staffordshire NHS Trust (City General), Newcastle Road, Stoke on Trent ST4 6QG

Ms Eleanor Main BSc BA MSc MCSP SRP
Physiotherapy Research Co-ordinator, Institute for Child Health, Physiotherapy Department, Great Ormond Street Hospital for Children NHS Trust, 30 Guilford Street, London WC1N 3EH

Mr James A McGuigan MB BAO FRCS
Consultant Thoracic Surgeon, Northern Ireland Regional Thoracic-Surgical Department, Royal Victoria Infirmary, Grosvenor Road, Belfast BT12 6BA

Mrs Pam Morgan DIP COT SROT
Amputee Support Co-ordinator, North Staffordshire Hospital, NHS Trust, Haywood Hospital, High Lane, Buslem, Stoke on Trent, Staffordshire ST6 7AG

Mr Richard H Morgan MD FRCS MB BCh
Consultant Vascular and General Surgeon, North Staffordshire NHS Trust (City General), Newcastle Road, Stoke on Trent, Staffordshire ST4 6QL

Mr Graham N Morritt MBBS FRCS(Ed) FRCP(Ed)
Consultant Cardiothoracic Surgeon, Cardiothoracic Unit, South Tees Acute Hospitals NHS Trust, Marton Road, Middlesborough, Cleveland TS4 3BW

Dr John C Mucklow MD FRCP
Consultant Clinical Pharmacologist, North Staffordshire NHS Trust (City General), Newcastle Road, Stoke on Trent ST4 6QG

Mrs Sue Neill MCSP SRP
Senior Physiotherapist, Transplant Team, Wythenshaw Hospital, South Moor Road, Wythenshaw, Manchester M23 9CT

Dr Charles FA Pantin MA PhD MRCP FRCP
Consultant Physician, Department of Respiratory Medicine, North Staffordshire NHS Trust, Newcastle Road, Stoke on Trent, Staffordshire ST4 6QG

Mrs Annette Parker MCSP SRP
Deputy Trust Physiotherapist, Taunton & Somerset Hospital, NHS Trust, Mosgrove Park Hospital, Taunton, Somerset TA1 5DA

Miss Marilyn Place MEd MCSP DipTP SRP CertEd
Head of School of Physiotherapy, Keele University, Keele, Staffordshire ST5 5BG

Mrs S Ammani Prasad
Senior Respiratory Physiotherapist, Great Ormond Street Hospital, Great Ormond Street, Bloomsbury, London WC1N 3JH

Dr Gavin Russell MD FRCP
Consultant Renal Physician, Department of Nephrology, North Staffordshire NHS Trust (Royal Infirmary), Princes Road, Hartshill, Stoke on Trent, Staffordshire ST4 7LN

Mrs Leslie Russell DSc SRD
Superintendent Dietician, Department of Dietetics, North Staffordshire NHS Trust (Royal Infirmary), Princes Road, Hartshill, Stoke on Trent, Staffordshire ST4 7LN

Mrs Sandy Robertson MSc MCSP DipTp Cert Ed SRP
Lecturer at the School of Physiotherapy, Keele University, Keele, Staffordshire ST5 5BG

Dr Sally Singh PhD MCSP
Pulmonary Rehabilitation Co-ordinator, Department of Respiratory Medicine and Thoracic Surgery, The Glenfield Hospital NHS Trust, Groby Road, Leicester LE3 9QP

Dr Barry Smith TD MB ChB FRCA
Consultant Anaesthetist, Anaesthetic Department, North Staffordshire NHS Trust (City General), Newcastle Road, Stoke on Trent, Staffordshire ST4 6QG

Mrs Mandy Smith MCSP SRP
Deputy Superintendent Physiotherapist, North Staffordshire NHS Trust (Royal Infirmary), Princes Road, Hartshill, Stoke on Trent, Staffordshire ST4 7LN

Prof Tom Treasure MD MS FRCS
Professor of Cardiothoracic Surgery, St George's Health Care, Blackshaw Road, London SW17 0QT

Miss Laura Yeo MA MCSP
Physiotherapist
Maryland Drive
Singapore

SECTION 1

PHYSIOLOGY AND ASSESSMENT

1

AH Kendrick

PHYSIOLOGY OF RESPIRATION

CHAPTER OUTLINE

- **Structure and function of the lungs**
- **Composition of inspired and alveolar gas**
- **Ventilation**
- **Diffusion**
- **Perfusion**
- **Ventilation-perfusion**

- **Gas transport**
- **Control of ventilation**
- **Acid-base balance**
- **Respiration during sleep**
- **Respiration during exercise**
- **Other functions of the lung**

INTRODUCTION

The main function of the respiratory system is the exchange of oxygen and carbon dioxide: oxygen is delivered from the atmosphere to cells, and carbon dioxide from cells to the atmosphere. Oxygen is required in the production of adenosine triphosphate (ATP), which provides a common energy source for various cellular activities including the synthesis of chemicals, and muscular contraction. The byproducts of ATP production include water and carbon dioxide.

To achieve gas exchange, a closely interrelated system is required. The lungs exchange oxygen and carbon dioxide between the atmosphere and the pulmonary circulation, called external respiration. Internal respiration is when the exchange of oxygen and carbon dioxide occurs at the cellular level between the systemic circulation and the cell. The circulatory system links these two respiratory systems.

This chapter describes the normal physiology of the respiratory system. The detail is broad but can be applied to both children and adults, and, unless stated otherwise, applies to the resting state. No description of disease processes or their effects is presented.

STRUCTURE AND FUNCTION OF THE LUNGS

The lungs consist of branching tubes that become narrower, shorter and more numerous with increasing distance from the trachea. The trachea divides into the right and left main bronchi, which then divide into lobar and then segmental bronchi. Branching continues until the terminal bronchioles are reached. Terminal bronchioles are the smallest airways without alveoli. Up to this point, the airways play no part in gas exchange but simply transport inspired air from the atmosphere to the gas-exchanging units, or alveoli. The respiratory system volume exclusive of alveoli constitutes the anatomical dead space (V_{anat}). From here, the airways divide into respiratory bronchioles, which have small groups of alveoli opening off their walls. Finally, the alveolar ducts, which are completely lined with alveoli, are reached. This branching is important as it increases the total cross-sectional area of tissue available for gas exchange, and slows air flow down so that the movement of gas by diffusion only.

The diffusion of oxygen and carbon dioxide occurs across the blood–gas interface, where the alveolar–capillary membrane separates the alveolar air from the pulmonary capillary blood (Figure 1.1). There are about 300 million alveoli in the adult human lung, giving a total surface area of 85 m² and a lung volume of 4.25 litres. As an approximation, the cross-sectional area of all the alveoli combined is about the size of a tennis court.

Blood flow to the lungs comes from the pulmonary circulation. Blood leaves the right ventricle of the heart via the pulmonary artery, which then divides into pulmonary capillaries that drain into the pulmonary veins, and on to the left atrium. The pulmonary capillary network is very dense and has the appearance of an almost continuous sheet of blood.

COMPOSITION OF INSPIRED AND ALVEOLAR GAS

Atmospheric air is a mixture of gases. Those of interest are oxygen and carbon dioxide. The composition of inspired gas at sea level remains fairly constant (Table 1.1). Inspired air at sea level or at altitude contains 20.93% oxygen. However, at sea level, atmospheric pressure (P_B; barometric pressure) is about 101 kPa while at the summit of

Mount Everest it is about 32 kPa. Thus, inspired PO_2 (P = partial pressure) decreases from 19.8 kPa to 5.4 kPa.

During inspiration, fresh gas from the atmosphere enters the airways, adding to and diluting the gas in the lungs. On completion of inspiration, the dead space contains atmospheric gas while the alveoli contain a constantly changing mixture from atmospheric gas to alveolar gas, as oxygen is removed and carbon dioxide is added. On expiration, the first gas to leave the lungs is atmospheric gas, then alveolar gas. Towards the end of expiration, the gas mixture is similar to that of alveolar gas.

VENTILATION

Ventilation is the exchange of air between the lungs and the ambient air (Figure 1.2). If the total volume of each breath during normal breathing, or tidal volume (V_T), is 500 ml and the breathing frequency 15 breaths/min, then total ventilation will be 7500 ml/min. However, if 150 ml of the tidal volume is the anatomical dead space and therefore not taking part in gas exchange, the alveolar ventilation (V_A) will be 5250 ml.

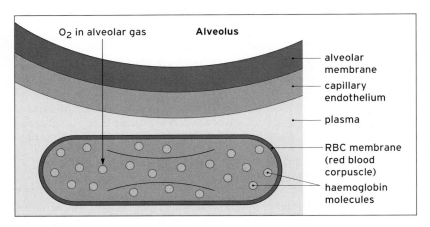

O₂ in alveolar gas   **Alveolus**

- alveolar membrane
- capillary endothelium
- plasma
- RBC membrane (red blood corpuscle)
- haemoglobin molecules

Figure 1.1 Schematic representation of the barriers across which oxygen travels before combining with haemoglobin.

Table 1.1 Partial pressure in the respiratory tract and in blood and tissues, and the effects of altitude on atmospheric gas pressures.

Partial pressure (in kPa) of oxygen and carbon dioxide at various points along the respiratory tract and in blood and tissues, and the effects of altitude on atmospheric gas pressures		
	Oxygen	**Carbon Dioxide**
Atmospheric air at sea level	21.0	0.0
Moist inspired air	19.8	0.0
Alveolar air	13.3	5.3
Arterial blood	12.0	5.3
Venous blood	5.3	6.0
Mitochondria	0.7	6.0+
Summit of Mount Everest	5.4	0.0

For alveolar ventilation to occur, the chest wall and lungs must have forces applied to them so that the system can be moved and any resistance to movement overcome. These forces are generated by the contraction of the respiratory muscles.

LUNG VOLUMES

Before describing the muscles and mechanics of ventilation, a brief overview of static lung volumes and capacities is presented.

During normal breathing, the amount of gas inspired and expired is referred to as the tidal volume (V_T). At the end of a tidal breath out, the volume of air remaining in the lungs is the functional residual capacity (FRC). When a person breathes in fully, total lung capacity (TLC) is reached. When a person breathes out fully, the volume of air remaining in the lungs is the residual volume (RV). The difference between TLC and RV is the vital capacity (VC); this may be forced or relaxed.

INSPIRATION

The most important muscle of inspiration is the diaphragm. When the diaphragm contracts, the abdominal contents are forced downwards and forwards, and the vertical dimensions of the thoracic cavity increase. The transverse diameter of the thorax also increases, since the rib margins are lifted and moved outwards. During tidal breathing, the diaphragm moves about 1 cm while during heavy exercise this excursion may be about 10 cm.

When the external intercostal muscles contract, the ribs are pulled upwards and forwards thereby increasing both the lateral and anteroposterior diameters of the thorax. The scalene and sternocleidomastoid muscles of the neck are accessory muscles that have little activity during rest, but may contract vigorously during heavy exercise.

EXPIRATION

Although normal resting expiration is described as 'passive', this is not the case. Inspiratory activity continues during most of expiration, acting as a brake to expiratory flow. The important muscles of active expiration include the internal intercostals, rectus abdominus, transversus abdominus and internal and external oblique. When these muscles contract, the diaphragm is pushed upwards. During vomiting, defaecation and coughing, these muscles contract forcibly.

PRESSURE-VOLUME RELATIONSHIPS OF LUNGS AND CHEST WALL

When the chest wall is opened, two observations can be made. First, the lungs collapse inwards. Therefore the lungs must be being held in a stretched state when attached to the chest wall. When this attachment is broken, the force holding the lungs stretched is released and the lungs, which are elastic structures, collapse inwards. A simple analogy is an elastic band. To stretch and then keep an elastic band stretched, force is applied and maintained, but when this force is removed the band returns to its normal resting state. The second observation is that the chest wall expands outwards, and therefore the chest wall must be being pulled inwards by adhesion to the lungs.

These observations provide important information about the elastic state of the lungs and the chest wall. While both function as a combined unit, it is easier to describe them separately.

LUNG COMPLIANCE

As the lung is an elastic structure, it needs a force to be applied to expand it from its resting state to the point of maximal distension. A simple analogy is a balloon. When a balloon is deflated it contains virtually no air, and a large force has to be applied to overcome the initial resistance to expansion (this is a similar scenario to the lung, where force is applied to initiate its inflation). Once this initial force has been applied, further force is needed to increase the volume of air in the balloon. Initially, this force is not very great, and the balloon expands easily but gradually. As the balloon expands further, greater force is required to increase its volume, until the balloon

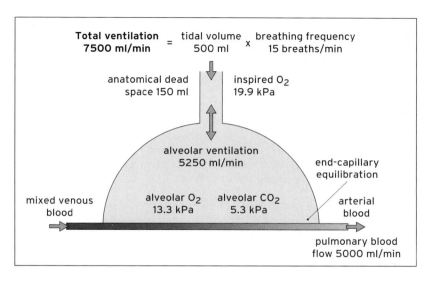

Figure 1.2 Schematic representation of the process of ventilation at the alveolar/capillary level.

Total ventilation 7500 ml/min = tidal volume 500 ml x breathing frequency 15 breaths/min

anatomical dead space 150 ml

inspired O_2 19.9 kPa

alveolar ventilation 5250 ml/min

end-capillary equilibration

mixed venous blood

alveolar O_2 13.3 kPa

alveolar CO_2 5.3 kPa

arterial blood

pulmonary blood flow 5000 ml/min

bursts. These pressure–volume changes are described by compliance (C), which can be applied to the lung, chest wall or respiratory system. Initially the balloon is compliant as there is a large change in volume for a given change in pressure, but as the maximum volume of the balloon is reached, the volume change for the same magnitude of pressure change is much smaller, so the balloon is less compliant.

CHEST WALL COMPLIANCE

The chest wall consists of the rib cage, intercostal muscles, diaphragm and abdomen. The pressure–volume relationship of the chest wall is alinear below FRC but essentially linear above FRC. Unlike the lung, the pressure–volume curve of the chest wall is negative at RV, indicating that the chest wall is under compression and below its unstressed position. Its unstressed position is where the curve crosses the volume axis, at about 70% of TLC.

The lungs and chest wall move together. The changes in volume of the chest wall and of the lungs are identical because of the coupling of the two by the molecular cohesion of pleural fluid.

Pressure–volume relationships influence volumes and capacities. The FRC has no active regulation, and is determined by the passive mechanical relationships of the lungs and chest wall. It is the point where the pressures of the chest wall (negative) and the lungs (positive) are of equal magnitude, but of opposite sign, so the net pressure is zero.

TLC is limited by the expansion of the lungs, not the chest wall. At TLC, the compliance of the chest wall (C_{CW}) is high with the curve having a steep slope, while the compliance of the lung (C_L) is lower, the curve being flatter. Therefore, further expansion of the lungs is not possible.

At RV, C_L is steep, so compliance is high, while C_{CW} is flatter, compliance therefore being less and the chest wall stiffer. Thus, compression of the chest wall limits expiration and determines RV.

SURFACE TENSION

Surface tension is generated because of the small diameter of the 300 million alveoli and the presence of an interface between air in the alveoli and the tissue. The alveoli are lined with fluid. Fluid molecules have a greater molecular attraction between themselves than that between molecules of liquid and gas. Thus, as with a soap bubble, the surface area tries to become as small as possible. To reduce surface tension, surfactant is secreted by cells lining the alveoli. Surfactant is a phospholipid substance containing dipalmitoyl phosphatidyl choline, which aligns itself on the surface of the alveoli with its hydrophobic and hydrophilic ends together. These oppose the normal attracting forces between surface molecules, thereby reducing surface tension.

Physiologically, surfactant increases C_L and reduces the work of breathing. It also stabilises the alveoli, which are inherently unstable structures. Alveoli are not all the same size, so without the stability provided by surface tension throughout all alveoli, smaller alveoli would collapse and form bigger alveoli. Finally, surfactant keeps the alveoli dry by preventing movement of fluid from the capillaries to the alveoli.

PRESSURE GRADIENT BETWEEN ATMOSPHERE AND ALVEOLI

For air to enter and exit alveoli, a pressure gradient must exist between the atmosphere and the alveoli. Alveoli do not expand themselves; they are simply passive structures which require the application of an external force. This force is provided by the muscles of inspiration, which contract, resulting in an increase in the volume of the alveoli and a decrease in alveolar pressure (P_A).

RESPIRATORY CYCLE

At the end of expiration, when the glottis is open and there is no air flow, the atmospheric pressure (P_B) equals P_A. The respiratory muscles are relaxed and inactive.

When the inspiratory muscles contract there is an additional outward force (P_{mus}) which is transmitted through the pleural space to the alveoli, which expand. Increasing alveolar volume decreases P_A with respect to the atmosphere. Thus, air flows down the pressure gradient from the mouth to the alveoli.

At the end of a tidal inspiration there is no air flow, so P_A equals P_B. The recoil of the chest wall and the lungs is more positive. As there is no air flow, all the actively applied pressure is used to overcome the elastic forces and to maintain the increased volume of the chest wall and lungs.

Expiration begins when the inspiratory muscles begin to relax. There is less muscle activity, but the same chest wall recoil pressure. Air flow is directed from alveoli to atmosphere down a pressure gradient, so P_A must be positive.

AIRWAYS RESISTANCE

Air flow along a tube requires a pressure difference between the two ends. This difference depends on the rate and pattern of air flow. In regions of the lung where the air flow rate is low, air flow is laminar, whereas in regions where it is high, air flow is turbulent. Transitional air flow occurs at airway branches. Turbulent air flow is associated with greater resistance to air flow, which is generally observed in the larger airways. In the peripheral airways, air flow is less, so laminar air flow occurs.

THE WORK OF BREATHING

Work is done to inflate the lungs from FRC to V_T, and is the product of the change in pressure and the change in volume. For a given change in volume, work is proportional to the change in pressure required to overcome both elastic and resistive work.

Elastic Work of Breathing

Elastic work of breathing overcomes the elastic recoil of the chest wall and lungs, and surface tension of the alveoli. During inspiration, work is performed to move the lungs and chest wall.

Resistive Work of Breathing

Resistive work of breathing overcomes both tissue and airways resistance. Tissue resistance contributes about 20% of the total resistance. To overcome the resistive work of breathing, additional pressure, above that needed to overcome the elastic work of breathing, is required.

Mechanical Power from the Respiratory Muscles

During tidal breathing all the work is done by the inspiratory muscles. The amount of work required varies with the level of ventilation and the breathing pattern, e.g. it is greater for nasal breathing than for mouth breathing, as the resistance to breathing is greater through the nose than through the mouth. During exercise, more effort is required, particularly at levels of ventilation greater than 50 litres/min.

Minimum Effort of Breathing

At rest, the frequency of breathing (f_b) is between 12 and 20 breaths/min, with an average V_T of 0.5 litres. There is, however, an optimal f_b where the energy expenditure is least. By increasing V_A, the optimal f_b increases, thus maintaining the minimum level of mechanical work required. This is true for levels of ventilation from 5 to 35 litres/min and for breathing frequencies from 5 to 20 breaths/min.

DIFFUSION

The movement of gas across the air–blood barrier takes place by passive diffusion, i.e. a gas moves down a pressure gradient from high to low pressure. The rate of diffusion also depends on surface area, membrane thickness and the properties of both the tissue and the gas. The diffusion of a gas is not an infinitely rapid process.

The time available for gas exchange depends on pulmonary capillary blood flow (Q_C) and pulmonary capillary blood volume (V_C). At rest, if Q_C is 5 litres/min (83.3 ml/s) and V_C 70 ml, the time an erythrocyte spends in the pulmonary capillaries will be 0.84 s (70/83.3). Since Q_C and V_C both vary, the time ranges from 0.75 s to 1.2 s. During exercise, Q_C can reach 30 litres/min (500 ml/s) and V_C can reach 200 ml, so the time decreases to about 0.4 s. Within these time constraints, gases must diffuse across the alveolar–capillary membrane.

OXYGEN

The partial pressure of oxygen in the mixed venous blood rises quickly, reaching equilibrium with the alveolar partial pressure (P_AO_2) within 0.25 s. Oxygen moves easily across the alveolar–capillary membrane and into the erythrocytes, where it combines with haemoglobin. A point is reached when haemoglobin becomes saturated with oxygen. Thus, the PO_2 in the blood will rise and eventually equilibrate with P_AO_2. Oxygen is therefore perfusion limited at rest. Exercise decreases the time the blood remains within the capillaries, but the time does not fall below that required for equilibrium to occur.

CARBON DIOXIDE

Carbon dioxide diffuses from the pulmonary capillary blood into alveoli. Under normal conditions, the partial pressure of carbon dioxide in the mixed venous blood is 6.0 kPa and in the alveolar gas 5.3 kPa and equilibration occurs in about 0.25 s. Carbon dioxide is also perfusion limited.

PERFUSION

For gas exchange to occur, the lungs must be perfused adequately. This is provided by the pulmonary circulation, which directly affects the ability of the lungs to exchange gases.

CARDIAC OUTPUT AND BLOOD PRESSURE

The volume of blood ejected during each contraction of the heart is the stroke volume (V_S) and ranges from 40 ml to 80 ml. The total volume of blood pumped every minute is the product of V_S and cardiac frequency (f_C) and is the cardiac output (Q), so $Q = V_S \times f_C$. An important point is that if f_C falls then V_S must increase to maintain Q. On average, the adult Q is about 5.0 litres/min, of which about 75% is in the systemic circulation, 15% in the heart and 10% in the pulmonary circulation.

Cardiac output directly influences blood pressure. When the ventricles contract, the pressure inside them increases, and decreases when they relax. This rise and fall in blood pressure corresponds to the phases of the cardiac cycle. With an increase in blood pressure in the ventricles, the blood is forced out into the aorta and pulmonary arteries. The maximum pressure generated is the systolic pressure. The lowest pressure remaining in the arteries, after the ventricles have relaxed, is the diastolic pressure. In the systemic circulation, the systolic/diastolic pressures in the arteries are 120/80 mmHg, whereas in the pulmonary circulation the pressures are 30/20 mmHg (Figure 1.3).

PULMONARY CIRCULATION

The pulmonary circulation is a low pressure, low resistance system. The mean pulmonary artery pressure (P_{PA}) is 15 mmHg, which falls to a mean of around 5 mmHg in the left atrium (see Figure 1.3). The pulmonary circulation has a resistance about 10 times lower than that of the systemic circulation.

The V_C is about 70 ml, which is spread over a vast array of thin-walled interconnecting vessels and takes all the Q_C. It achieves this by having arterioles as resistance vessels, which are in a dilated state. Clearly, it is important the blood vessels carefully regulate their size since the distribution of blood to the various lobes and segments depends on the resistance in the vascular tree.

Pulmonary vascular resistance (PVR) decreases as Q_C increases. The reasons for this are that the capillaries are not fully distended at rest. As Q_C increases, the pulmonary pressure increases and the vessels increase in diameter, thus lowering resistance. Furthermore, at rest, the capillaries are not fully perfused. As Q_C increases the pulmonary vascular pressures, so more blood vessels are recruited. Recruitment and distension of the pulmonary capillaries during exercise increases V_C from about 70 ml to about 200 ml.

VENTILATION-PERFUSION

One important area for consideration is the matching of ventilation to perfusion. Three criteria must be satisfied before gas exchange can take place. First, the alveoli must be ventilated, secondly, the alveoli must be perfused and, thirdly, ventilation must match perfusion.

VENTILATION-PERFUSION RATIO

The ventilation–perfusion ratio (V_A/Q_C) is the ratio of ventilation (V_A) to perfusion (Q_C) for a single alveolus, a group of alveoli or the whole lung. For the whole lung, the V_A/Q_C ratio is the alveolar ventilation divided by the pulmonary blood flow, and has a value of approximately 1.0. This suggests perfect matching, but this is not the case in the real lung as not all alveoli behave in the same manner. The distribution of ventilation and perfusion varies for different parts of the lung, giving a spread of V_A/Q_C ratios.

REGIONAL DIFFERENCES IN VENTILATION

The lung is not uniformly ventilated. Regional differences occur in the upright lung, mainly due to gravitational effects. The upright lung is a self-supporting structure, with each level of the lung being supported by the layer above it, so the mass of tissue pulling downwards increases from base to apex. Consequently, the lung is more expanded at its apex than at its base, resulting in a twofold increase in volume from base to apex.

LOCAL DIFFERENCES IN VENTILATION

Local differences in ventilation may be more important than regional differences. Local differences are not determined by gravity but by the local airways resistance and the compliance of the airways. The greater the resistance, the longer the alveoli will take to fill properly. Airways resistance can be affected by the local P_ACO_2.

REGIONAL DIFFERENCES IN PERFUSION

Since the pressures in the pulmonary circulation are lower than in the systemic circulation, gravity affects the distribution of blood flow. Furthermore, the pressure distribution throughout the lung is important as the P_{PA}

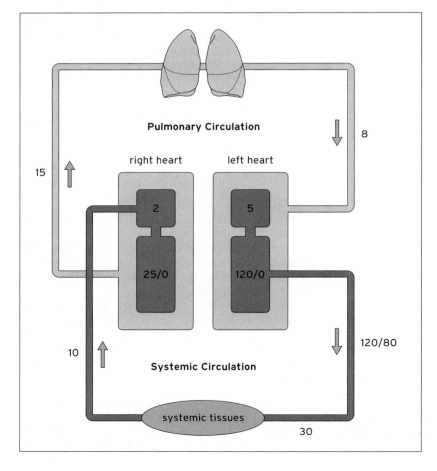

Figure 1.3 Systolic and diastolic pressures (mmHg) and mean blood pressure (mmHg) within the pulmonary and systemic circulations.

affects the distribution of blood. There is a greater blood flow at the lung base and Q_C has a fivefold increase from base to apex.

LOCAL DIFFERENCES IN PERFUSION

In the pulmonary circulation, P_AO_2 affects the distribution of blood flow. Under hypoxic conditions a decrease in blood flow to underventilated alveoli may occur. Hypoxia causes an increase in the PVR, thus raising pulmonary artery pressure (P_{PA}). Depending on the severity of the hypoxia, P_{PA} may increase twofold, resulting in an improvement in V_A/Q_C distribution.

A number of external factors alter the distribution of blood flow within the lung. These include body position and exercise. In the supine position, gravity affects the whole of the lung equally, so Q_C is evenly distributed throughout the lung. During exercise, P_{PA} increases, as does pulmonary venous pressure, but to a lesser extent. The result is that underperfused capillaries are recruited.

VENTILATION-PERFUSION RATIOS OF THE UPRIGHT LUNG

So far the distribution of ventilation and perfusion as separate entities has been described. In reality, they must combine for gas exchange to take place. As the perfusion of the lung base is greater than the ventilation, the V_A/Q_C ratio is less than 1.0. There is a gradual increase in the V_A/Q_C ratio as Q_C decreases faster than the ventilation. At about the third rib, the V_A/Q_C ratio becomes unity. Thereafter, ventilation exceeds perfusion, so the V_A/Q_C ratio is greater than 1.0.

GAS TRANSPORT

The cardiovascular system exists to ensure that nutrients and waste products are delivered to and removed from respiring tissues. Thus, oxygen is a nutrient and carbon dioxide a waste product. Oxygen combines with haemoglobin passing through the pulmonary capillaries and is transported, via the systemic circulatory system, to the respiring tissues where it is rapidly released. Conversely, carbon dioxide is transported from the tissues to the lungs where it is excreted to the atmosphere.

BLOOD, ERYTHROCYTES AND HAEMOGLOBIN

Blood is an important substance and has many roles; these include supplying food in a dissolved state from the gut, removing waste products of metabolism, stabilising water levels and body temperature, allowing gas exchange between the external and the internal environment, and forming a barrier to invasion by harmful substances.

The primary function of the erythrocyte is to transport haemoglobin. Its intense red colour is due to a high haemoglobin content, about 33 g/100 ml of erythrocytes. This high percentage of the erythrocyte volume for haemoglobin is achieved by a lack of intracellular structures and organelles. Each erythrocyte is a biconcave disc

of about 7 μm diameter, and has a volume of 87 μm³; it measures about 2 μm in the thickest part to less than 1 μm at its centre. The biconcave shape is functionally important as the large surface area favours the exchange of oxygen with the surrounding plasma, while reducing the distance between the surface and the haemoglobin molecule. The erythrocytes are easily deformed, and can pass through the narrow capillaries in tissue and lungs without being damaged. Since all the haemoglobin is transported within the erythrocyte, the oxygen capacity of the blood is determined by the number of erythrocytes. There are about 5×10^6 erythrocytes per ml of blood, which, for a circulating blood volume of 70 ml/kg gives a total of 350×10^9 erythrocytes per kilogram.

Haemoglobin has a large capacity for oxygen, with each molecule carrying four oxygen molecules. Haemoglobin releases oxygen upon demand, loads and unloads oxygen very quickly over the range of PO_2 found in tissues, and alters its binding affinity with oxygen when demands for oxygen alter. Additionally, it is involved in transporting carbon dioxide and hydrogen ions (H^+) and contributing to the buffering activity of the body (see page 15).

OXYGEN STORES

Oxygen is stored in the body in four forms—as a gas in the lungs, dissolved in tissue fluids, as oxyhaemoglobin in blood, and as oxymyoglobin in muscle. Compared with carbon dioxide, the stores of oxygen are extremely small and must be continually replenished. About 98% of oxygen stored is bound to haemoglobin.

OXYHAEMOGLOBIN DISSOCIATION CURVE

Each molecule of haemoglobin (Hb) carries four oxygen molecules, with one attached to each of the four haem units of the molecule. Thus:

- $O_2 + Hb_4 \rightleftharpoons Hb_4O_2$
- $O_2 + Hb_4O_2 \rightleftharpoons Hb_4O_4$
- $O_2 + Hb_4O_4 \rightleftharpoons Hb_4O_6$
- $O_2 + Hb_4O_6 \rightleftharpoons Hb_4O_8$

The combination of oxygen with haemoglobin occurs due to minute changes in the structure of the haemoglobin molecule, and accounts for the sigmoidal shape of the oxyhaemoglobin curve (Figure 1.4). The reaction takes less than 0.01 s. The relationship between PO_2 and oxygen saturation (SaO_2) is the result of the chemical reactions that occur between oxygen and each haem group. Oxygenation of the first haem, at low PO_2, increases the affinity of the other haem groups. The steepest part of the curve represents the binding of two more oxygen molecules, and the upper flat portion is the loading of the final oxygen molecule.

PHYSIOLOGICAL SIGNIFICANCE OF THE OXYHAEMOGLOBIN CURVE

The upper flat portion of the oxyhaemoglobin curve ensures that SaO_2 remains high and fairly constant, while allowing for variations in PO_2. This provides an excellent safety zone for the loading of oxygen in the lungs. For example, if the partial pressure of arterial oxygen (PaO_2) is 13.3 kPa, the SaO_2 is 97.4%. If the PaO_2 falls to 9.3 kPa, the SaO_2 will be 94.1%. Thus, for a 30% fall in PO_2, only a 3.4% fall in SaO_2 occurs, which is insignificant.

FACTORS THAT SHIFT THE OXYHAEMOGLOBIN DISSOCIATION CURVE

A number of factors alter the position but not the shape of the oxyhaemoglobin curve.

pH and Carbon Dioxide

The H^+ concentration ($[H^+]$) (pH) of the blood changes throughout the body. In the tissues, blood entering the capillaries has a $PaCO_2$ of 5.3 kPa, a pH of 7.40, a PaO_2 of 13.3 kPa and an SaO_2 of 97%. As blood passes along the capillary, carbon dioxide moves from the respiring tissues into the blood. The PCO_2 rises to 6.13 kPa, and pH decreases to 7.2. The curve moves to the right, reducing the affinity of haemoglobin for oxygen, and hence liberating oxygen to the tissues by passive diffusion.

When the blood enters the pulmonary capillaries, the reverse occurs. Carbon dioxide is discharged into the alveoli, pH increases and the curve shifts to the left. This increases the affinity of haemoglobin for oxygen, and so oxygen readily combines with haemoglobin.

Temperature

During exercise, the temperature of metabolising tissues increases and the curve shifts to the right. This enhances the release of oxygen, which is important as the blood will be flowing through the muscle capillaries faster.

2,3-Diphosphoglycerate (2,3-DPG)

Erythrocytes contain large amounts of 2,3-DPG—a metabolic intermediary formed by the erythrocytes during anaerobic metabolism. 2,3-DPG binds loosely with subunits of the haemoglobin molecule, thereby reducing the affinity of haemoglobin for oxygen. The concentration of 2,3-DPG increases in hypoxia and with pH.

OXYGEN CASCADE

So far, the overall principles of oxygen transport and the effects of various external factors upon it have been discussed. This section considers the transport and delivery of oxygen from the atmosphere to the mitochondria.

At sea level, dry atmospheric air has a PO_2 of 21.2 kPa. When this air enters the conducting airways it becomes humidified at 37°C, and the PO_2 falls to 19.9 kPa. Dilution of the oxygen in the gas within the airways and alveoli further reduces the PO_2 to about 13.3 kPa. By the time the blood arrives at the capillaries, the PO_2 has fallen to about 6 kPa. In the intracellular fluid, the PO_2 ranges from 0.5 kPa to 3.0 kPa. These stepped reductions in PO_2 form the oxygen cascade. Alteration in the inspired air, alveolar air or alveolar gas exchange may result in hypoxia.

Inspired Air

The PO_2 of inspired air decreases with increasing altitude. At sea level, the inspired PO_2 is about 19.8 kPa, which, at the summit of Mount Everest, decreases to 5.4 kPa.

Alveolar Air

Alveolar PO_2 is determined by alveolar ventilation and oxygen uptake. Alveolar hypoventilation results in a decrease in PO_2 and hence a decrease in blood PO_2.

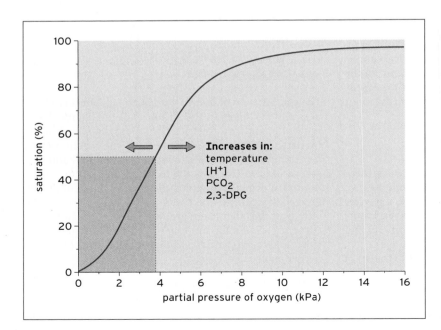

Figure 1.4 The oxyhaemoglobin dissociation curve. The curve shows the effects of pH, partial pressure of carbon dioxide (PCO_2), temperature and 2,3-diphosphoglycerate (2,3-DPG) on its position.

Alveolar Gas Exchange

An abnormality in alveolar gas exchange produces a large oxygen gradient between the alveolar gas and the blood. This may be caused by regional differences in V_A/Q_C relationships or increased diffusion resistance in the alveolar–capillary membrane.

This last step is of clinical relevance. The alveolar–arterial PO_2 difference ($P_{A-a}O_2$) in a young person should not exceed 2 kPa, rising to around 5 kPa in an elderly person. An increased $P_{A-a}O_2$ is the commonest cause of arterial hypoxaemia, and is an important step in the oxygen cascade.

TRANSPORT OF CARBON DIOXIDE

Carbon dioxide is produced by the mitochondria at a rate of about 200 ml/min. Normally, the quantity transported is 40 ml/litre of cardiac output, so a cardiac output of 5.0 litres/min will give a carbon dioxide output of 200 ml/min. This is just the tip of the iceberg. In reality, for a $PaCO_2$ of 5.3 kPa, the arterial blood will have a total carbon dioxide concentration of approximately 480 ml/litre with mixed venous blood having 520 ml/litre (480 + 40). The reason so much carbon dioxide is bound up is simply that carbon dioxide in blood and other body fluids is linked with the maintenance of the [H⁺] of the extracellular and intracellular fluids. This must be closely regulated to allow enzymes to function properly.

The carbon dioxide produced by mitochondria must diffuse out of the cell and, via the circulation, be released into the alveoli where it is excreted to the atmosphere. The carbon dioxide diffuses down a diffusion gradient with the mitochondria having the highest PCO_2 and the atmosphere having the lowest PCO_2. Carbon dioxide is carried by the blood in four forms—solution, carbonic acid, bicarbonate ions (HCO_3^-) and carbamino groups. The bulk is carried as carbonic acid and HCO_3^-.

Carbonic Acid

In solution, carbon dioxide combines with water to form carbonic acid (H_2CO_3):

$$CO_2 + H_2O \rightleftharpoons H_2CO_3 \rightleftharpoons H^+ + HCO_3^-$$

The reaction is slow (<5 s) in the plasma, but much faster (milliseconds) inside the erythrocyte where the enzyme carbonic anhydrase is present. Carbonic acid rapidly dissociates into H^+ and HCO_3^-. This occurs spontaneously and does not require any enzymes.

HCO_3^-

To prevent an accumulation of HCO_3^- within the erythrocyte, the HCO_3^- diffuses out into the extracellular fluid, while chloride (Cl⁻) diffuses in the opposite direction therefore maintaining electrical neutrality. The H^+ on the other hand combines with the very large quantities of haemoglobin within the erythrocytes, and to a lesser extent with various plasma proteins. The bulk of carbon dioxide is carried in this manner, accounting for about 90% of carbon dioxide carried.

The relationship of total carbon dioxide concentration and PCO_2 is shown in Figure 1.5. The position of the line depends on the saturation of venous oxygen (SvO_2). The higher line is for mixed venous SvO_2, the lower for SaO_2.

CONTROL OF VENTILATION

Breathing is an action spontaneously initiated within the central nervous system (CNS). A cycle of inspiration and expiration is automatically generated by neurones located in the brainstem. However, this cycle can be modified, altered or temporarily suppressed by various mechanisms.

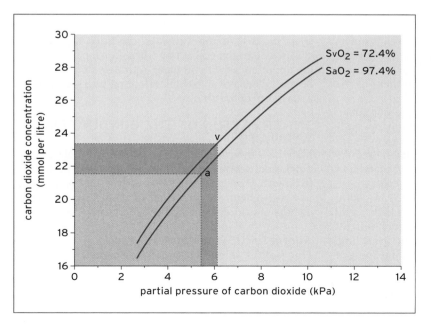

Figure 1.5 Carbon dioxide equilibrium curve of whole blood. The total carbon dioxide concentration (mmol/litre) is plotted against the partial pressure of carbon dioxide (PCO_2). The relationship is approximately linear over the range of PCO_2 presented. The two curves are for mixed venous blood and for arterial blood.

The system must fulfil three criteria: to maintain, through involuntary controls, a regular rhythmic breathing pattern; to adjust V_T and f_b, so that V_A meets the demands of cellular gas exchange; and to adjust the breathing pattern in various activities, such as speech, that use the same muscles.

Under most circumstances, breathing is controlled so finely that the PaO_2 and P_ACO_2 remain essentially constant. To achieve this, the system has three control pathways. The PCO_2 is the principal pathway, controlling the rate and depth of breathing on a breath-by-breath basis. Under certain circumstances, such as acclimatisation to altitude, the second pathway, the PO_2 pathway, can override the PCO_2 pathway. In addition, a third pathway is required to allow all the ancillary actions, such as talking, swallowing and coughing, to break through the normal pattern of breathing, and to try to match breathing to the expected voluntary or behavioural activity. In essence there are two controllers—the metabolic controller serving basic body needs, and a behavioural controller that temporarily overrides the metabolic controller. The overall control of breathing is complex, involving controllers, effectors and sensors.

BRAINSTEM AND SPINAL PATHWAYS

Neurones located in two areas of the brainstem—the pons and medulla oblongata—are responsible for the normal automatic process of tidal breathing, and form the principal 'controller' of breathing.

Classically, parts of the medulla have been described as 'respiratory centres', which included the inspiratory centre, the expiratory centre, the pneumotaxic centre and the apneustic centre. It is now accepted that these areas are poorly defined groups of neurones with various components. Three neurone pools (A, B and C) are located in the medulla and a single pool—the pneumotaxic centre (P)—in the pons. Pool A neurones roughly equate to the classic 'inspiratory centre'. Since pool B also sends inputs to the accessory muscles of breathing, this pool is also an inspiratory centre. However, it is not that clear cut because of other input. There is probably no equivalent of the classical apneustic centre.

Neurones in pool A (dorsal respiratory group) contain upper motor neurones. Axons from these neurones partially cross and project along the spinal cord to the lower motor neurone pools of the phrenic nerve (diaphragm) and the intercostal muscles. These neurones receive excitatory stimuli from the central and peripheral chemoreceptors.

Some of the output from pool A connects to pool B (ventral respiratory group) neurones, which send neurones down the spinal cord to the accessory muscles of breathing. The pool also receives input from lung stretch receptors and chest wall proprioceptors. Some of the output from pool B activates pool C neurones (nucleus retroambiguus) which, when stimulated, have an inhibitory effect on pool A. Neurones in pool P (pontine respiratory group) stimulate pool C and inhibit pool A neurones. Inputs to pool P probably come from the higher centres.

INNERVATION OF THE RESPIRATORY MUSCLES AND UPPER RESPIRATORY TRACT

The respiratory muscles and upper respiratory tract are innervated with nerve fibres and specialist receptor cells. The complete network contributes to a wide variety of neural events that serve to protect the airways or influence the rate and depth of breathing.

The diaphragm is innervated by the phrenic nerves, which are the only motor nerves to supply it.

The internal and external intercostal muscles are innervated by the intercostal nerves. These nerves also supply other muscles. The upper respiratory tract consists of a number of different structures—the larynx, oropharynx, nasopharynx, nose and mouth. The motor neurones innervating these muscles are located in the medulla, and innervate the muscles of the upper airways and bronchi through the cranial nerves. The muscles are activated just before the major muscles of inspiration are activated resulting in dilation of these airways before inspiration.

The importance of this dilation cannot be overstressed during inspiration. The inspiratory flow rate is dependent on the force generated by the inspiratory muscles, and on the resistance and compliance of the system. The overall efficiency of the system is greatly enhanced by the abduction of the vocal folds and the consequent decrease in airway resistance.

In expiration, the expiratory flow rate is dependent on the recoil and mechanical properties of the system. The duration of expiration is greater than the time required for the passive collapse of the system to FRC. Thus, in spontaneous, quiet breathing, expiratory flow is slowed by post-inspiratory contraction of the inspiratory muscles and by an increase in upper airways resistance due to partial closure of the laryngeal airway. These braking mechanisms are important as without them expiratory flow rate would be much higher, with possible effects on both gas exchange and control of breathing.

INNERVATION OF THE CONDUCTING AIRWAYS

Many cells in the conducting airways are controlled by the autonomic nervous system, which regulates involuntary functions. There are three systems—the adrenergic (sympathetic) system, the cholinergic (parasympathetic system) and the non-adrenergic–non-cholinergic (NANC) system.

Adrenergic (Sympathetic) System

Fibres of the adrenergic system leave the CNS from the thoracic and lumbar regions of the spinal cord. The neurotransmitter is usually norepinephrine (noradrenaline) but may also be epinephrine (adrenaline). Adrenergic nerves secreting noradrenaline innervate mucous glands, blood vessels and the airways. Few adrenergic nerves directly supply airway smooth muscle but they probably do alter airway tone indirectly. Many β-adrenoceptors are found in normal bronchial smooth muscle, and stimulation of them may lead to a reduction in the smooth muscle tone and to bronchodilation.

Cholinergic (Parasympathetic) System

The airways are innervated by the cholinergic system through the vagus nerve. Tonic parasympathetic activity maintains a mild but continuous degree of airway smooth muscle tone. This activity predominates in the major airways, decreasing towards the peripheral conducting airways. Cholinergic nerves innervate the mucous glands, as well as being involved in a variety of other reflex actions in the lungs. The postganglionic axons use the neurotransmitter acetylcholine, which is rapidly inactivated by the enzyme acetylcholinesterase, so the effect of cholinergic activity is short-lived and local. The released acetylcholine binds to receptors on the airway smooth muscle, and leads to constriction of the muscle.

Non-adrenergic–Non-cholinergic (NANC) System

The NANC system is subdivided into inhibitory and stimulatory systems. The neurotransmitters involved in this system have not been fully identified, so the significance of this system is unclear. The efferents from the NANC inhibitory system cause relaxation of airway smooth muscle. Constrictor activities of the NANC stimulatory system have been observed.

RHYTHMICITY OF BREATHING

The resting breathing pattern shows some variability in volume and duration of individual breaths. Inspiration is about one-third and expiration about two-thirds of the total breath time. Breath-by-breath changes at rest tend to occur in the opposite direction, such that a large V_T is associated with a reduced f_b and vice versa. Overall, however, total ventilation shows much less variability than either V_T or f_b.

FUNDAMENTAL STIMULUS FOR BREATHING–CHEMORECEPTOR CONTROL

V_T is controlled so that P_ACO_2 is maintained within a narrow band and does not vary by more than 0.3 kPa (5%) for more than a few minutes, regardless of conditions. Fortunately, the system is not so sensitive that very small variations in PCO_2 result in large variations in V_T or f_b. To maintain PCO_2 within this narrow band, the system has central and peripheral chemoreceptors which respond to changes in the chemical composition of the liquid surrounding or within them. In particular, these chemoreceptors are sensitive to changes in the respiratory gases and in H^+ composition.

Central Chemoreceptors

The trigger that generates inspiration is the accumulation of carbon dioxide or H^+ in the brain. The central chemoreceptors are involved in the second-by-second control of ventilation, and are located on or close to the surface of the medulla. Each central chemoreceptor is surrounded by extracellular fluid and responds rapidly to changes in the $[H^+]$ of the fluid. This is achieved by the cerebrospinal fluid (CSF) having a low buffering capacity. Consequently, responses to changes in the $[H^+]$ of the CSF are greater than responses to changes in blood for the same PCO_2. The response of these receptors is straightforward. An increase in $[H^+]$ stimulates ventilation while a decrease inhibits it. The mechanism is as follows:

- When P_ACO_2 rises, carbon dioxide rapidly diffuses across the blood–brain barrier into the CSF from the cerebral blood vessels.
- The carbon dioxide slowly combines with water to form H_2CO_3, which dissociates into H^+ and HCO_3^-.
- There is a rapid increase in $[H^+]$ in the CSF.
- The increased $[H^+]$ causes the central chemoreceptors to transmit signals to neurone pool A, resulting in an increase in V_A.
- By increasing V_A, the P_ACO_2 and the PCO_2 in the CSF are reduced.
- As the PCO_2 in the CSF decreases, so does the $[H^+]$, resulting in a decrease in stimulation of the central chemoreceptors, and a decrease in V_A occurs.

Peripheral Chemoreceptors

Peripheral chemoreceptors respond to decreases in PaO_2 and in $[H^+]$, and to increases in P_ACO_2. They are located in the carotid bodies at the division of the common carotid arteries, and in the aortic bodies above and below the aortic arch. Both respond to PO_2 and PCO_2, but only the carotid bodies respond to changes in $[H^+]$.

When activated by a low PaO_2, afferent (sensory) signals are transmitted to the neurones in pool A, which are stimulated, and efferent (motor) signals are transmitted to the respiratory muscles, causing ventilation to increase.

REFLEX MECHANISMS

Innervation of the airways is entirely autonomic. In the upper respiratory tract, the tracheobronchial tree and the respiratory muscles present many reflex mechanisms.

Apnoea

Apnoea can be induced by odours and irritants in the nose, and by water applied to the face. Breathing tends to stop at or close to FRC, with the inspiratory muscles relaxing. The apnoeic response prevents water or gas from entering the respiratory tract.

Sneezing

Most people experience sneezing either from mechanical stimulation or from a wide variety of chemical irritants.

The respiratory changes are an initial deep inspiration followed by a forced expiration against a closed glottis. The larynx appears to constrict, but when both the larynx and pharynx open, the subsequent forced expiration takes place via the nose and mouth.

Sniffing

Irritants and odours entering the nose can cause sniffing, in this case probably a reflex action. It is believed that there is increased air flow towards the olfactory mucosa, with each sniff being between 50 ml and 75 ml. Sniffing is also often used to clear the nose of mucus and obstructions, and in such cases is probably consciously induced.

Swallowing

Swallowing is probably initiated from many sites in the upper respiratory tract. Response to mechanical stimulation or the presence of water promotes swallowing. During swallowing of water or food, the activity of the diaphragm, chest wall and abdomen is inhibited. The action of swallowing is complex and includes the closure of the larynx and movement of the pharynx, larynx and epiglottis, with possible involvement of the accessory muscles within this region. The closure of the larynx prevents food from entering the lower respiratory tract.

Cough Reflex

The result of a cough is a forceful movement of respiratory muscles to effect the reflex. Generally, there is an initial deep inspiration that enhances the subsequent expiratory effort, not only mechanically, but also by activation of the pulmonary stretch receptors.

Expiration Reflex

Mechanical stimulation of the vocal cords does not cause coughing, but produces a transient expiratory reflex. This reflex is presumably to prevent entry of foreign bodies into the lower respiratory tract. The reflex consists of a brief expiratory effort, but without a preceding inspiration, which may then be followed by coughing or apnoea. The absence of an inspiration before expiration prevents aspiration of material that touches the vocal folds.

Stretch Receptors

Stretch receptors in the tracheobronchial tree and lungs are responsible for the Hering–Breuer inflation reflex. Increased output from these receptors during inspiration switches off inspiration, while their discharge lengthens the respiratory pause during expiration. Additionally, they can cause tracheobronchial smooth muscle to relax, and thus dilate the airways. The receptors appear to respond to changes in tension in the airway wall and can display both static and dynamic properties. They are located throughout the tracheobronchial tree as far as respiratory bronchioles and alveolar ducts.

Irritant Receptors

Irritant receptors rapidly adapt to a stimulus and provide protective reflexes to the tracheobronchial tree. Mechanical and chemical stimulation causes them to fire. Increases in V_T and/or air flow cause increased discharge, as does the presence of a wide variety of other stimuli causing irritation and inflammation of the airways.

Moderate Inflation and Deflation Reflex

The pulmonary reflexes are those of moderate inflation and deflation, the stretch receptors providing volume information. These reflexes have little influence on resting breathing, but once a threshold volume is achieved (>1 litre) the inspiratory off-switch of the stretch receptors determines V_T and the inspiratory time. Lung inflation also decreases airway smooth muscle tone, producing a bronchodilator effect, so reducing airways resistance and facilitating increased ventilation. Deflation of the lungs causes a reflex increase in f_b and a decrease in V_T. Minute ventilation increases and P_ACO_2 may decrease.

Airway Defence Reflexes

Airway defence reflexes provide a protective function for the airways and lungs. Sensitive areas in the upper airways are the first line of defence when irritants are inhaled. The result may be coughing, sneezing, rapid and shallow breathing, bronchoconstriction or increased airway secretion. This may be accompanied by substernal sensations of rawness and tickling.

There will generally be a reduction in V_T, and in inspiratory and expiratory time. These decreases are probably due to a reduction in the central threshold for the Hering–Breuer reflex, i.e. the stretch receptors in the lungs trigger the end of inspiration at smaller volumes. Inputs from the irritant receptors may trigger augmented breaths or sighs. Additional input from the peripheral chemoreceptors may be made in the presence of hypoxia.

RESPIRATORY SENSATION

Hyperventilation and apnoea can be voluntarily produced and maintained within limits. In addition, there are numerous sensations, some pleasant and others not so, that reach consciousness. Unpleasant sensations include chest tightness and shortness of breath. Most people are able to perceive changes in volume, pressure and added loads in relation to breathing.

INFLUENCES OF HIGHER CENTRES

Higher centre control of ventilation is an important part of the behaviour-related activities of humans. Crying, laughing, talking, singing and swallowing are all part of this higher centre control that takes place somewhere in the cerebral cortex.

One of the best examples of higher centre control is breath-holding. This results in the cessation of V_T, and can occur for less than a minute or can be prolonged for more than 10 minutes. The length of time the breath is held is determined by the motivation of the subject, the initial lung volume and the alveolar gas tensions at the commencement of the breath-hold. The end point is determined by the increase in PCO_2 and the decrease in PO_2, after which the subject has such an urge to breathe that breath-holding is concluded. The duration of a breath-hold can be prolonged by inhalation of 100% oxygen and/or by hyperventilating for one minute before breath-holding. In the case of hyperventilation alone, the end point is determined by the PO_2 as the PCO_2 is low. When 100% oxygen is inhaled, the end point is determined by the PCO_2.

ACID-BASE BALANCE

Several systems exist to maintain the acidity of the body fluids within defined ranges. This tight control is important since reaction rates that are catalysed by enzymes are often affected by small changes in acidity. Additionally, acidity can have significant effects on the excitability of the nervous system, resulting in coma or death.

Many chemical reactions in the body produce or absorb protons—one major source being H^+ ions that are formed from the reaction of carbon dioxide with water. Excess carbon dioxide and H^+ ions are removed by the lungs and the kidneys, respectively. While the lungs are a fast response system, the kidney is somewhat more sedate in its response. To maintain the $[H^+]$ in the short term, buffer systems prevent the $[H^+]$ changing too much.

pH

So far acidity and alkalinity as $[H^+]$ have been discussed. The problem with $[H^+]$ is that the values are very small. An alternative is to use the term pH (Table 1.2), which is defined mathematically as:

$$pH = -\log_{10}[H^+]$$

NORMAL VALUES

The average plasma acid–base composition remains stable from day to day and is not greatly affected by normal diet or activity. Normal ranges are given in Table 1.2.

BODY BUFFER SYSTEMS

The addition of large amounts of H^+ to the body would result in a significant change in the pH if buffer systems were not available. Buffer systems assist the kidneys and lungs in maintaining pH within the narrow limits required. The buffer systems, which include HCO_3^-, phosphate and proteins (including haemoglobin), mop up excess acid or base. The bicarbonate buffer system is the main system since HCO_3^- is readily available in large quantities.

ACID-BASE DISTURBANCES

Acid–base disturbances are classified using two variables—P_ACO_2 and $[HCO_3^-]$. P_ACO_2 changes are of respiratory origin, whereas $[HCO_3^-]$ changes are of metabolic origin. The four primary acid–base disturbances are shown in Table 1.3 and can be monitored using a simple acid–base diagram (Figure 1.6).

Respiratory Acidosis

Respiratory acidosis occurs when P_ACO_2 is elevated. P_ACO_2 rises when elimination of carbon dioxide lags behind the production of carbon dioxide, and may occur for a variety of reasons (Table 1.4).

Respiratory Alkalosis

Respiratory alkalosis occurs when P_ACO_2 is decreased, and indicates alveolar hyperventilation. The normal regulation of ventilation can be overridden by a variety of disorders, as well as by voluntary control (see Table 1.4).

Metabolic Acidosis

Metabolic acidosis can be produced by the addition of H^+ or the loss of HCO_3^-. It can result from an inability to

Units	Mean	Range
Normal acid-base values for adults		
pH	7.40	7.36-7.44
$[H^+]$ mmol/litre	39.80	35.8-43.8
$PaCO_2$ kPa	5.47	4.97-6.00
PaO_2 kPa @ 40 yr	12.60	10.5-14.70
$[HCO_3^-]$ mmol/litre	24.80	22.6-27.0
SaO_2 %		94.0-97.5

Table 1.2 Normal acid-base values for adults.

	The four primary acid-base disturbances		
Primary disturbance	**Primary alteration**	**Secondary response**	**Mechanism of secondary response**
Respiratory acidosis	Increase in P_ACO_2	Increase in plasma $[HCO_3^-]$	Acid titration of the tissue buffers
A transient increase in acid excretion occurs coupled with sustained enhancement of HCO_3^- reabsorption by the kidney			
Respiratory alkalosis	Decrease in P_ACO_2	Decrease in plasma $[HCO_3^-]$	Alkaline titration of the tissue buffers
A transient suppression in acid excretion occurs coupled with sustained reduction in HCO_3^- reabsorption by the kidney			
Metabolic acidosis	Decrease in plasma $[HCO_3^-]$	Decrease in P_ACO_2	Alveolar hyperventilation
Metabolic alkalosis	Increase in plasma $[HCO_3^-]$	Increase in P_ACO_2	Alveolar hypoventilation

Table 1.3 The four primary acid-base disturbances.

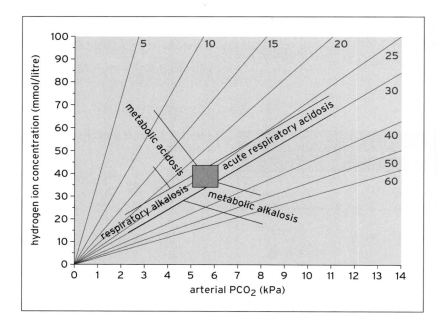

Figure 1.6 The acid-base diagram.
The diagram shows the significant bands of metabolic and respiratory acid-base disturbances. The central shaded area indicates the normal range.

excrete the dietary H^+ load or from an acute increase in the H^+ load, because of the addition of H^+ or the loss of HCO_3^- (see Table 1.4). Acute increases in H^+ load can overwhelm the renal excretory capacity, resulting in H^+ retention and hence metabolic acidosis.

Metabolic Alkalosis

Metabolic alkalosis is characterised by a decrease in $[H^+]$ and an increase in plasma $[HCO_3^-]$. A compensatory increase in P_ACO_2 is produced by a decrease in V_A (see Table 1.4).

RESPIRATION DURING SLEEP

VENTILATORY CONTROL

Understanding of ventilatory control during sleep is incomplete, but many respiratory problems occurring during sleep are related to abnormal control of ventilation.

During wakefulness, there is significant control of ventilation, which is driven by the respiratory control centres. This control disappears with sleep onset. Ventilation decreases by about 10% to 15% and the P_ACO_2 rises by between 0.4 and 1.1 kPa. There is a reduction in muscle tone, which reduces the activity of the intercostal and other respiratory muscles. The muscles of the pharynx relax, thereby narrowing the opening of the pharynx and increasing airway resistance. This has potentially serious implications, possibly leading to obstructive sleep apnoea. In addition, the hypoxic and hypercapnic ventilatory response may be reduced in some stages of sleep.

BREATHING PATTERN

The breathing pattern observed during sleep depends on the nature of the sleep. Periodic breathing may be observed during unsteady non-rapid eye movement (NREM) sleep. There is a gradual decrease in V_T followed by either a reduction in ventilation (hypopnoea) or a cessation of ventilation (apnoea). This pattern persists while sleep oscillates between arousal and light sleep. In deep sleep, periodic breathing does not occur.

In steady NREM sleep, the breathing pattern is very regular, both in the magnitude of V_T and f_b. The minute ventilation decreases (decreased V_T) due to a decreased ventilatory drive and an increase in the upper airway resistance.

Breathing during a burst of REM sleep has been described as irregular, with sudden changes in f_b and V_T. At the first eye movement of an REM burst, there is a sudden decrease in V_T followed by a gradual increase. The level of ventilation, when compared with wakefulness, appears to be variable.

RESPIRATION DURING EXERCISE

So far the physiology of the respiratory system under resting conditions has been described. As we do not remain under resting conditions throughout our lives, it is important to understand how the system is affected under conditions of stress, such as exercise.

Under resting conditions, the lung functions to maintain the levels of oxygen saturation and partial pressure

Table 1.4 Causes of respiratory and metabolic acidosis and alkalosis in normal subjects.

Causes of respiratory and metabolic acidosis and alkalosis in normal subjects	
Acidosis	**Alkalosis**
Respiratory	
Drugs–opiates, sedatives	High altitude residency
Cardiac arrest	Fever
Extreme obesity	Anaemia
Asphyxia	Subarachnoid haemorrhage
Metabolic	
Salicylate ingestion	Vomiting
Ethylene glycol ingestion	Administration of $NaHCO_3$
Methanol ingestion	
Lactic acidosis	
Diarrhoea	

within very narrow defined bands of normality. It is an inefficient system with a large reserve capacity. The cardiovascular system is similar. Within the tissues that are routinely used in exercise, such as lower limb muscles, there tends to be a greater number of mitochondria per unit volume than in muscle that plays a limited role in exercise, e.g. forearm and neck musculature.

The musculoskeletal system allows skeletal muscle contraction, achieved by the conversion of stored chemical energy into kinetic energy. The total integration of excitation–contraction necessary is controlled by the CNS, which attempts to deliver co-ordinated impulses to the muscles, thus triggering muscle contraction by the appropriate muscle groups. Furthermore, the CNS determines the outcome of the performance by control of the intangible component of performance, namely motivation. In addition to the CNS, the autonomic system regulates many components of the system that need to respond to the increasing demands of exercise, e.g. by increasing cardiac frequency and redistributing blood flow.

It is useful to have access to facilities for the assessment of exercise capacity or performance. There are many occasions when the clinical history and resting lung function studies do not lead to a clearcut diagnosis. To this end, an exercise test may well provide the missing piece of the jigsaw.

BIOENERGETICS

During exercise, resting oxygen consumption can increase from around 0.25 litres/min to in excess of 3.0 litres/min, this rise being in proportion to the actual intensity of exercise. To attain these high levels of oxygen consumption, energy must be created within the mitochondria. This energy is in the form of ATP. The reaction is, however, oxygen dependent, and so the increased rate of utilisation of oxygen that occurs with exercise must be matched by increased delivery of oxygen from the atmosphere to the mitochondria. For carbon dioxide, the reverse is the case. There is an increase in carbon dioxide production, which must then be rapidly removed from the cell and released to the atmosphere. Thus, the lungs, circulation and muscle systems must all work in harmony if the individual is to be able to achieve a high level of exercise.

ATP is produced during both aerobic and anaerobic metabolism. Six ATP molecules are gained during the catabolism of glucose to pyruvate during glycolysis. Two are produced in the glycolytic pathway, and the remaining four in the mitochondria. The tricarboxylic acid cycle, which takes place within the mitochondria, produces a further 30 ATP molecules, giving a total of 36 ATP molecules.

The production of 36 ATP molecules is based on the utilisation of carbohydrate as glucose. Other sources of energy can also be utilised. Theoretically, protein can be used although this is unlikely during exercise. Fat, as palmitate, is used, but cannot be utilised anaerobically. Thus, as the intensity of exercise increases, the use of fat will decrease. This leaves carbohydrate to be used increasingly as the intensity of exercise increases, or during prolonged exercise. This partly explains why marathon runners eat large quantities of pasta the night before a race as it provides a rapid energy source, maintains blood glucose and gives sufficient glycogen energy reserves.

The quantitative measure of exercise intensity is oxygen uptake (VO_2). As the energy demands of exercise increase, production of ATP cannot be sustained by aerobic metabolism alone. Therefore, ATP production continues, but anaerobically. Generally this occurs at about 50% of the maximum VO_2 (VO_{2max}). Above this point, oxygen is still consumed, and ATP is produced by both the aerobic and anaerobic pathways. During anaerobic metabolism, lactic acid is produced. Lactic acid leaves the cells and enters the bloodstream where it becomes dissociated almost completely. It is buffered mainly by the carbonic acid–bicarbonate system.

The point at which lactate production can be detected is termed the anaerobic threshold (AT). Since an acid is being produced and transported in the blood, metabolic acidosis develops and pH begins to decrease. The normal regulatory control mechanism for this is to increase the level of ventilation, thus causing a compensatory respiratory alkalosis. The result of these effects can be demonstrated using a simple progressive exercise test (Figure 1.7). The subject cycles for 1 minute at increasing workloads up to maximum. Measurements of ventilation (V_E), VO_2 and production of CO_2 (VCO_2) are made throughout. Initially, as the workload increases, V_E, VO_2 and VCO_2 increase linearly. When the anaerobic threshold is reached, the VCO_2 increases disproportionately to the increases in VO_2. The reason for this increase in VCO_2 is that not only is metabolically produced carbon dioxide being excreted but there is additional carbon dioxide generated by the bicarbonate buffering of lactate. For a short period of increasing exercise intensity, the V_E increases proportionally with the increase in carbon dioxide, called isocapnic buffering. As exercise intensity increases further, ventilation begins to exceed the rate of increase in VCO_2, so causing the P_ACO_2 to decrease, called respiratory compensation.

PULMONARY ADAPTATIONS TO EXERCISE

V_E, V_T and f_b all significantly alter with increasing exercise intensity. Ventilation increases from approximately 6 litres/min at rest to in excess of 150 litres/min in elite athletes. This increase is linear up to about 50% to 60% of maximal VO_2, after which the effects of anaerobic threshold take effect. Thereafter, V_E increases at a much faster rate.

In normal subjects, the increase in V_E is primarily due to an increase in V_T. Breathing frequency also increases with increasing exercise intensity, but at a more gradual rate. However, when V_T has reached maximum, the rise in ventilation is continued by a more rapid increase in breathing frequency.

The ventilatory changes described so far relate to total ventilation. To maintain adequate gas exchange, V_A is important. Up to about 75% of maximum VO_2, V_A increases linearly with increasing VO_2 and VCO_2. Above this point, V_A

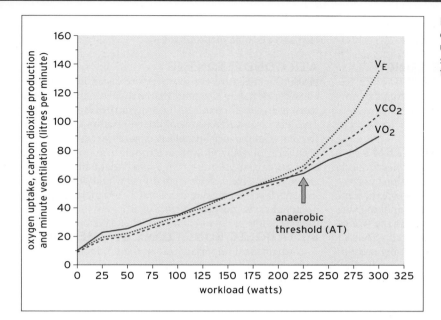

Figure 1.7 The relationship of exercise intensity to oxygen uptake in a normal healthy male subject. As the workload increases, the oxygen uptake increases linearly.

increases at a much greater rate. It is at this point of respiratory compensation that P_ACO_2 begins to decrease.

ACID-BASE BALANCE DURING EXERCISE

The regulation of H^+ within the cell and body fluids, and the role of the ventilatory and renal systems in the maintenance of acid–base balance, has already been described. During increasing levels of exercise, the regulation of H^+ becomes progressively more difficult since H^+ increases due to both carbon dioxide production and lactic acid formation. Lactate can rise to values as high as 30 mmol in short intermittent maximal exercise.

Alveolar oxygen remains constant up until about 50% of maximal VO_2, gradually rising thereafter. Arterial oxygen does the opposite, so the $P_{A-a}O_2$ difference increases. This probably reflects the increased pulmonary blood flow which limits the time spent by the red blood cells in the pulmonary capillaries to equilibrate the alveolar gas.

Blood lactate increases during exercise from the point of the AT onwards. Concomitant to this increase is a reciprocal decrease in plasma HCO_3^- levels. The lactate produced results in an approximately equimolar decrease in HCO_3^- in an attempt to balance the acid production. However, the lactate production from AT onwards tends to outstrip the effects of HCO_3^-. The result is an increase in $[H^+]$ and hence a decrease in pH. Subjects can develop a significant metabolic acidosis, with the pH falling as low as 6.8 during exhausting exercise. In active muscle, the pH is even lower, falling to around 6.4 at the point of exhaustion. The side effects of such a low pH are nausea, headache and dizziness, and pain in the exercising muscle groups!

On cessation of exercise, there is a continuing decrease in P_ACO_2, $[HCO_3^-]$ and pH until about 2 minutes post-exercise, after which these values begin to return towards normal resting levels. These effects probably occur due to the continuing increased level of post-exercise ventilation and the relatively high levels of perfusion of the recovering muscle.

INTEGRATION OF METABOLIC, CARDIOVASCULAR AND VENTILATORY SYSTEMS

The transfer of oxygen and carbon dioxide between the mitochondria and the air requires a finely balanced and co-ordinated interaction of cardiovascular, respiratory and cellular metabolic activity. Just because VO_2 increases from 0.50 to 5.0 litres/min, i.e. an increase of 10 times the resting value, it does not mean that the cardiovascular or oxygen extraction system increases its rate of activity by the same magnitude. Indeed, the cardiac output may increase from 5 to 30 litres/min, i.e. an increase of 6 times the resting value, while oxygen extraction can increase threefold from 50 to 150 ml/litre.

Oxygen transport is dependent on a series of linked, interactive mechanisms, which must work together to achieve the desired result (Figures 1.8A and B). A failure in any one of these linkages results in an impediment to oxygen transport and therefore results in submaximal performance. The removal of carbon dioxide is also dependent on a series of linked mechanisms, from the production of carbon dioxide in the cell to its final expiration in the lungs.

The flow diagrams illustrate that in some cases a limitation in one part of the chain may or may not be reduced if another part of the chain compensates. If V_T is reduced there will be higher than expected increase in cardiac output, thus maintaining the venous oxygen level. However, a reduction in V_T will result in a buildup of carbon dioxide since the other parts of the chain will be able to compensate to a very limited extent only. Thus, the position of ventilation in the chain affects the magnitude of the response of the compensatory mechanisms.

OTHER FUNCTIONS OF THE LUNG

The respiratory system has other functions that are not fully understood. These include defence mechanisms, air conditioning and metabolic functions.

PULMONARY DEFENCE MECHANISMS
Over a 12-month period an adult human breathes around 4.2 million litres of air that may contain infectious micro-organisms, hazardous dusts or chemicals. Exposure to contaminants may be voluntary, e.g. cigarette smoking, or involuntary, e.g. breathing contaminated air in the workplace or outdoors. Clearly, many pulmonary and systemic infections, inflammatory lung disorders and malignancies can result from exposure to airborne agents. Generally, the lungs manage by using a number of defence mechanisms, the main one being mucociliary clearance. Cough, sniffing and bronchoalveolar clearance are additional mechanisms.

Mucociliary clearance starts in the nose. The clearance of secretions in the nose is effected mainly by the mucus being swept backwards to the throat where it is swallowed or expelled. Below the larynx, the mucociliary escalator is responsible for the production and clearance of mucus. This escalator extends from below the larynx down to the 16th airway generation, after which it is replaced by bronchoalveolar clearance involving surfactant and alveolar macrophages.

AIR CONDITIONING
Humidification and the temperature of ambient air vary considerably. It is essential that the alveoli are protected from even small changes in temperature and humidity. The very large surface area of the respiratory tract and, in particular, of the nasal passages, ensures virtually complete equilibration to 37°C. At this temperature, water vapour exerts a partial pressure of 6.3 kPa. Adequate humidification is important, since cold, dry air would dehydrate the mucous layer, increasing its viscosity, and thereby slowing or stopping the flow of mucus.

METABOLIC FUNCTIONS OF THE LUNG
The lung has an important role in the production, storage and release of substances used either locally or elsewhere in the body. Probably the best example is the production of surfactant. Hormones and various vasoactive substances and proteases are also dealt with by the lungs.

ACKNOWLEDGEMENTS

I would like to thank Nicola Allaouat, Senior Medical Technical Officer, and Elizabeth Timms, Physiotherapist from the Respiratory Department, Bristol Royal Infirmary, for their advice in the preparation of this chapter.

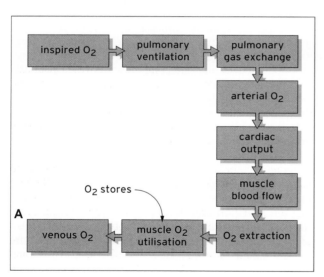
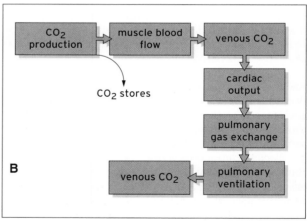

Figure 1.8 (A) and (B) represent the interactive mechanisms of oxygen and carbon dioxide transport.

GENERAL READING

Kendrick AH, Catterall JR. *An introduction to respiratory physiology – basic principles and clinical examples.* Oxford: Butterworth-Heinemann; 1996.
Nunn JF. *Applied respiratory physiology,* 4th ed. Oxford: Butterworth-Heinemann; 1993.
Staub NC. *Basic respiratory physiology.* New York: Churchill Livingstone; 1991.
West JB. *Respiratory physiology – the essentials,* 5th ed. Oxford: Blackwell Scientific; 1995.
West JB. *Ventilation/blood flow and gas exchange,* 5th ed. Oxford: Blackwell Scientific; 1990.

2

SJ Connellan

LUNG FUNCTION TESTING/CHEST ASSESSMENT

CHAPTER OUTLINE

- **Tests of ventilatory function**
- **Tests of gas exchange**
- **Exercise testing**
- **Clinical application of lung function tests**

- **Physiotherapy approach to the assessment of medical respiratory conditions**
- **Gathering information**
- **Subjective assessment**
- **Objective assessment**

INTRODUCTION

It is unusual for a specific lung function test to diagnose a disease. At best, a series of tests may place a lung disorder into one of several categories, and when other features such as history, physical examination, radiology and pathology are added to the equation, a possible diagnosis is considered. Most requests for tests will include a provisional diagnosis. When the most appropriate tests have been selected, further hurdles must be overcome before any reliable results can be obtained. The patient must be able to co-operate fully, and there is no substitute for an experienced, sympathetic but firm technician to ensure that maximum performance has been achieved; a rushed estimate of total lung capacity (TLC) in a claustrophobic and panicking, body box-bound patient is of no use to anyone. The technician must have the right to question the advisability of a test on a particular day as the patient may have become too ill to co-operate or may be recovering from fractured ribs or even recent surgery.

Finally, it is essential that the equipment used is serviced regularly and reliably calibrated.

The main uses of the lung function test are:

- To help define more clearly the type of functional disorder.
- To measure the natural progression (or regression with therapy) of the disorder by serial testing.
- To decide on the feasibility of thoracic surgery.
- To measure the degree of respiratory failure, which will include assessment for long-term oxygen therapy.

If the brain is functioning normally, a breath begins with contraction of the inspiratory muscles, enlarging the thorax, lowering intrathoracic and pleural pressures, enlarging the alveoli and airways and expanding alveolar gas, so reducing its pressure below atmospheric. Air at atmospheric pressure must flow into the thorax where it is conducted to, and diffuses into, the alveoli. At any one moment, approximately 100 ml of desaturated blood, with a strong affinity for oxygen, is spread over an area of 70 m^2 (the area of the pulmonary capillary bed) separated from air by a membrane which is 0.2 μm thick. Oxygen from alveolar air diffuses rapidly across the alveolar–capillary membrane and is finally chemically combined with haemoglobin molecules within circulating red blood cells. Carbon dioxide diffuses in the opposite direction and is eliminated in expired gas.

Appreciation of these steps in respiration is important in helping to understand how a specific lung function test may pinpoint a particular malfunction of the respiratory system.

Three broad categories of testing are considered:

- Tests of ventilatory function.
- Tests of gas exchange.
- Exercise testing.

TESTS OF VENTILATORY FUNCTION

Tests of ventilatory function measure the 'bellows' action of the thoracic cage and lungs, detecting any abnormal interference in the free flow of air from atmosphere to alveoli and back.

Figure 2.1 shows how TLC is broken down into its various volumes. Their size and relationship to each other give clues to underlying functional disorders. When deciding whether a particular volume is normal for an individual, height, age and sex need to be taken into consideration. The predicted TLC for a petite elderly woman may be half that expected for a tall young man. If the value obtained is more than 1.7 standard deviations from the predicted, it is very likely to be abnormal.

During normal resting ventilation, air moves gently back and forth in a tidal manner, and the total volume of each breath is called the tidal volume (V_T). The largest volume of air that can be inspired from the end point of the tidal expiration is called the inspiratory capacity (IC), and the largest volume that can be expired after full inspiration is called the vital capacity (VC). The lungs cannot collapse to an airless state because of the compliance of the thoracic cage, and there is always some residue of gas, the residual volume (RV). At the end of a tidal expiration much more air remains in the lungs and this is called the functional residual capacity (FRC). This is the neutral position of the respiratory system, at which point the inward recoil of the lungs is exactly balanced by the outward recoil of the chest wall.

All these volumes, apart from RV and FRC, can be measured by a spirometer. TLC can be derived by adding IC and FRC (see Figure 2.1).

The two most commonly used methods of measuring TLC are the helium dilution method and whole body plethysmography.

HELIUM DILUTION METHOD

When using the helium dilution method, the patient breathes into a closed circuit spirometer containing a mixture of gas with a known concentration of helium. The patient is switched into the system at the end of a normal expiration, and this mixture gradually equilibrates with the gas in the lungs. Oxygen is added and carbon dioxide is absorbed, maintaining a stable FRC.

When the helium concentration has stopped falling (the helium having been diluted by increasing lung volume), the patient takes a full inspiration and this IC is added to the FRC (derived from a simple equation) to give the TLC.

Equilibration between spirometer and lungs is achieved within 5–10 minutes in most normal subjects, but in severe airways obstruction mixing is much slower because of poor ventilation distribution, and this may make it more difficult to estimate the point at which equilibration has been achieved.

WHOLE BODY PLETHYSMOGRAPHY

Whole body plethysmography involves the patient sitting in an airtight box and attempting to inspire against an occluded airway. This results in a reduced intrathoracic pressure and a rise in the pressure of gas within the box (body plethysmograph).

This latter pressure change is proportional to the change in intrathoracic volume, which can be estimated.

Whole body plethysmography measures all gas within the thorax, which may include emphysematous bullae, hiatus hernia or pneumothorax. When there is an uneven ventilation distribution with generalised air flow obstruction or a large poorly communicating bulla, the TLC estimate by helium dilution may be much less than the plethysmographic estimate, the discrepancy being greater the more severe the disorder.

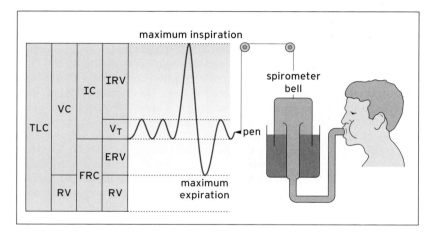

Figure 2.1 Total lung capacity (TLC) with spirometric recording of its subdivisions tidal volume (V_T) and vital capacity (VC). IRV = inspiratory reserve volume; ERV = expiratory reserve volume.

Tests of Forced Expiration

One of the simplest tests of forced expiration was the Snider match test in which patients were considered to have a serious impairment of ventilatory function if they were unable to blow out a lighted match held 15 cm from the mouth. All variations on this theme have in common the same manoeuvre, i.e. a deep full inspiration followed by expulsion of air from the lungs with the maximum force possible.

PEAK EXPIRATORY FLOW RATE (PEFR)

The peak flow sustained over a 10 ms period after the beginning of a forced expiratory manoeuvre can be measured using a Wright's peak flow meter (or the more commonly used, inexpensive, mini-Wright meter). From a position of full inspiration, air is forcibly expired across a pivoted vein (Wright's) or a lightweight piston (mini-Wright), both of which are spring-loaded and encased. The displacement of the vein or piston is proportional to maximum flow rate.

This is a highly effort dependent test but in practice and with education it is very reproducible. It utilises one piece of equipment, which should be available not only to the hospital doctor, nurse and physiotherapist but also to the general practitioner, practice nurse and, of course, the patient. It is one of the simplest ways of measuring lung function and is particularly useful for measuring serial changes in airways obstruction over periods of time.

In spite of this, many general medical wards do not have such a meter though they would find it inexcusable to be without a sphygmomanometer.

FORCED EXPIRATORY VOLUME IN 1 SECOND

The forced expiratory volume in 1 second (FEV_1) can be obtained by measuring the change in expired volume against time using a spirometer (Figure 2.2). When a forced expiration is started from full inspiration, i.e. TLC, flow rises rapidly to peak value and then, because of progressive airways narrowing due to a combination of high pleural pressure compressing the airways and a lowering of lung volume with reduction in elastic recoil of the lung, there is a rapid fall off of flow rate to zero when residual volume is reached and no more air can be expelled. In normal people this usually takes about 4 s and the full volume expired is the forced vital capacity (FVC). The volume expired in the first second of the manoeuvre is the FEV_1, and this is usually at least 75% of the FVC (see Figure 2.2).

The FEV_1 and PEFR are well correlated but the FEV_1 does measure average flow rate over a larger lung volume than the PEFR. Both FEV_1 and PEFR are the most widely used and reproducible measures of forced expiration.

Most modern spirometry in lung function departments relies on dry rolling seal systems but one of the most commonly used spirometers (vitalograph) uses the principle of a wedge bellows system. One of the advantages of this method, as opposed to some of the more modern hand-held digital printout spirometers, is that the technician can see the spirogram tracing as it is produced, and this makes it easier to ascertain whether the patient's technique and effort is satisfactory. A single measurement with no visual feedback and no encouragement is a waste of time.

FLOW VOLUME LOOPS

If, instead of plotting the FVC manoeuvre as volume against time, the maximum flow rate is plotted against changing lung volume, it is possible to record the maximum expiratory flow–volume (MEFV) curve. If this is followed immediately by a full forced inspiration to TLC, the maximum inspiratory flow–volume (MIFV) curve can be measured, which completes the flow volume loop (Figure 2.3). This enables the maximum flow rates to be recorded not only at large lung volumes near TLC but also at small volumes near RV, at which point flow through

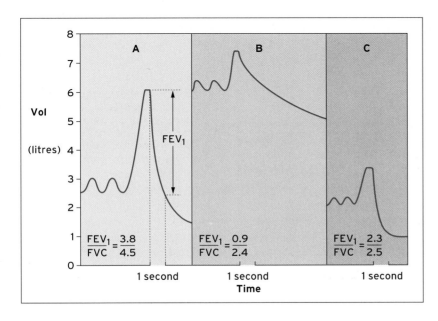

Figure 2.2 Spirometric patterns of (A) normal forced expiration, (B) airways obstruction and (C) lung restriction.

smaller airways will predominate. The shape of the MIFV curve is quite different, as there is no sudden flow limitation on inspiration in normal people, and peak flow occurs about midway up to TLC.

Airways Resistance

The major site of resistance to air flow during normal breathing is in the larger central airways. Measurement of airways resistance is more sensitive to changes in large airways, and relatively insensitive to changes in smaller airways. It is possible, therefore, for there to be extensive disease present in the peripheral airways before a significant increase in total airways resistance occurs. To measure resistance, the pressure difference between mouth and alveoli (the driving pressure), and the simultaneous flow rate need to be ascertained. This is achieved with the patient sitting in a body plethysmograph.

The measurement of airways resistance is a more sensitive test of airway calibre than FEV_1 but it is less reproducible. It also avoids the need for a full inspiration and forced expiration, which can in itself cause bronchoconstriction in asthmatics and, therefore, is preferred by some workers when assessing dose–response studies using bronchodilators or bronchoconstrictors.

Compliance

Compliance is a measure of elasticity or, in the case of the lung, distensibility or stiffness. The stiffer the lungs, the greater the external force (pressure) required to produce a given increase in lung volume. Compliance is measured by plotting changes in intraoesophageal pressure (which is an approximation of intrapleural pressure) against changes in lung volume. This pressure is obtained by positioning a thin-walled balloon in the lower third of the oesophagus, connected by a catheter to a pressure transducer. From the FRC position the patient inspires a measured volume of air, at which point the breath is held while transpulmonary pressure (mouth pressure–oesophageal pressure) is measured. Several measurements are made between TLC and FRC and the pressure–volume curve is constructed, the slope of which gives compliance. The lower the value of the compliance, the stiffer the lungs. Compliance is related to lung volume. Specific compliance is the ratio of compliance over FRC and is independent of age and sex.

TESTS OF GAS EXCHANGE

For efficient respiratory gas exchange, the major processes of lung ventilation, diffusion across the alveolar–capillary membrane and lung perfusion, should all be intact. Normal distribution of the inspired air depends on an adequate thoracic cage 'bellows' action followed by unimpaired flow through the bronchial tree to the lung periphery where molecular diffusion into the alveolar compartment takes place. The efficiency and uniformity of ventilation can be assessed by measuring nitrogen concentration at the mouth while breathing 100% oxygen. If gas mixing is perfect, the expired nitrogen concentration will fall by the same proportion with each breath, but in generalised airways obstruction, washout is much slower and more uneven. The single breath nitrogen test or closing volume is a variation in which single full inspiration of 100% oxygen is followed by a slow full expiration with monitoring of nitrogen concentration at the mouth. Initially the expired air comes only

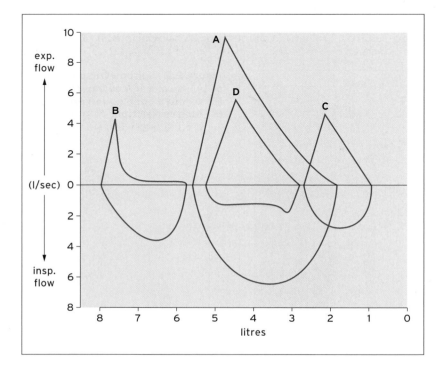

Figure 2.3 Schematic representation of (A) maximum flow volume loops in normal people, (B) severe air flow obstruction, (C) lung restriction, and (D) upper airways obstruction.

from the more central airways, and contains pure oxygen. Nitrogen concentration then rises rapidly as alveolar gas is mixed in with the expirate. Following this the concentration of nitrogen remains almost constant during the third phase of expiration unless there is poor ventilation distribution, in which case instead of seeing a plateau a slope of increase in concentration is seen. The greater this gradient the greater the inequalities of ventilation. This is because better ventilated alveoli (with lower nitrogen concentrations) tend to empty before less well ventilated alveoli. Towards the end of expiration the nitrogen concentration rises more sharply (phase 4). This is attributed to closure of airways, commencing at the lung bases and rising progressively up the lung as RV is approached. The sudden increase in nitrogen concentration is seen because the more distended alveoli in the upper lung zones have received relatively less oxygen during the preceding inspiration. They, therefore, contribute a disproportionately larger nitrogen concentration of the expirate once the airways supplying the low nitrogen basal alveoli start to close. Phase 3 may become so steep, however, that phase 4 may not be clearly identifiable. The slope of phase 3 has been used as a research technique for detecting early airways disease. The volume over which phase 4 occurs is called the closing volume, which is the lung volume at which closure of dependent airways begins. Closing volume increases with age and in association with abnormalities such as air flow obstruction and cardiac failure (see Figure 2.4).

Oxygen and carbon dioxide cross the alveolar–capillary membrane by diffusion. Molecules of oxygen have to cross the alveolar epithelium, interstitium, endothelium, blood plasma and red cell membrane before they chemically combine with haemoglobin (see Chapter 1). Carbon monoxide is also avidly taken up by haemoglobin, and serves as a useful inhaled gas in estimating the ease of transfer across the barriers—the carbon monoxide

transfer factor (T_LCO). The patient takes a VC breath of carbon monoxide and helium, holds the breath for 10 seconds and then exhales. As helium is not taken up by the pulmonary blood, this gives the dilution of the inspired gas with alveolar gas and thus the initial alveolar PCO. It is possible, using a simple equation, to calculate the volume of carbon monoxide taken up per minute, per mmHg alveolar PCO, i.e. T_LCO. As a bonus, the helium dilution technique also gives an estimate of the alveolar volume or, at least, that volume that the inspired carbon monoxide 'sees' while the breath is held.

In a patient with generalised airways obstruction, this volume will be much less than the true alveolar volume because of the impaired distribution of the inspired volume, and carbon monoxide transfer will also be reduced because of the reduced area 'seen'. To allow for this reduced volume effect, the transfer coefficient (or transfer factor divided by the alveolar volume obtained during the test) is estimated. This helps to differentiate between a real reduction in carbon monoxide transfer or a reduction solely due to the carbon monoxide being presented to an abnormally small volume or surface area. The patient who has had a pneumonectomy may have a perfectly functioning single lung but the transfer factor will be reduced by about 50% because of the halving of the TLC. The transfer coefficient, or KCO as it is known, corrects for this volume effect. The transfer factor is determined by the thickness and area of alveolar membrane and the size of the pulmonary–capillary volume, and how well ventilation is matched to pulmonary perfusion. It will therefore be affected by such diverse disorders as anaemia, pneumonectomy, emphysema and pulmonary embolus.

EXERCISE TESTING

In the same way that any piece of machinery cannot be considered fully tested until maximally stressed, the lungs

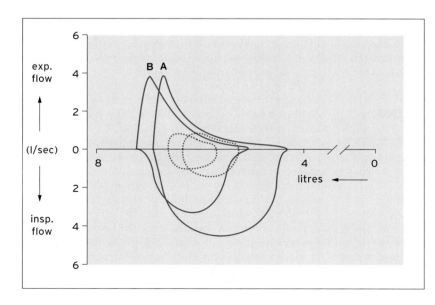

Figure 2.4 Tidal and maximum flow-volume curves in a patient with severe air flow obstruction, before and after treatment.

and heart need to be stressed with exercise to assess their efficiency. Minor dysfunction which is not apparent at rest may come to light on exercise. Asthma may be induced, known disability graded and myocardial insufficiency diagnosed and, on occasions, an objective assessment will contrast with the patient's own expectation of exercise performance.

Whatever the choice of exercise, a doctor should be present with resuscitation equipment to hand, and the patient should always be able to stop the test if symptoms become distressing.

In those patients already known to be moderately limited by respiratory disease, a simple walking test will be able to grade severity.

The 12 minute walking test (McGavin, 1976) and subsequent 6 minute variation are tests of free corridor walking in which the patient is asked to cover as much distance as possible during a defined period, with stops for a breather when necessary. At least two practice walks are required to improve subsequent reproducibility of the tests, and, like most exercise studies, motivation is an important factor. Free walking can be replaced by treadmill walking at a fixed rate and zero gradient for 12 minutes in a more controlled environment, and with continuous ECG monitoring. In more sophisticated testing using a treadmill or cycle ergometer, either with a progressively increased workload or at a steady state of exercise, tidal volume, ventilation, heart rate, ECG, oxygen consumption and carbon dioxide output, can be monitored continuously. In this way, the overall capacity to perform exercise can be assessed and compared with predicted values. If arterial blood is also sampled during exercise, information on the efficiency of pulmonary gas exchange can be obtained. If dyspnoea on exertion is due to respiratory rather than cardiac disease, the patient will tend to stop near to maximum predicted voluntary ventilation or even exceed this without reaching predicted maximum heart rate. The interpretation of such tests is not always clear.

Running on a treadmill for 6 minutes with regular monitoring of PEFR is one way of diagnosing exercise-induced asthma, a typical response being a slight rise in PEFR during exercise and a marked drop after exercise, usually reaching lowest levels about 4 minutes after stopping. This is one of the few diagnostic tests of lung function.

CLINICAL APPLICATION OF LUNG FUNCTION TESTS

This section considers specific examples of respiratory disorders, and the associated abnormalities of lung function.

AIR FLOW OBSTRUCTION

Patients with asthma, emphysema (with or without chronic bronchitis), bronchiectasis and cystic fibrosis may all be demonstrated as having variable degrees of air flow obstruction. Asthma is the one condition in which the degree of obstruction may vary spontaneously or with treatment by more than 20%. However, any of these conditions may have a reversible component demonstrated by response to a bronchodilator.

ASTHMA

One of the simplest ways of demonstrating reversible air flow obstruction is by measuring the percentage increase in FEV_1 or PEFR after taking an inhaled bronchodilator. If this is >20% (some would accept 15%) asthma is a likely diagnosis. Another approach, particularly in more chronic severe air flow obstruction, is to monitor PEFR during a course of high dose corticosteroids, which may result in a mean rise of PEFR of 20% and may also enhance the acute response to the bronchodilator. In some cases of asthma the diagnosis may be missed, unless daily PEFRs are recorded to reveal the typically increased diurnal variation often accompanied by early morning 'dips' in PEFR. There may be other 'dips' specifically associated with, for example, exposure to an allergen/irritant at work. Typical patterns may also be seen during recovery from an acute attack of asthma. This is often observed during a course of high dose corticosteroids, and a gradual rise in PEFR may be accompanied by transient and troublesome morning 'dips'.

In an acute attack of asthma there is widespread narrowing of airways with bronchospasm, mucosal oedema, inflammation and mucous plugging of small airways. These changes result in reductions in maximum expiratory flow rates (decreased PEFR, FEV_1/VC and MEFV flow rates). Airways resistance increases and as the narrowed airways close off even during tidal expiration, the patient tends to breathe at a higher lung volume to try to keep the airways open for as long as possible during expiration. This results in a higher FRC and RV with some restriction of the VC. TLC is elevated as a result of widespread air trapping behind closed airways. Ventilation distribution becomes very uneven and poorly matched with perfusion, resulting in impaired pulmonary gas exchange. Initially, the increase in total ventilation will offset the fall in PO_2; however, with more severe air flow obstruction, the increase in total ventilation might not be maintainable. As the patient tires from the exhausting work of breathing, the PO_2 might suddenly start to drop with a corresponding rise in PCO_2. Without intensive therapy, including assisted ventilation, death may follow rapidly.

In chronic stable asthma there may be persistent findings of hyperinflation with increased TLC and decreased FEV_1/VC and VC, but T_TCO is usually normal when corrected for lung volume, i.e. KCO.

Many asthmatics will volunteer that certain things, such as cold air, exercise, paint fumes or specific allergens, trigger off their asthma, and diagnostic tests may be based on these facts. Challenging the patient with increasing amounts of inhaled histamine or cold dry air and noting the point at which the FEV_1 falls by 20% will give an estimate of the non-specific bronchial responsiveness of the airways (Cockroft et al., 1977). The lower the concentration required the more 'twitchy' the airways.

Under careful supervision, with an overnight stay in hospital, the patient can be challenged with a nebulised solution of suspected allergen, a fall of greater than 15% being taken as an asthmatic reaction. These latter tests are not for the casual, inexperienced investigator.

CHRONIC OBSTRUCTIVE PULMONARY DISEASE

Chronic obstructive pulmonary disease (COPD) is an all embracing term which in current usage includes chronic bronchitis with an obstructive element and/or emphysema. It suggests less variability of air flow obstruction with no periods of normality. This can, of course, happen in long-standing asthma but COPD is usually associated with a long history of smoking.

Chronic Bronchitis

Chronic bronchitis is defined in terms of sputum production, and reflects mucous hypersecretion in the airways. Any associated air flow obstruction can be assessed by using the forced expiratory spirogram or MEFV curve as already described.

Emphysema

Emphysema is a pathological diagnosis, but lung function testing in combination with high resolution thoracic computerised tomography (CT) scanning can result in a reasonably confident diagnosis. Emphysema is characterised by a breakdown of alveolar walls with consequent dilation of distal air spaces and destruction of some of the pulmonary–capillary bed. This results in loss of lung elasticity and a reduced area for gas exchange. As in severe asthma, there will be reductions in all forced expiratory flow rates (Figures 2.3 and 2.4). This flow limitation, seen early in forced expiration, is the result of dynamic compression of airways which have lost elastic support from surrounding lung and may also be more 'floppy' due to loss of elasticity of airways walls. In addition, there may be increased mucus with inflammation and narrowing of small airways. This tendency to early expiratory airways closure may occur during tidal breathing, and the patient has to 'climb up' a TLC until tidal breathing is at a point where expiration can be fuller without early airways closure. This results in a higher FRC and RV; TLC is also increased as a result of air trapping. The VC in severe air flow obstruction, particularly in emphysema, is better assessed by avoiding forced expiration by getting the patient to breathe out slowly from TLC, thus avoiding the much earlier flow limitation due to dynamic airways compression. This is called the relaxed or slow VC (SVC) and the difference between this and the FVC gives some indication as to the severity of obstruction.

There is often a large discrepancy between the FRC measured by helium dilution and the body plethysmographic estimate, the former being an underestimate because of poorly ventilated areas. The larger RV tends to reduce the 'room' left within the TLC for the VC, which becomes more restricted as emphysema worsens.

A recognised response to bronchodilators in emphysema is one of lung deflation (Connellan and Morgan, 1982). The FRC, RV and possibly TLC, decrease and there may be a small increase in tidal volumes. There are greater increases in FVC and peak inspiratory flow rate (PIFR) than in PEFR and FEV_1 (see Figure 2.4). Although the improvements in FEV_1 and PEFR may be disappointing, the patient may feel less dyspnoeic, presumably as a result of the reduced FRC putting inspiratory muscles at a better mechanical advantage and reducing the work of breathing.

Gas exchange is markedly impaired in emphysema contrary to the usual findings of normal or raised T_LCO in stable asthma. The surface area of normal lungs approaches that of a tennis court, and in emphysema this may be reduced to the side lines, particularly if a large non-ventilated bulla is compressing surrounding lung. If damage to the pulmonary–capillary bed and poor distribution of ventilation (badly matched with perfusion) is added to this it can be appreciated how distressing it must be for the emphysematous 'pink puffer' to maintain near normal arterial blood gases at the expense of hyperventilation at high lung volumes with an increased work of breathing. Some patients with chronic bronchitis and air flow obstruction have smaller increases in TLC and tend not to hyperventilate, 'accepting' the high PCO_2 and low PO_2 with subsequent drift into pulmonary hypertension and right-sided heart failure. These are know as 'blue bloaters', i.e. cyanosed and oedematous. The stimulus to breathe in these patients is hypoxaemia and this might be removed if the concentration of inspired oxygen delivered to the patient is too high, the overall result being a reduction in ventilation and a rapid rise in PCO_2, a fall in arterial pH, coma and death.

UPPER AIRWAYS OBSTRUCTION

So far the effects of generalised airways obstruction have been considered, but a narrowing of the larger more central airways at any point from the main bronchi up to the pharynx will also cause characteristic functional abnormalities. The flow volume loop will help to localise the lesion to below (intrathoracic) or above (extrathoracic) the thoracic inlet. In the example shown in Figure 2.3 there is a sharp early cut off of inspiratory flow caused by a narrowing in the upper trachea. The rapid initial flow of air across the narrowing results in a fall in pressure immediately below the lesion, and this negative pressure (Bernoulli effect) tends to suck the walls together cutting off flow for an instant and setting up a vibration as air is forced through. This vibration produces the characteristic noise of stridor. The PEFR is also reduced and often more blunted than shown (see Figure 2.3). There is usually a high airways resistance with a relatively normal FEV_1, and the VC may be well preserved.

SLEEP APNOEA SYNDROME

In the sleep apnoea syndrome, episodes of upper airways obstruction may occur as a result of enhancement of the pharynx due to such conditions as obesity, malformations of the mandible or enlarged tonsils or adenoids. Pharyngeal muscular tone is reduced further during the rapid eye movement (REM) portion of sleep, and the resulting episodic pharyngeal closure during inspiration (the common snore is a less severe form) results in variable degrees of upper airways resistance and obstruction. If severe enough it may be associated with transient arterial hypoxaemia, pulmonary hypertension and cor pulmonale. Sleep will tend to be fragmented with frequent arousal, and sleep deprivation will result in day-time hypersomnolence.

The characteristic features of this syndrome have been discovered by recording the EEG, nasal and oral air flow, oxygen saturation and chest and abdominal wall movement during sleep. Absence of air flow, oxygen desaturation and vigorous, out of phase, chest and abdominal wall movement, suggest obstructive sleep apnoea. If air flow and chest/abdominal wall movement are absent for more than 10 seconds, this suggests central apnoea and results from a transient lack of drive to breathe. This latter form of apnoea is much less common but it is also recognised that both central and obstructive patterns may occur in the same patient (Guilleminault *et al.*, 1976).

LUNG RESTRICTION

Diseases which restrict expansion of the lungs are characterised by a reduced VC and TLC. This may result from increased lung stiffness, pleural disease, reduced skeletal mobility or an abnormal neuromuscular apparatus.

Lung Fibrosis

Interstitial and alveolar wall thickening with collagen deposition both serve to stiffen up the lungs. Increased radial traction on the airways may actually increase airways calibre for a given lung volume. VC and FEV_1 will both be reduced (FEV_1 to a lesser extent) and the $FEV_1/VC\%$ is typically supernormal. The maximum flows as demonstrated by the MEFV curve tend to be greater than normal (see Figures 2.2 and 2.3). TLC and RV are reduced (RV to a lesser extent) and the RV/TLC ratio is typically high. Abnormally high pressures are required to distend the lungs, i.e. compliance is decreased. Patchy inequalities in ventilation and perfusion, in addition to thickening of alveolar walls and a reduction in the pulmonary–capillary bed, result in impaired carbon monoxide transfer. Estimation of the KCO will help to determine how much of the impairment is a result of the reduced surface area for gas exchange. Arterial blood gases typically show reduced oxygen and carbon dioxide tension. The hypoxaemia is mild at rest but may fall dramatically on exercise. The diffusing capacity for carbon monoxide may be measured during exercise and usually doubles or trebles in normal people but remains low in interstitial lung disease. The breathing pattern tends to be rapid and shallow in more severe cases, and high resting respiratory frequency achieves a minute ventilation in spite of the small tidal volume. Dyspnoea tends to be inversely related to VC, and the response to a trial of high dose corticosteroids can be assessed by serial measurements of VC.

Chest Wall Restriction

Anything which limits chest wall expansion will result in a restrictive ventilatory defect with reduction in lung volumes, although TLC may be normal. If there is no associated lung abnormality, gas transfer, although reduced, will be normal or high when corrected for lung volume, i.e. KCO. Skeletal disease (scoliosis, ankylosing spondylitis), neuromuscular disease (motor neurone disease, myasthenia gravis, muscular dystrophy) and pleural disease (thickening or effusion) will all cause restrictive defects. Long-standing restriction may result in areas of atelectasis which, if widespread, may result in reduced lung compliance. The limited tidal volume, atelectasis and lung stiffness in more severe disease will result in arterial hypoxaemia and subsequent ventilatory failure with arterial hypercapnia.

Acute neuromuscular disease such as Guillain–Barré syndrome may require daily monitoring of spirometry to detect progressive ventilatory failure, requiring transfer of patients to the Intensive Care Unit.

Combined Restrictive and Obstructive Pattern

Any disease process of the lung parenchyma which also scars and narrows airways may produce a mixed restrictive and obstructive ventilatory defect with reductions in TLC, FEV_1, FEV_1/VC and T_TCO. Sarcoidosis is a good example of such a condition in which lung fibrosis may be associated with narrowing of small airways and even localised large airways stenoses (the latter may produce an additional feature of upper airways obstruction).

Pulmonary oedema may also result in a mixed picture caused by fluid, narrowing small airways and stiffening of the lungs. The phrase 'all that wheezes is not asthma' is a reminder that pulmonary oedema may present with symptoms predominantly of air flow obstruction. In long-standing mitral stenosis with chronic pulmonary venous congestion and ultimate lung fibrosis, there is reduction in lung compliance, VC and FEV_1/VC with a tendency to elevation of RV as a result of airways narrowing and a stiffening of alveolar walls.

It is important to note that some chronic conditions with airways obstruction may also show additional restrictive ventilatory defects. Patients with cystic fibrosis are likely to suffer with nutritional deficit resulting in reduced muscular mass. If this affects the respiratory muscles chest expansion and the power of coughing will be reduced, which in turn will compound the problems of sputum retention. Patients on long-term steroids may suffer additional ventilatory restrictive defect due to respiratory muscle atrophy.

Respiratory Failure

There is an inverse relationship between the partial pressures of arterial carbon dioxide ($PaCO_2$) and alveolar ventilation. The lower the ventilation the higher the $PaCO_2$. When the $PaCO_2$ rises above normal the patient is in ventilatory failure and there is a concomitant drop in PaO_2. In acute ventilatory failure, the rise in $PaCO_2$ results in a drop in arterial pH (respiratory acidosis). In the chronic situation the kidneys will compensate by retaining bicarbonate (HCO_3^-) and this may partially correct the low pH (compensated respiratory acidosis). Other mechanisms which compensate for low PaO_2 include changes in cardiac output and the oxygen dissociation curve, and an increase in haemoglobin levels. In the acute impairment of gas exchange (as a result of ventilation/perfusion mismatching) as seen in severe asthma, pulmonary emboli or oedema, there will be a lowering, initially, of both PaO_2 and $PaCO_2$. As the patient tires and is unable to maintain an adequate minute ventilation in response to the abnormal gas exchange, alveolar ventilation drops and $PaCO_2$ rises as ventilatory failure supervenes. This sequence of events may follow any sustained severe impairment of respiratory function whether it be due to severe air flow obstruction or lung restriction.

Pre-operative Assessment

Lung function testing may help in deciding whether to proceed to surgical removal of a lobe or lung. Some patients will be excluded easily on the basis of severe air flow obstruction. In others it may help to have additional information on regional ventilation and perfusion by use of radio-isotope lung scanning. In occasional patients with lung cancer, a surprisingly large defect in both ventilation and perfusion may be found on the side of the tumour. This may indicate mediastinal node involvement and an increased risk of inoperability. It also follows that the effect of a pneumonectomy on overall lung function can be more easily gauged when the lung affected by tumour has already been demonstrated to have little ventilation or perfusion, i.e. contributing little to the existing lung function. An FEV_1 of less than 50% of the predicted value or an elevation of $PaCO_2$ are indications that, whatever the surgery contemplated, associated risks will be much higher. Lung function is but one of many factors to be taken into consideration in the decision to operate. Simple exercise testing may complement other measurements when formulating this decision.

Finally, it should always be remembered that dyspnoea is a very complex sensation, the perception of which may vary greatly from one individual to another. Not only can the awareness thereof be heightened in certain neurotic patients (see Chapter 10), but it can also be precipitated by excess circulating thyroxine in thyrotoxicosis or by progestogenic hormones in pregnancy.

PHYSIOTHERAPY APPROACH TO THE ASSESSMENT OF MEDICAL RESPIRATORY CONDITIONS

The purpose of assessment is twofold—it enables the therapist to determine the patient's problems, and to obtain a precise database which can be used as a baseline for future reference. The patient's problems may be classified as those which are a problem to the patient and those which need treatment. Discussion following assessment ensures understanding and agreement between the therapist and patient which leads to an accurate, prioritised problem list. From this list an appropriate management programme can be planned.

Assessment may be divided into three main areas:
- Gathering information.
- Subjective assessment.
- Objective assessment.

Assessment should not be considered as a one-off procedure at the start of treatment but rather as an ongoing process, where the patient's status is continuously monitored and reassessed throughout any interaction.

GATHERING INFORMATION

Initially, the therapist should review the patient's medical notes and diagnostic test results to obtain information about current status, the nature and severity of the disorder and any factors which may influence physiotherapy management. Other members of the multidisciplinary team may often prove to be a rich source of information.

Normally, data in the medical notes are recorded in a standardised format which make it easier to extract relevant information. Essential patient details such as name, address, hospital number and diagnosis should be recorded in the physiotherapy treatment notes. Next, the notes are summarised to include relevant information with regard to medical history, history of present complaint, social history, family history, drug history and examination findings of the major systems, including results of appropriate investigations, e.g. blood gas analysis, lung function tests, chest X-rays and ECGs. It should be remembered that relevant information is any factor contributing to the present situation and anything which may affect patient management. The closely integrated function of the respiratory and cardiovascular systems often means that respiratory disease precipitates changes in the cardiovascular system and *vice versa*. This is particularly true in chronic respiratory conditions. Special note, therefore, must be made of any cardiovascular disorders as these may influence the patient's overall condition and management. Musculoskeletal and neurological disorders may also have a bearing on management, and this should be noted.

Often the notes of patients with chronic respiratory conditions contain an overwhelming amount of information. In this instance the most recent admission notes should be reviewed, referring to earlier notes if appropriate and/or time allows.

INVESTIGATIONS/DIAGNOSTIC TESTS

Of the investigations performed it is essential to review blood gas analysis and HCO_3^- or acid–base balance. These results provide critical information about the patient's current respiratory status, and enable the therapist to determine the severity of the current disorder and the urgency of intervention required.

Review of the partial pressure of oxygen in arterial blood (PaO_2) and arterial oxygen saturation (SaO_2) indicates the level of oxygen in the blood. Oxygen supply is fundamental to normal cell, tissue and system function. A reduction in oxygen levels means not only that system function may be impaired but also that the nature of any intervention must be carefully considered. Most physiotherapeutic interventions increase oxygen consumption and this must be weighed against the overall safety of the patient and any potential benefit derived from the treatment.

Details of blood gas analysis are covered in Chapter 1; however, normal values and a basic overview of how these values change in the different stages of respiratory disorders are given in Table 2.1.

Present and past chest X-rays are viewed, alongside the radiologist's report if available, to reveal current radiological changes and the progression of changes over a period of time. Any disorders detected can be confirmed, and further information gathered, in the following subjective and objective assessments.

Detailed information on lung function tests is given on page 22 onwards.

The information gathered provides an overview of the patient before questioning. In the instance of a severely ill/breathless/distressed patient it may be the only information that can be gathered without further distressing the him or her. The following subjective assessment would be considerably modified in this case.

SUBJECTIVE ASSESSMENT

The subjective assessment enables the therapist to obtain the patient's perspective of his or her disorder and to confirm and elaborate upon existing data. It is essential to identify what the patient considers to be the most important concern at that time. It is also the therapist's first contact with the patient, and the impression created will affect any further interactions. The subjective assessment should therefore be considered as an opportunity to establish a good working relationship with mutual respect.

The assessment should take the form of a structured conversation not a formal interview, where relevant information is elicited in a relaxed manner. Open questions are more effective for gaining a fuller picture, and often additional relevant information, not included in the medical notes, may be obtained. However, closed questions may be of use if a specific yes/no answer is applicable (Holt, 1995).

Initial questioning seeks to gain background information and information concerning the patient and his or her lifestyle; later, more specific questions about the patient's symptoms are asked. It is often appropriate to begin the subjective interview with the question 'What is the main problem?'

It may be helpful for those who have trouble remembering which topics should be covered during the subjective assessment to devise a mnemonic to aid memory. A written list of questions always runs the risk that the student/clinician concentrates more on the paper than the patient (Clarke, 1986). The following mnemonic is simply an example:
How Do People Pay For Only A Small Smoke?

where **H** is the History of present complaint, **D** the Drug history, **P** the Past medical history, **P** Physiotherapy, **F** the Family history, **O** the Occupational history, **A** Allergies, **S** the Social history, and **S** the Smoking history.

	Blood gas analysis and acid–base balance in respiratory disorders				
	Normal values	Early acute disorder/hyper-ventilation may lead to respiratory alkalosis		Later acute disorder may lead to respiratory acidosis	Chronic disorder may lead to compensated respiratory acidosis
pH	7.35–7.45	→	↑	↓	→
PaO_2	12–14 kPa	↓	↓	↓	↓
$PaCO_2$	4.5–6.5 kPa	→	↓	↑	↑
HCO_3^-	22–26 mmol/litre	→	→	→	↑
Base excess	−2 to +2	→	→	→	↑
Saturation	97–98%	↓	↓	↓	↓

→, within normal range;

↑, increased above normal range;

↓, decreased below normal range.

Table 2.1 **Blood gas analysis and acid–base balance in respiratory disorders.**

The questions do not have to be asked in any specific order. Where possible try to establish a smooth, logical progression from one area to another.

POSITION OF THE PATIENT

For the subjective assessment patients are encouraged to be in a position which they find most comfortable.

HISTORY OF PRESENT COMPLAINT

Clarify the sequence of events which have led to the hospital admission or the treatment referral.

DRUG HISTORY

Note all the drugs the patient is and has taken, both now and at the time of admission, the dose, length of time for which they have been prescribed and the mode of delivery. The action, dose and side effects of any unfamiliar drugs can be looked up in a current *British National Formulary* or *Mimms*.

Does the patient understand why he or she is taking the medication and have any side effects been experienced? Clarify the patient's perception of the effectiveness of the drugs taken. It should be noted that poor technique in the administration of certain respiratory drugs, e.g. inhaler therapy, inhibits delivery and hence effectiveness of the drug.

MEDICAL HISTORY

Medical history should encompass all relevant facts regarding the patient's previous illnesses, including any surgery and/or previous hospital admissions and management.

PHYSIOTHERAPY

Has the patient had physiotherapy treatment in the past? If so, when and for what? What type of treatment was received and was it of any value? Patients' perceptions of past therapeutic interventions are invaluable when planning further treatment.

FAMILY HISTORY

Do any relatives suffer from the same disorder? Are there any diseases which have been prevalent among immediate family members, e.g. any history of lung disease or a high incidence of heart disease?

OCCUPATIONAL HISTORY

An occupational history may be relevant if the patient has had an occupation that could predispose to a respiratory or vascular condition, e.g. working in a dusty or smoky environment. Continued working in an adverse environment should be discouraged if at all possible. Social workers may be able to help in negotiating with the employer a change in role.

ALLERGIES

Is the patient aware of any allergies to food, drugs or external agents such as pollen or house dust mites? Can they be avoided?

SOCIAL HISTORY

It is important to note the type of accommodation the patient lives in; for example, is it all on one level or is the bathroom upstairs? Does the patient share accommodation with anyone and how physically able is that person? Does the patient live alone, and does he or she have support from family, friends, neighbours or an outside agent such as a home help?

Particular note should be made of patients' ability to shop and cook for themselves, hence maintaining an adequate diet. Many patients with chronic respiratory diseases are malnourished due to a poor intake or hypermetabolism, which is particularly so in patients with COPD (Mowatt-Larsen and O'Brown, 1993). Remember that chronically breathless patients experience difficulty with eating and are often malnourished.

One way of eliciting an overall impression of the way in which the disorder affects the patient's lifestyle is to ask the patient to describe a typical day from waking in the morning to going to bed at night. In this way incidences which have become second nature to the patient, but which may be of major significance, may be elicited. How does the disorder affect social interactions? Breathlessness may limit hobbies and social outlets and this often leads to isolation and depression.

SMOKING HISTORY

Smoking is closely linked with both respiratory and cardiovascular disorders so information about any smoking history is essential. In addition, remember to check if the patient lives or works with people who smoke. Recent evidence shows that non-smokers are also at risk if living or working in a smoky environment. Does the patient have a history of smoking and if so determine frequency, form (pipe, cigar, un/filtered cigarettes), duration and tar content of the tobacco used. Has the patient given up smoking; if so, when? Physiotherapists play a key role in changing smoking habits and are often involved in education associated with health promotion.

The initial questioning helps to develop a rapport with the patient and once a baseline of general information is established, questions more specifically related to respiratory symptoms may be asked. The following mnemonic may aid memory:

Chronic Chests Will Behave Oddly

where **C** is **C**ough and sputum, **C** **C**hest pain, **W** **W**heeze, **B** **B**reathlessness and **O** **O**ther symptoms.

COUGH AND SPUTUM

Cough is protective in nature: its function is to clear the airways of irritant and potentially damaging substances. Questioning relates to the nature and productivity of the cough. Does the patient have a cough? If so, is it effective? Cough may be affected by pain, weakness, fatigue or drugs. How long has the cough been present and when is it most noticeable? Has it recently changed in nature or become more persistent? Is the cough productive and if the answer is affirmative, what colour is the sputum and how much is expectorated each day?

The colour of sputum gives an insight into the nature of the disorder, e.g. green sputum can represent *Staphylococcus aureus*. With a respiratory infection, patients usually produce mucopurulent or purulent sputum. Airways irritation results in clear mucoid sputum, and in smokers this may be flecked with black. The patient may describe haemoptysis (blood stained sputum), which could be attributable to the rupture of a small blood vessel, mucosal ulceration or, if in large quantities, carcinoma of the bronchus, pulmonary embolus or lung contusion. White frothy sputum, sometimes pink (containing red blood cells), is produced with pulmonary oedema. Thick sputum is difficult to clear and may indicate that the patient is dehydrated.

CHEST PAIN

Chest pain may vary in intensity and origin but, if present, it must always be managed appropriately. Patients are often anxious about chest pain, and physiotherapists should give psychological support alongside the prescribed drug or physical management. Questioning will elicit the site and distribution plus the nature of the pain. The following systems may precipitate pain: the cardiovascular system; the pulmonary system; the digestive system; and the musculoskeletal system. The most common causes are:

- Cardiac, e.g. angina pectoris—a constricting pain commonly radiating into the left arm and the jaw. It is caused by cardiac ischaemia. Exercise may precipitate angina. Also, pericarditis—a retrosternal pain often exacerbated by respiration.
- Pulmonary, e.g. pleuritic—a sharp and stabbing pain, aggravated by deep breathing but not tender on palpation. This may be associated with a pulmonary infection, pneumothorax or pulmonary embolism. Also, tracheitis—a raw central chest pain, aggravated by coughing. Tumours may give rise to any type of chest pain, depending upon the location.
- Digestive, e.g. oesophageal reflux—a retrosternal burning worse on lying down and leaning forwards.
- Musculoskeletal, e.g. a dull ache around the costal margin as a result of muscular strain following excessive coughing. Rib fractures give rise to a sharp localised pain, worse on deep breathing and extremely tender on palpation. Exercise extreme caution on palpating a potential fracture site, in particular in pathological rib fractures associated with cancer.

WHEEZE

Wheeze is produced by air flow through narrowed airways: it always increases the work of breathing. Wheeze may occur not only in the presence of bronchospasm but also with stridor due to foreign body inhalation, for example, and if mucosal oedema and/or retained secretions are present. Try to differentiate between the noisy breathing often associated with retained secretions, and a true wheeze which is often musical. If a wheeze is present determine any precipitating factors such as dust or pollen, as this may indicate asthma. The presence of both inspiratory and expiratory wheeze indicates severe airways narrowing such as caused by copious tenacious secretions. Wheeze may be identified both on listening at the mouth and/or on auscultation.

BREATHLESSNESS

A patient's personal experience of breathlessness is termed 'dyspnoea'. Dyspnoea is therefore subjective in nature. It must be differentiated from observed breathlessness which may be characterised as:

- Tachypnoea, i.e. a rapid rate.
- Hyperpnoea, i.e. a rapid rate associated with exercise.
- Hyperventilation, i.e. increased ventilation with no apparent cause.

Questioning to ascertain precipitating and easing factors, the mode of onset and progression will give insight to the nature of the breathlessness. For example: is it associated with the onset of infections; does it occur at a certain time of the year or following contact with known allergens? The severity of breathlessness will be indicated by the patient's functional and exercise limitations.

Specifically, the therapist should ask about nocturnal breathlessness, e.g. How many pillows do you sleep with at night? Patients who give a history of breathlessness on lying flat suffer from orthopnoea; those who wake with breathlessness experience paroxysmal nocturnal dyspnoea. Orthopnoea is a result of a poorly functioning left ventricle in association with pooling of blood in the pulmonary circuit. On lying there is increased venous return and re-distribution of stored blood within the pulmonary vascular beds. This increases pulmonary hypertension and results in pulmonary oedema, which interferes with gaseous exchange.

Paroxysmal nocturnal dyspnoea may simply occur if a patient with orthopnoea who usually sleeps propped up on a number of pillows, slides into a more recumbent position. However, patients who experience orthopnoea/paroxysmal nocturnal dyspnoea caused by cardiovascular problems may also have respiratory disorders.

In a patient with a respiratory disorder, nocturnal breathlessness may occur in the supine or slumped position. Two factors are responsible for this. Firstly, a reduction in functional residual capacity (FRC) occurs as a result of the abdominal contents elevating the diaphragm and collapsing the lung bases. Secondly, if the diaphragm is fatigued its action may be compromised due to the increased workload required to displace the abdominal contents. Both of these situations result in reduced gaseous exchange.

OTHER SYMPTOMS

Specific enquiries about headaches, body weight and night sweats may help in the process of clinical diagnosis.

Headaches, especially in the morning, may indicate carbon dioxide retention. Increased $PaCO_2$ causes cerebral vasodilation, which raises the pressure of cerebrospinal fluid and leads to headaches (Henderson, 1994).

A rapid reduction in body weight without intention is often associated with advanced carcinoma.

Finally, night sweats are typical of pulmonary tuberculosis (TB). The incidence of TB appears to be increasing in specific population groups, for example in immunosuppressed individuals (Brewis, 1993), and with the advent of new drug-resistant strains of the TB bacillus (Hough, 1996).

This completes the subjective assessment. The next stage is patient examination or the objective assessment.

OBJECTIVE ASSESSMENT

Physical examination of the patient forms the basis of the objective assessment, and includes the results of physical testing. Such examination determines the degree to which the respiratory disorder and/or disorders of other systems affect normal functioning. It is essential that this information is taken into consideration when defining an appropriate problem list and management programme. An accurate and comprehensive examination provides an objective database which serves as a reference point from which progress and outcome measures can be determined.

Initially, note drips, drains and the percentage of any supplemental oxygen. Review the patient's charts at the bedside noting temperature, heart rate and rhythm, blood pressure, peak flow and fluid balance. Record both the current values and the trend of these parameters as this gives valuable insight into the progression or otherwise of any disorder. A raised temperature is usually indicative of a source of infection, for example of respiratory origin, urinary tract, a wound or septicaemia. Any instability of the cardiovascular system as indicated by abnormal rate, rhythm and/or blood pressure must be evaluated before physiotherapeutic intervention. Also an assessment of the medication the patient requires can show whether the patient's cardiovascular or haemodynamic status requires support.

POSITIONING OF THE PATIENT

Examination is best carried out with the patient adequately undressed and sitting at an angle of 45 degrees. However, if this position is not suitable, the patient should be allowed to choose a more comfortable one, e.g. sitting in a chair. Ensure that the patient is warm and adequately covered to preserve modesty.

Objective examination of the patient with a respiratory disorder begins with a general observation followed by a detailed examination of body areas, commencing with the lower extremities. This allows the patient to get used to being touched on more acceptable areas before handling the more intimate area of the chest.

Examination comprises observation, palpation and physical testing. In order to perform an effective and efficient examination these three skills are combined to promote a logical, smooth progression through the examination with minimum disturbance to the patient.

GENERAL/FACIAL OBSERVATION

If possible, observe patients' facial expression before making contact as often their behaviour alters once they are aware of being observed. This gives an indication of the level of alertness and psychological state, for example the degree of anxiety or distress. In addition, a true assessment can be made of any degree of breathlessness.

Look more specifically for signs of central cyanosis and pursed lip breathing. The lips, oral mucosa and tongue may show central cyanosis, a blueness of the tissues. If present it may indicate reduced oxygen content in the arterial blood; however, this must be verified by the patient's PaO_2 and/or SaO_2. Care must be exercised in this assumption as patients with anaemia may not appear cyanosed in the presence of reduced oxygen levels, whereas patients with polycythaemia may appear cyanosed with only minimal reduction in oxygen levels.

A phenomenon sometimes seen in patients with airways obstruction is pursed lip breathing. Expiration through pursed lips creates a resistance to expiratory flow and hence the back pressure created serves to keep floppy airways from closing. Although this may increase overall air flow (Webber and Pryor, 1993) it also increases the work of breathing.

UPPER AND LOWER EXTREMITIES

Examination of the extremities is focused on assessment of the cardiovascular and musculoskeletal systems.

The function of the cardiovascular system is evaluated with regard to skin colour, texture and temperature, presence of pulses and swelling.

Poor blood flow as a result of partial obstruction or low blood pressure, e.g. as caused by atheroma or poor cardiac output, may result in peripheral cyanosis, which is distinct from the central cyanosis described above. Again this is a result of reduced arterial oxygenation, but in the peripheries it is produced by the slow flow of blood through the capillary beds allowing greater extraction of oxygen from the blood. Cooler extremities and poor/absent peripheral pulses are also associated with a decreased arterial supply. Testing of temperature changes is more accurately performed using the dorsum of the fingers of one hand, moving proximal to distal along the length of the digit. Reduction of blood flow over a period of time leads to trophic changes of the skin and poor skin condition.

Swelling of the feet and ankles may be unilateral or bilateral. A unilateral swelling may be the result of trauma or venous obstruction (deep vein thrombosis). Traumatic swelling is quite firm on palpation due to the proteinous nature of the exudate, and may be associated with bruising. However, bilateral swelling may result from two mechanisms as identified by Henderson (1994). Firstly, peripheral oedema associated with ascites, hepatomegaly and raised jugular venous pressure (JVP) indicates a rapid onset of right ventricular failure following an acute respiratory episode, e.g. acute obstructive pulmonary disease or COPD. The mechanism underlying this is hypoxaemia causing pulmonary arteriolar vasoconstriction which in turn leads to pulmonary hypertension. This suddenly increases the workload on the right ventricle, causing failure. Secondly, ankle swelling, in the absence of right ventricular failure, is a result of hypoxaemia and hypercapnoea which impairs kidney function causing fluid retention. The upright posture in humans coupled with the effect of gravity means that tissue oedema will be more evident in the dependent regions, i.e. the feet and ankles. Patients confined to bed will have sacral oedema.

Clubbing of the toes (and fingers) is recognised by increased curvature of the nail bed and loss of the angle of the nail bed. The aetiology remains unknown. Sudden onset of clubbing is associated with carcinoma while a more insidious onset is associated with long-term respiratory sepsis or cardiac disease.

Observation and palpation of muscle bulk and tone should correlate with the level of activity established in the subjective assessment.

ABDOMEN

In normal breathing the movement of the abdominal wall reflects the changing position of the diaphragm and its effect on abdominal contents: on inspiration the abdominal wall moves outwards, and falls back on expiration. This is a passive process. In patients with airways obstruction the abdominal muscles are actively contracting during the expiratory phase in an attempt to force air through narrowed airways. However, this serves only to increase further the work of breathing (Ninane *et al.*, 1992) and does not result in enhanced respiratory flow. Palpation of the abdomen confirms abdominal muscle activity.

Patients with diaphragmatic weakness may demonstrate paradoxical abdominal movement. In this instance, accessory muscles increase thoracic size resulting in inspiration due to a decrease in intrathoracic pressure. The decrease in pressure, coupled with an ineffectively contracting diaphragm, causes an upward movement of the diaphragm and the abdominal wall falls inwards. On expiration, the raised intrathoracic pressure forces the diaphragm downwards pushing the abdominal wall outwards.

It should be remembered that in the obese patient the enlarged abdomen offers resistance to the downward movement of the diaphragm so reducing basal ventilation (Hough, 1996).

Finally, violent changes in pressure associated with frequent coughing may result in inguinal hernia. If present and unrepaired, manual support by the patient will make coughing more comfortable.

CHEST AND NECK

Begin with a general observation of the chest and neck, noting overall shape and respiratory movements.

Observation of the shape and symmetry of the thorax may give an insight into the nature of the respiratory disorder. Respiratory problems may be caused by an abnormal thoracic shape, e.g. kyphoscoliosis interfering with normal mechanics or, conversely, an altered thoracic shape

may be a result of a respiratory disorder, e.g. the hyperinflated barrel chest.

Initially, observation and measurement of the respiratory rate, depth and pattern should be made without the patient's knowledge, as an awareness of this may influence these three parameters.

Respiratory rate and depth should be noted. A normal respiratory rate is between 12 and 18 breaths/min. A rate of over 40 breaths/min is classed as tachypnoea whereas a reduced rate of breathing is termed hypopnoea. An increased rate is always associated with an increased work of breathing and may or may not result in a reduction in $PaCO_2$, depending on the patency of the airways and depth of respiration. A slow rate of normal/reduced volume is associated with a raised $PaCO_2$.

A normal breathing pattern at rest is regular with active inspiration and passive expiration. The inspiratory to expiratory ratio (I:E) is approximately 1:2. Any deviation from this is less efficient and may lead to increased work of breathing and altered blood gases. Patients with airways obstruction may demonstrate an increase in expiratory time, altering the I:E ratio up to 1:3 or 1:4.

At the neck observe the JVP and the level of activity of the accessory muscles.

The JVP is estimated by looking at the level of the column of blood in the jugular veins, i.e. the neck veins. When the bed end is elevated to 45 degrees, the patient's neck veins may only just be visible above the clavicle. Elevation of venous pressure may distend these vessels up to the level of the jaw. The JVP is measured in centimetres from the sternal angle. The measurement is not a direct measurement from the sternal angle to the level of distension; it is determined from a line projected horizontally from the level of venous distension to dissect a perpendicular line projected upwards from the sternal angle. With the patient at 45 degrees, the normal JVP is 3–4 cm; any reading above this measurement is abnormal. Normally, the JVP is expressed as the height above the normal reading, e.g. +1, +2. It should be noted that in a normal person in the supine position the neck veins are distended.

A raised JVP may indicate:

- A failing right ventricle, where the right ventricle in not emptying effectively.
- Hypervolaemia, i.e. an increase in circulating fluid volume.
- Generation of high pressures in the thorax on expiration. In respiratory disorders where there is obstruction to expiratory flow the high pressures generated on expiration may compress the soft vein walls and impede flow into the right ventricle, raising the JVP. The negative intrathoracic pressure of inspiration allows the veins to empty. In this instance, therefore, the JVP varies with breathing.

Activity in the accessory muscles of respiration is an indication of increased work of breathing: activity at rest is always abnormal. The accessory muscles lift the upper chest and increase sternal lift in an attempt to enlarge thoracic size and improve ventilation. However, improvement in ventilation is achieved at the expense of an increased breathing workload associated with increased oxygen consumption.

To palpate the trachea, lightly place the thumb and fingers on either side of the trachea just above the suprasternal notch. The trachea should be centrally positioned. A shift from the midline may indicate collapse, pneumothorax, lung tumour or a large pleural effusion. Loss of lung volume causes a shift of the trachea towards the side of the collapse whereas pressure from a pneumothorax, lung tumour or large pleural effusion forces the trachea towards the opposite side.

To estimate the patient's level of hydration, place the fingers in the axillae. The axillae should be warm and moist; if dry, this indicates dehydration (Eaton *et al.*, 1994). Sputum clearance is more difficult in a patient with dehydration.

Certain chronic respiratory disorders, e.g. COPD, and episodic respiratory disorders, e.g. asthma, lead to hyperinflation of the thorax. Hyperinflation of the thorax produces specific physical changes, which may be observed and/or palpated on examination. They may be broadly categorised as:

- An elevation of the upper thorax and shoulder girdle leading to sculpturing and a short tracheal length. Sculpturing is a draping of the skin over the bony structures of the shoulder girdle and accessory muscles emphasising the fossae. In addition, the normal distance between the thyroid cartilage and the suprasternal notch, approximately four fingers in breadth, is lessened making the tracheal length appear shorter.
- A loss of the bucket handle movement and increased sternal lift. The expansion of the thoracic cage is at the limit of its bucket handle action making it appear that the patient has lost the bucket handle movement of the ribs. Further thoracic expansion causing inspiration occurs as a result of overuse of the accessory muscles which, by their distal attachment, produce an increase in the pump handle movement or sternal lift.
- A flattened diaphragm which leads to tracheal tug, displacement of the apex beat and indrawing of the costal margins. Hyperinflation causes the normally domed structure of the diaphragm to become flattened, drawing down the central tendon which in turn pulls down the mediastinum. The mediastinal contents are also moved downwards so displacing the heart, and the apex beat moves downwards from the 5th left intercostal space. Tracheal tug is produced by any further downward action of the diaphragm pulling on the trachea via the mediastinum. Patients demonstrate a sharp downward movement of the thyroid cartilage on inspiration. Finally, the altered angle of pull of the diaphragm causes an indrawing of the costal margin on inspiration.

A change in the patient's position is now needed as access to all aspects of the patient's chest is required for the following techniques of physical testing. Sitting on the edge of the bed or upright in a chair is the position of choice for effectively palpating any areas of tenderness, expansion, auscultation and percussion.

Palpate any areas of tenderness to ascertain cause if possible.

Palpation of chest movement gives an indication of lung expansion. The apical sections of the upper zones, the anterior aspects of the middle zones and the posterior aspects of the lower zones are tested. While these three positions roughly correspond anatomically to the upper, middle (lingula) and lower lobes, it is impossible to determine accurately the degree of expansion in these lobes due to the extent of bronchial distortion which may be present in some respiratory conditions, e.g. segmental or lobar collapse.

Apical
Facing the patient, place the fingertips firmly around the base of the neck overlying the upper fibres of trapezius and place the thumbs on the sternal end of the clavicle. The fingertips become the fixed point.

Anterior Aspects of the Middle Zone
Facing the patient, place the fingertips in the axillae and, applying tension on the underlying skin, span the thumbs towards the midline. Again the fingertips become the fixed point.

Posterior Aspects of the Lower Zone
Standing behind the patient, place the fingertips up towards the axillae and, applying tension on the underlying skin, span the thumbs towards the spine in the midline. Again the fingertips become the fixed point.

Once the hands are in position, ask the patient to take a deep breath. Observing the movement of the thumbs away from the midline indicates the degree, quality and symmetry of movement. Loss of movement and asymmetry is abnormal.

Auscultation
Auscultation is the process of listening to chest sounds using a stethoscope. Interpretation of these sounds, linked with other assessment findings, enables the therapist to determine problems more precisely. In addition, auscultation is a useful tool to measure outcomes of physiotherapy intervention. However, recent literature has demonstrated confusion caused by variations in terminology, and has highlighted inaccuracies and inconsistencies in the interpretation of lung sounds (Brooks *et al.*, 1993). It is an inexact science and will probably remain so until the advent of a computerised, diagnostic stethoscope (Jones, 1995).

Only the basic principles of auscultation are given here, as it is beyond the scope of this chapter to give a detailed description.

The technique of auscultation is performed by listening with the diaphragm side of the stethoscope. When listening to the patient's chest, the therapist should visualise the underlying lung structure—a surface indication of the extent of the lungs, and the position of the lobes, fissures and segments. Therefore the sounds heard may be localised to a specific anatomical region, unless areas of anatomical distortion are evident on chest X-ray, e.g. collapse. Precision facilitates more accurate assessment findings and treatment planning.

Classically, auscultation involves listening in one position and comparing with the sounds over a reciprocal position on the opposite side, following a logical pattern around the chest. However, the number of positions normally suggested is often unrealistic in the clinical setting. Each auscultation point requires a moderately deep breath through an open mouth but because patients with respiratory disorders are often too distressed or breathless to be able to perform this, a full procedure might not be possible. Practically, therefore, the lungs are divided into three zones. These are:

- The upper zone, extending down to the level of the fourth rib.
- The middle zone, extending to the level of the sixth rib.
- The lower zone, extending to the base of the lung.

Auscultation is focused on the anterior, posterior and, where possible, lateral aspects of these zones. Auscultation findings from these zones, which very roughly correspond to the upper, middle and lower lobes, should be translated to represent the underlying anatomical structures as indicated above.

Breath sounds heard on auscultation are either generated in the trachea and large airways or transmitted across lung tissue to the chest wall.

The breath sounds heard on listening over the chest wall are generated by turbulence in the trachea and large airways only. Air flow in the smaller airways is laminar and silent. Transmission of the generated sound across normal lung tissue causes a damping down or attenuation of the high frequency, altering the nature of the sound when heard over the chest wall. Listening over the trachea and comparing with the sounds heard at the posterior aspects of the lower zones (posterior segments of the lower zones) demonstrates the degree of the damping effect or attenuation as sounds travel through lung tissue.

Both the generation and transmission of breath sounds may be altered by respiratory disorders.

Generation of the sound in the trachea and large airways depends on the amount of turbulence produced. Where a patient is unable to take a deep breath, e.g. in the presence of pain or muscle weakness, there is reduction in air flow, reduced turbulence and a reduction in the generation of breath sounds. In patients with narrowed upper airways, e.g. sputum retention, airway narrowing speeds up the air flow and increases the turbulence, resulting in increased generation of breath sounds. These abnormal, generated breath sounds are then transmitted to the chest wall with a correspondingly altered sound.

Transmission of generated sound may be altered depending upon the condition of the underlying lung tissue. Air is a poor conductor of sound and it is the presence of air in lung tissue which is responsible for attenuation or damping. Therefore a lung with a greater number of air spaces present, e.g. as found in emphysema, results in increased attenuation, so much so that at times it is difficult to hear anything at all

at the chest wall. Conversely, in the presence of consolidation where there is no air, the generated sounds are transmitted across the lung tissue with little or no attenuation. In this instance the sounds heard over the chest wall are close to those heard over the trachea and are called bronchial breath sounds. It should be noted that on occasion the term 'transmitted breath sounds' is used to indicate the presence of bronchial breath sounds. This is misleading as all breath sounds heard at the chest wall are transmitted.

Transmission of breath sounds to the chest wall may be altered in two other ways. Firstly, a local reduction in breath sounds may be representative of bronchial obstruction. Obstruction of a bronchus by a plug of sputum or a bronchial carcinoma, for example, prevents breath sounds being transmitted. This is true even over a patch of consolidation. Secondly, fluid or air in the pleural cavity also affects transmission of breath sounds. Large volumes of air reduce transmission of sound waves whereas a wall of fluid reflects the sound waves back away from the chest wall. Therefore over an area of pleural effusion or a pneumothorax, there are absent or reduced breath sounds.

Added sound may consist in crackles, wheezes or a pleural rub.

Crackles are short explosive sounds which occur on pressure equalisation across either narrowed airways or collapsed alveoli. Airways are usually narrowed due to secretions, oedema, bronchospasm or altered anatomical structure ('floppy' airways) and alveoli collapse as a result of poor ventilation.

Crackles may be heard during inspiration and expiration. During inspiration, crackles may occur early, at midpoint or late, or at all three stages. The principle underlying the timing of their occurrence is based on compliance, as compliant areas of the respiratory tract open before less compliant ones. Therefore the more compliant the structure the earlier the crackle will occur. For example, floppy airways which occur in COPD are extremely compliant: they open easily and pressure equalisation along the airways occurs early in the inspiratory cycle. Floppy airways are therefore characterised by early inspiratory crackles.

Narrowed airways are less compliant and opening is signalled by early to mid-inspiratory crackles. This is often indicative of secretions and/or oedema, e.g. in conditions such as bronchiectasis and chronic bronchitis.

Late inspiratory crackles occur with the opening of poorly compliant, stiff respiratory bronchioles and alveoli in pathological conditions such as pulmonary oedema, pneumonia and pulmonary fibrosis.

Expiratory crackles are the result of air forcing its way through obstructed airways, and signify retained secretions.

Wheezes are generated by air flowing through narrowed/obstructed airways causing vibration of the walls. Wheezes may occur on both inspiration and expiration, and in the presence of oedema, sputum, bronchospasm and floppy airways. Widespread air flow obstruction is characterised by a polyphonic wheeze, which is a musical note of many frequencies, whereas a localised obstruction is indicated by the presence of a monophonic wheeze, i.e. a single musical note.

A pleural rub is a localised sound heard in pleurisy. Hough (1996) describes this sound as being 'like boots crunching on snow, stronger on inspiration than expiration'. If present, it is invariably associated with pain.

Finally, voice sounds may be heard through a stethoscope—vocal resonance—or felt by the hand placed over the chest wall—vocal fremitus. Speech transmitted through lung tissue is subject to the same influences as generated breath sounds.

In normal lungs, as a result of attenuation, speech is low pitched and indistinct, whereas consolidated lung transmits speech accurately: this is termed bronchophony. Whispering pectoriloquy is the accurate transmission of whispered speech across consolidated lung tissue. It is associated with bronchial breath sounds.

Percussion of the chest is a useful assessment technique which is performed by tapping on the chest wall in an attempt to evaluate the underlying structure. It helps to localise lung disease and is also useful in patients whose ventilatory effort is so poor that use of the stethoscope is negated. Percussion findings linked with those of auscultation often help therapists to determine more accurately the nature of the lung disorder.

Percussion is performed by placing a finger over an intercostal space and tapping it sharply with the middle finger of the other hand near the base of the terminal phalanx. Similar areas on both sides are compared.

A resonant note is present over normal lung tissue which contains air, while the large volume of air present over a pneumothorax produces a hyperresonant note. Conversely, where there is no air a dull percussion note is elicited such as in the presence of atelectatic, consolidated lung tissue or a pleural effusion.

Finally, specific tests to estimate exercise tolerance may be performed in the chronic stages of a disorder. The 6 minute distance test (Butland *et al.*, 1982) or the shuttle walk test (Singh *et al.*, 1992) are appropriate. Results from exercise testing give an accurate reference point from which success of a rehabilitation programme can be estimated and, in the long term, the effects of progression of the disease process may be evaluated.

Position of the Patient

On completion of the objective assessment, the patient is returned to an appropriate resting position, with easy access to personal effects. Ensure that an appropriate drink is available.

INTERPRETATION OF ASSESSMENT FINDINGS

Following completion of the assessment, the findings are considered, interpreted and evaluated. Individual findings should not be considered in isolation but viewed and evaluated in the light of all the information gathered. From these deliberations a problem list is constructed which is discussed with the patient and then revised in order of priority. On occasion the therapist's and patient's perceptions of the problems may differ, but it is essential that agreement is reached before the objective setting, to ensure patient compliance with treatment.

Realistic short- and long-term objectives, which should be measurable, are formulated; short-term objectives often relate to current clinical features whereas long-term objectives relate more to activities of everyday living.

The detailed treatment plan is aimed at achievement of the stated objectives.

An accurate and comprehensive assessment is the most crucial aspect of physiotherapy intervention. It enables the therapist to determine the patient's problems and plan an effective and efficient management programme. The baseline measurements obtained from the assessment serve as reference points by which the outcomes of physiotherapy intervention may be judged.

In addition, assessment identifies those patients for whom physiotherapy intervention is of little or no value or, more importantly, where treatment implementation may be dangerous.

REFERENCES

Brewis RAL. *Lecture notes on respiratory disease*, 4th ed. Oxford: Blackwell Science; 1993:115.

Brooks D, Wilson L, Kelsey C. Accuracy and reliability of 'specialised' physical therapists in auscultating tape-recorded lung sounds. *Physiotherapy Canada* 1993, **45(1):**21-24.

Butland RJA, Gross ER, Pang J *et al.* Two, six, and twelve minute walking test in respiratory disease. *BMJ* 1982, **284:**1607-1608.

Clarke D. Planning for the patient. *Senior Nurse* 1986, **4(5):**23-24.

Cockroft DW, Killian DN, Mellon JJA, Hargreave FE. Bronchial reactivity to inhaled histamine: a method and clinical survey. *Clin Allergy* 1977, **7:**235-273.

Connellan SJ, Morgan N. The effects of nebulised salbutamol on lung function and exercise tolerance in patients with severe airflow obstruction. *Br J Dis Chest* 1982, **76:**135-142.

Eaton TD, Bannister P, Mulley GP, Connolly MJ. Axillary sweating in clinical assessment of dehydration in ill elderly patients. *BMJ* 1994, **308(6939):**1271.

Guilleminault C, Tilkian A, Dement WC. The sleep apnoea syndrome. *Am Rev Med* 1976, **27:**465-484.

Henderson A. Chronic respiratory failure. *Practitioner*. May, 1994, **238:**345-350.

Holt PR. Role of questioning skills in patient assessment. *Br J Nurs* 1995, **4(19):**1145-1148.

Hough A *Physiotherapy in respiratory care*, 2nd ed. London: Chapman & Hall; 1996.

Jones A. A brief overview of the analysis of lung sounds. *Physiotherapy* 1995, **81(1):**37-42.

Mowatt-Larsen CA, Brown RO. Specialised nutritional support in respiratory disease. *Clin Pharm* 1993, **12(4):**276-292.

Ninane V, Rypens F, Yernalt JC, De Troyer A. Abdominal muscle use in patients with chronic airflow obstruction. *Am Rev Resp Dis* 1992, **141(1):**16-21.

Singh SJ, Morgan MD, Scott S, Walters D, Hardman AE. The development of the shuttle walking test of disability in patients with chronic airway obstruction. *Thorax* 1992, **47(12):**1019-1024.

Webber AB, Pryor JB. *Physiotherapy for respiratory and cardiac problems*. Edinburgh: Churchill Livingstone; 1993.

GENERAL READING

Anderson A. ABGs—six easy steps to interpreting blood gases. *Am J Nurs* 1990, **90(8):**42-45.

Gibson GJ. *Clinical tests of respiratory function*. Macmillan Press: London; 1984.

Hurray JM, Saver CL. Arterial blood gas interpretation—improving perioperative skills. *AORNJ* 1992, **55(1):**180-185.

McGavin CR, Gupta SP, McHardy GJR. Twelve-minute walking test for assessing disability in chronic bronchitis. *BMJ* 1976, **1:**822-823.

Pride NB. The assessment of airflow obstruction. Review article. *Br J Dis Chest* 1971, **65:**135.

Webber BA, Pryor JA. *Physiotherapy for respiratory and cardiac problems*. Edinburgh: Churchill Livingstone; 1996.

West JB. *Respiratory physiology—the essentials*, 3rd ed. Oxford: Blackwell Scientific; 1985.

West JB. *Respiratory physiology—the essentials*, 5th ed. Baltimore: Williams and Wilkins; 1995.

West JB. *Pulmonary pathophysiology—the essentials*, 2nd ed. Baltimore: Williams and Wilkins; 1983.

West JB. *Respiratory physiology—the essentials*, 5th ed. Baltimore: Williams and Wilkins; 1997.

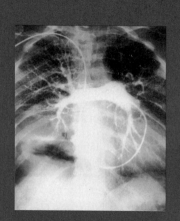

3 S M Greaves

IMAGING OF THE CHEST

CHAPTER OUTLINE

- **Techniques including computerised tomography scan, ultrasound**
- **The normal chest radiograph**
- **The abnormal chest radiograph**

INTRODUCTION

This chapter aims to introduce the physiotherapist to chest imaging, concentrating primarily on those diseases most frequently encountered. It will deal mainly with the interpretation of plain chest radiographs but more advanced imaging techniques such as computerised tomography (CT) and magnetic resonance imaging (MRI) will also be discussed.

TECHNIQUES

CHEST RADIOGRAPHY

Plain chest radiographs are often the first radiological investigation in the diagnosis of chest and heart disease, and are the most commonly performed imaging study.

The standard chest radiographic projection is an erect postero-anterior chest radiograph taken in full inspiration (Figure 3.1). The patient is positioned with the front of the chest against the imaging plate, and the X-ray beam passes from posterior to anterior.

Patients who are too ill to be taken to the radiology department require radiographs taken at the bedside with mobile equipment. It is difficult consistently to produce high quality portable examinations with conventional equipment, and image quality is frequently poor. The imaging plate must be positioned against the patient's back and the X-ray beam passes from front to back producing an antero-posterior chest radiograph. The diverging X-ray beam passing from front to back magnifies the size of anterior structures such as the heart and anterior mediastinum, often leading to difficulties in interpretation. Portable supine radiographs cause additional diagnostic difficulties. Redistribution of pulmonary blood flow to the upper zones is normal in the supine patient but may be misinterpreted as pulmonary congestion. Pleural effusions will layer posteriorly, and are less conspicuous than on erect radiographs. Finally, a pneumothorax may not be appreciated as air accumulates anteriorly and medially at the lung bases rather than over the apex of the lung (Figure 3.2).

Lateral radiographs are very useful in localising disease identified on the postero-anterior view. Depending on the policy of the imaging department, a lateral radiograph may be routinely taken at the same time as the postero-anterior view, or obtained only in special circumstances.

FLUOROSCOPY

Fluoroscopy enables real time imaging of a patient using X-rays and an image intensifier. In the chest, its main applications are to view diaphragmatic motion and to guide interventional procedures such as fine needle lung biopsy and insertion of central venous catheters and cardiac pacemakers.

ULTRASOUND

Ultrasonography utilises high frequency sound waves to image tissue. Ultrasound is transmitted through the body wall to the area of interest, and reflected echoes from objects are detected and used to create an image.

Ultrasonography is frequently used to image the heart (echocardiography) as the motion of the cardiac walls, the valves and the blood can easily be studied. It is useful in the detection and characterisation of pleural diseases, particularly pleural effusions (Figure 3.3), and often helpful in guiding pleural and pericardial fluid aspiration, pleural biopsy and drain placements. As ultrasound is not transmitted by air, it is generally not used for guiding percutaneous lung biopsy, although in certain circumstances peripheral lung lesions may be localised using this technique.

COMPUTERISED TOMOGRAPHY (CT)

A CT scanner uses a narrow beam of X-rays to generate a cross-sectional image of the patient. The patient usually lies supine in the scanner, and an intravenous injection of iodinated contrast may be given. Intravenous contrast increases the density of blood, making it brighter on CT and thus enabling the differentiation of vessels from other structures such as lymph nodes. During the examination, the X-ray beam rotates around the patient very quickly and is recorded by an array of detectors. The computer reconstructs a digital image, which represents a 'slice' of the patient. The thickness

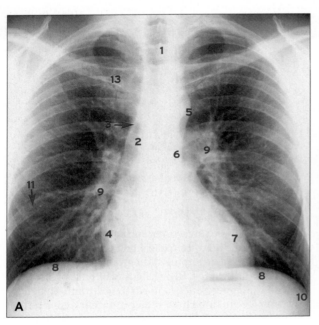

A

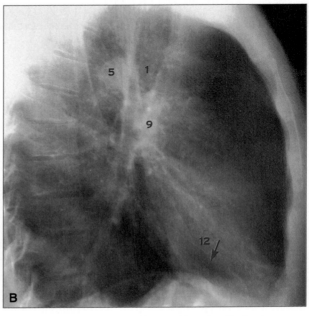

B

Figure 3.1 (A) Normal postero-anterior and (B) lateral chest radiographs. 1, trachea; 2, right main bronchus; 3, superior vena cava; 4, right heart border; 5, aortic arch; 6, left main bronchus; 7, left heart border; 8, diaphragm; 9, pulmonary artery; 10, lateral costophrenic angle; 11, minor fissure; 12, major fissure; 13, clavicle.

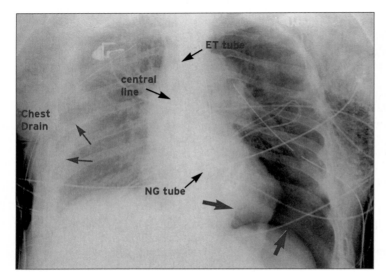

Figure 3.2 Portable chest radiograph demonstrating appearances of a right pleural effusion and a left pneumothorax in the supine position. The right pleural effusion is layering posteriorly and seen tracking into the major fissure (small blue arrows). Air from the left pneumothorax is seen accumulating medially and at the left base depressing the left hemidiaphragm (large blue arrows). An endotracheal tube, a nasogastric tube, a right central venous line and bilateral chest drains have been inserted.

of this slice can be varied depending upon the clinical investigation but typically a thickness of 8–10 mm is sufficient. Information from CT scanners is manipulated to show soft tissue, lung or bone to best advantage, and usually several sets of images are provided for review.

Spiral or helical CT has resulted from recent technical developments in CT scanner technology. Spiral CT enables continuous scanning as the patient moves through the scanner, resulting in a reduced examination time and production of a block of scan data rather than individual slices. The information acquired is then reconstructed into a similar set of image slices as conventional CT. Spiral CT offers several advantages including improved enhancement of vessels with smaller volumes of contrast, and the ability to produce high quality multiplanar and three-dimensional images.

CT scans expose the patient to a large amount of radiation and therefore are a secondary imaging technique. The most common uses for thoracic CT are detailed in Table 3.1.

High resolution computerised tomography (HRCT) is a modification of the conventional CT technique enabling visualisation of tiny lung structures. This is achieved primarily by obtaining very thin CT slices that are typically 1–1.5 mm

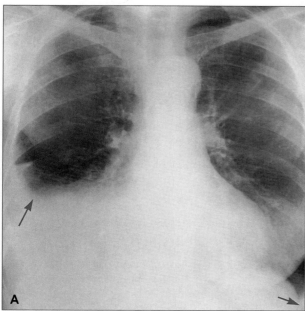

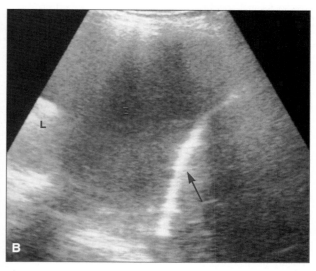

Figure 3.3 Bilateral pleural effusions in a patient with metastatic breast carcinoma.
(A) Postero-anterior chest radiograph demonstrates a moderate-sized right and a tiny left pleural effusion (arrows). **(B)** Ultrasound of the right effusion before drain placement. The effusion (E) is seen as a dark region between bright collapsed right lower lobe (L) and the hyperechoic band representing the diaphragm (arrow). **(C)** Pleural effusion with pneumothorax. Note the definite straight lines of the effusion when there is air in the hemithorax.

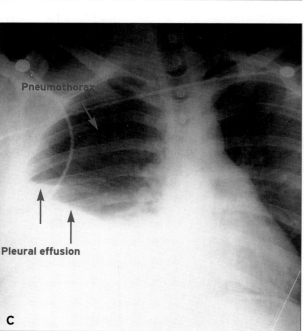

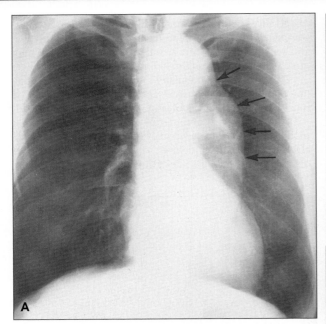

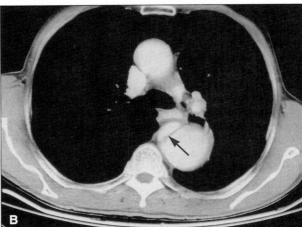

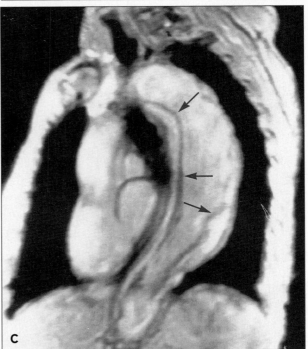

Figure 3.4 Aortic dissection limited to the descending aorta. (A) Postero-anterior chest radiograph. The descending thoracic aorta is markedly dilated (arrows). **(B)** Contrast enhanced spiral computerised tomogram demonstrates the dissection flap (arrow) within the descending thoracic aorta. **(C)** Sagittal oblique magnetic resonance image allows visualisation of the dissection (arrows) in multiple planes without the need for intravenous contrast or ionising radiation.

Common indications for thoracic computerised tomography
Staging primary lung carcinomas
Further evaluation of an abnormal or equivocal chest radiograph
Detection of pulmonary metastases
Diagnosis of aortic dissection
Diagnosis and characterisation of interstitial lung disease
Guiding interventional procedures

Table 3.1 Common indications for thoracic computerised tomography.

thick. HRCT is superior to plain radiography and conventional CT in diagnosing and evaluating diffuse lung diseases such as cryptogenic fibrosing alveolitis, bronchiectasis and sarcoidosis.

MRI

MRI scanners contain a powerful magnet that generates a strong magnetic field. Patients are positioned within the scanner and exposed to short bursts of radio waves, called radiofrequency (RF) pulses, in specific sequences. The motion of protons within the body's tissues is altered by the RF pulses and when left to return to their original state they emit RF signals of their own. These are detected by the scanner and used to construct a cross-sectional image of a slice of tissue. The main advantages of MRI over CT scanning are the lack of ionising radiation, the ability to produce an image in any plane, and improved contrast between different tissues. MRI is well established in the diagnosis of cardiac, aortic and mediastinal disease (see Figure 3.4c). At present, due to technical factors, MRI is of little value in imaging lung parenchyma.

VENTILATION–PERFUSION RADIONUCLIDE LUNG IMAGING (V/Q SCAN)

Ventilation–perfusion radionuclide lung imaging (V/Q scan) is performed in the nuclear medicine department, and is useful in the diagnosis of pulmonary embolism. The symptoms and clinical signs of pulmonary embolism are frequently non-specific, and chest radiographs are often normal or non-diagnostic. Occasionally, more convincing chest radiographic evidence may be seen such as a wedge-shaped, peripheral opacity representing a region of pulmonary infarction.

The V/Q scan is non-invasive, safe and easy to perform. Images of lung perfusion and ventilation are produced via a gamma camera. Perfusion in the lung is assessed by giving the patient an injection of tiny radiolabelled (99mTc)

particles. These lodge in the microvasculature of the lung, and the number of particles lodged is directly proportional to the pulmonary blood flow to that region. Subsequently the patient breaths a radioactive gas (typically krypton 81m or xenon 133) and a ventilation image is obtained (Figure 3.5).

In pulmonary embolism, vessels are typically occluded by emboli resulting in perfusion defects. These areas usually ventilate normally. If this classic picture of ventilation–perfusion mismatch occurs then the diagnosis of pulmonary embolism is made. If the V/Q scan is normal then it can be safely assumed that pulmonary embolism has not taken place. Unfortunately, many patients with suspected pulmonary embolism have V/Q scans that are non-specific and that neither confirm nor exclude the diagnosis. In these patients it may be appropriate to proceed to a pulmonary angiogram (Figure 3.6).

ANGIOGRAPHY

Angiography is the radiographic examination of a vascular structure using an injection of iodinated contrast. The contrast is given via a catheter that has usually been introduced via a femoral artery or femoral vein, and guided to the vessel under examination. Positioning of the catheter is optimised with the aid of fluoroscopy, and imaging of the contrast within the vessel recorded using either cine film, a rapid serial film changer or digital acquisition. The majority of arteries can be studied using this technique; in the chest this includes the pulmonary arteries, the coronary arteries and the bronchial arteries (see Figure 3.6). Once the vessel has been accessed and imaged, interventional radiology may play a part in patient treatment. Identifiable narrowing of vessels (stenoses) can then be dilated by small balloon catheters (angioplasty), embolic materials can be injected to control bleeding, and large collections of thrombus, for example in the pulmonary arteries, can be mechanically and chemically broken down.

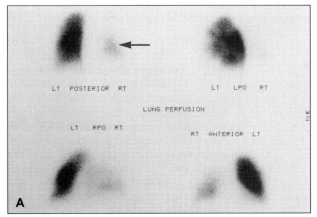
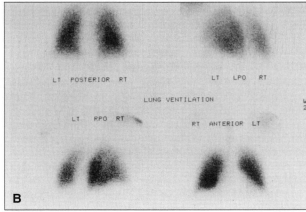

Figure 3.5 Pulmonary embolism on V/Q scan. (A) Perfusion lung scan demonstrates markedly decreased perfusion in the right lung. **(B)** Ventilation lung scan. Both lungs are seen to ventilate normally.

THE NORMAL CHEST RADIOGRAPH

On first looking at a chest radiograph, the patient's name, date of the examination and the side marker should all be checked. The projection of the radiograph, i.e. antero-posterior, postero-anterior or supine, should be noted and the radiographic technique should be satisfactory. Assessment of the patient's position should be made as patient rotation can produce distortion of mediastinal contours and increased lucency of one hemithorax.

Inexperienced viewers of chest radiographs must have a systematic approach to avoid missing significant abnormalities. All structures should be evaluated including the bony thorax, mediastinum, hila, diaphragms and lungs (see Figure 3.1). Areas in which lesions are commonly missed such as the lung apices, behind the heart, and beneath the diaphragms are well worth a second look.

Previous chest radiographs are often helpful in establishing the time course of a disease. For example, a nodule or mass that was not present 4 weeks previously is far more likely to represent infection than malignancy.

CHEST WALL

Both breasts should be identified in women. Rib borders should be defined except in the mid and lower thorax where their bony flanges produce more indistinct margins. Calcification of rib cartilages is common and increases with increasing age. The thoracic spine is usually straight on postero-anterior chest radiographs, and demonstrates a minor anterior concavity on lateral examinations. On the lateral projection, vertebral bodies should become apparently less dense as the eye moves downward. Any increase in density implies intrathoracic disease.

LUNGS

Pulmonary vessels and bronchi are primarily responsible for the lung markings seen on chest radiographs. These structures taper from the hila into the lung periphery, and discrete vascular markings are not usually identified within 1–2 cm of the pleural surface.

The fissures are the contact points between the visceral pleura of the lobes. The minor (horizontal) fissure separates the right upper lobe from the right middle lobe and can be identified on the postero-anterior chest radiograph. It is horizontally oriented and typically lies at the level of the anterior fourth rib. The major (oblique) fissures separate the upper from the lower lobes and can be identified only on the lateral radiograph. They begin at approximately the level of the fifth thoracic vertebral body, and extend antero-inferiorly, usually along the line of the sixth rib, to contact the diaphragm (see Figure 3.1).

THE HILA

The hila are composed of the pulmonary arteries, the upper lobe pulmonary veins, the major bronchi and lymph nodes. The first two structures are primarily responsible for the hilar opacities seen on the chest radiograph, as the bronchi are filled with air and normal lymph nodes are too small to contribute significantly. The left hilum appears slightly higher than the right as the left pulmonary artery lies above the left main bronchus. The hila should be of approximately equal size and an obvious increase in density of one implies an abnormality of the hilum itself or of lung anterior or posterior to it.

MEDIASTINAL CONTOURS OF THE DIAPHRAGM AND HEART

Structures producing the cardiomediastinal contours on the frontal chest radiograph are illustrated in Figure 3.1. The hemidiaphragms form smooth curves marginating the inferior border of the thorax. In the majority of people, the right hemidiaphragm is slightly higher than the left and both diaphragmatic contours and the lateral costophrenic angles should be clearly defined. Mediastinal and diaphragmatic

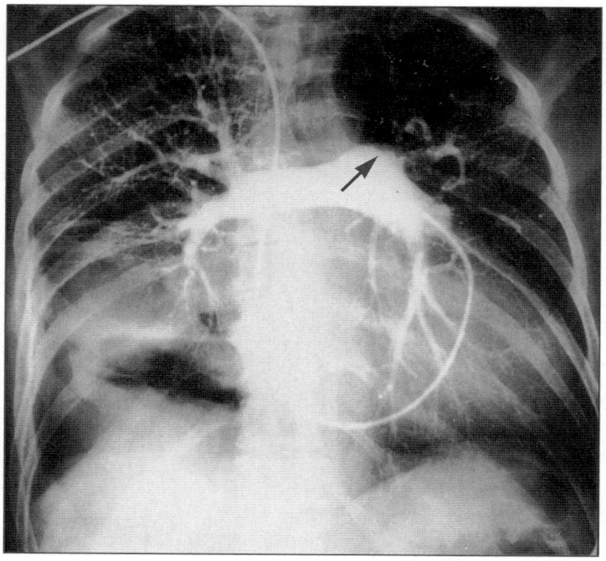

Figure 3.6 Pulmonary embolism confirmed by a pulmonary angiogram. A filling defect representing thrombus lies within the left upper lobe pulmonary artery (arrow).

interfaces are important both in identifying abnormal enlargement of mediastinal and cardiac structures and in localising abnormalities within the lungs. Usually the interfaces are seen clearly as they are bordered by air in the lungs. If the adjacent lung is consolidated or collapsed the usual mediastinal or diaphragmatic border will not be seen. If disease is present within the right middle lobe the right heart border will be obscured; if it is within the lingula the left heart border will not be seen. Similarly, disease in the left lower lobe will obliterate the left hemi-diaphragmatic contour. Consolidation in the right lower lobe produces right basal opacification, but the right heart border remains clearly defined (Figure 3.7).

THE ABNORMAL CHEST RADIOGRAPH

It is not possible to provide a complete account of the radiological features of all thoracic diseases but an attempt has been made to include those that the physiotherapist may come across in practice.

CHEST WALL

A mastectomy will result in asymmetry of soft tissues of the chest wall. This may be misinterpreted as abnormal lung lucency on the same side as the mastectomy or as lung disease on the opposite side. Previous thoracic surgery is often implied by deformed or absent ribs, and destroyed ribs may be secondary to primary or secondary malignancy. Thoracic trauma may result in rib fractures, most commonly the fourth through to the 10th. Fractures of the first three ribs imply major blunt trauma and are often associated with tracheobronchial and vascular damage. Fractures of the 10th, 11th and 12th ribs are often associated with liver, spleen or kidney injury.

LUNGS

Very many diseases can result in abnormal lung appearances, and it helps to have some system to try and narrow the possibilities down to a manageable number. An important initial step is to decide whether there are areas of increased density or abnormal lucency within the lungs.

Increased Lung Density
Consolidation

Airspace consolidation refers merely to filling of the alveoli with either oedema fluid, blood, pus or cells. Consolidation typically manifests as ill-defined 'fluffy' pulmonary opacities that rapidly coalesce. Filling of alveoli with little involvement of the airways results in the bronchi becoming visible as lucent tubes within predominantly opacified lung. This phenomenon is known as an air bronchogram. Many diseases can cause pulmonary consolidation, the commonest of which are discussed below.

Pneumonia. This can be caused by a variety of micro-organisms, and the airspaces become filled with an inflammatory exudate. The radiological features are the same as those described for all airspace diseases, namely homogeneous consolidation of lung with air bronchograms (see Figure 3.7). Pneumonia can be classified according to its radiological distribution. Lobar pneumonia is caused by disease in the distal airspaces, and is classically limited to one lobe. Bronchopneumonia occurs when the small airways are infected and disease subsequently spreads to involve the adjacent airspaces. Typically, multifocal, patchy airspace consolidation is seen on the chest radiograph. Certain micro-organisms, notably viruses and atypical bacteria, can result in interstitial rather than airspace disease, and this is discussed further below.

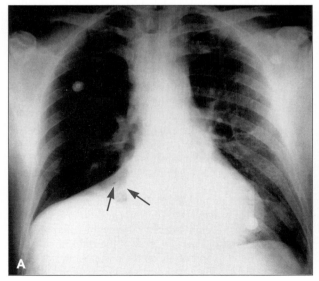

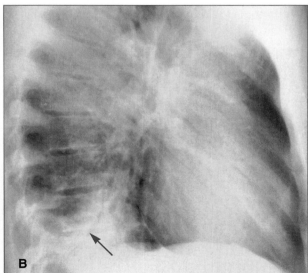

Figure 3.7 (A) Collapse and consolidation of right lower lobe with a visible right heart border (B). This localises the disease to the right lower lobe. Note the air bronchogram on the lateral and postero-anterior views (arrow).

Aspiration pneumonia. This results most often from inhalation of oropharangeal secretions or stomach contents. Typically, there is patchy airspace consolidation that may reflect the position of the patient at the time of aspiration (the posterior portions of the upper and lower lobes are commonly affected). The radiographical appearance may be indistinguishable from cardiac failure or pneumonia.

Cardiogenic pulmonary oedema. This is frequently the result of left ventricular failure. Raised pressures within the pulmonary veins and arteries result in dilation of these vessels (pulmonary congestion). As the heart fails further, oedema fluid is squeezed out from the veins into the lung interstitium. The lung vessels become hazy and indistinct and fluid in the interstitium produces interstitial (septal) lines on chest radiographs. As pressures continue to rise, fluid passes from the interstitium into the airspaces. Radiographically this is seen as poorly defined airspace disease that is particularly marked in the perihilar regions (Figure 3.8). While the heart size may be normal, it is usually increased and small pleural effusions are common.

Adult respiratory distress syndrome (ARDS). This follows a variety of insults including sepsis, trauma, shock and aspiration, and is a serious disease with a mortality rate of over 50%. It is characterised by tachypnoea, shortness of breath, hypoxaemia and pulmonary function tests consistent with 'stiff' lungs. Initially, chest radiographs may be normal but patchy airspace disease develops 12 to 48 hours after injury. This rapidly progresses to widespread airspace consolidation of both lungs. Institution of ventilation with positive end expiratory pressure may apparently decrease the amount of airspace disease, increase the lung volumes and be complicated by the development of pulmonary interstitial emphysema. This may falsely be interpreted as improvement in the patient's condition. While ARDS may be difficult to differentiate from cardiogenic pulmonary oedema, important distinguishing features may be present. In ARDS the heart size is usually normal, pleural effusions are uncommon, and pulmonary vessels remain undistended and well defined.

Pulmonary haemorrhage. Trauma is probably the commonest cause of pulmonary haemorrhage; others include pulmonary infarction, tumours, bronchiectasis, pulmonary vasculitis and infection. All forms of pulmonary haemorrhage will result in airspace consolidation similar to that described above.

Collapse

Collapse or atelectasis of lung indicates loss of volume of pulmonary parenchyma without significant filling of the airspaces. It most commonly arises from airways obstruction. Many things may cause airways obstruction ranging from primary and secondary carcinomas to mucous plugs and bronchial trauma. Extrinsic compression may be secondary to enlarged lymph nodes or mediastinal masses. Radiographically, there are several chest signs of lung collapse (Table 3.2).

Collapse of an entire lung. This is usually secondary to obstruction of its main bronchus and is most common on the left. The chest radiograph typically shows opacification of the affected hemithorax with marked displacement of the mediastinum to that side (Figure 3.9). The contralateral lung overinflates and may herniate across the midline. The diaphragm elevates but this is usually appreciated on the left only due to the position of the stomach bubble.

Collapse of the right upper lobe. This results in elevation of both the right hilum and the minor fissure. The lateral view reveals anterior displacement of the right major fissure. With extensive right upper lobe collapse the lobe may become inseparable from the right superior mediastinum. If this happens the only clue to its presence will be gained from elevation of the right hilum, tracheal shift to the right and compensatory overinflation of the right middle and lower lobes.

Collapse of the left upper lobe. This occurs antero-superiorly, and tracheal deviation and left hilar elevation can frequently be identified. The collapsed lobe produces a veil-like opacity over the upper left hemithorax (Figure 3.10). Unlike right upper lobe collapse, its lateral margin is ill defined fading gradually into the normal lung. On a lateral chest radiograph the left major fissure moves anteriorly paralleling the anterior chest wall and the collapsed left upper lobe is seen as a region of increased density anterior to the fissure.

Collapse of the right middle lobe. This is diagnosed when the minor fissure is displaced inferiorly and there is obliteration of the normal right heart border by the collapsed lobe (Figure 3.11A). Complete collapse of the right middle lobe may be difficult to appreciate on the postero-anterior radiograph as the lobe is small and secondary signs such as compensatory overinflation are usually not prominent. The triangular opacity that represents the collapsed right middle lobe is usually more obvious on the lateral view projected over the heart (Figure 3.11B).

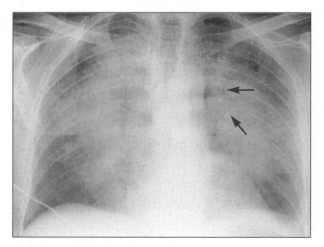

Figure 3.8 Cardiogenic pulmonary oedema. Poorly defined, homogeneous airspace disease is most marked in the perihilar region. Faint air bronchograms can be seen (arrows).

Radiographic changes indicating lung or lobar collapse

Displacement of fissures

Increase in lung density

Crowding of vessels

Shift of the mediastinum to the affected side

Hilar displacement

Elevation of the diaphragm on the affected side

Approximation of ribs

Compensatory overinflation of the remaining lung

Table 3.2 Radiographic changes indicating lung or lobar collapse.

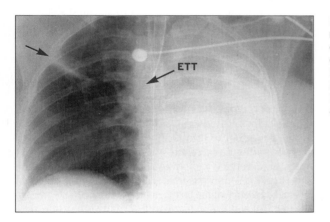

Figure 3.9 Collapse of the left lung secondary to malposition of an endotracheal tube (ETT). The ETT extends into the right bronchus intermedius beyond the origins of both the left main and the right upper lobe bronchi. There is complete opacification of the collapsed left lung with displacement of the mediastinum to the left. Early collapse of the right upper lobe (arrows) can also be seen.

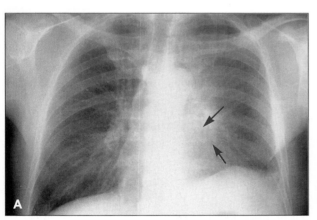

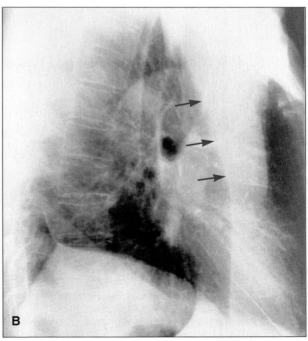

Figure 3.10 Collapse of the left upper lobe secondary to bronchogenic carcinoma. (A) Veil-like opacification of the left upper thorax with obscuration of the left heart border (arrows) on the postero-anterior radiograph. **(B)** On the lateral view, the left major fissure moves anteriorly and the collapsed left upper lobe is seen as an opacity anterior to this (arrows). The retrosternal lucency represents the right lung which has herniated over the midline.

Collapse of both lower lobes. This is similar to right middle lobe collapse radiographically. The lobes collapse downwards, posteriorly and medially towards the spine. The collapsed lobe is seen as a wedge shaped opacity with its apex at the hilum (see Figure 3.7A). On the lateral view, the oblique fissure moves posteriorly and the collapsed lobe is seen as a region of increased opacity projected over the lower thoracic spine. Left lower lobe collapse results in obliteration of the left hemidiaphragm; the left heart border remains clearly marginated. On the right the appearances are similar to right middle lobe collapse but the right heart border can be clearly seen.

Interstitial disease

The interstitium is the connective tissue framework of the lung. This surrounds and supports the bronchi and pulmonary vessels, extends in from the pleura as fibrous strands, and comprises a portion of the alveolar wall. Thickening of the interstitium usually produces fine lines or a reticular (net-like) pattern on chest radiographs.

There are many causes of interstitial disease, most of which cannot be differentiated using plain radiography alone. HRCT can often limit the differential diagnosis, and in some instances appearances are so characteristic as to enable a specific diagnosis to be made.

The commonest cause of acute interstitial disease is interstitial pulmonary oedema, followed by infection. Viral and atypical bacteria such as mycoplasma can cause inflammation of the bronchial walls and pulmonary interstitium producing an interstitial pneumonia.

Interstitial disease that is little changed from month to month is frequently a result of some form of pulmonary fibrosis. Pulmonary fibrosis typically results in a reticular pattern of interstitial disease, and is usually associated with some loss of lung volume. With end stage disease, the lung architecture is so destroyed that normal lung parenchyma is replaced with thick-walled cysts; this is termed honeycombing (Figure 3.12). There are innumerable diseases that can cause pulmonary fibrosis ranging from sarcoidosis to rheumatoid arthritis. Idiopathic pulmonary fibrosis (cryptogenic pulmonary fibrosis) is one of the commonest causes.

Nodules

Lung nodules can range in diameter from a few millimetres to several centimetres and are caused by either infection, granulomatous disease (such as sarcoidosis) or malignancy. By convention, nodules greater than 3 cm in maximum diameter are termed masses. Multiple small nodules scattered throughout the lungs produces miliary shadowing on the chest radiograph. One disease typically associated with this type of lung opacity is miliary tuberculosis. Multiple nodules that vary in size and shape are frequently caused by metastases.

The majority of solitary nodules greater than 3 cm (masses) represent primary lung carcinoma. CT can be very useful in the staging of lung carcinoma, and in identifying occult metastases not visualised on the chest radiograph.

Decreased Opacification (Increased Lucency)

Before definitively diagnosing abnormal lucency of the lungs, a number of things should be excluded. An overexposed radiograph may result in apparent hyperlucent lungs, and rotated radiographs often produce unilateral hyperlucency. A previous mastectomy will result in apparent increased lucency of the ipsilateral hemithorax due to the relative lack of soft tissue compared with the other side.

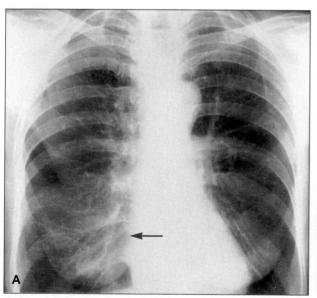

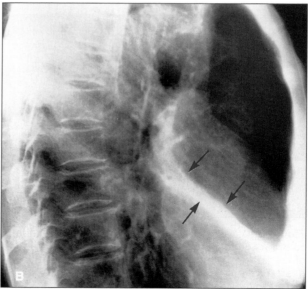

Figure 3.11 Complete collapse of the right middle lobe secondary to a mucous plug. (A) The right heart border is indistinct on the postero-anterior chest radiograph. **(B)** The collapse is more easily appreciated on the lateral projection overlying the heart (arrows).

Chronic obstructive pulmonary disease (COPD)

Emphysema. This is a common cause of increased lucency of the thorax. Destruction of the alveoli and their capillary beds combined with overinflation of the lungs produces a generalised reduction in lung density. In severe emphysema the diaphragms are depressed and flattened, there is an increase in the antero-posterior diameter of the chest and in the retrosternal clear space, and there is loss of the normal vascular branching pattern (Figure 3.13A). Bullae may produce focal areas of increased lucency and are frequently seen in patients with more severe emphysema.

HRCT is a more accurate way of diagnosing and assessing the extent of emphysema than plain chest radiographs. Lung destruction can be clearly seen as focal areas of very low attenuation contrasted with areas of more normal lung (Figure 3.13B).

Chronic bronchitis. The radiographic appearances in chronic bronchitis are similar to those found in emphysema with hyperinflated, lucent lungs but the lungs look 'dirtier' with increased bronchovascular markings.

Asthma. This is characterised by reversible airways obstruction. Most patients with asthma have a normal chest radiograph although hyperinflated lungs and bronchial wall thickening may be seen in some.

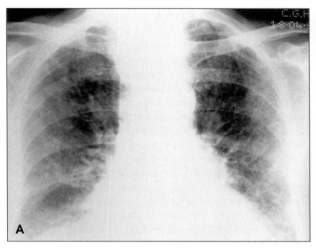

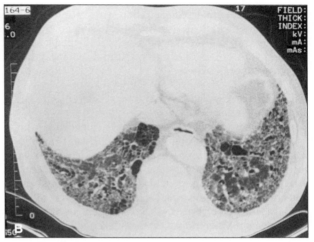

Figure 3.12 Idiopathic pulmonary fibrosis. (A) Extensive fibrosis is seen as a coarse network of lines that is most marked peripherally and at the lung bases on the chest radiograph. **(B)** The fibrosis can be seen in much greater detail on the high resolution computerised tomogram. Normal lung architecture has been destroyed and replaced with a cystic reticular pattern.

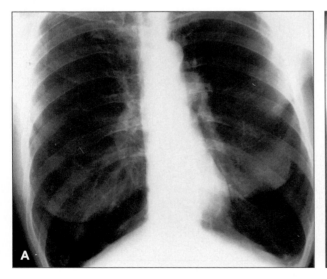

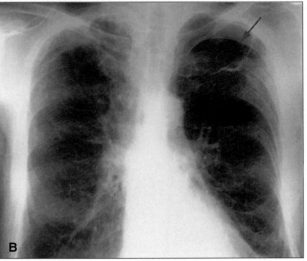

Figure 3.13 Severe emphysema. (A) The diaphragms are flattened, the antero-posterior diameter of the chest is increased and there is loss of the normal vascular pattern. **(B)** There is bulla formation (arrow).

Pneumothorax

A pneumothorax results from air gaining access to the pleural space, and may be caused by the rupture of small, subpleural blebs or bullae. Lungs that are abnormal such as in emphysema, cystic fibrosis and pulmonary fibrosis, are more susceptible. Trauma, particularly iatrogenic (such as in central venous line insertion), is another common cause. On a chest radiograph a pneumothorax usually appears as a well-demarcated, visceral pleural line paralleling the thoracic wall (Figure 3.14). No lung markings are present peripheral to this line, and the underlying lung exhibits varying degrees of collapse depending on the size of the pneumothorax. Occasionally, due to a ball valve effect, there is an inexorable increase in size of the pneumothorax with each inspiration. This is called a 'tension pneumothorax' and is a life-threatening emergency. Mediastinal structures are characteristically displaced to the opposite side, and the ipsilateral diaphragm is depressed or even inverted.

ABNORMAL AIRWAYS
Bronchiectasis

Bronchiectasis refers to irreversible bronchial dilation, and usually develops as a consequence of airways infection where damage to the airway wall initiates a vicious circle of recurrent infections, each resulting in further structural damage. Causes are many but include respiratory infections in childhood, congenital abnormalities of the airways and cilia, and cystic fibrosis. Chest radiographs, while often non-specific may, demonstrate the thickened airway walls as parallel linear structures ('tramlines') or as end-on ring shadows. If the bronchi are very dilated, cystic areas with fluid levels may be present. Bronchography in which contrast material is introduced directly into the bronchial tree has been replaced by HRCT in the vast majority of cases.

HRCT clearly demonstrates dilated bronchi, bronchial wall thickening, and fluid or mucus within the abnormal airways.

Cystic Fibrosis

Cystic fibrosis is an autosomal recessive condition in which the main problem is inadequate hydration of mucus, producing abnormally viscid secretions. The lungs are normal at birth but frequent and prolonged respiratory infections result in extensive damage. Typical radiographic abnormalities include hyperinflated lungs, bronchial wall thickening, bronchiectasis, scarring and areas of atelectasis (Figure 3.15).

ABNORMAL PLEURA
Pleural Effusion

The potential space between the visceral and parietal pleura contains 10–15 ml of fluid. A pleural effusion results from the accumulation of an increased amount of pleural fluid, and at least 175 ml of fluid has to be present to be seen on a postero-anterior chest radiograph. Lateral chest radiographs are more sensitive to smaller amounts of pleural fluid (50 ml), and lateral decubitus radiographs can detect as little as 2 ml. The commonest causes of pleural effusions are congestive cardiac failure, bacterial pneumonia and malignant disease. They are also common in the post-surgical patient. Pleural effusions typically result in a homogeneous opacity localising at the lung bases if the patient is upright. The diaphragmatic contour and lateral costophrenic angle are obliterated, and the upper border of the fluid is usually well defined with a lateral meniscus concave towards the lung (see Figure 3.3a). Many critically ill patients have radiographs in the supine position, and redistribution of the fluid along the posterior chest wall can make pleural effusions difficult to appreciate (see

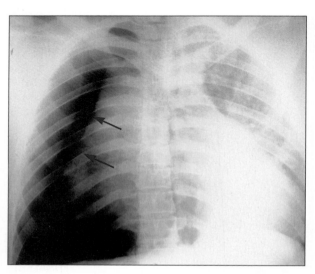

Figure 3.14 Right pneumothorax. The visceral pleura can be identified as a fine line paralleling the right costal margin (arrows).

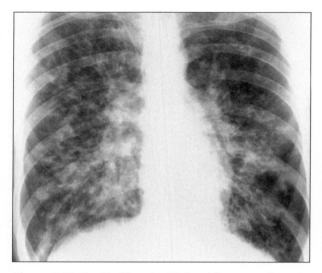

Figure 3.15 Cystic fibrosis. Bilateral linear, cystic and nodular shadows represent bronchiectasis and peribronchial inflammation. The lungs are hyperinflated.

Figure 3.2). Typically, there is a homogeneous increase in lung opacification with obliteration of the lateral costophrenic angle and diaphragmatic contour. In contrast to parenchymal consolidation, the bronchopulmonary markings are still visible. Fluid may pool over the apex of the lung, forming an apical cap.

If the pleural space becomes partially obliterated with adherence of visceral and parietal layers, loculated effusions can occur. Loculated pleural effusions and empyemas usually have sharply defined contours that are convex to the lung.

Pleural Thickening

Thickening of the pleura may be focal or diffuse, and results in a band of soft tissue density paralleling the chest wall medial to the ribs. Pleural thickening may calcify particularly if secondary to asbestos exposure, tuberculosis or haemothorax. Malignant pleural disease such as that found in mesothelioma often produces lobulated pleural thickening that may extend to involve mediastinal pleura. The volume of the affected hemithorax is typically reduced and there may be an associated pleural effusion.

ABNORMAL MEDIASTINUM
Mediastinal Masses

A variety of primary and secondary neoplasms can produce masses in the mediastinum. In the majority of cases these can be detected on plain postero-anterior and lateral chest radiographs; however, CT is almost invariably used to localise and characterise the lesion further.

Mediastinal Emphysema

The commonest cause of mediastinal emphysema is traumatic alveolar rupture due to asthma, mechanical ventilation, coughing or trauma. Air enters the

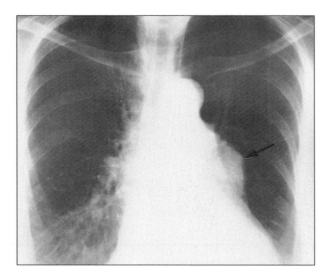

Figure 3.16 Thymoma. The postero-anterior chest radiograph shows an abnormal left mediastinal contour (arrow).

pulmonary interstitium and tracks to the mediastinum. On chest radiographs the air is seen as multiple linear lucencies within mediastinal soft tissues. Air may extend into soft tissues of the neck and the chest wall, and is frequently seen outlining the inner surface of the mediastinal pleura.

ABNORMAL HEART AND PULMONARY VASCULATURE

The chest film is often the first imaging technique requested to investigate cardiac symptomatology, and is also frequently used to follow patients with known heart disease. The cardiac contour should be evaluated for changes in size and shape together with an assessment of pulmonary vasculature.

Cardiac Enlargement

Although cardiac measurement using plain chest radiographs is imprecise, the cardiothoracic ratio is widely used:

Cardiothoracic ratio = maximum width of the heart on the postero-anterior chest radiograph/ maximum diameter of the thorax above the costophrenic angles

If this ratio is greater than 0.5, the heart is generally taken to be enlarged.

Cardiac Contours

It may be possible in certain circumstances to recognise specific chamber enlargements secondary to changes in cardiac and mediastinal contours on the chest radiograph. Enlargement of the left atrium may result from mitral valve disease, left ventricular failure and left atrial myxoma (Figure 3.17). One of the earliest signs of a large left atrium is a double right heart border. As the left atrium enlarges still further the left main bronchus elevates, the carina becomes widened, and sometimes the left atrial appendage becomes visible as a hump below the left main bronchus. Enlargement of the right atrium may be difficult to appreciate as there is a wide range of normal variation in its appearances. The right atrial border may be prominent and displaced by several centimetres to the right of the spine. Causes of right atrial enlargement include tricuspid valve disease and atrial septal defects. Displacement of the left ventricular border to the left, inferiorly or posteriorly, implies enlargement of the left ventricle. There are many causes of left ventricular enlargement including ischaemic heart disease, hypertension and aortic stenosis.

Enlargement of the right ventricle may result in uplifting of the cardiac apex. On the lateral view the enlarged right ventricle fills in more than one-third of the retrosternal space. Causes of right ventricular enlargement include pulmonary arterial hypertension and atrial septal defects.

Pulmonary Vasculature

Pulmonary vasculature may be abnormally increased or decreased. It may be increased in cardiac failure (see

Figure 3.17), in high output states such as thyrotoxicosis, and in left-to-right cardiac shunts (atrial and ventricular septal defects). Decreased pulmonary vasculature is often difficult to appreciate but may be seen in congenital heart disease with a right-to-left shunt, thromboembolic disease and primary lung disease such as in severe emphysema (see Figure 3.13).

Pneumopericardium

Pneumopericardium usually results from trauma or from recent cardiac surgery. Rarely it may result from ventilation-induced barotrauma. Pneumopericardium can be difficult to distinguish from pneumomediastinum but is much less common except in post-operative cardiac patients. Pneumopericardium usually is seen as a single band of gas that outlines the heart and does not extend into the superior mediastinum or neck.

Pericardial Effusion

An enlarged cardiac shadow can result from accumulation of fluid within the pericardial sac. The heart is typically flask shaped. Damping of cardiac motion by the surrounding fluid produces a sharp cardiac outline on the chest radiograph. Rapidly accumulating effusions will result in an increasing cardiac size on serial chest radiographs. The presence of a pericardial effusion can easily be confirmed with an echocardiogram.

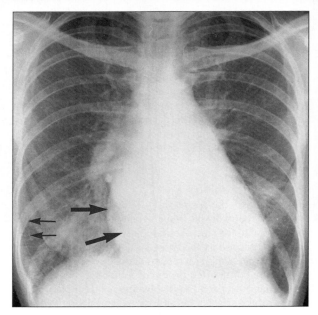

Figure 3.17 Mitral valve disease. Mild cardiac enlargement with a double right heart border due to left atrial enlargement (large arrows). The upper lobe vessels are dilated indicating pulmonary venous hypertension. Septal lines representing interstitial oedema lie peripherally at the lung bases (small arrows).

GENERAL READING

Corne, Carroll, Brown and Delaney, *Chest X-rays made easy*. *Chest radiology/plain film patterns/differential diagnosis*. London: Mosby International.

Langes and Start, *Radiology of chest diseases*. Theme Medical. Armstrong, Wilcox, Dee and Hansell. *Imaging of diseases of the chest*. London: Mosby International.

4 ELECTRO-CARDIOGRAPHY

G Buchanon & M Smith

CHAPTER OUTLINE

- Basic electrophysiology
- Conduction in the normal heart
- Components of the ECG
- Paper
- Recording the ECG
- Common rhythms and dysrhythmias
- Atrial or supraventricular tachycardia
- Myocardial infarction and ischaemia
- Examples of other ECGs
- Exercise electrocardiography
- Echocardiogram

INTRODUCTION

The aim of this chapter is to introduce the physiotherapist to the basic electrophysiology of an electrocardiogam (ECG), and to help in the recognition of common cardiac rhythms. Any cardiac rhythm that depresses the patient's blood pressure is dangerous and sometimes life threatening, so it is important that the physiotherapist is able to recognise the clinical signs and also the ECG trace on the monitor. Cardiac drugs are covered in Chapters 5 and 9. In assessing the rhythm it is important to establish if the patient is on any medication that may affect the ECG.

BASIC ELECTROPHYSIOLOGY

At rest, when the heart muscle is not contracting, the electrical charge is positive on the outside of each cell membrane but negative inside. This is because there is a predominance of positive ions on the outside of the membrane. The cells are said to be polarised, and depolarisation of the cells causes muscle contraction. Depolarisation occurs when ions (initially sodium and later calcium) move across the membrane rendering the inner state more positive. The sequence of this procedure from cell to cell causes muscle fibres to contract in synchrony resulting in the pumping action of the heart. Normally, depolarisation and repolarisation continue and result in the contraction and relaxation of heart muscle, respectively. Any abnormal changes in the membrane environment can affect the contraction of the muscle, its frequency and regularity.

Anatomically, there are organised cells that depolarise spontaneously, e.g. the sino-atrial (SA) node. The SA node initiates the heart beat and is called the pacemaker. In a human adult, the normal cardiac rate is approximately 70 beats/min.

The changing electrical status across the cell membranes causes voltage changes within the heart muscle, and these voltage differences can be detected at skin level and measured with electrodes placed on the skin. The results can be recorded by using the ECG, giving the ECG rhythm strip.

CONDUCTION IN THE NORMAL HEART

Preceding each mechanical contraction, a wave of depolarisation spreads through the heart. This begins at the SAN, situated at the junction of the superior vena cava and the right atrium, and travels through the right and left atria arriving at the atrio-ventricular (AV) node, sited near the atrio-ventricular junction of the right atrium. After a short delay, the impulse is transmitted to the bundle of His, which lies in the anterior interventricular septum, and reaches the Purkinje fibres in the endocardial surface of the heart via the right and left bundle branches (Figure 4.1). The contraction of the ventricles is simultaneous whereas those of the atria show a slight time difference.

Any damage along this pathway leads to heart block, e.g. bundle branch block (see page 58).

COMPONENTS OF THE ECG

P WAVE
The P wave represents atrial depolarisation (Figure 4.2). It is measured from the beginning of the deflection to a point where the wave joins the baseline. Its duration is between 0.08 and 0.12 s.

P-R INTERVAL
The P–R interval represents the time lapse of the impulse travelling from the SA node through the AV node on its way to the ventricles (see Figure 4.2). There is no muscle contraction during this event and its duration is between 0.12 and 0.2 s.

QRS COMPLEX
The QRS complex represents the depolarisation of the ventricles (see Figure 4.2). Normally, the deflections are rapid and the duration is between 0.08 to 0.10 s. Usually, the R wave is the upward deflection whereas the Q and S waves are downward deflections.

S-T SEGMENT
Following completion of ventricular depolarisation, there is a period of electrical inactivity represented by the S–T segment (see Figure 4.2). The segment is not normally more than 0.5 mm above or below the baseline or isoelectric line.

T WAVE
The T wave represents ventricular repolarisation in preparation for the next cycle (see Figure 4.2).

U WAVE
The U wave represents late repolarisation after the T wave, and is of little use in interpreting dysrhythmias but needs to be recognised so as not to confuse it with other components (see Figure 4.2).

PAPER

It is the fundamental principle of ECG machines that the paper used is of a standard square size and runs at a standard rate. Each large square is the equivalent of 0.2 s , with five large squares per second or 300 per minute, at normal running speed. Twenty-five small squares are included in each large square and so each of the the former is equivalent to 0.04 s.

The normal running speed for recording an ECG is 25 mm/s (see Figure 4.2). To establish the patient's heart rate simply count the number of large squares between two consecutive R waves (for ease of assessment) and divide 300 by the number calculated; for example, if there are five squares the patient's heart rate is 60 beats/min. In irregular rhythms such as atrial fibrillation, the rate may vary from 70 to 200 beats/min (see page 56).

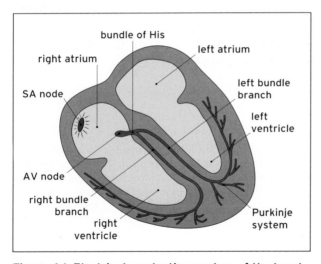

Figure 4.1 Electrical conduction system of the heart.

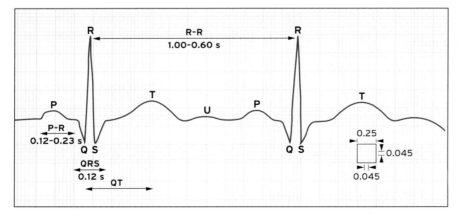

Figure 4.2 Principal time intervals of the electrocardiogram. Figures stated for the Q-T interval relate to a heart rate in the range 60 to 100/min.

RECORDING THE ECG

The 12 lead ECG assesses different areas in and around the heart to detect any anomalies of cardiac structures. The 12 leads include three standard leads, three unipolar limb leads and six chest or precordial leads. Each lead incorporates two electrodes measuring the potential or voltage difference between them. The positive electrode detects the electrical impulse from the heart and the 'neutral' electrode completes the electric circuit and offers the direction of pathway for the impulse. The ECG monitor (M) placed in the circuit detects electrical activity (Figure 4.3).

STANDARD LEADS

Lead I
The exploring electrode is attached to the left arm and the neutral electrode to the right arm.

Lead II
The exploring electrode is attached to the left leg and the neutral electrode to the right arm.

Lead III
The exploring electrode is attached to the left leg and the neutral electrode to the left arm.

Figure 4.3 Electrocardiograph leads.

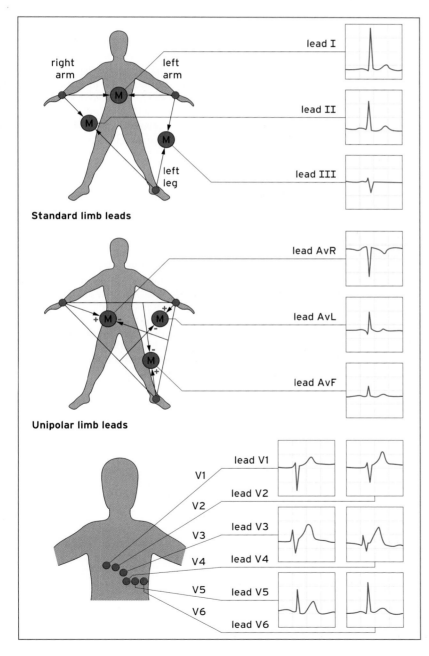

UNIPOLAR LEADS

The unipolar leads are arranged so that the exploring electrode is on the right leg and the neutral electrode on all the other limbs:

- Lead AvR is attached to the right arm.
- Lead AvL is attached to the left arm.
- Lead AvF is attached to the left leg.

Where 'A' represents augmented, as the voltages are very low and need to be increased to be comparable with the voltages from the other leads.

Lead AvR assesses the right side of the heart, lead AvL, the left side of the heart and lead AvF, the inferior aspect of the heart. These leads give a vertical cross-sectional view of the heart.

The chest leads are placed on the thorax at specific positions (see Figure 4.3) and give a horizontal cross-sectional view of the heart. The leads are named V1 to V6; V1 and V2 assess the right ventricle, V3 and V4 the interventricular septum and V5 and V6 the anterior and lateral aspect of the heart. For example, if a patient suffers an anterior, inferior infarct, changes occur in the leads that look at these areas, i.e. leads AvL, AvF, V5 and V6. This is grossly simplified but gives an idea of the principle. Further changes are discussed on page 59.

COMMON RHYTHMS AND DYSRHYTHMIAS

SINUS RHYTHM

Normal rhythm originating from the SA node is sinus (Figure 4.4A). The R–R interval is regular and the rate can vary between below 60 beats/min (sinus bradycardia; Figure 4.4B) and above 100 beats/min (sinus tachycardia; Figure

4.4C). The former is common in fit individuals or during rest or sleep, and the latter is common after exercise. Medication, e.g. β-blockers, can induce bradycardias as can some medical conditions such as hyperkalaemia (high serum potassium).

Sinus dysrhythmia is not unusual in infants and adolescents where the R–R interval is irregular but there is a P wave.

ATRIAL FIBRILLATION

In atrial fibrillation, the heart rate is irregular with an unequal R–R interval (Figure 4.5). The ventricular rate varies between 70 and 170 beats/min and the ECG trace shows fibrillation or an irregular isoelectric line and typically there are no P waves because the atrial rate is so fast (400–1000 times the ventricular rate). Here the atria are not contracting well and there are multiple ectopic (abnormal) foci causing the quivering of the atria. The AV node allows some of the stronger impulses to be conducted, giving the ventricular rate.

If the atrial rate is not too high, patients are relatively asymptomatic but the common symptoms of atrial fibrillation are palpitations and dizziness. Common causes are ischaemia, e.g. post myocardial infarction, valve disease, especially mitral, rheumatic heart disease and thyrotoxicosis.

ATRIAL FLUTTER

In atrial flutter, the ventricular rate varies between 45 and 55 beats/min but the atrial rate is high at around 200 beats/min (Figure 4.6). Here there is an irritable ectopic focus firing at a rate of 250–400 beats/min with a ventricular contraction every second, third or fourth impulse causing atrial flutter with 2:1, 3:1 or 4:1 block, respectively. On the ECG, there are many P waves in between the QRS waveform. The cause of atrial flutter is usually organic heart disease, and because of the reduced ventricular rate there is a danger of reduced

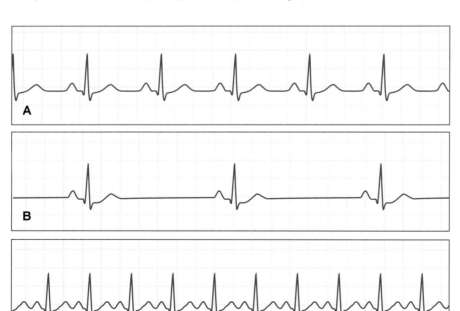

Figure 4.4 (A) Sinus rhythm, (B) sinus bradycardia and (C) sinus tachycardia.

cardiac output and left ventricular failure. Patients are aware of palpitations, and treatment method includes carotid sinus massage, direct current (DC) shock and drugs, e.g. digoxin.

ATRIAL OR SUPRAVENTRICULAR TACHYCARDIA

In atrial or supraventricular tachycardia (Figure 4.7), the heart rate is fast—too fast to originate from the SA node—but begins above the ventricles (hence supraventricular). The P waves are not identifiable, the R–R rate is regular and the duration of the QRS complex is normal which distinguishes the rhythm from some ventricular tachycardias. The danger with this rhythm is the potential to depress the cardiac output and therefore treatment must be rapid. Treatment methods include anti-arrhythmic therapy such as amiodarone or DC shock.

VENTRICULAR TACHYCARDIA

Ventricular dysrhythmias are dangerous as they tend to lower the patient's blood pressure with poor ventricular contraction and low cardiac output (Figures 4.8A and B). Ventricular tachycardia and fibrillation can lead to asystole, which causes death. Treatment is in the form of resuscitation (see Chapter 6).

Ventricular tachycardia is recognisable by its fast regular ventricular rate (150–250 beats/min) with a QRS duration of greater than 0.12 s. It may be difficult to distinguish the P waves or the T waves and the P–R interval is not measurable.

VENTRICULAR FIBRILLATION

Ventricular fibrillation occurs with completely chaotic electrical activity in the heart (Figures 4.9A and B). No coherent contraction occurs and this is the commonest cause of cardiac arrest. Ventricular fibrillation may occur without

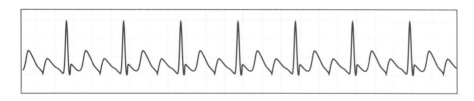

Figure 4.5 **Atrial fibrillation.**

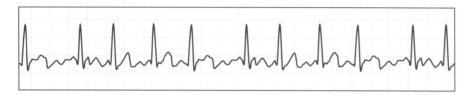

Figure 4.6 **Atrial flutter.**

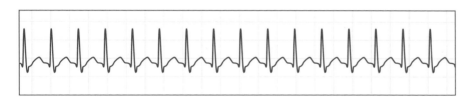

Figure 4.7 **Supraventricular tachycardia.**

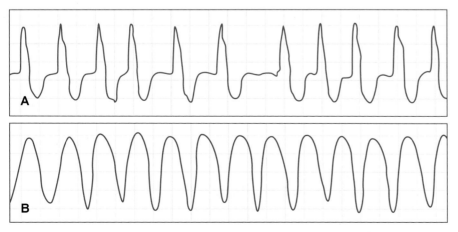

Figure 4.8 **(A and B) Examples of ventricular tachycardia.**

warning, follow a ventricular ectopic beat, especially if it is very premature, or degenerate from ventricular tachycardia. On the ECG there are no identifiable P waves or QRS complexes. There is no measurable P–R interval, and the rate cannot be determined accurately. Cardiopulmonary resuscitation must be instituted immediately while waiting for electrical defibrillation.

HEART BLOCK

As mentioned earlier, if there is a disturbance in the conduction mechanism of the heart this causes heart block. There are three common types of heart block:

First Degree Heart Block

In first degree heart block there is a delay in the impulse reaching the AV node from the SA node but the rhythm does not affect the patient and therefore no treatment is needed (Figure 4.10). The rate is not really affected and the only discrepancy is a longer than normal P–R interval (greater than 0.2 s). Common causes include ischaemic heart disease or myocardial infarction.

Second Degree Heart Block

If the ventricles do not respond to atrial stimuli, the P wave is not followed by a QRS complex. In second degree heart block there is blocked atrial conduction of varying frequency so not every P wave is followed by a QRS complex (Figure 4.11). If there are two P wave deflections to every ventricular deflection, this is known as 2:1 block. There

may be 3:1 or 4:1 blocks, and so the larger the block the slower the heart rate. On the ECG there are frequent P waves with fewer QRS complexes. If the rhythm is causing the patient symptoms such as dizziness or syncope (fainting), the treatment of choice is a pacemaker. If the rhythm has been caused by drug therapy, e.g. digoxin toxicity, then the drug must be reviewed and still the choice of treatment is a temporary pacemaker until the rhythm is rectified, especially if there is a concern that the block will become complete heart block.

Third Degree or Complete Heart Block

In complete heart block there is no relationship between the atria and the ventricles, with the SA node still producing impulses at approximately 70 beats/min but with complete dissociation from the ventricles, which have their own rate of approximately 33 beats/min (Figure 4.12). The ventricular rate is established either at the atrio-ventricular junction, giving a narrow QRS complex, or below the junction, giving a wide, bizarre QRS complex. The patient shows the symptoms of poor cardiac output and needs a pacemaker.

BUNDLE BRANCH BLOCK

Structurally, in bundle branch block there is a disturbance in the intraventricular conduction, and so typically the QRS complex is wide (greater than 0.1 s). There are normal P waves and P–R intervals, and the heart rate is normal as governed by the SA node. Because there is a discrepancy in the contraction time of the ventricles (which normally

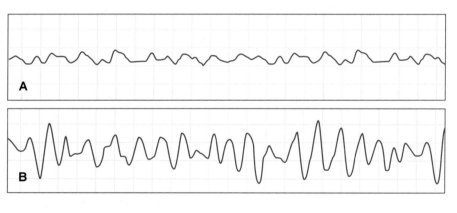

Figure 4.9 (A and B) Examples of ventricular fibrillation.

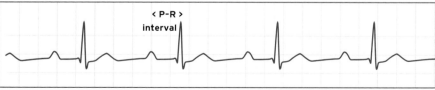

Figure 4.10 First degree heart block with long P-R intervals.

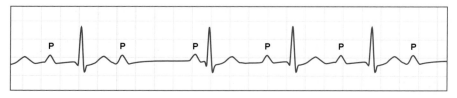

Figure 4.11 Second degree heart block.

contract simultaneously), the complex is wide and often with two peaks on the R wave. Depending on which leads demonstrate the changes it can be established if the block is a left or right bundle branch block.

MYOCARDIAL INFARCTION AND ISCHAEMIA

By definition, a myocardial infarction is an incident where heart muscle becomes devoid of its blood supply rendering the muscle necrotic with eventual fibrosis of the area. Ischaemia refers to the muscle having an impaired blood supply but not completely cut off from that supply. Details of the pathophysiology are described in Chapter 9. If a full thickness of heart wall, commonly the left ventricle, is depleted of its perfusion, the resultant condition is referred to as a transmural infarction as opposed to a subendocardial infarction, where a percentage of the wall is affected. The latter tends to be a zonal lesion and the former a regional lesion.

The changes that occur on the ECG depict the changing state of the myocardium (Figure 4.13):
- Within minutes or hours, the S–T segment becomes elevated in the leads facing the infarction.
- Within hours or days, there is development of broad and/or deep Q waves with R wave reduction and an inverting T wave. N.B. Abnormal Q wave is the definitive diagnosis for a transmural infarction.
- Within a week or more, there is a return of the S–T segment to baseline but the other signs remain.
- Months later, there is a possible gradual return of the T wave but persistent abnormal Q wave or QS complex.

LOCATION OF THE INFARCT

Based on the appearance of the abnormal Q wave or QS complex in the individual leads, and the relationship of the leads to the various portions of the ventricular wall, the site of the infarction can be localised as follows:
- Extensive anterior myocardial infarction—abnormal Q waves in leads I, V1–V6 and AvL.
- Anterolateral myocardial infarction—abnormal Q waves in leads V1 to V3.
- Inferior myocardial infarction—abnormal Q waves in leads II, III and AvF.
- True posterior myocardial infarction—abnormal R waves in leads V1, V2 or occasionally V3 or V4.

Again, this is oversimplified but gives the basics for interpretation of ECGs.

EXAMPLES OF OTHER ECGs

The following are examples of situations where a physiotherapist may be asked to see a patient with clinical signs, e.g. shortness of breath; the ability to interpret the ECG is of great use to establish that the problem is not a physiotherapeutic one.

PULMONARY EMBOLUS
In the acute stage of pulmonary embolism, if the embolus is of sufficient size to cause right-sided heart strain there may be right bundle branch block or inverted T wave and/or S–T depression in V1 to V3.

VENTRICULAR HYPERTROPHY
In left ventricular hypertrophy there are abnormally large R waves (greater than five large squares of the ECG paper) in leads V4 and V6 as is the case in right ventricular hypertrophy, showing large R waves in V1 and V2. This may be accompanied by signs of heart muscle strain such as S–T depression and/or T wave inversion in V5 and V6 in left ventricular hypertrophy and V1 to V3 in right ventricular hypertrophy.

PERICARDITIS
In the acute phase of pericarditis there is S–T elevation in all leads except AvF and V1 (which may show S–T depression). In the later stages there is T wave inversion in multiple leads.

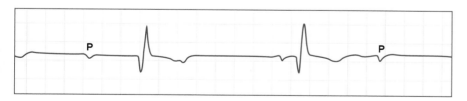

Figure 4.12 Complete heart block.

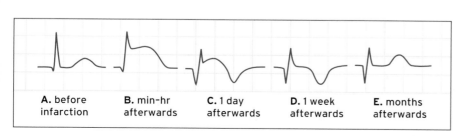

| A. before infarction | B. min–hr afterwards | C. 1 day afterwards | D. 1 week afterwards | E. months afterwards |

Figure 4.13 Transmural myocardial infarction. Sequence of electrocardiographic changes in a lead facing the infarction.

BRAIN DAMAGE

In brain damage, the possible explanation for abnormalities in the ECG is altered autonomous tone to the heart. Typical findings on the ECG are deep inverted or tall upright T waves and Q–T interval prolongation with prominent U waves. Autopsy shows no abnormality of the myocardium.

COPD

Patients with severe respiratory disease with pulmonary hypertension may show ECG signs in keeping with right-sided heart strain similar to those found in pulmonary embolism.

Described below are some common investigative procedures employed in the general hospital to help in the diagnosis of cardiac problems. Details of the more specialised equipment available are given in Chapter 7.

EXERCISE ELECTROCARDIOGRAPHY

The aim of exercise electrocardiography is to elicit signs of ischaemia by exercising the patient on either a bike or a treadmill while attached to a 12 lead monitor. The changes in S–T shape will establish that there is a reduced blood supply to areas of the myocardium or, in the case of a patient with myocardial infarction, that there is a lack, or existence, of a collateral blood supply. Untoward effects of the exercise test are angina, severe shortage of breath and dizziness; in the presence of significant changes in the ECG, the test should be stopped.

If the test is found to be positive, i.e. there are significant changes in the leads, then further examination, such as cardiac catheterisation, to establish the true extent of the coronary stenosis, will be considered with the view to operate. Details of the build-up to surgery are covered in Chapter 7.

ECHOCARDIOGRAM

By using ultrasound, the anatomy and dimensions of all cardiac structures can be studied. Valve defects, ventricular hypertrophy, septal defects, hypokinesia (slow movement) or akinesia (no movement) of the ventricles are a few of the diagnoses that can be made using ultrasonography.

Ultrasonography is a non-invasive tool that can also be employed via an oesophageal probe to study the posterior structures of the heart.

CONCLUSION

This chapter gives a broad outline of the recognition of common dysrhymias and their clinical presentation. In the acute setting, especially in Intensive Care, it is very important that the physiotherapist is able to recognise diverse effects of the physiotherapy treatment and to alert the medical team to the problem if, while studying the monitor, an irregularity appears. Similarly, if the physiotherapist is examining the patient and has access to the ECG, it is good practice to be able to assess him or her or at least to recognise that there is an abnormality present. Recognition of anti-arrhythmic drugs is also important as this will establish the stability of the patient and whether physiotherapy intervention at that stage is recommended.

GENERAL READING

Levick JR. *Introduction to cardiovascular physiology*, 2nd ed. Oxford: Butterworth-Heineman; 1995.
Hampton JR. *ECG made easy*, 5th ed. Churchill Livingstone; 1977.
The heart. Opie. Grune and Stratton.
Goldschlager N, Goldman M. *Principles of clinical electrocardiography*, 13 ed. Appleton & Lange; 1989.

Gray, Huon, Dawkins, Keith, Simpson and Morgan. *Lecture notes on cardiology*. Oxford: Blackwell Science; 1998.
Steine E, Xenakis T. *Rapid analysis of arryhmias: A self study programme*, 2nd ed. Lea and Febiger; 1992.

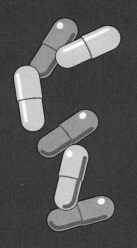

5 JC Mucklow

DRUG THERAPY

CHAPTER OUTLINE

- Drugs used in the treatment of heart failure
- Drugs used in the treatment of hypotension
- Drugs used in the treatment of angina
- Drugs used in the treatment of hypertension
- Drugs used in the treatment of cardiac dysrhythmias

- Drugs used in the treatment of asthma
- Drugs used in the treatment of respiratory failure
- Antimicrobial agents used in the treatment of acute respiratory tract infection
- Antimicrobial agents used in the treatment of chronic respiratory tract infection

INTRODUCTION

Most patients who need physiotherapy will be taking one or more drugs, either for the condition requiring physiotherapy, e.g. analgesics, antibiotics, or for a pre-existing disease or illness, e.g. anti-anginal agent, bronchodilator. If you are familiar with the drugs that have been prescribed for your patient, you will be able to take their effects into account when deciding on the need for treatment and the patient's stability for treatment, and be able to assess the outcome of that treatment. Drugs such as muscle relaxants and analgesics will have effects that complement physiotherapy while sedatives and cough suppressants may have effects that interfere with the patient's ability to co-operate. Other drugs such as anti-Parkinsonian agents and anti-anginal agents may simply reveal the existence of an underlying medical condition (not always immediately apparent from the patient's medical record) which could have an important bearing on how you plan and carry out treatment.

You do not need a detailed knowledge of pharmacology to be able to interpret your patient's drug chart. But you do need to value what it can tell you, so that you refer to it as part of your routine when you assess your patient. You should also know where you can find information about those drugs whose names you do not recognise. Never assume that a drug is irrelevant to your treatment plan until you have satisfied yourself that you know why it has been prescribed and what effects it is likely to have. There should be a reference source, e.g. *British National Formulary* (BNF), on every hospital ward and in every general practitioner's surgery, and there should also be a copy in every physiotherapy department. This text will tell you a great deal about the drug your patient is taking.

This chapter is not intended to be comprehensive. It sets out to cover a selection of drugs that you will commonly encounter in your patients' drug charts, using as headings those medical conditions they are intended to correct, relieve or prevent.

DRUGS USED IN THE TREATMENT OF HEART FAILURE

Heart failure occurs when the cardiac output, i.e. the volume of blood expelled from the heart each minute, is insufficient to provide for the body's needs. It can occur suddenly, for example, because of damage to the heart muscle due to a myocardial infarction (heart attack), or due to a dysrhythmia (disturbance of heart rhythm). More often it occurs gradually because of progressive heart disease, when many of its symptoms and signs result from the body's attempts to compensate for the low cardiac output. The kidney retains more salt and water to enlarge the circulating blood volume and to support the blood pressure, which leads in turn to leakage of fluid across capillaries and causes swelling of the skin, lungs and other internal organs (congestive cardiac failure).

The symptoms of heart failure include generalised oedema, weight gain caused by fluid retention, shortness of breath and loss of appetite, coupled with marked fatigue due to low cardiac output. Aside from those forms of drug treatment directed at the underlying cause of heart failure, such as anti-arrhythmics or anti-hypertensives, there are three ways in which drugs can help. They can:

- Increase salt and water excretion by the kidney, e.g. diuretics.
- Enhance the heart's contractility, e.g. positive inotropic drugs.
- Reduce the workload of the heart by reducing arterial resistance (afterload) or the volume of venous blood returning to the heart (preload) or both, e.g. vasodilators.

DIURETICS

Diuretics inhibit the re-absorption of salt and water by the kidney tubule. There are two main types: thiazide diuretics and loop diuretics.

Thiazide Diuretics

Thiazide diuretics act on the proximal and distal convoluted tubule of the nephron but are of limited effectiveness in the treatment of cardiac failure, except in mild cases. Examples include bendrofluazidemethiazide (bendrofluazide), chlortalidone, cyclopenthiazide and hydrochlorthiazide. At higher dosage, thiazide diuretics inhibit the tubular secretion of glucose and uric acid (predisposing to the development of diabetes mellitus and gout) and have unfavourable effects on blood lipids (triglycerides and cholesterol), although these effects are negligible at low dosage.

Loop Diuretics

Loop diuretics, such as bumetanide and furosemide (frusemide), act on the loop of Henle. They are more effective than thiazides and play a vital role in the treatment of most patients with cardiac failure. They can be given by mouth and by injection, and daily dosage is adjusted according to the response, as judged by urine output, weight loss or disappearance of oedema.

In the course of inhibiting tubular re-absorption of sodium, thiazides and loop diuretics also inhibit re-absorption of potassium. This can lead eventually to hypokalaemia (a low plasma potassium concentration), which is particularly likely to occur in patients with generalised oedema. Potassium depletion can be prevented by using a potassium-sparing agent, such as amiloride, spironolactone or triamterene. These drugs act on that part of the distal tubule where sodium is reabsorbed in exchange for potassium, under the influence of the mineralocorticoid hormone, aldosterone. By antagonising this exchange process, sodium excretion is enhanced while potassium excretion is reduced. In patients taking angiotensin-converting enzyme (ACE) inhibitors (see below), potassium-sparing agents are unnecessary and the combination can cause dangerous hyperkalaemia (a high plasma potassium concentration).

POSITIVE INOTROPIC DRUGS

A positive inotropic drug, or inotrope, increases myocardial contractility (the force of heart muscle contraction). Inotropes fall into three groups: cardiac glycosides, e.g. digoxin; sympathomimetics, e.g. dobutamine; and phosphodiesterase inhibitors, e.g. enoximone.

Cardiac Glycosides

Cardiac glycosides enhance contractility by facilitating the activity of heart muscle fibres, but this is only one of several effects that they have on cardiac function. They are more commonly used to slow the heart rate in patients with atrial fibrillation, and are no longer a first-line treatment in heart failure where the rhythm is regular, because other drugs are relatively more effective and safer to use.

Digoxin is the agent most commonly used, sometimes by intravenous infusion but usually by mouth. The range of daily dosage that is both effective and safe is narrow (125–500 μg) and depends on individual patient age, body weight and kidney function, so dosage must be chosen and adjusted carefully. Too high a dose can cause nausea, vomiting, mental confusion or dangerous dysrhythmias. Digoxin is slowly eliminated from the body, and recovery from excessive dosage can take a week or more. Because the effects of digoxin are difficult to measure directly, its serum concentration is sometimes used to check that the chosen dose is correct.

Sympathomimetics

Sympathomimetics mimic the effects of autonomic adrenergic (sympathetic) nervous stimulation of the heart, and stimulate β-adrenoceptors situated on the surface of heart muscle fibres. The most commonly used sympathomimetic inotrope is dobutamine, which increases the force and, to a lesser extent, the rate of myocardial contraction. It is given by intravenous infusion, the rate of which is increased until the cardiac output, measured directly or as reflected by the blood pressure, is sufficient to maintain vital organ blood flow without an unacceptable acceleration of heart rate. Dobutamine is used to support the heart after cardiac surgery or myocardial infarction, and in patients with septic shock. Treatment usually continues for 24–48 hours, until the heart recovers sufficiently to sustain an adequate output unsupported.

Another drug commonly used in the same circumstances, and in the same way, is dopamine; this has similar effects on the heart but protects the kidney against the effects of hypotension (low blood pressure)—it acts on dopamine receptors to maintain renal blood flow in the face of intense generalised arterial vasoconstriction. Infused dopamine has to be administered via a long intravenous catheter to prevent leakage around the infusion site and tissue damage. The dose must be carefully adjusted—at high dosage, dopamine stimulates α-adrenoceptors and increases vasoconstriction, even in the kidney.

Phosphodiesterase Inhibitors

Phosphodiesterase inhibitors, such as enoximone and milrinone, inhibit the deactivation of cyclic adenosine monophosphate (cAMP), one of the intracellular messengers that translate muscle stimulation into contraction. Given by intravenous injection or infusion, these drugs have a sustained effect on myocardial contractility but are reserved for patients with acute heart failure occurring, for example, after cardiac surgery, or in chronic heart failure that has failed to respond to conventional measures. There is no evidence that their use, which requires specialist supervision, improves survival.

DRUGS THAT REDUCE CARDIAC WORKLOAD

ACE Inhibitors

ACE inhibitors act on the enzyme that converts angiotensin I (an intermediate compound derived from the intrarenal hormone, renin) to angiotensin II, a highly potent vasoconstrictor. By reducing vasoconstriction, these drugs reduce peripheral arterial resistance and lower diastolic blood pressure, hence their value as antihypertensive drugs (see below). By reducing peripheral resistance, they increase cardiac output and have therefore become the mainstay in the treatment of chronic cardiac failure. If started soon after a myocardial infarction, they also reduce mortality in this condition.

The first dose of an ACE inhibitor can cause an abrupt fall in blood pressure. Patients with heart failure should take the first dose lying down and have their blood pressure carefully measured for the first 2 hours. These drugs can also impair renal function, especially when there is severe stenosis (narrowing) of both renal arteries, and renal function should be monitored carefully for the first few weeks of treatment while the daily dosage is being increased. Numerous other unwanted effects can occur but are uncommon. One worth mentioning, because it is often undiagnosed, is a persistent dry cough that occurs in 10–15% of patients and usually means that the drug has to be withdrawn. ACE inhibitors in common use include captopril, enalapril, perindopril, quinapril and ramipril.

Directly Acting Vasodilators

Directly acting vasodilators, such as hydralazine, also reduce afterload; hydralazine has been used together with long-acting nitrates in the treatment of chronic cardiac failure. This regimen is less effective than treatment with an ACE inhibitor but may be useful as an alternative in selected patients.

DRUGS USED IN THE TREATMENT OF HYPOTENSION

In clinical settings where blood pressure falls acutely as a result of peripheral vasodilation and a fall in peripheral resistance, e.g. septic shock and anaphylactic shock, initial management involves attempts to expand the circulating blood volume with intravenous infusions of crystalloid, e.g. saline, or of colloid, e.g. Haemacel, Gelofusin solutions, but this approach may not suffice; drugs that constrict peripheral arterioles may be required for a while to sustain blood pressure and maintain organ blood flow while the cause of the problem, e.g. generalised infection, is being treated.

SYMPATHOMIMETIC DRUGS

Norepinephrine (noradrenaline) constricts most peripheral arterioles, and this effect leads to a reflex slowing of heart rate; it is given by intravenous infusion via a central venous catheter to raise blood pressure in patients with shock (acute hypotension), usually as a second-line treatment after volume expansion alone has proved insufficient.

Adrenaline stimulates the myocardium, constricts the blood supply to the skin, and causes bronchodilation; it is used only for the treatment of anaphylactic shock (an acute allergic reaction comprising circulatory collapse with bronchoconstriction) or during cardiopulmonary resuscitation following a cardiac arrest.

DRUGS USED IN THE TREATMENT OF ANGINA

Angina pectoris, commonly known as angina, occurs when the supply of oxygen to the heart muscle fails to match that required for effective contraction, usually because one or more coronary arteries are narrowed by atheroma. Although it can occur at rest, angina commonly occurs when cardiac work is increased by exertion, resulting in a cramp-like pain in the front of the chest that is relieved in a few minutes if the person rests. Angina that occurs frequently for the first time, becomes suddenly worse after a period of stability, or recurs at rest, is known as unstable angina.

NITRATES

Organic nitrates, e.g. glyceryl trinitrate, isosorbide dinitrate and isosorbide mononitrate, relax smooth muscle in the walls of arterioles and venules, causing them to dilate. Although it used to be thought that they relieved angina solely by dilating coronary arteries, most of their beneficial effect in fact results from dilation of peripheral blood vessels, which reduces cardiac work. Isosorbide dinitrate and isosorbide mononitrate are taken regularly by mouth to prevent attacks of angina. Glyceryl trinitrate (GTN; nitro-glycerine) is largely ineffective when swallowed and has to be administered to allow absorption across the mucosal lining of the mouth (sublingual or buccal tablets, oral spray), or through the skin (adhesive patch). GTN is absorbed sufficiently rapidly from within the mouth that it can be used either to relieve an attack of angina or to prevent one that is imminent. All nitrates cause a throbbing headache if given in a high enough dosage, and patients vary in their ability to tolerate this unwanted effect.

β-BLOCKERS

β-Blockers inhibit the response of β_1-adrenoceptors in the heart to stimulation by sympathetic nerve activity or circulating epinephrine (adrenaline). They limit the increase in heart rate during exercise and reduce myocardial contractility. β-Blockers have been the mainstay of the medical management of angina since they were first introduced in the 1960s. Taken daily, they increase the amount of exertion that is possible before angina occurs. Examples of β-blockers include atenolol, bisoprolol, metoprolol, nadolol, oxprenolol, propranolol and timolol.

Unfortunately, reducing the heart rate during exercise can cause unacceptable fatigue. Other unwanted effects of β-receptor inhibition include bronchoconstriction and coldness of the hands and feet. Bronchoconstriction occurs because of β_2-receptor inhibition in the bronchial smooth muscle. β-blockers can also trigger or worsen an attack of asthma. Although some β-blockers, e.g. atenolol, bisoprolol and metoprolol, inhibit β_1-receptors selectively, none are safe in patients with asthma. Because they depress cardiac function, β-blockers should generally not be used in patients with heart failure except under specialist supervision.

CALCIUM CHANNEL BLOCKERS

Calcium channel blockers relax smooth muscle by inhibiting the transport of calcium into muscle cells. Dihydropyridines (amlodipine, isradipine, nicardipine, nifedipine) exert their effects mainly on arteriolar smooth muscle, and have minimal direct effects on the heart. Some examples of calcium channel blockers are dihydropyridines, verapamil and diltiazem.

Verapamil acts predominantly on the cardiac muscle to reduce myocardial contractility and also impairs cardiac conductivity (the conduction of electrical impulses through the heart), thereby slowing heart rate; its effect on arteriolar smooth muscle is relatively less than that of the dihydropyridines. Diltiazem relaxes arteriolar smooth muscle to a lesser extent than the dihydropyridines and has less effect than verapamil on cardiac contractility and conductivity.

All these drugs reduce the frequency and severity of angina if taken regularly. Blood pressure falls, especially during treatment with a dihydropyridine. The side effects of these drugs depend on their sites of action. Dihydropyridines cause palpitation, flushing and headache as the heart responds to a fall in blood pressure, and can also cause troublesome oedema of the lower legs.

Verapamil's commonest unwanted effect is constipation. Diltiazem is generally better tolerated as its effects are more evenly distributed. All calcium channel blockers, especially verapamil, can depress heart function and worsen cardiac failure.

POTASSIUM CHANNEL ACTIVATORS

The only drug available in this category at present is nicorandil. This drug facilitates the entry of potassium into vascular muscle cells and dilates peripheral arteries; it also acts rather like a nitrate to dilate peripheral veins. Taken regularly, nicorandil is as effective in the treatment of angina as any of the alternatives. Its unwanted side effects include headache and flushing.

Patients with angina commonly need a drug from one of these groups to prevent attacks and to improve exercise tolerance. When using drugs together it is important to bear in mind their side effects, so as to minimise the likelihood of intolerance. Thus, β-blockers should not be used with verapamil, as their combined effects could depress myocardial contractility excessively. Similarly, using dihydropyridines together with either nitrates or nicorandil could cause intolerable headache or flushing. There is little evidence that using more than two drugs together improves the clinical response.

DRUGS USED IN THE TREATMENT OF HYPERTENSION

Although hypertension can occur as a consequence of an underlying disease or condition, 95% of patients affected have essential hypertension for which no curable cause can be found. Hypertension is defined as persistently raised blood pressure, where the systolic pressure exceeds 140 mmHg and/or the diastolic pressure exceeds 90 mmHg. It is categorised with reference to the diastolic pressure as either mild (90–99 mmHg), moderate (100–119 mmHg) or severe (equal to or greater than 120 mmHg). The higher the pressure, the greater is the risk of stroke, myocardial infarction, renal failure or cardiac failure, and the greater is the imperative to introduce and to continue drug treatment. Nevertheless, lifestyle changes play an important part in the management of the condition, and mild hypertension will often respond to non-pharmacological measures alone.

Drugs that reduce blood pressure do so by reducing cardiac output, peripheral arterial resistance or both. Many of the drugs used to treat hypertension are also valuable in the treatment of other cardiovascular conditions, as detailed in the previous section.

β-BLOCKERS

All β-blockers lower blood pressure, reduce heart rate and myocardial contractility, and they also reduce the secretion of renin by the kidney, thereby lessening the production of angiotensin II, which causes vasoconstriction. The side effects of β-blockers have already been described.

THIAZIDE DIURETICS

Thiazides lower blood pressure initially by reducing circulating blood volume. However, their effect is sustained even after blood volume returns to normal within a few months of starting treatment, probably by relaxation of vascular smooth muscle.

ACE INHIBITORS

ACE inhibitors reduce blood pressure by inhibiting the production of angiotensin II. Although blood pressure may fall abruptly after the first dose, it does not have to be monitored as carefully during the first few hours in patients with hypertension as it does in patients with heart failure, and symptoms can usually be avoided by starting treatment with a small dose at bedtime.

CALCIUM CHANNEL BLOCKERS

Dihydropyridines, verapamil and diltiazem are all effective as antihypertensive drugs, especially dihydropyridines.

α-BLOCKERS

Drugs that inhibit the effects of autonomic adrenergic (sympathetic) stimulation at peripheral α-adrenoceptors, reduce vasoconstriction and lower peripheral arterial resistance. Examples include doxazosin, indoramin, prazosin and terazosin. Like ACE inhibitors, although for different reasons, these drugs can cause blood pressure to fall abruptly after the first dose, which should be small and taken at bedtime. Unwanted effects of α-blockers include drowsiness, dry mouth, nasal congestion, urinary frequency and postural hypotension (a symptomatic fall in blood pressure on standing up).

As in the drug treatment of angina, one drug alone may not be completely effective in reducing the blood pressure to below the target level (140/90 mmHg) and two or more drugs may be used together. Whereas combining two drugs from the same pharmacological group is of no value, two drugs from different groups can interact very favourably and cause fewer unwanted effects than using a high dose of a single drug.

DRUGS USED IN THE TREATMENT OF CARDIAC DYSRHYTHMIAS

The normal cardiac rhythm depends on the generation of an electrical impulse in the sino-atrial (SA) node located in the right atrium of the heart, which is then conducted via the atrio-ventricular (AV) node, at the junction between the atria and the ventricles, to the ventricles themselves, thereby completing atrial emptying and triggering ventricular muscle contraction. Dysfunction in any part of the pathway will impair conduction of the impulse and lead to heart block. However, most anti-arrhythmic drugs are given to prevent or control excessive electrical activity arising within or outside the conducting system. Such rhythm disturbances are classified broadly as supraventricular (arising in the SA node, atrium or AV node) or ventricular (arising in the ventricle).

Anti-dysrhythmic drugs are categorised most usefully according to whether they are effective in the suppression or prevention of supraventricular dysrhythmias, ventricular dysrhythmias, or both.

DRUGS THAT SUPPRESS SUPRAVENTRICULAR BUT NOT VENTRICULAR DYSRHYTHMIA

Cardiac glycosides, such as digoxin, have already been mentioned in the context of heart failure. They prolong the atrio-ventricular refractory period (the interval following conduction of each cardiac impulse before the next can be conducted), and limit the extent to which supraventricular disturbances of rhythm (supraventricular ectopic beats or tachycardia, atrial flutter, atrial fibrillation) can dictate the frequency of ventricular contraction. Digoxin is the drug of choice for established atrial flutter or fibrillation. However, in patients who are susceptible to transient (paroxysmal) supraventricular disturbances of cardiac rhythm, digoxin does not prevent their occurrence.

The most effective drug in the management of paroxysmal supraventricular tachycardia is adenosine. Given rapidly by intravenous injection into a large vein, it usually restores sinus rhythm within a matter of minutes, and is useful when one cannot decide whether a rapid tachycardia is supraventricular or ventricular in origin. Adenosine can give rise to facial flushing, chest pain, dyspnoea, bronchospasm or a choking sensation, but its effects are short lived.

Verapamil, the calcium channel blocker, inhibits conduction of the cardiac impulse via the AV node and slows the ventricular response to supraventricular arrthymias. It can be given by mouth or by intravenous injection, but should be avoided if there is any doubt that a tachycardia is supraventricular, or if the patient has already been treated with a β-blocker, as it can profoundly impair ventricular contraction in these circumstances.

DRUGS THAT SUPPRESS SUPRAVENTRICULAR AND VENTRICULAR DYSRHYTHMIAS

Amiodarone is a most useful drug in the treatment of all forms of paroxysmal tachycardia, atrial flutter and atrial or ventricular fibrillation, and causes little or no depression of myocardial contractility. It can be given either by mouth or intravenous injection, the route being determined by the urgency of the situation. It would probably be the drug of choice in all tachydysrhythmias were it not for its potential to have serious unwanted effects.

Amiodarone contains iodine and can disturb thyroid gland function, giving rise to either overactivity (thyrotoxicosis) or underactivity (hypothyroidism), and making biochemical tests of thyroid gland function difficult to interpret. The drug can also cause phototoxic skin reactions, and patients are advised to apply a wide spectrum sunscreen to protect the skin against ultraviolet and visible light. Amiodarone causes the appearance of microdeposits in the cornea, although these seldom interfere with vision. More seriously, amiodarone can cause inflammatory changes in the lungs (pneumonitis) leading to shortness of breath or cough, and can also impair conduction in peripheral nerves (peripheral neuropathy).

β-Blockers attenuate the effects of sympathetic stimulation on cardiac conductivity and reduce the heart rate in paroxysmal or sustained tachycardia.

Disopyramide impairs both cardiac conductivity and contractility. It is useful for controlling tachydysrhythmias that occur soon after myocardial infarction. It can be given by mouth or by intravenous injection. Its unwanted effects arise chiefly from its antimuscarinic activity, which mimics the effect of autonomic parasympathetic stimulation, and resembles the effects of atropine (dry mouth, dilation of the ocular pupil, impaired bladder emptying).

Flecainide is effective in the prevention of symptomatic ventricular dysrhythmias, junctional tachycardias (arising at the atrioventricular junction) and paroxysmal atrial fibrillation. Less used nowadays is quinidine, another versatile agent for the prevention of paroxysmal tachydysrhythmia. Both flecainide and quinidine depress myocardial contractility and can themselves cause serious dysrhythmias; they should be used only under specialist cardiological supervision.

The final drug in this category is propafenone, useful for preventing ventricular and some supraventricular dysrhythmias, which also has weak β-blocking activity and can cause bronchoconstriction in patients with asthma or chronic obstructive pulmonary disease (COPD).

DRUGS THAT SUPPRESS VENTRICULAR BUT NOT SUPRAVENTRICULAR DYSRHYTHMIAS

The drug of first choice for the management of ventricular dysrhythmias occurring soon after myocardial infarction is lignocaine (lidocaine), which must be given by intravenous injection or infusion as it is ineffective when taken orally. Lignocaine suppresses ventricular ectopics and tachycardia, and reduces the risk that these will lead to ventricular fibrillation. If given in too high a dosage, lignocaine depresses the central nervous system (CNS) and can cause convulsions. It also depresses myocardial contractility.

Mexiletine has effects similar to those of lignocaine but has the advantage that it is also effective when given by mouth, although this sometimes gives rise to nausea and vomiting. It is useful in patients in whom symptomatic ventricular dysrhythmias continue to occur for more than a few days after a myocardial infarction.

DRUGS USED IN THE TREATMENT OF ASTHMA

Asthma is the reversible reduction of bronchial calibre by a combination of bronchial muscle spasm, bronchial wall oedema and increased secretion of tenacious mucus. Its major symptoms are cough, wheezing and shortness of breath. Drugs that relieve these symptoms do so either by relaxing bronchial smooth muscle (bronchodilators) or by reducing inflammation in the bronchial mucous membrane, e.g. corticosteroids, sodium cromoglycate (cromolyn sodium).

BRONCHODILATORS

The most widely used bronchodilators are β_2-stimulants, which stimulate β_2-adrenoceptors on the surface of bronchial smooth muscle cells, leading to muscle relaxation. Common examples include fenoterol, rimiterol, salbutamol (albuterol) and terbutaline. Although some of these drugs can be given by intravenous injection or by mouth, they are no more effective when given by these routes than by inhalation. In the routine everyday management of asthma, they are most conveniently taken using a metered dose inhaler, but correct technique is important because no more than 10% of an inhaled dose remains adherent to the bronchial lining after inhalation, the rest being swallowed. Young children and elderly people often find a breath-actuated inhaler or a dry powder inhaler easier to use.

All these drugs are equally effective; a single dose produces partial or complete relief of symptoms within 15 minutes, and remains effective for 4–6 hours. In acute severe asthma, salbutamol or terbutaline is usually given via a nebuliser, driven by air or oxygen, over about 15 minutes, at intervals dictated by the severity.

Salmeterol is a long-acting β_2-stimulant that does not relieve symptoms immediately, but which has a sustained bronchodilator effect when taken regularly via a metered dose inhaler. It is currently recommended for asthmatics who have not responded adequately to combined effects of regular treatment with a conventional β_2-stimulant and an inhaled corticosteroid.

Unwanted effects of β_2-stimulants depend largely on the route of administration. Given by mouth, by injection or via a nebuliser, the drugs commonly cause a fine muscle tremor (because of β_2-receptor stimulation in skeletal muscle) and can cause peripheral vasodilation, palpitation and headache (because of β_2-receptor stimulation in arterial smooth muscle). These symptoms seldom occur after using a metered dose inhaler unless dosing is very frequent.

ANTICHOLINERGIC BRONCHODILATORS

Anticholinergic bronchodilators, such as ipratropium bromide and oxitropium bromide, antagonise the effects of cholinergic (parasympathetic) autonomic stimulation of the bronchial smooth muscle, causing relaxation. They are rather less effective than β_2-stimulants in patients with asthma, but in patients with COPD, in whom β_2-stimulants are often poorly tolerated, anticholinergic bronchodilators can be extremely useful. Their effect takes longer to appear (peak effect after about 30 minutes) but lasts longer (6–8 hours), and it is generally unnecessary to take more than two doses in a day. These drugs can also be given by nebuliser and have a useful additive effect when combined with β_2-stimulants in patients with acute severe asthma.

THEOPHYLLINE

Although theophylline is effective as a bronchodilator in the treatment of asthma, it is not altogether clear how it works; it may also have anti-inflammatory and bronchoprotective effects. It is given either by mouth or intravenously, by injection or infusion (combined with ethylenediamine as aminophylline). Unwanted effects include abdominal discomfort, nausea and vomiting, but higher doses can cause cardiac dysrhythmias, convulsions and coma. The dose of theophylline has to be adjusted carefully because the range of dosage that is both effective and safe is narrow. Optimal use of theophylline requires measurement of the plasma concentration of the drug.

ANTI-INFLAMMATORY DRUGS

Corticosteroids are the most effective agents capable of inhibiting the inflammatory reaction that leads to mucosal oedema and mucous secretion. They are given most commonly by inhalation, using a range of devices similar to those used to deliver β_2-stimulants, and are introduced in asthmatics who find it necessary to use a β_2-stimulant inhaler more than once every day. They must be taken regularly to be effective and seldom produce a response when given by this route until 36–48 hours after treatment has begun. Their maximal effect may not be apparent for 1–3 months. Examples include beclomethasone, budesonide (also available for administration via a nebuliser) and fluticasone.

The unwanted effects of inhaled corticosteroids occur chiefly because of deposition of the drug on the lining of the mouth and throat (oral thrush), and on the larynx (hoarseness). Topical delivery of corticosteroids, like that of β_2-stimulants, is relatively inefficient, 90% of a dose being swallowed. At higher dosage enough can be absorbed across the intestinal wall to suppress the production of natural corticosteroid (hydrocortisone) by the adrenal glands, and to adversely affect bone mineralisation. Because of the potentially serious nature of these effects, once the daily dose exceeds 800 µg, the dose should be administered via a large volume spacer device to minimise the amount swallowed.

In acute severe asthma, topical delivery of corticosteroid becomes unreliable and treatment is best given by mouth (prednisolone) or by injection (hydrocortisone) for 7–10 days until recovery is sufficient to allow the topical route to be resumed. Severe asthmatics may need to take prednisolone continually, keeping the dose as low as possible to minimise unwanted effects that include adrenal suppression, osteoporosis, diabetes, hypertension and bruising.

In children with asthma, the introduction of corticosteroids should be delayed, if possible, to minimise any possible effects on growth, although this is much less likely to occur if inhaled corticosteroids are used.

Where asthma is primarily an allergic reaction, sodium cromoglycate or nedocromil sodium may reduce bronchial wall inflammation and reduce the number and severity of attacks. These drugs inhibit the release of inflammatory mediators but are less effective than inhaled corticosteroids. Sodium cromoglycate can also help to reduce exercise-induced asthma if the dose is taken half an hour in advance.

DRUGS USED IN THE TREATMENT OF RESPIRATORY FAILURE

The term respiratory failure implies that the partial pressure of oxygen in the arterial blood (PaO_2) has fallen below 8 kPa, with or without an associated rise in the partial pressure of arterial carbon dioxide ($PaCO_2$) above 6.4 kPa. In patients with advanced COPD, this state of affairs can be permanent, and may not merit any drug treatment in addition to bronchodilators and intermittent courses of antibiotic therapy. However, respiratory effort in such patients is driven by hypoxia. When gas exchange is compromised acutely in patients with COPD, the administration of oxygen therapy removes this drive, respiratory effort is reduced, and $PaCO_2$ rises, causing drowsiness. Assisted ventilation may be necessary, but as an interim measure, or in those in whom assisted ventilation is inadvisable, other measures can be used. Reducing the concentration of inspired oxygen can improve matters, but it may be necessary to give a respiratory stimulant, such as doxapram, by intravenous infusion.

Doxapram stimulates carotid chemoreceptors, increasing their sensitivity to carbon dioxide in the blood. At higher doses it stimulates the respiratory centre in the brain and has a non-specific stimulant effect on the CNS. It may arouse drowsy patients sufficiently to increase respiration, improve co-operation with physiotherapy, and facilitate expectoration of sputum. It is seldom given for more than 24 hours, and may alert patients sufficiently to remove the need for assisted ventilation. The drug's effects should be monitored by repeated arterial blood gas analysis. It causes an increase in heart rate and blood pressure and can also cause dizziness. Higher doses cause hyperactivity and tremor of skeletal muscles other than those involved in respiration, which limit patient tolerance.

ANTIMICROBIAL AGENTS USED IN THE TREATMENT OF ACUTE RESPIRATORY TRACT INFECTION

The management of an acute infection of the respiratory tract depends on its clinical severity and the micro-organism(s) likely to be involved. The type of micro-organism found is influenced by the part of the respiratory tract affected, the pre-existing health of the respiratory tract, and where the infection was acquired. For example, acute bronchitis is usually caused by a virus; in a previously fit adult, secondary bacterial infection is uncommon and seldom requires antibiotic therapy, whereas in a patient with pre-existing COPD, secondary bacterial infection is likely to occur and would usually be treated promptly with an antibiotic. The antibiotic used in the treatment of acute pneumonia acquired in hospital differs from that used for infections acquired outside hospital (Table 5.1).

5

Table 5.1 lists the bacteria likely to be responsible for infections affecting different parts of the respiratory tract in circumstances such as these, and the antibacterial agents that are commonly used against them. Many of these agents are effective when given by mouth. Intravenous therapy is indicated only if the patient is severely ill, frail and elderly, immunocompromised, unconscious, or unable to swallow. Wherever possible, oral treatment is substituted once body temperature falls and clinical recovery is clearly underway. In the treatment of pneumonia, the course of antibiotic is usually continued until at least 3 days after the temperature has fallen to normal. In infective exacerbations of COPD, treatment is usually continued until the sputum is mucoid.

ANTIMICROBIAL AGENTS USED IN THE TREATMENT OF CHRONIC RESPIRATORY TRACT INFECTION

Bronchiectasis (chronic dilation of the bronchi) resulting from childhood infections of the lung or bronchial obstruction, allows bronchial secretions to accumulate in the bronchial tree and leads to frequent secondary bacterial infection. The organisms responsible are those that cause acute respiratory tract infection, but bacterial resistance is more likely to occur and the choice of antibiotic must be based on the results of sputum microscopy and culture and antibiotic sensitivity testing. In most patients a 10 day course of antibiotics combined with postural drainage and appropriate physiotherapy is sufficient.

Cystic fibrosis is an inherited disorder in which impaired excretion of chloride and water across mucosal surfaces results in the presence of thickened mucosal secretions, increased susceptibility to infection and progressive lung damage (bronchiectasis, fibrosis and cyst formation). In childhood, the commonest infecting organism is *Staphylococcus aureus*, whereas in adults *Pseudomonas aeruginosa* increasingly dominates. Although physiotherapy is the cornerstone of management, acute exacerbations must be treated promptly using antibiotics that are not commonly used in less chronic lung infections. Popular regimens include ceftazidime, or azlocillin

Micro-organisms commonly responsible for lower respiratory tract infections	
Bacteria	**Antibacterial agent**
Infective exacerbations of chronic obstructive pulmonary disease (secondary bacterial infection)	
Haemophilus influenzae *Streptococcus pneumoniae*	Amoxicillin, co-amoxiclav (amoxicillin/ clavulanic acid) or parenteral cephalosporins
Community-acquired pneumonia	
Streptococcus pneumoniae	Benzyl penicillin (penicillin G), amoxicillin or erythromycin
Haemophilus influenzae	Amoxicillin or co-amoxiclav (amoxicillin/clavulanic acid)
Staphylococcus aureus	Flucloxacillin
Klebsiella	Gentamicin or cefuroxime
Mycoplasma pneumoniae	Erythromycin or oxytetracycline
Legionella pneumophila	Erythromycin or oxytetracycline
Chlamydia B	Oxytetracycline
Hospital-acquired pneumonia	
Streptococcus pneumoniae	Co-amoxiclav (amoxicillin/clavulanic acid) or cefuroxime
Staphylococcus aureus	Flucloxacillin
Haemophilus influenzae	Co-amoxiclav (amoxicillin/clavulanic acid) or cefuroxime
Klebsiella	Gentamicin or parenteral cephalosporin
Pseudomonas aeruginosa	Gentamicin or parenteral cephalosporin
Anaerobes	Metronidazole

Table 5.1 Micro-organisms commonly responsible for lower respiratory tract infections, and antibacterial agents to which they are usually sensitive.

with gentamicin, but the development of bacterial resistance often necessitates use of aztreonam, ticarcillin/clavulanic acid, piperacillin, imepenem/cilastatin or tobramycin. Courses of treatment should continue for at least 10 days.

MUCOLYTICS

Mucolytics are often prescribed to reduce sputum viscosity and aid expectoration in patients with chronic bronchitis or asthma. Whereas agents such as carbocisteine (carbocysteine) and mecysteine may make sputum less viscid, there is little evidence that they are superior to steam inhalation in aiding expectoration. Dornase-alpha (DNase) is a genetically engineered version of a naturally occurring enzyme that cleaves extracellular DNA and which is present in very high concentration in purulent bronchial secretions. It is administered by jet nebuliser and reduces the viscosity of sputum in patients with cystic fibrosis. In some patients it has led to a worthwhile improvement in lung function. It is extremely expensive.

GENERAL READING

Downie G, Mackenzie J, Williams A. *Pharmacology and drug management for nurses*. Edinburgh: Churchill Livingstone; 1995.
Grahame-Smith DG, Aronson JK. *Oxford textbook of clinical pharmacology and drug therapy*, 2nd ed. Oxford: Oxford University Press; 1992.

Hopkins SJ. *Drugs and pharmacology for nurses*, 11th ed. Edinburgh: Churchill Livingstone; 1992.
Young LY, Koda-Kimble MA. *Applied therapeutics: the clinical use of drugs*, 6th ed. Vancouver: Applied Therapeutics; 1995.

SECTION 2

ADULT MANAGEMENT

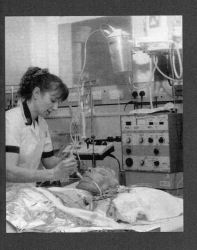

6

A Adams, V Ball, G Brett, J Eddleston, G Russell & L Russell

THE INTENSIVE CARE UNIT

CHAPTER OUTLINE

- Patient selection
- Respiratory failure
- Humidification
- Cardiovascular failure
- Renal failure
- Monitoring systems

- Therapeutic beds
- Resuscitation
- Role of the ICU nurse
- Physiotherapy management
- Role of the dietician

INTRODUCTION

This chapter will cover the Intensive Care Unit (ICU) scenario with a breakdown of the reasons for admission onto the unit, common organ failures and their treatment, methods needed to monitor the patients and resuscitation. The specialist beds employed in ICUs are also covered as they are becoming an important addition to the care of the critically ill patient. Finally, the chapter discusses the roles of clinicians in the management of patients: the doctor, the nurse, the dietician and the physiotherapist, and includes a breakdown of the physiotherapy management of specific disorders met in the ICU.

INTENSIVE CARE

Intensive care has been defined as a 'service for patients with potentially recoverable diseases who can benefit from more detailed observation and treatment than is generally available in the standard wards and departments' (Petros *et al.*, 1995). Unfortunately this definition is too broad for clinical practice and includes both high dependency care and intensive care.

The provision of intensive care and high dependency care requires quite different resources. Human and financial resources, the nature and complexity of equipment required and the intensity and type of care provided are quite different in the two environments. Only intensive care will be discussed here.

Intensive care medicine consumes a large fraction of healthcare resources. It is estimated that 1–2% of the hospital budget in the UK (Bion, 1994) is spent treating critically ill patients. It is therefore of utmost importance that clinicians select those patients who are most likely to survive.

Prognostic scoring systems capable of predicting mortality have become an integral part of critical care practice and play an important role in ICU-based research by facilitating patient stratification based on objective evaluation of illness severity at time of presentation and over the initial hours following commencement of therapy. None is sensitive enough to predict a particular outcome for a particular patient. The Acute Physiology and Chronic Health Evaluation (APACHE) scoring system was the first such system (Table 6.1).

The launch of APACHE in 1981 was a landmark since it represented the first time that a quantitative evaluation of severity of disease had been introduced into the intensive care environment. The system was cumbersome to apply and was designed using a subjective method to weight several variables determined by a panel of experts to be the most important. The variables included were

Acute Physiology and Chronic Health Evaluation (APACHE) II scoring system (score=A+B+C)
A **Clinical variable (detection of variance from normal)** Temperature Mean arterial pressure Heart rate Respiratory rate Oxygenation with respect to concentration of inspired oxygen Arterial pH Serum sodium Serum potassium Serum creatinine (double score if in acute renal failure) Haematocrit White blood cell count Glasgow Coma Score Serum bicarbonate A score of 0–4 is given to each variable (these sums are additive)
B **Age of patient** <44   0 points 45–54   2 points 55–64   3 points 65–74   5 points >75   6 points
C **Chronic health points** A patient must have severe organ insufficiency to gain any points in this category. Patients score 2 points for elective surgery and 5 points for a non-operative condition or emergency surgery.

Table 6.1 Acute Physiology and Chronic Health Evaluation (APACHE) II scoring system.

temperature, heart rate, mean arterial blood pressure, plasma sodium, potassium, creatinine, arterial pH, partial pressure of arterial oxygen (PaO_2) with reference to the inspired oxygen concentration, serum bicarbonate, haematocrit and white blood cell count. A score of 0–4 is attributed to each variable (abnormally low and high results score, respectively). In addition the age of the patient, abnormal Glasgow Coma Score (GCS—a scoring of eye opening, best verbal response and best motor response, 3 being minimum and 15 maximum), and chronic health status of the patient are weighted. The higher the score the greater is the severity of the illness.

In 1984, Le Gall *et al.* showed that an abbreviated version of the original APACHE score performed with similar effectiveness. This system, known as the Simplified Acute Physiology Score (SAPS) has been widely used, especially in France and many other European countries. As is true with the APACHE system, the values of the variables chosen to compute the score reflect the worst level in the first 24 hours in the ICU. In 1985 a new version of APACHE, known as APACHE II, was published. This addition required the selection of a primary diagnosis. The APACHE II system used a logistic regression equation to compute the

probability of death for each patient. Since then APACHE II has been the most widely used system in the world.

Using a completely different approach based on the selection of the most influential variables by logistic regression, Teres developed a model in 1982 for estimating the probability of mortality for ICU patients. This model eventually evolved into the Mortality Probability Model (MPM) in 1985, and was refined in 1988. The system was built on three unique time periods—on admission, at 24 hours and again at 48 hours after entry onto the ICU.

Recently new versions of the three systems have been released (APACHE III, SAPS II and MPM II), each offering real improvement, but none stands out as being clearly superior (Dinh-Xuan *et al.*, 1995).

Distinction must be made between these predictive prognostic scoring systems for a heterogeneous group of patients and a score that is capable of predicting outcome for a particular patient. ICU outcome is rarely a direct result of the evolution of the disease that precipitated admission. Rather, the most common cause of ICU morbidity and mortality is the development of progressive physiological dysfunction in organ systems remote from the site of the primary disease process, a phenomenon widely termed the multiple organ dysfunction syndrome. Several such scoring systems have now been developed, providing an objective measure of the severity of organ dysfunction at the time of ICU admission, quantifying any subsequent deterioration over the course of the individual patient's ICU stay and correlating the progressive score with mortality. The most recent score proposed was that described by Marshall *et al.* in 1995 (Table 6.2). Dysfunction in the respiratory system (PaO_2/FiO_2 ratio), renal system (serum creatinine μmol/litre), hepatic system (serum bilirubin μmol/litre), cardiovascular system (blood pressure and heart rate), haematological (platelet count) and central nervous systems (CNS; GCS) was graded and scored. This group has succeeded, in their own unit, to correlate a particular score to mortality. They have verified its accuracy in over 700 patients and although not perfect it is a major step forward in quantifying mortality with a deterioration in organ function.

RESPIRATORY FAILURE

Critical illness always impacts on the function of the respiratory system. Consequently, respiratory insufficiency is the most common reason for requesting advice from an intensive care clinician. More often than not, as expected, cardiovascular instability is also apparent. Critical care medicine has evolved over the past two decades into a speciality with extensive multidisciplinary skills. The 'old' vision of the role of the ICU being solely to provide ventilatory support for critically ill patients certainly is no longer an accurate representation of its functions.

DEFINITION

Hypoxia has historically been defined as a condition characterised by the clinical signs of cyanosis. As the use of arterial blood gases became widespread, hypoxia came to signify a condition of low PaO_2. Traditionally, respiratory failure has been subdivided into two types:

- Type I: PaO_2 <60 mmHg (8 kPa), $PaCO_2$ normal or low.
- Type II: PaO_2 <60 mmHg (8 kPa), $PaCO_2$ >55 mmHg (7.2 kPa).

Patients with type II respiratory failure are typified as the so-called blue bloaters. This very small subset of patients represents the only group in whom injudicious application of oxygen therapy results in dangerously elevated hypercarbia. Historically, this increase in $PaCO_2$ has been attributed to a blunted or absent hypoxic respiratory drive. Recent work has cast doubt on this theory and suggested that changes in physiological dead space are sufficient to account for the observed hypercarbia (Gauger *et al.*, 1996).

Requests for intensive care facilities for these patients are rare. Often acute exacerbations of their respiratory function are a direct result of an acute infective event, and provision of invasive respiratory support for these patients is then questionable.

Patients with type I respiratory failure, on the other hand, form the overwhelming population in whom supplemental oxygen therapy and respiratory support are both indicated and more often than not appropriate. It is not uncommon for these patients to develop significant hypercarbia before the introduction of ventilatory support, and this clinical scenario must be differentiated from that of patients with chronic obstructive pulmonary disease (COPD) and a hypoxic respiratory drive. Exhaustion is the commonest reason for hypercarbia in this latter population, and as such is a late and ominous finding.

Inadequate gas exchange can result from a multitude of causes, ranging from CNS depression (head injury, drug

The Multiple Organ Dysfunction Score					
Organ system	0	1	2	3	4
Respiratory (PaO_2/FiO_2 ratio)	>300	226-300	151-225	76-150	<75
Renal (serum creatinine) μmol/litre	<100	101-200	201-350	351-500	>500
Hepatic (serum bilirubin) μmol/litre	<20	21-60	61-120	121-240	>240
Cardiovascular (PAR)	<10	10.1-15.0	15.1-20.0	20.1-30.0	>30.0
Haematological (platelet count $\times 10^9$/litre)	>120	81-120	51-80	21-50	<20
CNS (Glasgow Coma Score)	15	13-14	10-12	7-9	<6

Cumulative score is additive from the six organ systems, and related to mortality.
PAR, pressure adjusted rate, i.e. heart rate × mean blood pressure/central venous pressure.

Table 6.2 **The Multiple Organ Dysfunction Score.**

overdose) through neuromuscular disorders (myasthenia gravis, Guillain–Barré, other myopathies/neuropathies) and musculoskeletal malfunction (flail chest, ruptured diaphragm) to direct pulmonary pathology (infective process, exacerbation of asthma, pneumonitis, pulmonary embolism, acute lung injury, cardiac induced pulmonary oedema). It is important to recognise impending problems early so that evasive action can be instituted to minimise complications.

ACUTE LUNG INJURY

In 1967, Ashbaugh and colleagues reported a series of 12 patients with acute onset of tachypnoea, hypoxia, decreased respiratory system compliance, and diffuse pulmonary infiltrates on chest X-ray. Four years later this constellation of signs and symptoms was officially called the adult respiratory distress syndrome (ARDS).

Since that time the defining features of ARDS have evolved, and although there is no uniformly accepted clinical definition there is sufficient agreement among clinicians in the UK that certain criteria must be met to make the diagnosis of ARDS (Baum *et al.*, 1989). These criteria are:

HYPOXIA
Defined as a PaO_2/FiO_2 of <200 (regardless of positive end-expiratory pressure level). For example, for a patient with a PaO_2 of 200 mmHg receiving 100% oxygen, the score in this instance would be 200.

CHEST RADIOGRAPH
Bilateral diffuse infiltration seen on frontal chest X-ray.

PULMONARY ARTERY OCCLUSION PRESSURE
Pulmonary–capillary wedge pressure (PCWP) of <18 mmHg. The presence of a pulmonary artery flotation catheter (Figure 6.1) is essential not only for diagnosis but also for patient management to ensure that there is no cardiac component to the hypoxia (cardiac failure and hypotension both influence oxygenation).

AT RISK DIAGNOSIS
There are certain patients who have a particularly high chance of developing ARDS. These patients usually fall into one of a number of categories including those with sepsis, pancreatitis, inflammatory bowel disease, abdominal trauma, pulmonary aspiration of gastric contents, chest trauma (e.g. fractured ribs), fat embolism from long bone fractures, head injury, poisoning, high volume blood product transfusion and chemotherapy.

The prevalence of patients with ARDS in any ICU will depend to a certain extent on the medical and surgical sub-specialities available within the hospital. Overall figures within the UK are scant, but in the USA it is estimated that 150 000 patients are affected annually (Baum *et al.*, 1989). Mortality rates from ARDS have decreased somewhat over the past two decades but still remain near 40%. Intractable hypoxia, despite modern ventilatory techniques and adjuvant therapy such as inhaled nitric oxide, accounts for only 20% of the deaths. By far the commonest cause of death is multiple organ failure and sepsis. This reinforces the point that ARDS is the pulmonary manifestation of a systemic illness.

There is still much uncertainty as to the exact sequence of events and their relative importance in the development and maintenance of the inflammatory response in ARDS. However, it is clear that the body's own cellular inflammatory cascade response is of paramount importance. Much time, effort and considerable financial resources have been deployed searching for a new therapeutic treatment for ARDS, all to no avail. Agents capable of blocking selective parts of the systemic inflammatory response have been tried. Refinements of conventional ventilatory techniques would also appear unlikely to offer significant impact on outcome. The problems associated with both volutrauma and barotrauma (extra-alveolar air) and oxygen toxicity are still of immense practical importance in clinical practice.

MANAGEMENT OF RESPIRATORY FAILURE

The management of respiratory failure can be broadly divided into non-invasive and invasive support.

NON-INVASIVE SUPPORT
Face Mask
The simplest technique of increasing inspired oxygen concentration is to use a face mask. Facemasks are divided into variable and fixed performance devices.

Variable performance masks
The actual inspired oxygen concentration achieved with a variable performance device depends on the flow rate of oxygen, the presence of holes in the side of the mask, and the breathing pattern of the patient. It is important to realise that the holes in the side of the mask are designed to entrain air, thus reducing the oxygen concentration delivered to the patient. This is necessary because the patient's peak inspiratory flow rate (about 30 litres/min in this population) is much greater than the oxygen delivery rate, which is in the region of 4–10 litres/min. The actual oxygen concentration achieved is heavily dependent on the patient's breathing pattern.

Fixed performance devices
In their simplest form, oxygen passes through a 'venturi' which entrains a volume of air 10 times greater than the amount of oxygen supplied. Each mask has a specific entrainment ratio, thereby ensuring that a predictable concentration of oxygen reaches the patient. These devices can produce concentrations up to 60% but are more commonly used, in practice, to supply oxygen at lower concentrations, such as 28%, to patients with COPD.

High Flow Therapy

Devices which accurately mix oxygen and air are being increasingly used for supplemental oxygen. They require piped oxygen and air supplies which are available in ITUs and high dependency units (HDUs). An oxygen electrode measures the inspired oxygen concentration and combined air/oxygen flows of up to 50 litres/min are used. The provision of this particularly large flow rate necessitates the presence of a reservoir bag within the circuit.

Continuous Positive Airway Pressure (CPAP)

This mode of support permits the preservation of a pre-selected positive pressure to be present throughout the respiratory cycle. Continuous positive airway pressure (CPAP) is determined by the choice of valve (usually 2.5–10 cmH$_2$O). Flow rates up to 50 litres/min can be generated with the new high flow circuits. CPAP can be applied either through the use of a tight fitting face mask (Figure 6.2) or nose mask, or in conjunction with an endotracheal tube or tracheostomy. The use of CPAP and biphasic positive airway pressure (BiPAP) in the early stages of respiratory failure may obviate the patient requiring formal intubation and ventilation, and for the longer stay ITU patient this latter application used in conjunction with pressure support in the initial stages of the weaning process is invariably an essential part of the transition from full mechanical ventilation to no ventilatory support.

CPAP increases lung surface area for gaseous exchange by increasing the lung volume at the end of expiration (functional residual capacity, FRC) and reducing atelectasis (lung collapse at alveolar level), thereby improving oxygenation by reducing ventilation/perfusion (V/Q mismatch and intrapulmonary shunting). In addition, chest wall and pulmonary compliance may improve such that the work of breathing will be diminished.

Unfortunately, CPAP can be unsuccessful in preventing the requirement for mechanical ventilation in some patients. The reasons for this can be split into technical failures, inability of the circuit to provide adequate inspiratory flow rates to match the patient's demand, thereby increasing the work of breathing, and progressive deterioration in pulmonary pathology.

Because of the tight fitting nature of the masks, pressure areas do develop in some patients, particularly over the bridge of the nose. In addition, for a group of patients the experience of a CPAP mask can be frightening due to the claustrophobic sensation invoked.

Non-Invasive Positive Pressure Ventilation

There is great interest in this field of assisted ventilation, particularly for the large group of patients who are admitted annually with exacerbation of COPD. Conventional ventilation of these patients is fraught with pitfalls. Instead attention has focused on techniques of non-invasive ventilation using either positive pressure delivered by a nose mask or face mask, or negative pressure cuirass (Hayek ventilator).

Positive Pressure Ventilation

The simplest form of this mode of ventilation is the use of the Bird Corporation Mark 8 respirator. It is patient triggered and will deliver a positive pressure breath. A nebuliser for inhalational therapy is incorporated.

Mouth pieces are routinely used in practice instead of masks. This form of ventilation necessitates full co-operation from the patient in terms of both the level of consciousness and also the physical strength and ability to initiate the breath. In reality this means that there must be an intact neuromuscular pathway, intact and mobile rib cage, and the absence of a myopathy. Its popularity has largely waned. This has occurred because it has been surpassed by the use of continuous modes of non-invasive respiratory support.

Another more recently introduced form of positive pressure non-invasive ventilation is BiPAP. This form of ventilation, as the name suggests, will provide bi-phasic positive pressure in the airway throughout the ventilatory cycle. Nose or face masks can be used. The clinician selects the pressure support for inspiration and the positive end-expiratory pressure (PEEP). The device is flow triggered by the patient. In comparison with CPAP, the

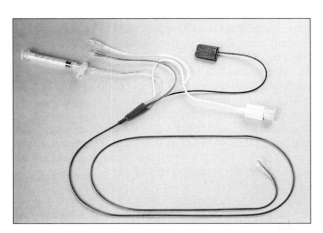

Figure 6.1 Pulmonary artery flotation catheter.

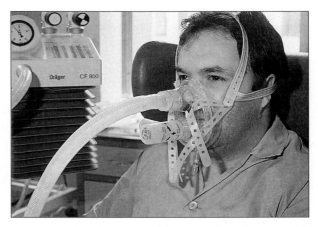

Figure 6.2 Continuous positive pressure airway mask.

resistance to ventilation is much reduced and hence patient acceptance is much higher.

Improvements in mask texture and design have reduced the incidence of pressure sores.

Hayek Oscillator

The Hayek oscillator (Figure 6.3) consists of a plastic cuirass (available in different sizes) which connects via wide bore tubing to a power unit consisting of two pumps—a vacuum pump which creates a baseline negative pressure with a second pump superimposing oscillating pressures (Hardinge *et al.*, 1995; Petros *et al.*, 1995). There are four variables which can be altered during the use of the machine: frequency of oscillation, ratio of inspiratory to expiratory time, and inspiratory and expiratory pressures. By altering these variables different mean negative chamber pressures and different spans of pressure can be created (where span is the difference between maximum inspiratory and maximum expiratory pressure). Expiration is actively controlled and does not rely on passive lung recoil.

Frequency of oscillations currently employed range from 30 per minute (0.5 Hz) to >120 per minute (>2 Hz). The principle of ventilation is dependent on the selected frequency. Below 2 Hz the oscillator acts as a conventional ventilator giving maximal ventilation at 0.25–0.5 Hz and a span of 30–40 cmH$_2$O. However, as the frequency approaches 2 Hz the ventilator behaves more like a high frequency oscillator, presumably achieving oxygenation by molecular diffusion. Clearance of mucus has also been shown to be enhanced at higher frequencies such as 3–17 Hz, possible due to a reduction in sputum viscosity and enhancement of ciliary clearance. This has been confirmed by our own experience when using 5 Hz oscillations.

The Hayek oscillator also significantly increases FRC at increasing negative extrathoracic pressures. When used in synchrony with conventional positive pressure ventilation it may be possible to reduce the peak inspiratory pressure and PEEP, both of which have been implicated in causing lung parenchymal damage. Its role in patients with ARDS is still to be established.

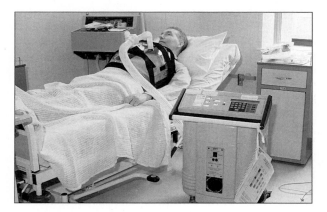

Figure 6.3 Hayek oscillator.

INVASIVE SUPPORT (ARTIFICIAL VENTILATION)

The initiation of mechanical intermittent positive pressure ventilation first requires the patient to be intubated either with an endotracheal tube or a tracheostomy tube, if oral intubation is anticipated to be impossible. The use of conscious intubation with a fibreoptic laryngoscope would be normal practice now if difficulty is anticipated. Tracheostomies are normally reserved for latter placement in those patients in whom weaning from ventilation is anticipated to be protracted and difficult.

It is conventional practice within the UK that patients are intubated unconscious. Although obviously humane, this adds to the potential risks associated with the procedure. It is therefore essential that every member of the team attending the patient is well versed in his or her role. The sedative drugs may precipitate profound hypotension, intubation will almost certainly be difficult, and the larynx may be obscured from view by sputum, oedema, structural pathology or gastric contents which have passively regurgitated into the oropharynx. Ventilation is initiated manually at first and then swiftly changed to mechanical.

The earliest devices for artificial ventilation were designed for apnoeic patients. Thus the frequency of artificial ventilation was rigidly controlled at a pre-set level, and the ventilators were unable to adapt to any spontaneous respiratory activity. This tended to discourage weaning. Also, patients who were not apnoeic frequently attempted to inhale against closed inspiratory valves, causing distress and creating a subatmospheric pressure that increased the gastro-oesophageal pressure gradient, and sometimes caused regurgitation. However, over four decades ventilators and their modes of ventilation have evolved to match patients' individual requirements such that the morbidity of ventilation is minimised.

The potential for positive pressure breaths to injure the lungs has long been appreciated. The best known form of injury occurs when positive pressure breaths grossly overinflate the lungs and result in pneumothorax, pneumomediastinum, subcutaneous emphysema, and other forms of 'volutrauma' or 'barotrauma'. The mechanism for this type of injury is thought to be actual alveolar rupture into the perivascular space with subsequent dissection of air into the mediastinum, pleura and other locations. The risk of stretch injury probably begins to rise when transalveolar pressure exceeds the normal maximum of 30–40 cmH$_2$O. Lung injury is initially characterised by alveolar–capillary inflammation. At higher transalveolar pressure, lung injury is manifest by alveolar rupture. Of note is that this injury may be most pronounced in previously healthy lung units. This is because diffuse lung injury is often quite heterogeneous, i.e. certain lung units are severely injured and atelectatic while other units remain relatively normal. Thus positive pressure ventilation delivered to the airways may only minimally inflate abnormal units but may grossly overdistend and consequently injure the healthier units. Conventional mechanical ventilation goals, to aggressively recruit and ventilate abnormal lung units with distending pressures in excess of 30–40 cmH$_2$O, therefore, may run the risk of overdistending (stretching) and injuring the remaining healthier units.

POSITIVE END EXPIRATORY PRESSURE (PEEP)

PEEP maintains above atmospheric pressure at the end of expiration and increases FRC. In some pulmonary pathologies, FRC is reduced causing refractory hypoxaemia due to intrapulmonary shunting, and therefore PEEP is effective in the management of these conditions. Complications associated with the use of PEEP include overdistention of the alveoli resulting in increased intrapleural pressures that may decrease venous return and therefore cardiac output.

LUNG PROTECTIVE VENTILATORY STRATEGIES

Minimising PEEP

Since PEEP is the baseline pressure, it determines baseline alveolar volume. Minimising PEEP, however, requires trade-offs. Alveoli that do not collapse provide better gas exchange and thus a lower FiO$_2$ requirement. High concentrations of oxygen in neonates have been implicated in the development of retinal (retrolental fibroplasia) and pulmonary (bronchopulmonary dysplasia) complications. In adults it has been much more difficult to separate the toxic effects of oxygen from the initial pulmonary pathology.

Appropriate PEEP is probably in the 5–15 cmH$_2$O range. Prolonging the inspiratory time can also be used as an alternative to additional PEEP if mechanical recruitment seems optimal. A longer inspiratory time has two effects. First, there is a longer mixing period and exposure of capillaries to gas filled alveoli. A second effect is the prevention of complete lung emptying because of consequently shorter expiratory times. This is the phenomenon of air trapping and produces 'intrinsic' PEEP . It is well known that intrinsic PEEP functions much like applied PEEP in its effects on FRC and lung volumes and in its negative effect on cardiac performance. Using longer inspiratory times must therefore be done with caution and careful monitoring of air trapping.

Minimising Tidal Volume (V_T)

The second component of alveolar distension is tidal distension. Historically, delivered tidal volumes (V_T) were often recommended to be as high as 15–20 ml/kg. This, however, was a reflection of practice in anaesthesia before the development of PEEP when large tidal volumes were required to overcome atelectasis. Lowering V_T to 6–8 ml/kg will clearly reduce alveolar pressures and distension. Alveolar ventilation can be maintained up to a point by increasing the respiratory frequency. Ultimately, however, rapid rates cannot compensate for the loss of V_T. Under these circumstances, alveolar ventilation and arterial pH will fall, and arterial PCO$_2$ will rise. This hypercapnia is often referred to as 'permissive hypercapnia' and pH with this strategy has been reported to fall below 7.0. The effects of normoxic hypercapnia under these circumstances are only beginning to be understood. In general, however, humans seem to tolerate an arterial pH of 7.15 and PaCO$_2$ of 10.33 kPa quite well. The rate at which the PaCO$_2$ is allowed to rise should probably be <1.33 mmHg/h so as to permit the intracellular pH to adjust. The patient's respiratory drive will require to be suppressed and it is our experience that sedation needs are increased and the introduction of a muscle relaxant is almost always required.

Patient Compliance with Ventilation

The degree of sedation that a patient requires to obtain maximal ventilatory performance and minimal pressure/V_T swings depends on the mode of ventilation and individual patient characteristics. In the weaning modes the requirement for sedative drugs reduces and ultimately disappears but when full ventilation is required a fine balance must be struck between sedation and suppression of respiratory drive and cough reflex. A balanced approach is always better. In addition there is a group of patients in whom muscle relaxant drugs are required. This is because the underlying pathology dictates, e.g. patients with head injuries in whom management of intracranial pressure (ICP) necessitates the abolition of any further increases in venous pressure, for instance by coughing or oxygenation, is so precarious that the provision of muscle relaxation may aid pulmonary compliance.

MODES OF VENTILATION

There are a variety of ventilators available nationally and the methods of ventilation are either volume cycled or pressure cycled. The former cycle is achieved by pre-setting the patient's V_T, and the latter is achieved by altering the V_T to maintain a pre-set airway pressure. The airway pressure scale measures the resistance offered to the inspired volume of oxygen, and normally this value is between 20 and 30 cmH$_2$O. Situations that raise the airway pressure suggest obstruction to the incoming flow, e.g. ventilator tube kinking, patient coughing against the inspiratory cycle of the ventilator, patient biting the endotracheal tube, bronchospasm, major airways obstruction and stiff lungs. Situations that lower the airway pressure include disconnection of the patient from the ventilator, loss of volume through a leaking endotracheal tube cuff, and air escaping through a chest drain in the situation of a bronchopleural fistula. The latter situation is ideal for pressure-cycled ventilation as the V_T will alter to accommodate the air leak. Patients who are at risk of barotrauma, e.g. pneumothorax because of poor lung compliance, are also good candidates for pressure-cycled ventilation. Pressure-controlled ventilation is discussed later.

Controlled Mandatory Ventilation

Controlled mandatory ventilation (CMV) is not generally used because there is no allowance for the patient to interact with the ventilator. A pre-set V_T is delivered a pre-determined number of times per minute. Only patients who are electively paralysed and sedated are on CMV.

Intermittent Mandatory Ventilation

In intermittent mandatory ventilation (IMV), the patient receives a pre-set number of breaths from the ventilator but can still initiate and receive additional breaths if they wish. IMV was an enormous advance in the 1970s but has been surpassed by synchronised IMV (SIMV).

Synchronised Intermittent Mandatory Ventilation (SIMV)

The goal of SIMV is to synchronise the mandatory breaths from the ventilator with respiratory effort from the patient. The volume of each mandatory breath is identical but the inspiratory pressure required to achieve each breath will vary. This mode is classified as flow limited, volume cycled. The variation in inspiratory peak airways pressure can on occasion produce deleteriously high alveolar pressures, and hence may jeopardise alveolar integrity. There are many clinicians who now feel that this mode of ventilation may well not be ideal for patients with worsening respiratory failure.

If the patient fails to trigger the mandatory breath in a pre-determined period, the ventilator delivers its mandatory breath of its own accord. It is customary to add inspiratory pressure support to the non-mandatory breaths which the patient initiates. This is essential in the majority of patients to ensure an acceptable volume for each breath. Without such support the V_T would be variable, very small, and such a respiratory pattern would ultimately be counterproductive because the work of breathing would be excessive. Weaning from mechanical support would be both time and financially consuming, and particularly unpleasant for the patient. Such pressure support for non-mandatory breaths is essential for all modes of ventilation where the patient has the ability to trigger a breath.

A pressure augmented breath will be terminated when the pre-set inspiratory pressure 'target' is achieved. This 'target' is progressively reduced as weaning from mechanical ventilation proceeds until ultimately it is unnecessary. In addition, as a safety feature, a breath will be terminated if the ventilator detects expiratory effort by the patient.

Initiation of both a mandatory- and pressure-supported breath usually relies on the detection by the ventilator of a pressure drop within the breathing circuit. Consequently there will be a time delay before gas flow is available to the patient. In an attempt to overcome this time delay, improve patient comfort, reduce work of breathing and, ultimately hopefully, hasten the weaning process, certain manufacturers have incorporated in addition the 'flow by' system into such modes of ventilation. A constant pre-selected flow of gas is delivered to the circuit during the expiratory phase. Access to this reservoir of gas requires not a pressure change within the circuit but instead the detection of flow.

Pressure-Controlled Ventilation

The concept of pressure-controlled ventilation (PCV) encompasses the vision of a pressure-controlled rather than volume pre-set breath (Rappaport *et al.*, 1994). Consequently the volume of each breath depends on the pre-set pressure limit and the patient's pulmonary compliance at that time, all other things being equal. This mode of ventilation is also characterised by having an 'adjustable' flow. It is this adjusting flow feature of the pressure-limited breath that probably accounts for the improved patient–ventilator synchrony and comfort reported.

It is postulated that the initial rapid and then decelerating flow pattern associated with PCV may mix and distribute gas differently from a constant flow pattern (as is found in volume-cycled ventilation). In addition, the decelerating flow would appear to result in a 'square' airway pressure pattern. In practice, a lower peak airway pressure for the same V_T seems to occur with this mode of ventilation compared with constant flow volume-cycled ventilation.

In practice it must be noted that if there is a sudden deterioration in pulmonary compliance, e.g. after the development of a pneumothorax or collapse of one lobe of the lung, there will be an instantaneous reduction in V_T and this will have serious implications for oxygenation and arterial pH.

Much research into PCV is being done but the initial reports are favourable in patients with severe lung injury, a most difficult group to treat and in whom the mortality rate approaches 40%.

High Frequency Ventilation

There are three different types of high frequency ventilation (HFV) (Rouby, 1990): high frequency oscillation (HFO), high frequency positive pressure ventilation (HFPPV) and high frequency jet ventilation (HFJV). HFO has been extensively studied by physiologists but still remains an experimental method of mechanical ventilation. Up to now, only HFPPV and HFJV have received defined clinical applications.

HFPPV and HFJV, which are very similar, deliver small V_T (between 1 and 5 ml/kg) at high frequencies (between 60 and 400/min) and require a specific ventilator characterised by a reduced internal volume and non-compliant ventilatory circuits. The commonest mode is HFJV.

Circuit for HFJV

Air and oxygen are supplied to the jet ventilator under a high pressure (4 × atmospheric pressure) and are mixed in a blender where there is a pressure drop of about 1 atmosphere. Therefore, the driving pressure of gases arriving at the jet ventilator is around three atmospheres. The gases are then pulsed, and as they pass through the ventilator there is further pressure reduction such that the operating driving pressure of the gas reaching the patient is often in the region of 1.5 atmospheres. Because most of the injection systems accelerate gases and produce gas entrainment, the V_T delivered to the patient is equal to the jet gas volume delivered by the ventilator plus the entrained volume. The 'entrainment' system is usually a high flow circuit with the appropriate PEEP valve in place. Expiration is passive. Consequently a contraindication to the use of HFJV would be air flow obstruction such as in status asthmaticus.

Measurement of minute ventilation is impossible and $PaCO_2$ is determined largely by driving pressure, entrainment volume, inspiratory time (%) and, to a much smaller extent, the respiratory frequency. It is claimed that this mode of ventilation should reduce peak airway pressures compared with conventional volume-cycled ventilation, thereby producing greater cardiovascular stability and lowering the risk of barotrauma. This has not been our own experience of the technique in patients with severe lung injury. It is, however, postulated to have a place in patients with bronchopleural fistulae where conventional ventilation may aggravate the leak through the fistula.

Humidification of the gases delivered to the patient, both through the jet and also from the entrainment circuit, is essential.

Biphasic Positive Airway Pressure (BiPAP)

One problem associated with PCV is that the flow valve on the ventilator remains closed at certain times in the ventilatory cycle, rendering spontaneous respiratory effort impossible. BiPAP (Baum *et al.*, 1989) is similar to PCV in that the ventilator alternates between a low pressure (PEEP) and a high pressure (inspiratory pressure). However, BiPAP allows unrestricted spontaneous breathing at any time in the respiratory cycle. This improves patient tolerance, especially when inverse inspiratory:expiratory ratios are being used, and means that less sedation should be required.

If supplementary spontaneous breaths are needed with pressure support this is possible but the patient must be placed in the BiPAP–SIMV mode to gain access to the pressure support facility.

NEW STRATEGIES FOR RESPIRATORY FAILURE

POSTURE MANIPULATION

Manipulation of posture may be of benefit to patients with 'critical' oxygenation secondary to severe lung injury. The explanation for an improvement in oxygenation may reside in part in alveolar recruitment of previously atelectic but now healthy lung (Kirkpatrick *et al.*, 1996). The change in posture can be particularly fraught, and great care should be taken to secure all intravenous/intra-arterial cannulae, the endotracheal/tracheostomy tube, chest drains, urinary catheters, and any other invasive monitoring.

EXTRACORPOREAL MEMBRANE OXYGENATION (ECMO)

See Chapter 20.

INTRAVASCULAR OXYGENATION (IVOX)

The intravascular oxygenator is a membrane oxygenator composed of multiple elongated hollow fibres that has to be implanted by surgical venotomy in the venae cavae (Sim and Evans, 1993). Design modifications, including a siliconised, heparin bonded, surface fibre coating, have reduced the systemic anticoagulation requirement and increased the functional longevity of a single device to 4 weeks. As presently configured, the performance of intravascular oxygenators has been disappointing, providing at best one-third to one-half of basal gas exchange requirements, with unpredictable improvements in oxygenation.

Data must be interpreted with caution as few centres have experience with large series of patients. Ultimately, however, IVOX may find applications beyond severe lung injury, for example, in patients with thoracic trauma, and post-surgery, by reducing stress on friable tissue and suture lines.

NITRIC OXIDE (NO) INHALATION

Pulmonary hypertension may complicate various chronic and acute pulmonary disorders, including ARDS. The treatment of pulmonary hypertension, irrespective of its aetiology, has always represented a formidable challenge for clinicians, the main difficulties stemming from the fact that no pulmonary vasodilator is actually devoid of systemic side effects. The 'ideal' pulmonary vasodilator must therefore be selective, having activity restricted to the pulmonary circulation. Knowing that nitric oxide (NO) is rapidly inactivated by haemoglobin, it has been hypothesised that NO, given by inhalation, could be such a selective pulmonary vasodilator (Dinh-Xuan *et al.*, 1995). After entering the airways, inhaled NO primarily reaches the pulmonary vascular smooth muscle through diffusion from alveolar spaces, thereby causing pulmonary vasodilation.

In practice, the theory has held (Dinh-Xuan *et al.*, 1995). In addition, inhaled NO has a unique ability to improve gas exchange, hence arterial oxygenation in both adults with ARDS and newborn babies with refractory hypoxaemia (Dinh-Xuan *et al.*, 1995). Thus, unlike infused prostacyclin, which dilates pulmonary vessels of ventilated as well as non-ventilated lung units, inhaled NO preferentially induces vasodilation only in the ventilated units (Dinh-Xuan *et al.*, 1995). As a result, ventilation/perfusion mismatching is reduced as shown by a decrease in intrapulmonary shunting, and gas exchange is improved as depicted by an increase in PaO_2/FiO_2.

The use of inhaled NO also improves right ventricular function in patients with ARDS (Dinh-Xuan *et al.*, 1995).

Inhaled NO undoubtedly has led to a recent, and dramatic, breakthrough in the way in which patients with ARDS are managed; at least when considering its specific and beneficial effects on pulmonary haemodynamics and gas exchange. However, as with other therapeutic advances, the outcome from large ongoing multicentre controlled trials is still awaited before inhaled NO can become universally accepted.

LIPOSOMAL PROSTAGLANDIN E₁ (PGE₁)

Acute inflammatory lung disease, i.e. ARDS, is characterised by increased pulmonary vascular permeability and interstitial oedema, accompanied by massive neutrophil infiltration into the lungs. Prostaglandin E_1 (PGE_1) can block platelet aggregation, down-regulate neutrophil-mediated inflammatory responses, and produce vasodilation. Unfortunately, no tangible clinical benefit has been identified from PGE$_1$ in patients with ARDS. Liposomal PGE$_1$ may, however, have something to offer as an adjuvant therapy in ARDS (Abraham *et al.*, 1996). The liposomal preparation differs by producing a greater inhibition of neutrophil activation and adhesion than that exhibited by free PGE$_1$. In addition, the liposomal product appears to permit higher doses of PGE$_1$ than is possible with the free drug, without being limited by clinically important hypotension.

This product certainly requires extensive evaluation but preliminary reports are suggestive of it having a possible adjuvant role to play in the management of patients with ARDS. Once again the role of the neutrophil in the pathophysiology of ARDS is in the limelight.

LIQUID VENTILATION WITH PERFLUROCARBON

In 1966, Clarke and Gollan demonstrated the adequacy of gas exchange in mice spontaneously breathing perfluorocarbon liquid. It has taken three decades for the technology to be attempted in humans, or to be more precise in children.

Perflurocarbons are unique, inert and colourless fluids that have the appearance and consistency of water. They are a remarkable class of compound, having one-quarter the surface tension, 16 times the oxygen solubility and three times the carbon dioxide solubility of water (Gauger *et al.*, 1996). The perflurocarbon currently under evaluation in humans (perflubron) is minimally absorbed across the alveolus and is eliminated from the lungs by evaporation. Liquid ventilation with perfluorocarbon has generally been performed by one of two techniques:

- 'Total' liquid ventilation, in which the lungs are completely filled with perfluorocarbon and ventilated using a 'liquid' ventilator with tidal volumes consisting entirely of the liquid.
- 'Partial' liquid ventilation, which requires partial filling of the lungs with perfluorocarbon and ventilation with gas tidal volumes using a conventional gas mechanical ventilator.

A 'liquid' ventilator appropriate for clinical use is not yet available.

The reports of the use of this technology describe it as in its infancy (Gauger *et al.*, 1996) and we must wait to see if there is a place for this supportive therapy in our treatment options for patients with severe intractable hypoxia.

ARTIFICIAL SURFACTANT

Despite the fact that surfactant has an established role in the infant respiratory distress syndrome, its use in adults with acute lung injury, i.e. ARDS, has so far been inconclusive. The benefits of surfactant therapy are theoretically substantial, particularly if introduced early in the course of the disease.

HUMIDIFICATION

Adequate humidification is required at all times to allow the functions of the respiratory tract to take place.

In health, inspired gas is warmed, filtered and moistened by the mucous membranes of the upper airways. Nose breathing allows 75% of the total water content of inspired gas to be attained before reaching the larynx, whereas with mouth breathing this reaches only 25% (Oh, 1990).

During periods of disease, or when mechanical ventilation is administered via an endotracheal airway or tracheostomy, bypassing the oropharynx, it is essential to provide artificial humidification.

The term humidity describes the water content of air and may by expressed as absolute or relative. Absolute humidity reflects the mass of water vapour per litre of gas and is measured in mg/litre. Maximum capacity is the maximum volume of vapour that a given volume of gas can carry at a particular temperature. As the temperature of gas increases, so does its ability to hold more vapour. When a gas reaches maximum capacity it is referred to as saturated. If the temperature of saturated gas drops, water will fall out of the gas as condensation. For example, at 37°C the maximum capacity of a gas is 44 mg/litre.

Relative humidity is the ratio of absolute humidity to the maximum capacity. Relative humidity is expressed as a percentage.

Normally, the upper airways warm gas to a temperature of 37°C and achieve maximum humidity at a point just below the carina. This optimum temperature allows 44 mg/litre absolute humidity to be achieved.

In an ICU, a wide variety of applications of humidity can be found, and the physiotherapist should play a leading role in ensuring optimum delivery of properly humidified gas to the patient.

When a patient is intubated with an endotracheal tube, and ventilated for any length of time, it is possible that adverse effects of inadequate humidification may occur. For example, if cold, dry anaesthetic gas bypasses the naso-oropharynx the relative humidity can fall to 50% or less (Oh, 1990). The effects of this can be very serious indeed and include damage to cilia and mucus-secreting glands and cellular damage at each level of the membrane. Mucosal ulceration and reactive hyperaemia may also occur. There is a proportional relationship between the duration of exposure to dry, cold anaesthetic gas and the time taken to recover (Ballard *et al.*, 1992).

These risks are minimised by effective humidification. The most common devices for delivery of humidification are:

- The heat and moisture exchanger.
- The heated respiratory humidifier.

Heat and moisture exchangers such as the Edith, Pall and Portex, utilise the principle of replication of the functions of the naso-oropharynx, utilising moisture obtained from condensation during expiration. The Edith contains a lithium chloride coated polypropylene sponge which is impregnated with chlorhexidine as a bacteriostatic agent. Heat and moisture exchangers are effective in short-term anaesthesia and provide an economical humidification device.

When a patient is admitted to an ITU with already thickened secretions or with traumatised lung tissue it can be more effective immediately to instigate a closed circuit heated humidifier system such as the Fisher and Paykel MR730.

These systems have the benefit of providing safe, convenient and cost-effective humidification. Gas is delivered fully saturated at core temperature and any 'rain out' condensation in the tubing is eliminated by the use of a heated wire in the delivery circuit. Another feature of excluding condensation is that any opportunity for bacteria to replicate and reach the patient is ruled out by disallowing any potential mode of transport from the unit to the patient.

Three main factors reduce the risk of nosocomial pneumonia by using this method. These are:
- Maintenance of a closed delivery system.
- Dry circuit.
- Conservation of the mucociliary transport system.

The risk of infection is further reduced by it being necessary only to change the circuit weekly, which provides less opportunity for bacterial infiltration.

Non-ventilated patients with endotracheal intubation, e.g. during weaning, are accommodated with the 'Swedish nose' type of heat and moisture exchanger, which is a device designed to fit over the end of an endotracheal or tracheostomy tube, and provide the facility for effective humidification. Oxygen is safely administered through these devices at low flow because of their characteristic of replication of the basic function of the naso-oropharynx.

Humidified gas can also be administered through a tracheostomy mask, and for this purpose the gas must be humidified at source by utilising one of the oxygen entraining types of unit such as the Inspiron, Multifit or Misty Ox. These all use elephant tubing thereby reducing condensation but are best used when the patient needs only short-term oxygen. For longer periods of gas administration heated devices should be used, e.g. the Hudson Aquatherm 3.

As with any application of heat, the risks must be carefully calculated and steps taken to minimise them. Modern humidification systems are alarmed at both the chamber and the patient ends of the system, and correct setting of these alarms will rule out any risk of hyperpyrexia or less than optimum delivery temperatures.

The Fisher and Paykel heat and moisture system allows gas to leave the chamber at 37°C (carrying 44 mg/litre of water vapour), the heated wire inside the delivery tubing then adds 2°C to the transported gas, which eliminates condensation, and then as the gas passes the probe at the patient end to be delivered to the airways, the temperature drops, ensuring 37°C and 44 mg/litre saturation as it passes the carina (see Figure 6.4).

Cold water bubble-through devices are still seen on various wards even though they are considered to be inefficient and provide a risk of microbiological contamination. Any hope of delivering humidification is lost by the fact that they utilise narrow bore tubing which causes condensation and rain out long before the gas reaches the patient.

The physiotherapist's role in humidification issues is one of identifying the optimum system of delivery to suit different situations, and the constantly changing requirements of the patient. Close working relationships with the anaesthetic department, nursing staff and medical technicians can help to ensure maximum efficiency in this essential element of respiratory care.

WEANING FROM VENTILATORY SUPPORT

The widespread introduction of HDUs throughout the UK has changed forever the case mix of patients being treated in ICUs. In our own unit, for instance, the severity of illness of our patient population changed dramatically over a short period of time, with the mean length of stay increasing from 4 to 7 days. No longer, or very infrequently, do we ever accept an elective post-theatre admission. Increasing lengths of stay bring with them other problems, unrelated to the pathological process resulting in the patient's admission, that might not be immediately apparent. These include drug dependence (benzodiazepams,

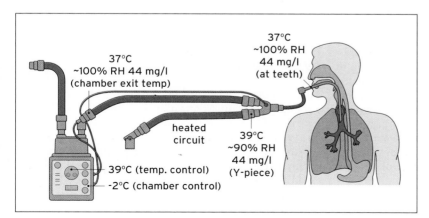

Figure 6.4 Humidification system. (RH; relative humidity)

37°C
~100% RH
44 mg/l
(at teeth)

37°C
~100% RH 44 mg/l
(chamber exit temp)

heated circuit

39°C
~90% RH
44 mg/l
(Y-piece)

39°C (temp. control)

-2°C (chamber control)

opiates), increased incidence of nosocomial infection, increased incidence of psychological sequelae and muscular weakness.

Muscular weakness in ICU patients can be a reflection of simple disuse of the muscle or may be due to a neuropathy or myopathy as a result either of the disease process *per se* (e.g. Guillain–Barrè), nerve compression due to positioning while unconscious (ulnar and common peroneal nerves are most vulnerable), drug therapy (there is an association between steroid muscle relaxants such as pancuronium and myopathy), or the multifactorial phenomenon of critical illness polyneuropathy. The prognosis for each differs.

Critical illness polyneuropathy is increasingly being recognised in ICU patients, tends to affect peripheral nerves only but not exclusively, and most patients make a complete recovery.

Weaning from mechanical ventilatory support should be undertaken only when:

- Inspired oxygen concentration is in the region of about 40%.
- The patient is stable both cardiovascularly and pulmonarily, e.g. tracheal secretions are minimal.
- Dysfunction in other systems such as neurological (raised ICP), renal and hepatic is expected neither to deteriorate as a consequence of the weaning process nor to adversely affect the likelihood of success.

In addition, long-stay patients will almost certainly require a tracheostomy to be performed in advance of the commencement of weaning. Now it is common practice for tracheostomies to be performed not by ear, nose and throat surgeons but by intensive care clinicians themselves using a percutaneous technique.

When compared with use of an endotracheal tube, the advantages of a tracheostomy in this patient population are:

- Increased comfort for the patient.
- Lower requirement for sedative drugs.
- Ease of mouth care.
- Reduction in sinusitis and oral infective complications.
- Reduction in anatomical dead space.

The weaning from mechanical ventilatory support is gradual, can take many days, and is coupled to a gradual reduction in the dosage of sedative drugs to minimise the risk of acute withdrawal syndrome. Weaning is undertaken in the majority of patients by slowly reducing in the first instance the number of mechanical breaths delivered by the ventilator, and then the pressure support added to each spontaneous breath initiated by the patient. Finally, the PEEP is reduced and ultimately withdrawn. In practice the decision when to decannulate depends on bulbar function, i.e. the strength of cough and gag reflexes, and the volume and nature of tracheal secretions.

No presentation of the management of respiratory failure would be complete without discussing the management of cardiovascular failure. Respiratory failure almost always has an impact on cardiovascular performance.

CARDIOVASCULAR FAILURE

Systemic blood pressure is the product of cardiac output and total peripheral resistance; an increase in either the total peripheral resistance or cardiac output will therefore usually be associated with increased blood pressure, unless of course a compensatory depression in the opposite variable governing the blood pressure occurs concurrently.

Cardiac output is defined as the product of heart rate and stroke volume (SV). SV, the amount of blood ejected with a single beat, is influenced by:

VENTRICULAR PRELOAD

Ventricular preload can be assessed as end-diastolic volume, and clinically measured by echocardiography. In practice, due to relative ease, clinicians assess end-diastolic filling pressures, such as the central venous pressure (CVP) for the right ventricle, and the PCWP for the left ventricle. End-diastolic filling pressures do not, however, relate to end-diastolic volume in any linear function, but rather exponentially. Therefore there are occasions when we must supplement our knowledge of end-diastolic filling pressures with echocardiography. If ‘ideal’ filling volumes are exceeded, pulmonary oedema will develop and hinder oxygenation.

VENTRICULAR AFTERLOAD

In practice, ventricular afterload is approximated by measuring the mean pressure that the ventricle is exposed to during ejection, or by calculating the appropriate vascular resistance, i.e. systemic or pulmonary vascular resistance. These resistances can be obtained from the use of a pulmonary artery flotation catheter (see Figure 6.1). These catheters are placed in a central vein, in the internal jugular, subclavian or femoral veins, and are then passed through the heart, with the help of an inflatable balloon, in the sequence of right atrium, right ventricle, pulmonary artery. The catheter is positioned distally in the pulmonary tree, ideally in the middle or preferentially the lower regions of the lung, and ultimately provides a measurement of end-diastolic left ventricular pressure in the majority of patients. The catheter has a thermistor incorporated at its tip which allows calculation of cardiac output using the Fick principle.

VENTRICULAR CONTRACTILITY

The inotropic state of the heart refers to the vigor of ventricular contraction when preload and afterload are both known and held constant. Contractility is the most difficult determinant of SV to measure accurately. Clinically, however, it is acceptable to define an increase in stroke volume output, as measured by the pulmonary artery flotation catheter, as a reflection of enhanced contractility when preload and afterload are held constant.

In the critically ill population, cardiovascular function can be impaired as a result of:

- A direct effect of the respiratory intervention, e.g. by increasing intrathoracic pressures mechanical ventilation will reduce ventricular preload by reducing venous return; PEEP exaggerates this phenomenon. Sedative drugs will reduce systemic vascular resistance and hence blood pressure.
- Increasing pulmonary vascular resistance, secondary to the pulmonary process. This will in turn have a negative influence on right ventricular afterload and ultimately SV.
- A direct 'depressive' effect of the disease process on ventricular contractility, e.g. systemic inflammatory response syndrome and the myocardial depressant factor.
- A direct effect of the disease process on systemic vascular resistance. In the majority of critically ill patients, systemic vascular tone is reduced.

MANAGEMENT OF CARDIOVASCULAR FAILURE

In the management of cardiovascular dysfunction it is important not only to preserve an appropriate mean blood pressure for the patient, thereby ensuring all organ beds receive a global flow within their current range of autoregulation, but also that cardiac output is appropriate for the present clinical condition of the patient. Unfortunately, an adequate global flow to any one organ does not signify that cellular function within any particular organ will be preserved. The splanchnic bed depicts this phenomenon better than most. The mucosal bed within the gut is vulnerable to a reduced flow, the effect of which could be the development of multiple organ failure and the increased mortality that this carries. To date the most sensitive measure of mucosal flow within the gut is obtained with the use of a tonometer. This device is placed in either the stomach or sigmoid colon. It has a silicone balloon at the tip which is permeable to carbon dioxide. An elevated $PaCO_2$ within the balloon in comparison with arterial carbon dioxide trends signifies poor mucosal blood flow.

In time, other devices will develop to allow us to assess more accurately cellular function within organs but for now we must make educated decisions based on mean blood pressure and global cardiac output.

MANIPULATION OF VENTRICULAR PRELOAD

In clinical practice, end-diastolic filling pressures trends are most commonly used to assess volume. Pressure obviously does not equate to volume, but one can use quite satisfactorily trends in pressure in response to fluid challenges to optimise ventricular filling, CVP for the right ventricle, and pulmonary artery occlusion pressure for the left side. On occasion this may not be sensitive enough, e.g. right ventricular dysfunction secondary to severe lung injury. At these times one often needs supplemental information gained from the insertion of an oesophageal Doppler probe, which can measure cardiac output. The impact on stroke volume following a fluid challenge can then be observed directly.

MANIPULATION OF VENTRICULAR AFTERLOAD

Adjusting systemic vascular resistance can be achieved either pharmacologically or mechanically. Several vasodilators are available for lowering systemic vascular resistance, e.g. glyceryl trinitrate (GTN), nitroprusside (and other direct smooth muscle vasodilators), calcium channel blockers, β_2-agonists, α_1-antagonists or even ganglion blockers. Some require intravenous administration only while others are oral preparations.

To elevate systemic vascular resistance, however, the most commonly used drug is noradrenaline. Systemic vascular resistance can also be elevated by the use of temporary assist devices such as the intra-aortic balloon pump (IABP). The IABP was first conceived in 1962, and has been very successful in supporting the failing left ventricle, usually following cardiopulmonary bypass. Counterpulsation is accomplished when the intra-aortic balloon is positioned in the descending aorta; the balloon is rapidly inflated in diastole concurrent with the closure of the aortic valve. With the onset of systole, the balloon is rapidly deflated, allowing the forthcoming ventricular ejection to pass unhindered. The mechanism of the balloon is twofold. First, by augmenting diastolic pressure, coronary blood flow and myocardial oxygen supply can be increased, thereby improving myocardial contractility. Secondly, the rapid balloon deflation just before systole reduces impedance of the left ventricle (see Chapter 7).

MANIPULATION OF VENTRICULAR CONTRACTILITY

Improvements in contractility can be achieved with drugs which possess β_1-agonist activity, e.g. isoprenaline or dobutamine, or through the use of drugs such as the phosphodiesterase inhibitors, enoximone or milrinone. These drugs have combined inotropic and vasodilator properties and are available only in the intravenous form.

MANAGEMENT OF CARDIAC DYSRHYTHMIAS

Dysrhythmias are particularly common in critically ill patients. They can be classified by their origin as either atrial or ventricular.

ATRIAL DYSRHYTHMIAS

The commonest atrial dysrhythmia in critically ill patients is atrial fibrillation. The loss of synchronised atrial contractions and the often rapid ventricular rate can impair cardiac performance. Treatment aims to convert the rhythm back to sinus. The choice here resides between cardioversion and pharmacological means. Aggravating factors should be treated, e.g. low serum potassium (hypokalaemia).

Direct Current (DC) Cardioversion

Direct current (DC) cardioversion is the treatment of choice if there is haemodynamic instability.

The DC shock is synchronised with the R wave of the electrocardiogram (ECG) to minimise the risk of a ventricular arrhythmia. DC cardioversion initially restores sinus rhythm in 70–90% of patients. Sedation requires to be increased in advance of the procedure, and a degree of muscle relaxation is essential.

Chemical Cardioversion

Chemical cardioversion can be achieved with drugs such as quinidine, disopyramide and procainamide but the most commonly used is amiodarone, which is becoming a popular choice for these atrial arrhythmias due to its high conversion rate back to sinus rhythm.

If conversion back to sinus rhythm is not possible, it is imperative that the ventricular rate is controlled. Digoxin is still the drug of choice for this purpose.

VENTRICULAR DYSRHYTHMIAS

Ventricular dysrhythmias are not uncommon in ICU patients. Once again aggravating factors such as hypokalaemia and hypomagnesaemia must be treated aggressively. The rhythm disturbances can range from single to multiple ectopics, and ventricular tachycardia to life-threatening ventricular fibrillation.

Management of the aggravating factors often abolishes the ectopic beats. Ventricular tachycardia and fibrillation require more aggressive management as defined by nationally adopted guidelines.

RENAL FAILURE

In acute renal faulure (ARF), there is a deterioration of renal function, often abrupt and rapid, resulting in the accumulation of waste materials; these include nitrogenous compounds, as measured by serum urea and plasma creatinine levels, which rise with progressive retention of these compounds. Furthermore, there is an inability of the kidney to regulate water and salt balance. This may result in complete cessation of urine output (anuria), a low output of urine (oliguria, <400 ml/24 h) or indeed a high output of dilute urine (polyuric ARF). The outcome is better the more urine output there is.

ARF can be classified simplistically into three categories: pre-renal, intrarenal and post-renal (Figure 6.5). Pre-renal and post-renal causes, if not corrected rapidly, may lead to the more severe form of intrarenal damage. This is the common type seen in intensive care, and usually requires dialysis support. However, a number of patients will have had clinical opportunities to avoid this progression and it is for this reason that discussion of pre-renal and post-renal causes appears in this chapter.

PRE-RENAL ARF

The major causes of pre-renal ARF are outlined in Table 6.3. Pre-renal failure is caused by some combination of low blood volume (hypovolaemia), low blood pressure (hypotension) and diminished renal blood flow. This leads to decreased renal perfusion without intrinsic damage to the renal tubules. The body responds to this by compensatory mechanisms aimed to correct the hypovolaemia or hypotension. There is stimulation of certain hormones (in the autonomic nervous system, adrenaline and noradrenaline, angiotensin II and vasopressin [antidiuretic hormone]), which results in peripheral vasoconstriction and stimulation of thirst. The effects on the kidney are to promote retention of salt and water by the kidney tubules with a resultant reduction in urine output. If the original problem is severe then glomerular filtration rate (GFR) falls and further enhancement of tubular fluid resorption occurs. Ultimately the body is attempting, by these mechanisms, to restore normal blood volume and pressure.

Pre-renal
low blood pressure
low blood volume

Renal
diseases of artery and vein

artery

vein

Renal
diseases of glomeruli, small blood vessels, tubules or interstitium

Ureter and Bladder
obstruction
e.g. stones, prostatic

Figure 6.5 Diagram of a kidney demonstrating areas of acute renal failure.

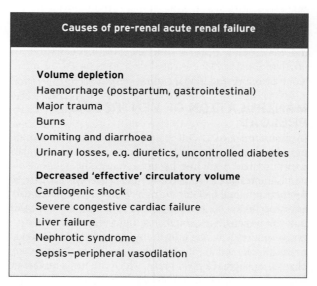

Causes of pre-renal acute renal failure
Volume depletion
Haemorrhage (postpartum, gastrointestinal)
Major trauma
Burns
Vomiting and diarrhoea
Urinary losses, e.g. diuretics, uncontrolled diabetes
Decreased 'effective' circulatory volume
Cardiogenic shock
Severe congestive cardiac failure
Liver failure
Nephrotic syndrome
Sepsis—peripheral vasodilation

Table 6.3 Causes of pre-renal acute renal failure.

Patients with a low blood volume will have a fast pulse, low blood pressure, dry mucous membranes, flat neck veins and decreased filling pressures. Those patients with cardiac output problems will have the above but increased filling pressures.

In pre-renal renal failure, therefore, there will be a low urine output, high urine specific gravity and osmolality, and low urinary sodium. The urine will be of small volume but concentrated because of the tubule resorption of sodium and water.

The clinician must rapidly replace fluid and blood losses, and restore blood volume and blood pressure in the patient with pre-renal renal failure, before renal tubules become damaged (intrarenal damage). Certain conditions (see Table 6.3) are associated with oedematous states (fluid overload), but because the central volume space is depleted, there is a low 'effective' circulatory volume, and the same conditions apply as in those who have true hypovolaemia. The low 'effective' volume is often the consequence of low plasma oncotic pressure because the low albumin and fluid are in the wrong compartment, i.e. the interstitial space instead of the central venous space.

INTRARENAL (INTRINSIC) RENAL FAILURE

The main categories of intrarenal (intrinsic) renal failure are shown in Table 6.4. The vast majority of cases are found following ischaemic or toxic injury to tubules, and this is often called acute tubular necrosis (ATN). Renal failure due to arterial disease is rare as it usually has to involve both kidneys. The most common cause follows atheroemboli, which are dislodged following interventional procedures, e.g. radiology or surgery. Diseases of glomeruli and small blood vessels are numerous and seldom seen in the ICU setting, and patients usually do not require ventilation. Causes of tubulointerstitial disease other than those of ischaemia and nephrotoxins are often difficult to diagnose and should always be borne in mind, e.g. infection or allergic inflammation.

ISCHAEMIC INTRARENAL RENAL FAILURE (ATN)

The only difference between ischaemic intrarenal renal failure and pre-renal renal failure is the severity of the insult that has resulted in hypoperfusion (hypotension, hypovolaemia). In this case damage to the renal tubules has been sufficiently severe that there is no immediate response to correction of the hypoperfusion. If this insult is very severe it can result in the death of the kidney (cortical necrosis), with no recovery. Where recovery is possible the time is quite variable, but usually 10 to 14 days; it may be as long as 4 to 6 weeks in more severe episodes. At the beginning, severe damage causes tubules to disintegrate and shed epithelium and cellular debris, resulting in casts which obstruct the tubules, causing back pressure from urine unable to flow through the tubules. Vasoconstriction and mesangial contraction in the glomeruli also occur, reducing GFR. This phase may be thought of as protective, by reducing function and allowing the kidney to heal. This component of injury lasts about 2 weeks, and subsequent recovery is associated with epithelial cell repair and regeneration of tubule cells. Urine output slowly increases and there may be a polyuric phase while the kidney adjusts to its concentrating function again. It is over this period of injury and recovery that the patient may require dialysis support (see page 89).

NEPHROTOXIC INTRARENAL RENAL FAILURE

The renal tubules and interstitium are very sensitive to toxins, which, in the same way as ischaemia causes damage, produces casts and obstruction to the tubules. Toxins may arise from within the interstitum and tubules (endogenous), e.g. myoglobin, a breakdown product of muscle which appears following rhabdomyolosis, a consequence of severe trauma and crush injuries. Uric acid crystals in the urine can cause tubular damage and this is often seen following rapid tumour lysis and large releases of uric acid. Patients being treated for cancer are protected by pretreatment with allopurinol, which

Causes of intrarenal (intrinsic) renal failure
Diseases of large renal blood vessels
Artery
Severe atherosclerosis
Thromboembolism
Thrombosis
Vein thrombosis
Disease of glomeruli and small blood vessels
Acute glomerulonephritis
Malignant hypertension
Pre-eclampsia and eclampsia

Small vessel thrombosis–haemolytic uraemic syndrome
                         –disseminated intravascular
                              coagulation

Diseases of renal tubule injury
i) Ischaemia–following pre-renal causes

ii) Nephrotoxin–exogenous, e.g. antibiotic,
                                    radiocontrast
                –endogenous, e.g. myoglobin,
                                    myeloma,
                                    uric acid

Diseases of interstitium
Infection–pyelonephritis
Inflammation–allergic interstitial nephritis

Table 6.4 Causes of intrarenal (intrinsic) renal failure.

reduces the amount of uric acid in the urine. Those patients with myeloma secrete light chain proteins, which are also toxic to tubules.

There may be toxins which are actually administered or consumed by the patient and hence are exogenous, e.g. antibiotics such as gentamicin, and anticancer agents such as cisplatin.

In ATN, urine volume and composition may be variable, depending on the phase. The urine specific gravity, osmolality and urine urea concentration are low, and the urine sodium fractional excretion of sodium high. This is because of tubular damage and failure of concentration of sodium and water, urine which does get through the kidney thus being dilute and containing sodium.

The management of this type of renal failure will be discussed later.

POST-RENAL RENAL FAILURE

Although it is not uncommon for one kidney to become obstructed, it would be unusual for renal failure to supervene, because the other kidney 'takes over' (Table 6.5). For both kidneys to be affected the obstruction is usually at the level of the bladder neck or below, a common cause being prostatic hypertrophy. Patients with one kidney only are obviously going to suffer adversely with obstruction at any level of the urinary pathway. Obstruction leads to back pressure of urine and dilation of the ureters and renal pelvis, eventually leading to hydronephrosis. It is important to relieve the obstruction and this requires co-operation between the radiologist, urologist and physician. At its simplest, urinary catheterisation may be all that is required. If the obstruction is higher than the bladder, then a tube from the exterior into the kidney urinary pelvis will need to be inserted under X-ray guidance, i.e. a nephrostomy. Once urine flow is re-established, the process of determining the diagnosis can begin and more effective long-term treatment offered, usually operative.

MANAGEMENT OF ARF

In the management of ARF, the most important requirement is to determine the cause; this will often be in the history, which may or may not be obtained from the family or relatives. Where a pre-renal cause such as low blood pressure is determined, it needs rapid correction to ensure reversibility of renal function, before more severe damage occurs. Where possible the patient should be well oxygenated, have circulating volume corrected and blood pressure restored to normal, and any possible nephrotoxins removed as quickly as possible. Prevention of the development of ATN from pre-renal renal failure is vitally important, as there is not a specific treatment for ATN. Treatment for ATN is primarily supportive until recovery occurs. It is this failure of an organ, and for the patient in the ICU an additional problem on top of often multiorgan ones, that has a serious effect on ultimate survival.

MANAGEMENT OF INTRARENAL (INTRINSIC) RENAL FAILURE (ATN)

After prevention, there is little encouragement that any specific treatment is of benefit in ATN. Agents have been used to augment kidney blood flow (low dose dopamine), relieve tubule obstruction by increasing urine flow (mannitol and frusemide), and reduce energy consumption by the kidney (frusemide), but unfortunately have not been demonstrated to produce consistent benefits for patients.

Complications of ARF

The complications of ARF are managed as they appear, and often dictate the need for dialytic support (Table 6.6). The most important problem is fluid overload as a consequence of decreased urine output. Conservative management can be practised, and the usual method in euvolaemic patients is to administer 30 ml of fluid plus the same amount of fluid as urine output of the previous hour (24 hours × 30 ml = 720 ml = obligatory losses from sweat and bowel). However, if the urine output is very low it allows very little capacity for the fluid requirements of a patient in the ICU setting, i.e. fluids for drugs, inotropes, nutrition, so in the anuric patient fluid overload can develop very quickly. In addition, patients are often fluid overloaded when they arrive in the ICU setting.

Serum potassium is a great danger for the patient, and rises in the anuric patient as the kidney is responsible for its excretion. Restricting potassium intake is helpful, but as potassium is released from damaged cells, it will continue to rise in most situations of ATN. Potassium binding ion exchange resins (calcium resonium) can be used, but are rarely helpful in the ICU context. Acute treatment with

Causes of post-renal renal failure	
Ureteric obstruction	
i) Inside lumen	Stones
	Sloughed renal papilla tumour
ii) Outside lumen	Retroperitoneal fibrosis
	Tumour spread
Bladder obstruction	
Prostatic hypertrophy	
Prostatic carcinoma	
Bladder carcinoma	
Urethral obstruction	
Congenital valves	
Stricture, e.g. gonococcal	
Phimosis	

Table 6.5 **Causes of post-renal renal failure.**

Complications of acute renal failure
Fluid overload
Electrolyte imbalance, e.g. high potassium, low sodium, high phosphate
Acid–base balance, e.g. development of systemic acidosis
Uraemia (raised urea and creatinine)
Poor nutrition (catabolic patients)

Table 6.6 Complications of acute renal failure.

insulin and glucose is helpful in stabilising the patient, but is only a short-term remedy.

Severe metabolic acidosis rapidly develops in the severely ill patient who is anuric, and impedes biological function. Sodium bicarbonate correction can be useful, but remains a difficulty in those patients with fluid restriction, and in those in whom the underlying cause for acidosis has not been corrected.

Patients with ATN develop anaemia as a consequence of a number of events. The kidneys fail to produce erythropoietin, which stimulates the marrow to produce haemoglobin. The uraemic state is associated with coagulation problems, which may cause bleeding. There is platelet dysfunction, which may add to the problems with bleeding. Red cell survival is shortened, and white cell function is affected. This means that there is a risk of infection—the greatest danger for patients with ATN. There is a high incidence and high mortality from infection. Host defence mechanisms are not very effective in uraemia, and patients in the ICU with ARF have numerous catheters and tubes in place providing the opportunity for infection and sepsis.

There are a number of ways of managing ARF which alleviate these complications as they develop.

CONSERVATIVE MANAGEMENT

Conservative management of ARF requires the clinician to take a number of steps to stabilise the patient, so that renal function can recover during that period. These steps include:
- Removal of any toxins where possible, e.g. stop gentamicin.
- Restoring correct fluid balance. If the patient is not fluid overloaded then give 30 ml of fluid (allow for insensible losses) and equivalent of urine output in previous hour. It is important to allow for losses through diarrhoea, burns and drains, and in this context the monitoring of CVP is helpful.
- Daily monitoring of electrolytes, especially potassium, with urea, creatinine and acid–base balance.
- Adequate nutrition, i.e. high calories and moderate protein intake are required at this stage. Nutrition is a very important aspect of ARF, as these patients are often highly catabolic and require calorie and nutrient replacement.

If the urine output does not increase sufficiently, then the decision to dialyse needs to be taken. In the ICU setting, the need for dialysis support often rests on the fact that large volumes of fluid need to be given (parenteral nutrition, drugs), and this often dictates an earlier approach to dialysis support than with conservative management.

DIALYSIS TREATMENT

It is not clear that early dialysis or type of dialysis favourably affects the outcome of patients with ATN. Low blood pressure difficulties and anoxia may accompany haemodialysis, although less often with more modern techniques. Therefore, dialysis is reserved for the treatment of symptoms and signs of uraemia, management of volume overload, and high potassium or acidosis refractory to conservative management; judgement will vary according to the patient.

Types of Dialysis (Table 6.7)

Peritoneal dialysis and haemodialysis in the ICU setting are gradually being replaced by continuous techniques of filtration and dialysis, i.e. continuous arteriovenous haemofiltration (CAVHF), continuous veno-venous haemofiltration (CVVHF), continuous arteriovenous haemodialysis plus haemofiltration (CAVHF/D) and continuous veno-venous haemodialysis plus haemofiltration (CVVHF/D). These techniques are simpler, need less monitoring, produce better cardiovascular stability, can be run by ICU staff and need no specialist renal unit staffing. However, there is no consistent study extant demonstrating clinical outcome benefits from these techniques, although a greater range of unstable patients can be treated.

Peritoneal dialysis

This technique is useful in unstable patients and in those with bleeding problems, or if other techniques are not available. A peritoneal catheter is inserted by stab technique into the lower abdomen, and directed into one or other paracolic gutter. Dialysis fluid is run in and out, allowing 1–2 hours' dwell time for equilibration of solutes across the peritoneal membrane. The peritoneal membrane acts as an artificial membrane, and solutes move down the concentration gradient, i.e. from blood with high urea and potassium concentrations to peritoneal dialysate fluid with no urea or potassium present. If excess fluid is to be removed, a more highly concentrated sugar solution is used

Types of dialysis
Peritoneal dialysis
Haemodialysis
Continuous modes of filtration
i) Continuous arteriovenous haemofiltration (CAVHF)
ii) Continuous veno-venous haemofiltration (CVVHF)
iii) Continuous arteriovenous haemodialysis plus haemofiltration (CAVHF/D)
iv) Continuous veno-venous haemodialysis plus haemofiltration (CVVHF/D)

Table 6.7 Types of dialysis.

in the dialysates so that fluid is drawn across the peritoneal membrane from the blood by the process of osmosis.

The major complication of this technique is peritonitis, particularly if poor technique is used or if the procedure carries on for a number of days. Occasionally, there may be extravasation of fluid into the interstitial spaces or puncture of organs or bowel with this technique. It is particularly hazardous if there has been previous abdominal surgery.

Haemodialysis

This is, by the nature of the technique, intermittent, and requires 3–4 hours for a session, possibly on a daily basis. It requires a specialist machine together with a renal nurse. A dialyser incorporates a semipermeable membrane of large surface area, down one side of which blood passes. Substances at a higher concentration in blood diffuse across the membrane into the dialysate and are removed (potassium, urea). Some substances are replaced by having a higher concentration in the dialysate fluid and the movement is in the opposite direction, e.g. calcium. If fluid is to be removed, then a negative pressure is exerted at the dialysate fluid end to draw fluid across the membrane (ultrafiltration). This enables some solutes to be dragged across with this flow of filtrate; this technique is termed convection. In haemodialysis, the majority of solute exchanges take place by slow diffusion, which is highly effective and often needs to be used in patients with a very high catabolic rate, where urea rises very sharply each day.

Haemofiltration/dialysis

Continuous haemofiltration requires either arteriovenous access (shunt; or catheters [in the femoral artery and vein]), or venous access (subclavian, internal jugular or femoral vein catheters). The former is driven by the blood pressure of the patient, the latter requires a blood pump to increase venous outflow from the patient and through the filter. The difference between techniques can best be represented by:
- CAVHF, i.e. continuous convective clearance.
- CVVHF, i.e. continuous convective clearance but using a blood pump.
- CAVHF/D, i.e. continuous convective plus diffusive clearance.
- CVVHF/D, i.e. continuous convective plus diffusive clearance but using a blood pump.

The last two techniques are the ones most often used in the ICU setting now.

Where large volumes of fluid need to cross the membrane to achieve a satisfactory exchange of solute, diffusion is more efficient at removing solute than convection.

In these techniques patients are continuously treated and close attention is required for fluid balance.

OUTCOME OF ARF

The mortality rate for acute intrarenal (intrinsic) renal failure is still very high (50%) in spite of all the advances in supportive care. This, however, may reflect a more ageing population and more cases of multiorgan failure being treated. Of those that survive, most regain good function; those few who do not (due to severe renal cortical necrosis) will require long-term haemodialysis treatment. Hence, it is important in the acute treatment phase of these patients that care is taken to preserve veins and arteries in case long-term dialysis is needed.

In summary, prevention and acute resuscitation is the best course to take in patients with ARF hence avoiding more sustained renal failure which will require supportive dialytic care. When dialytic care is required, it is best undertaken in a specialist centre, where there is a combined team of intensivists and renal physicians available to offer the best possible expertise.

MONITORING SYSTEMS

In ICUs, the need for minute by minute evaluation of the cardiovascular system is paramount in the assessment of patient stability. The monitors available are sophisticated and computerised, and allow easy analysis. Nurses, doctors, physiotherapists and other medical staff must be familiar with the monitors used in their units and trained according to the *Intensive Care Standards*.

The patient in intensive care will have several pieces of equipment attached to a monitor, so that a visual display of measurements is available, e.g. transducers, ECG leads, pulse oximetry probe and thermometer. Some monitors, e.g. Space Labs, are finger-touch controlled, so the clinician need only touch the screen to alter the parameters. Perhaps the most important parameters are the alarm settings. If the alarms sound, then the clinician's attention is drawn to the screen to see the discrepancy. The clinician still needs to value the importance of assessing the patient as an individual, and to look to the clinical signs of instability—the monitors should not therefore exclude clinicians' evaluation of the patient (Table 6.8).

THE MONITOR

The monitor screen above the patient will display:
- Blood pressure (BP).
- CVP.
- Heart rate.
- Pulmonary artery pressure (PAP).
- Oxygen saturation (SaO_2, SvO_2).
- Patient temperature.
- Intracerebral pressure (ICP, CPP) (if available).

OXYGEN SATURATION

Pulse oximetry (SpO_2) is an essential non-invasive method of monitoring arterial oxygen saturation. It provides an early and immediate warning of hypoxaemia and should be used for any patient at risk of hypoventilation or respiratory arrest. SpO_2 readings below 95% occur when the oxygen delivery system is inadequate to meet the needs of the tissues or cardiac output is poor, resulting in tissue hypoxia. It should be used in conjunction with other observations and monitoring and not used in isolation as other factors including artefact, vasoconstriction and abnormal haemoglobin may provide a false reading.

ECG MONITORING

Continuous ECG monitoring should be routine for any critically ill patient, allowing the early detection of rhythm and rate abnormalities. Alarms are set for individual requirements to alert staff at the earliest opportunity when problems occur. Some monitors have a facility enabling the alarms to be set automatically depending on the individual patient's readings. It is important for all staff working within the ICU to be able to recognise sinus rhythm, sinus tachycardia and sinus bradycardia in addition to the life-threatening rhythms of ventricular fibrillation, asystole, electromechanical dissociation and pulseless ventricular tachycardia. Any changes in the ECG that affect cardiac output and therefore blood pressure need immediate attention.

ARTERIAL PRESSURE MONITORING

Arterial cannulation is commonly used in patients in the ICU to provide access for arterial blood sampling and blood gas analysis; it is also used for arterial pressure monitoring in patients with unstable blood pressure, and for those patients on vasoactive drug therapy. A continuous display of the patient's blood pressure is used to assist in patient management, allowing the effect of inotropic or vasoactive therapy to be observed and altered as necessary. All staff involved in caring for the patient need to be aware of the hazards of invasive monitoring, which include the risk of cannula contamination, disconnection and therefore haemorrhage, thrombosis, peripheral embolisation and ischaemia of the digits. The arterial cannula cannot be used as an intravascular route for drugs.

CENTRAL VENOUS PRESSURE (CVP) MONITORING

The central venous cannula is inserted most frequently into the internal or external jugular vein or subclavian vein. The tip is situated approximately 2 cm above the right atrium in the superior vena cava. Central venous cannulation provides access for intravenous therapy, particularly for drugs which cause irritation to peripheral veins, e.g. strong potassium chloride, or for long-term damage that may be caused by the infusion of adrenaline or dopamine. When connected to a transducer, the CVP can be monitored providing an indication of the fluid status of the patient, the function of the right side of the heart and an evaluation of the response to vasoactive drugs. There are several causes of a rise in CVP including fluid overload, myocarditis, pulmonary hypertension and ventricular septal defect with left-to-right shunting. Hypovolaemia and vasodilation can cause a decrease in CVP. Complications include the risk of air embolism, pneumothorax, tamponade and haemorrhage during insertion, while the complications following insertion include infection and inaccurate readings which may be

Monitoring of ICU patient	
Frequency	**Data monitored**
Continuous	ECG, BP, temperature SaO_2, SvO_2 ICP, CPP
Hourly	Fluid intake/Urine output Dialysis input/output CVP, PAP, PCWP
>2 Hourly	Arterial blood gas analysis Blood sugar level Neurological status Skin status Cardiac output studies
>Daily	Blood chemistry Chest X-ray Microbiology Urinalysis

Table 6.8 Monitoring of ICU patient.

caused by a misplaced transducer or problems with the equipment. Normal CVP in the ventilated patient is between 6 and 12 cmH$_2$O.

PULMONARY ARTERY PRESSURE (PAP) MONITORING

Increasingly, the pulmonary artery catheter is used as a matter of routine in the management of critically ill patients (see Figure 6.1). It provides a measure of the function of the left and right side of the heart, tissue oxygen consumption and cardiac output. This information provides the necessary data to institute the required drug therapy for the patient. Inotropic therapy including adrenaline, noradrenaline and dobutamine can be managed more effectively with the data provided from the cardiac output studies as opposed to relying on the arterial blood pressure, CVP reading and heart rate.

The PCWP is recorded when the balloon-tipped catheter is inflated and the tip moves along with the blood flow to occlude a small pulmonary artery. The inflated balloon blocks the recording of pressure behind it in the pulmonary artery, allowing only the recording of pressures in the pulmonary capillaries in front of it. The PCWP reflects the left atrial pressure. Decreased PCWP may be caused by hypovolaemia from fluid loss or vasodilation. Increased PCWP can indicate an increased preload caused by fluid overload, increased systemic vascular resistance caused by vasoconstriction or systemic hypertension, or decreased contractility due to myocardial ischaemia, left ventricular failure and electrolyte imbalance. Normal wedge pressure is 12 to 15 cmH$_2$O.

Cardiac output can be measured by using the thermodilution technique. A measured amount of cold fluid (usually 10 ml on each of three successive occasions) is injected into the right atrial port of the catheter. A thermister at the tip of the catheter measures the temperature of the fluid as it passes the tip. A computer measures the cardiac output; the degree of warming indicates the contractility of the heart. The cardiac index is used as a measure which takes into account the cardiac output in relation to the surface area of the patient. The cardiac index, systemic vascular resistance, pulmonary vascular resistance, PCWP, and other cardiovascular monitoring provide an indication of the therapy required in terms of fluid management and inotropic support.

As with any invasive monitoring, use of the pulmonary artery catheter is not without risks. These include the risks associated with CVP lines, and additional problems which may occur including the possibility of spontaneous wedging of the balloon, balloon rupture, erosion of an artery, dysrhythmias, and valve trauma occurring on insertion or removal of the catheter.

BLOOD GAS ANALYSIS

Arterial blood gas sampling is required for the assessment of oxygenation and ventilation while also providing information on the acid–base state, adequacy of the circulation, and metabolic abnormalities. ICUs frequently have their own blood gas analysis machine thereby providing results and changes in treatment promptly. Samples of arterial blood are typically taken from the radial artery, less commonly from the femoral artery.

Normal values and variations from the normal are discussed in Chapter 2.

THERAPEUTIC BEDS

The frequent changing of body position is a recognised nursing procedure within the ICU, and has been for many years, in an attempt to reduce pressure on the skin and in the prevention of respiratory complications. The perceived advantages of regular changes in position include benefits for the pulmonary blood flow, ventilation, the mobilisation of secretions, pain relief, the prevention and treatment of pressure sores, burns and open wounds, reduction in venous stasis and reduced risk of venous thrombosis. The respiratory system is affected by immobility more than any other system and consequently the patient is affected by atelectasis and pooling of secretions which becomes a breeding ground for infection (Tapson and Fulkerson, 1991). Turning patients on a frequent basis helps to reduce atelectasis and promotes secretion clearance by using gravity to move the secretions from the lower airways to the upper airways where they can be removed.

PRESSURE SORES

Any acutely ill patient is at risk from pressure sores, and critically ill patients are more susceptible than most. Pressure sores occur when the skin and underlying structures are compressed, causing blood to be diverted and blood vessels forcibly constricted resulting in ischaemia and tissue anoxia. This impairs cellular respiration and causes cells to die.

COST OF PRESSURE SORES

The pursuit for methods of pressure sore prevention has increased following the publication of *The Health of the Nation* (Department of Health, 1991) in which it was estimated that pressure sores affect 6.7% of the hospital population, a figure thought by some to be higher (O'Dea, 1995). The cost of pressure sore prevention is estimated at £60m per year (Department of Health, 1991) although the real cost of pressure sores remains unknown. There have been numerous estimations ranging from £60m to £200m per year (Department of Health, 1993). The cost of treatment is high due to the extended hospital stay, the need for plastic surgery on severe pressure sores, the cost of dressings, and the potential cost of litigation which would increase costs considerably (cited by Department of Health, 1993). Providers are currently expected to set annual targets for an overall reduction in pressure sores of at least 5%. While there are many perceived advantages of the use of therapeutic beds, the one which is most frequently debated is their use in the prevention of pressure sores.

PRESSURE SORE PREVENTION

Most prevention strategies are based on risk assessment and reduction of that risk (Waterlow, 1991), and turning is the most commonly used method of reducing that risk, but not always possible, particularly in the critically ill patient. Various scoring systems for the assessment and prevention of pressure sores exist (Braden and Bergstrom 1988; Norton et al., 1962; Waterlow, 1991) although these need to be used in conjunction with clinical observation and not in place of it (Flanagan, 1995). None of these methods of risk assessment has been devised specifically for intensive care patients; however, they do provide a useful indicator. Generally, patients in intensive care are at high risk or very high risk of pressure sore development, as determined by the Waterlow (1991) assessment card which uses a number of predisposing factors to determine risk.

AN OVERVIEW OF THERAPEUTIC BED USE

The need for guidelines for the use of therapeutic beds and mattresses is recognised to ensure there is a sound scientific reason for the therapy, and the most effective use of limited resources (Crunden, 1994). There are numerous therapeutic beds and mattresses available on the market for purchase or for hire to assist in the relief of pressure and to assist in the turning of patients, and the range of products continues to grow. However, their effectiveness remains questionable as the majority of clinical trials are conducted by the manufacturers and not by healthcare professionals. Although research studies have been limited owing to the insufficient sample sizes and interpatient variability, some studies have demonstrated significant benefits.

Beds available include low air loss beds, low air loss turning beds, low air loss pulsating beds, low air loss beds providing percussion and vibration, turning tables and air fluidised beds. The array of beds available has resulted in some confusion as to their function and to their operation. An effective education programme for those operating the beds is essential.

The choice of bed will primarily depend upon the reason for use, which can be established from guidelines for practice or trust policies. Additionally, important considerations are cost, the support offered by the hire company or manufacturers in terms of education and in-service training for the multidisciplinary team, and technical support.

All beds are required to fulfil safety standards including the need to maintain patient safety and the safety of those who have the responsibility of changing the patient's body position and for bed operation. Dual controls are usually available for both the patient and carer to operate the position of the base, enabling it to be positioned at the most appropriate angle for the patient. Cot sides, weighing scales and the facility to insert an X-ray plate into the bed frame are integral in some models and it is essential that the bed can quickly be repositioned in the event of a cardiac arrest or other emergency.

AIR FLUIDISED THERAPY

The air fluidised bed consists of a tank of glass microspheres which are fluidised by the upward flow of warm, filtered air. This looks like liquid but is dry to touch. Air fluidised therapy was developed to alleviate the problems burns patients suffer including pain, sepsis, pressure sores, sleep deprivation, repeated surgery, and slow wound healing, and also for temperature control, exudate management and infection control. Since the bed will absorb fluid losses from the patient, it is important that these losses are considered when estimating the insensible loss, otherwise dehydration may occur. Air fluidised therapy enables patients to be nursed directly on skin grafts, and allows the body temperature to be controlled by altering the air temperature of the bed. The main disadvantages include difficulties in positioning the patient and problems with patients maintaining a sitting position, although the latter problem has been overcome to some extent by incorporating a back rest into some models including the SSI Uplift (Figure 6.6). Some patients dislike the sensation of weightlessness, and there have been reports of disorientation and a feeling of motion sickness from the therapy (Ryan, 1990).

LOW AIR LOSS THERAPY

Several low air loss beds which provide low pressure support from air filled cushions are currently available. Some low air loss beds provide pulsation which is designed to massage the skin and improve tissue perfusion. This is useful in the management of patients with reduced peripheral circulation, and patients with burns (Ryan, 1995). The low air loss bed has proved to be cost effective in reducing the incidence of pressure sores in critically ill patients (Inman, 1993), and promotes the healing of pressure sores in elderly patients (Mudler et al., 1994).

ROTATIONAL BEDS

Rotational beds include the low air loss turning bed which enables the patient to be turned from one side to the other to a maximum of 45°, and the turning table which rotates to a maximum of 62°. A physiotherapy bed, the Respicair (SSI) (Figure 6.7) has recently been introduced in the UK. This bed has percussion and vibration modes, and enables the patient to be rotated without the need for a physiotherapist to be present. The value of percussion or vibration to the dependent lung is yet to be proved.

Originally, kinetic therapy involved rotating the patient along the longitudinal axis from one lateral position to the other at degrees manually set by the operator; however, both types of bed can now be programmed automatically to rotate from one side or the other and at various angles to optimise the physiological effects. The table has now been extended for use in patients with chest, spinal or pelvic injuries.

Research on the Kinetic Treatment Table, which turns the patient to a 40° angle, has indicated a reduction in the incidence of pneumonia (Summer et al., 1989; Fink et al., 1990). Reduction in the length of stay on the

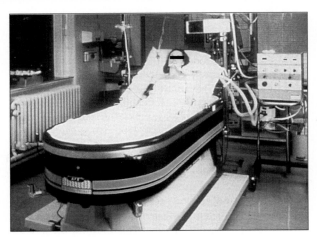

Figure 6.6 Air fluidised therapy bed.

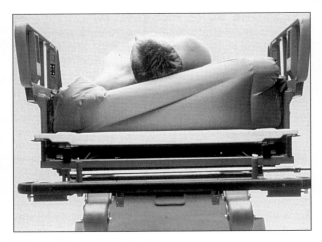

Figure 6.7 Rotating bed.

ICU or time ventilated is under debate. In a study by Choi and Nelson (1992) there was found to be no reduction in the length of stay; however, in an earlier study, length of stay was reduced by up to 5 days in patients suffering from COPD and sepsis (Kelley *et al.*, 1987). While the use of the turning table has been recommended for patients with head injuries (Mitchell, 1986) it is also considered to be a contraindication due to the potential rise in ICP (Kelley *et al.*, 1987; Gentilello *et al.*, 1988). The turning table was originally designed for spinal immobilisation. It requires a firm mattress and therefore does not provide pressure relief. One of the main disadvantages is that pressure damage can occur relatively quickly despite the patient's position being changed continually. Anxiety and tolerance of turning is reported to be problematic, particularly when sedation has been reduced, and in turn this may invoke cardiac arrhythmias (Kelley, 1987; Gentilello *et al.*, 1988; Summer *et al.*, 1989). The potential risk of lines and catheters being disconnected must not be overlooked, emphasising the importance of effective monitoring and the use of alarms in critical care.

RESUSCITATION

THE RHYTHMS OF CARDIAC ARREST

Cardiac arrest can be defined as 'the cessation of cardiac mechanical activity confirmed by the absence of a detectable pulse, unresponsiveness and apnoea (or agonal respirations)'. It can be associated with ventricular fibrillation, pulseless ventricular tachycardia, asystole, and electromechanical dissociation. The need for prompt recognition and diagnosis of a cardiac arrest to ensure the optimum prognosis for the victim is well established since after 2 minutes cerebral anoxic damage occurs (Resuscitation Council, 1994). It is essential that all healthcare professionals are familiar with the diagnosis and treatment of the rhythms of cardiac arrest as defined by the European Resuscitation Council (1994). Three algorithms, for ventricular fibrillation, asystole, and electromechanical dissociation respectively, provide a framework for treatment, assisting in the organisation required for dealing with the cardiac arrest and optimising the treatment. A brief overview of each cardiac rhythm type is provided but must be used in conjunction with the European Resuscitation Council guidelines (1994).

VENTRICULAR FIBRILLATION

Ventricular fibrillation results from unco-ordinated depolarisation throughout the myocardium causing a cessation of cardiac output. Delay to defibrillation is the most important determinant of the outcome of resuscitation when the patient is in a state of ventricular fibrillation (European Resuscitation Council, 1994). It is the most common rhythm of cardiac arrest, and prospects for survival decrease by at least 5% per minute even with effective life support. Asystole can occur within minutes of the onset of ventricular fibrillation. The longer ventricular fibrillation persists the more likely it is for the rhythm to deteriorate into asystole which has a lower success rate from resuscitation than ventricular fibrillation. Defibrillation is the primary treatment of choice in ventricular fibrillation and adrenaline the first line resuscitation drug. The length of time resuscitation is continued will depend upon the individual situation; however, so long as ventricular fibrillation persists resuscitation should not be abandoned.

ASYSTOLE

In asystole there is complete absence of electrical and mechanical activity, and the prospects of survival are poor. If it is difficult to determine if the patient is in asystole or ventricular fibrillation the algorithm for the latter should be pursued. The treatment of choice is adrenaline since defibrillation will not help in the treatment of asystole. If resuscitation time exceeds 15 minutes it is unlikely the patient will survive.

ELECTROMECHANICAL DISSOCIATION

In electromechanical dissociation there is a continuous waveform on the ECG; however, there is absence of mechanical activity and the patient is therefore pulseless. Causes include hypothermia, pneumothorax, pulmonary embolism, hypovolaemia, electrolyte imbalance and cardiac tamponade, and until the cause is treated muscular activity cannot resume. In electromechanical dissociation, while a diagnosis is sought, support can be given by providing airway management preferably from intubation, gaining intravenous access and administering adrenaline 1 mg.

DRUGS USED IN RESUSCITATION

ADRENALINE

Adrenaline 1 mg is administered in all types of cardiac arrest every 2–3 minutes. It is administered in an attempt to increase myocardial contraction, coronary blood flow, cerebral blood flow, systemic vascular resistance and arterial blood pressure. In asystole, an increased dose of 5 mg may be considered if the patient is not responding to treatment.

ATROPINE

Atropine 3 mg is administered in asystole. It antagonises the effect of the vagus nerve on both the sino-atrial (SA) node and the atrio-ventricular (AV) node, increasing sinus automacity and AV node conduction.

EQUIPMENT

Within the ICU, patients are usually already attached to monitoring equipment and have life support measures in progress. The aim in this environment is to prevent complications and therefore reduce the potential for cardiac arrest; however, inevitably some patients will succumb to this critical event. It is essential that equipment is available for rapid intervention and that staff working within the area are familiar with its function. Traditionally, medical staff manage the cardiac arrest in response to an urgent call from the nurses; however, more nurses are enhancing their practice skills and are able to perform advanced life support including airway management, defibrillation and the administration of resuscitation drugs, in addition to basic life support.

DEFIBRILLATORS

The array of defibrillators available on the market has resulted in some confusion and debate regarding the use of automated external defibrillators, and semi-automated and manual defibrillators. Studies have demonstrated that the ability of the automated and semi-automated defibrillators to detect rhythms is similar to that of trained personnel (Weaver, 1988). The need for extensive education is reduced with the use of automated defibrillators as, if a shockable rhythm is detected, the machine will alert the operator and automatically charge to 200 joules in the first instance. This is particularly useful in situations where there are a lack of skilled personnel able to defibrillate, for example, arrests occurring out of the hospital.

The automated and semi-automatic defibrillators are cardiac rhythm analysis systems that will sense and record the rhythm and if necessary deliver a shock. The fully automated mode requires the defibrillator pads to be attached and the defibrillator turned on, while the semi-automated or shock advisory mode requires the operator to initiate the automated external defibrillator to analyse the rhythm, and then deliver the shock on the indication of the automated external defibrillator. The operator is then in a position to discharge the defibrillator. Manual defibrillators rely entirely on the operator to make the correct diagnosis and discharge the defibrillator.

It is essential that the operator takes responsibility for the safety of all personnel involved. No one should be in direct contact with the patient or bed before discharging the defibrillator. Additionally, the defibrillator should not be discharged if there is a risk of contact with body fluids.

The paddles are normally placed over the apex of the heart and to the right of the sternum, beneath the right clavicle. The sternum should be avoided as bone impedes the current. Alternatively, if this position is unsuccessful the anterior/posterior position should be considered.

Special consideration should be given to:
- Pacemaker sites: these should be avoided by at least 12–15 cm.
- Patients on IABP: these can receive the shock with the IABP still switched on.
- Transdermal GTN patches: these must be removed to avoid explosion on delivery of the shock.

AIRWAY MANAGEMENT

Airway management is generally continuously controlled in intensive care, as most patients are already intubated and undergoing artificial ventilation. In such patients, 100% oxygen can be rapidly delivered via the endotracheal tube by increasing the delivery via the ventilator or by administering oxygen via a re-breathe bag or ambu bag for resuscitation purposes. Intubation protects the lungs from contamination with regurgitated stomach contents. It is essential that the following equipment is readily available for each patient:
- Guedal airways: these are sized by measuring the airway from the corner of the jaw to the centre point of the lip. A wrongly sized airway can push the tongue backward and obstruct the airway, or stimulate the vagus nerve and induce vomiting.
- Face mask.
- Re-breathe bag/reservoir bag.
- Mcgills forceps.
- Laryngoscope.
- Artery forceps.
- Introducer/bougee.
- Syringe 10 ml.
- Endotracheal tubes: in general of 7.0–8.0 mm width for females and 8.0–9.0 mm for males. Suction equipment including catheters, tubing and gloves.
- Stethoscope to assess air entry following intubation.

If attempts at intubation are unsuccessful they must be abandoned immediately and another method of airway management selected.

Although the endotracheal tube is the preferred method of airway control during cardiopulmonary resuscitation, the laryngeal mask is a valuable adjunct to airway management and has partially replaced the use of endotracheal intubation for anaesthetists in theatre. It offers a method by which the non-expert can effectively secure an airway and ventilate the patient. It is useful in emergency situations in which there are no personnel trained in intubation; however, within the critical care area its use does not take the place of oral or nasal intubation although it can be used as a temporary measure before intubation.

ACTIVE COMPRESSION DECOMPRESSION DEVICE

The active compression decompression device is undergoing evaluation for its effectiveness in resuscitation. It is dependent upon the venous return to the heart as a result of negative intrathoracic pressure generated during the decompression phase, which results in an increased ejected volume during the compression phase. As a result there are improvements to cerebral perfusion and ventilation

LEGAL AND ETHICAL ISSUES

It is essential that healthcare professionals are aware that a decision not to resuscitate a patient has been made or if circumstances have led to that decision being reviewed and reversed. Where appropriate this decision should be made in discussion with the patient, which is rarely possible in the ICU. Relatives, friends and the multidisciplinary team should be involved in discussions, although the ultimate decision is the responsibility of the clinician in charge. Good communication is essential if all relevant team members are to be informed of this. Unless there are specific instructions to the contrary documented in the medical records, a resuscitation attempt must be made.

EDUCATION

Research has shown that resuscitation skills are poor, that instruction is inconsistent and that theoretical knowledge and practical skills are limited. In a small study by Inwood (1995), the relationship between confidence and skills was demonstrated highlighting the need for annual resuscitation workshops to update both knowledge and skills. Education in basic life support is essential for all personnel working within the hospital environment, and for those working in critical care areas there is a need for familiarity with the *European Guidelines for Resuscitation* (1994). To ensure that optimum treatment is delivered, the algorithms need to be used as a guide to promote greater team work and understanding. It is essential that all staff who operate a defibrillator are familiar with the equipment and have the

opportunity for regular updates in using the equipment and managing life support scenarios. Clearly, staff need to be aware of specific instructions for individuals, e.g. 'Do not resuscitate' orders, national recommendations and hospital resuscitation policies.

THE ROLE OF THE CLINICIAN IN INTENSIVE CARE

Patient management in critically ill patients is of vast scope. It relies on staff, who have effective communication skills and the ability to work together as part of a large multidisciplinary team, to perform a highly skilled role whatever their professional background. It is essential that the needs of the patient and family are met, and that the patient is assessed holistically by the multidisciplinary team to meet the clinical requirements.

ROLE OF THE DOCTOR

The role of the intensive care clinician is to manage the patient's condition and to administer life support. This occurs in close conjunction with all other support groups, e.g. physiotherapy, pharmacy and dietetics. Patients can be admitted to the ICU under the specialism of the orthopaedic team, but their ventilatory requirements and general stability is cared for by the intensivist.

Patient selection for an intensive care bed is ultimately the responsibility of the consultant in charge of the ICU, and, equally, the decision to withdraw treatment is made in collaboration with the consultant under whom the patient was first admitted. Major decisions in the management of the patient's condition are the responsibility of the intensivist, and instructions concerning administration of drugs, changes in ventilatory requirements, haemodynamic measurement and the daily care of the patient are carried out by the nursing staff.

ROLE OF THE NURSE

ORGANISATION OF THE ICU
Patients of all ages are admitted to ICUs for numerous medical and surgical reasons, depending upon the speciality treatment undertaken in the hospital. Staffing for the unit requires one qualified nurse per patient on each shift as recommended in the *Guidelines on admission to and discharge from Intensive Care and High Dependency Units* (Department of Health, 1996).

Not all patients require one nurse at all times and some will require more than one; therefore patient dependency is assessed holistically by being scored between a maximum of 5 and a minimum of 0.5 for each of the following criteria:
- Respiratory.
- Cardiovascular.
- Fluid balance.
- Nutritional.
- Neurological.

- Musculoskeletal.
- Soft tissue.
- Psychological.
- Social and cultural.
- Communication.

Since there are 10 criteria, a maximum of 50 points can be awarded. A score of 40–50 indicates a patient dependency of one to two nurses, a score of less than 20 indicates a 0.5 nurse to patient dependency, and for those patients in between, a one to one nurse to patient ratio is required. This system is used in North Staffordshire.

Continuity of care is desirable, therefore effort is made to allocate a nurse who has cared for the patient, their family and friends previously. This promotes better communication between the nurse, patient and family and can lead to a more trusting and honest relationship, enabling the nurse to act as advocate for all concerned. Additionally, communication between the nurse and the multidisciplinary team is enhanced enabling them to work collaboratively in assessing, planning, implementing and evaluating care and treatment.

Consideration is given to the nursing staff dealing with critically ill patients constantly, as it can be exhausting coping with a patient's relatives and treating an unstable patient, in particular the dying, or young children and babies.

Nurses are the only care group present for the 24-hour period. Their responsibilities vary according to the role they have been employed to undertake; this will depend on their grade, the extent to which their roles have been developed, the type of ICU, the dependency of the patients admitted, and medical interventions. Following the production of the *Scope of Professional Practice* (UKCC, 1992) nurses are developing roles to improve the quality of patient care and treatment

through specialist training courses to enhance their skills, while also addressing some of the issues regarding the reduction of junior doctors' hours (NHSME, 1991). The skills needed in critical care include management of:

- The airway.
- Cardiac arrest.
- Arterial cannulation.
- Ventilation and weaning.
- ICP monitoring.
- Pulmonary artery catheter.
- Continuous dialysis, e.g. CVVHF.

These skills require comprehensive education and assessment in both theory and practice. Although the enhancing practice programme has yet to be formally evaluated, apparent benefits include improvements in the quality of care, greater job satisfaction for those performing the skills, decision making at a higher level, and improvements in the relationship between medical and nursing staff.

AIRWAY MANAGEMENT

Most patients in intensive care require airway management through either an oral or nasal endotracheal tube or tracheostomy (Figure 6.8). The advantages and disadvantages of each method can be seen in Table 6.9.

Tracheostomy through either the traditional surgical method or percutaneous method is usually reserved for patients who are to be ventilated for a prolonged period or in whom intubation has been unsuccessful. Normally, any patient intubated for 10 days and needing further intubation is a candidate for a tracheostomy. Regular suction through the endotracheal tube or tracheostomy tube, and assessment of the tenacity of the secretions, prevent obstruction of the

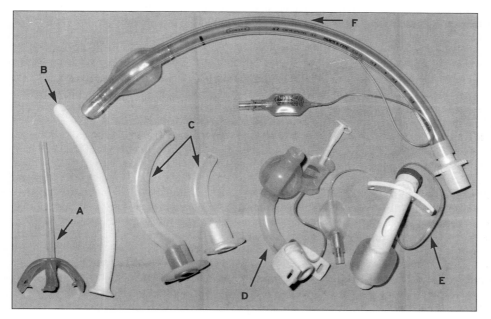

Figure 6.8 Various airways and ventilatory tubes. (A) Mini tracheostomy tube. (B) Nasopharyngeal tube. (C) Oral airways. (D) Tracheostomy tube. (E) Fenestrated tracheostomy tube. (F) Endotracheal tube.

Advantages and disadvantages of airway management techniques		
Method	**Advantages**	**Disadvantages**
Oral endotracheal tube (ETT)	Easier intubation	Difficult oral care Lip reading difficult High level of discomfort Gagging
Nasal endotracheal tube	Greater security than with oral ETT	Less discomfort than with oral ETT Easier access for oral care Lip reading easier More skill required for insertion
Tracheostomy	Percutaneous method can be performed on Intensive Care Unit Lip reading easier Tolerated better than other methods Reduced dead space facilitates weaning Oral hygiene Speaking tubes available	Theatre required for tracheostomy, requiring surgery Patients prone to chest infection Tracheostomy site infection

Table 6.9 Advantages and disadvantages of airway management techniques.

airway. In the absence of the physiotherapist and doctor, nurses need to be competent to perform this assessment and to recognise when a doctor or physiotherapist is required to treat the patient.

VENTILATION

Intensive care facilities are required to provide patients with the equipment to support ventilatory needs. Piped oxygen, air and ventilators, which have the capabilities to provide a variety of ventilatory modes to accommodate the individual needs of patients requiring both long- and short-term ventilation, are essential. To detect problems and signs of deterioration, continuous monitoring and observation are important.

FLUID MANAGEMENT

One of the nurse's responsibilities is the accurate administration of fluids prescribed by the medical staff and the recording thereof. All patients require early detection of fluid imbalance, which may present in a number of ways. While the nurse monitors the urine output by measuring it hourly, there are additional signs to be observed, including alterations in the cardiovascular status of the patient and electrolyte abnormalities. Tachycardia, hypotension, a low CVP, a low PCWP and oliguria indicate hypovolaemia. Physical signs are dryness of the mouth, sunken eyes and loss of skin elasticity. High urine osmolality, low urinary

sodium and raised haematocrit may also assist in the diagnosis. Fluid overload may not be as easily detected although physical signs will be noticeable. These include generalised puffiness, particularly apparent on the hands and fingers if the patient is wearing a ring. If the patient has been lying in a supine position, puffiness around the eyes, and facial swelling may be particularly noticeable where tapes have been used to secure the endotracheal tube. The haematocrit will be decreased indicating haemodilution, the heart rate rapid, and the urine volume and urinary sodium variable depending on the aetiology.

PHYSICAL AND PSYCHOLOGICAL CARE

SEDATION AND ANALGESIA
Most patients require some form of sedation and analgesia during their stay in the ICU (Aitkenhead, 1989). Sedation, analgesia and the occasional use of muscle relaxants are used to promote comfort, facilitate ventilation, improve tolerance to tubes and invasive procedures, and induce sleep (Bion, 1988; McMurray, 1991; Vinik and Kissin, 1991).

SEDATION
Over the past few years there has been a general trend for fewer patients in the UK to receive muscle relaxants (Reeve and Wallace, 1991). There is also an increasing number of patients who are cared for with less sedation, and there is some concern that this increases the amount

of stress patients suffer (Gow, 1995). A reduction in the sedation reduces the problems of prolonged weaning, hence reducing the length of stay on the ICU with its resulting cost implications.

By using sedation scoring, the patient continually receives the optimum amount of sedation, promoting appropriate levels of sedation and comfort. A sedation scoring system adapted from Laing (1992) is one example (Table 6.10).

The patient may require a bolus of sedation and/or analgesia before undergoing painful procedures, and treatment including physiotherapy. This requires careful planning by the nurse and the multidisciplinary teams involved. The correct choice of drugs is important and is dependent on the condition and the plan of treatment for the patient. Two examples of sedatives are given below.

Propofol

Propofol is a quick-acting non-cumulative sedative with a short halflife, and can be used when a patient is unlikely to require long-term ventilation. Propofol, however, is expensive and high in lipid content, and is unsuitable for patients requiring sedation for more than 72 hours.

Midazolam

For patients requiring long-term ventilation midazolam can be used although caution must be exercised — particularly in those patients with impaired liver and renal function, due to its accumulation.

PAIN ASSESSMENT

When considering patients' needs for sedation, their need for analgesia must also be determined. The use of recognised pain assessment scales is limited in intensive care where patients have communication difficulties. While the physiological signs of pain must be used as part of the assessment, including tachycardia, hyperventilation, hypo- and hypertension, other signs such as grimacing, muscle tension and increased airway pressures need consideration. Pain is an individual experience, and culture, age, gender and known pain threshold need to be examined when assessing pain in the patient who is unable to communicate. Commonly used analgesics include fentanyl, alfentanil and morphine via continuous infusion.

PHYSICAL CARE

Critically ill patients are entirely dependent upon the nurse to care holistically for their needs. The importance of general care to avoid the complications of bed rest caused by immobility, including pressure sores, respiratory infections and thrombosis, must not be underestimated. The patient is also at risk from the complications of invasive monitoring, infections of the eyes and mouth and malnutrition. The nurse needs to develop the knowledge and skills to prevent these complications, and to manage ventilation, monitoring and drug therapy while not overlooking the basic needs of patients to ensure their comfort and safety.

NORTH STAFFORDSHIRE HOSPITAL NHS TRUST
Directorate of Anaesthesia

RESUMÉ OF THE SEDATION SCORING FOR THE ASSESSMENT OF VENTILATED PATIENTS

SCORE	
1	Unmanageable, agitated, disoriented
2	Awake and oriented
3	Roused by voice or touch. The patient may require bolus sedation, as well as the background sedation cover prior to handling
4	Roused by voice or touch. The patient does not require bolus sedation and tolerates handling and procedures well
5	Sluggish level
6	Flat level
	Sedation levels 3 & 4 are ideal levels allowing the patients to tolerate treatments, general nursing care, physiotherapy and suction without compromising their ventilation or cardiovascular state
	Sedation levels 5 & 6 are only acceptable in certain cases, i.e.: a The patient who is receiving neuromuscular blocking agents b The critically ill unstable patient where heavy sedation is desirable
	To be used in conjunction with the *Intensive Care Unit Standard of Care in Sedation and Analgesia*

Table 6.10 Resume of the sedation scoring for the assessment of ventilated patients.

Although most patients require turning every 2–3 hours, patients need to be assessed individually and care delivered accordingly. Most critically ill patients are at risk of pressure sore development (Waterlow, 1991). Some patients cannot be turned due to their injuries or cardiovascular instability and therefore skin integrity needs to be maintained by using either therapeutic beds or mattresses.

PSYCHOLOGICAL CARE

During the critical period priority will be given to the patient's stability and the need to maintain life support; however, it is important that the patient's psychological needs are considered. The intensive care environment can be overwhelming for patients, visitors and, on occasion, staff. It is noisy, warm and often a hive of activity and the cause of sensory overload, sensory deprivation and sleep loss. Orientation of patients to their surroundings is an important role for the nurse in an attempt to assist in patients' understanding of the situation and reduce stress and anxiety. There is also a need to distinguish between day- and night-time by reducing care activities whenever possible, using subdued lighting and keeping noise to a minimum. Baker (1992) measured noise levels greater than 65 decibels (dB) in intensive care, a level which interferes with sleep and speech. While some patients are prepared for their critical care experience, particularly if they are transferred to the ICU post-operatively, many patients wake up in the unit psychologically ill-prepared and anxious. It is well documented that patients experience communication difficulties due to endotracheal tube attachment and, as a result of drug therapy, are often unable to convey their thoughts and feelings, pain and discomfort, thereby increasing stress levels (Pennock et al., 1994). While staff and visitors are able to benefit from breaks and days off, patients are not, some spending weeks in this environment. It is therefore essential that carers assess the needs of the patient and plan their care in the patient's best interests, considering physiological and psychological requirements. As patients progress to a lower dependency, they become more psychologically aware, with increased needs. This then calls upon the skills of the nurse to alleviate fear and frustration and, with communication difficulties, exasperation on both sides (Bergbom-Endberg and Haljamae, 1993).

ROLE OF THE PHYSIOTHERAPIST

The first visit to an ICU can be a disorienting experience for the novice physiotherapist. The patient is surrounded by an array of tubes, monitors, machines, flashing lights and bleeping noises, to such an extent it is sometimes difficult to see the person. Familiarity with the equipment and the environment diminishes the sensory overload, but remember the first impact felt by you, and therefore how your patient will be feeling.

This section will define the physiotherapist's role in the ICU. It will look at the common reasons for admission to intensive care, the effects of positive pressure ventilation, the adverse effects of prolonged immobilisation, assessment of the patient, physiotherapy treatment techniques, the hazards of physiotherapy intervention to the critically ill patient, and specific patient problems.

ADMISSION TO INTENSIVE CARE

The physiotherapist on the ICU will encounter a wide variety of patient pathologies, but the reasons for admission fall broadly into two categories—elective and emergency.

The planned admissions to intensive care consist of patients undergoing high risk surgery. These patients may require elective post-operative ventilation or monitoring of vital signs, e.g. to observe for cardiovascular instability or respiratory problems. Another group of patients electively admitted to intensive care following relatively minor surgery are those with a medical history indicating that the ensuing period may be problematic, e.g. a previous adverse reaction to anaesthesia or severe chronic lung disease. Those patients who require monitoring are more likely to be nursed on the HDU where the cost is considerably less than if an intensive care bed were to be used.

The non-elective admissions to intensive care are many and varied. Such patients' medical status before admission to the unit may not be known, and having had no preparation for the experience they are likely to be very frightened.

Not every patient admitted to the ICU will require physiotherapy treatment. Accurate assessment will establish any such need, but must also consider the problems associated with positive pressure ventilation and immobilisation. The role of the physiotherapist in prevention will be discussed later in the chapter. Assessment will ascertain if active treatment should be deferred until the patient's condition has stabilised.

EFFECTS OF POSITIVE PRESSURE VENTILATION

Positive pressure ventilation reverses the normal ventilation gradient and increases the perfusion gradient, resulting in a V/Q mismatch. The reversal of the ventilation gradient is due firstly to the positive pressure of the ventilator forcing the air/oxygen mixture into the areas of least resistance, i.e. the upper areas of the lungs; and secondly, to the diaphragm becoming passive, moving down in response to the pressure from the ventilator (Froese and Bryan, 1974). The result of these two effects is poor ventilation of the basal areas of the lungs, which become progressively atelectatic. The perfusion gradient is increased by ventilation because the positive pressure forces more of the pulmonary circulation to the dependent areas of the lungs. A minimum oxygen requirement of 30% is normally required to maintain a normal arterial oxygen tension caused by the V/Q mismatch. If high concentrations of oxygen are required to maintain tissue oxygenation, nitrogen washout occurs, i.e. the inert nitrogen that normally remains in the alveoli during gaseous exchange is lost causing micro-atelectasis. PEEP is used to decrease the oxygen requirement, by increasing the surface area available for gaseous exchange.

Intermittent positive pressure ventilation (IPPV) affects the work of breathing. It can greatly decrease the work of breathing of the exhausted patient in respiratory failure by reducing or eliminating the effort of the muscles of inspiration. Conversely, it can increase the work of breathing if the patient fights against the ventilator. In this situation:

- The patient may need to be sedated.
- The mode of ventilation needs to be synchronised with the patient's pattern of breathing.
- The patient is allowed to breath spontaneously.

Which option is chosen will depend on the general status of the patient.

The debilitated and immunosuppressed status of patients in intensive care makes them very susceptible to bacterial infection in the respiratory tract. Nosocomial pneumonia occurs in about 21% of all ventilated patients. Those at the highest risk of nosocomial pneumonia include patients:

- With medical chest pathology.
- Requiring ICP monitoring.
- With ARDS.
- Admitted during the winter months (Pingleton, 1988).

The secondary cause is the presence of an endotracheal or tracheostomy tube, irritating the respiratory tract to cause an increase in tracheobronchial mucous production, combined with a decrease in mucociliary clearance, which produces an environment perfect for colonisation by bacteria. In some units, patients will be routinely prescribed broad spectrum antibiotics to counter this risk, but the development of resistant strains of bacteria is changing the emphasis to using only specific antibiotics after a positive sputum sample.

Physiotherapists must play their part in prevention of infection—the importance of sterile technique during suctioning cannot be over emphasised. The potential for cross-infection from treating one patient after another without changing plastic aprons and thorough hand washing is very high. The use of latex gloves when handling some patients, e.g. patients positive to methicillin resistant *Staphylococcus aureus,* may be hospital policy. It is the individual's responsibility to understand and adhere to the hospital's policy.

IPPV increases intrathoracic pressure which impedes venous return to the heart. An increase in the resting heart rate is the compensatory mechanism, but if cardiac function is inadequate the cardiac output will fall. The application of PEEP can exacerbate this problem. Patients with a low cardiac output unable to maintain their blood pressure without inotropic support may not be able to tolerate physiotherapeutic input. This is because the heart cannot increase its output in response to the body's demand.

EFFECTS OF IMMOBILISATION
Prolonged immobilisation affects the musculoskeletal, cardiovascular, respiratory, metabolic and central nervous systems. The effect of prolonged bed rest on a critically ill patient can be devastating.

Inactivity can decrease muscle strength at a rate of up to 20% per week. For each successive week a further 20% reduction occurs (Sciaky, 1994). This means that a recovering patient sedated and ventilated for 4 weeks may have only 41% of muscle strength available at weaning, and after 8 weeks less than 17%. Mobilisation at the earliest opportunity facilitates successful weaning from mechanical ventilation.

Immobility causes a shift in body fluids to the thorax, which even in healthy subjects subjected to periods of supine lying cannot be overcome by performing vigorous exercise (Ross and Dean, 1989). Orthostatic intolerance occurs within hours, emphasising the importance of monitoring blood pressure in the upright position and taking graduated steps towards this position if the effects are profound. Exercise prescription must take into account the increased basal heart rate, decreased maximal heart rate, decreased vital capacity and V/Q mismatch. Compounded by the reduction in the haemoglobin content of blood, the patient's ability to exercise is reduced. Mobilisation sessions must initially be short and frequent to avoid fatigue.

Other effects of immobilisation include malnutrition, osteoporosis and psychosis. There is also an increased risk of venous thrombosis, pressure sores and joint contractures.

PSYCHOLOGICAL EFFECTS OF INTENSIVE CARE
Patients in intensive care, and their families, are subjected to severe physical and emotional stress. Fortunately the majority of patients will have total amnesia of their time on the ICU even if they were conscious and holding a conversation. Some patients have distorted dream-like memories, where their days merge into one another, while others have hallucinations. Fifteen per cent of patients develop serious psychological problems such as aggression, anxiety, emotional outbursts and personality changes, termed ICU psychosis. The use of powerful sedatives, sleep deprivation and the loss of the normal circadian cycle can leave the patient with a poor concentration span, agitated and unco-operative. Physiotherapists can reduce the negative impact of their treatment on patients by involving them in decision making even when semi-conscious, co-ordinating position changes with nursing procedures, and, most importantly, explaining everything to the patient in lay terms. If the procedure is likely to be distressing, e.g. manual hyperinflation, ask for the sedation to be increased during the treatment. The family will also need support and reassurance, the physiotherapist's role being explained and their involvement in the patient's care allowed. They need to understand the purpose of physiotherapy procedures which appear distressing, to be able to give informed consent to treatment or to deny it so as not to prolong suffering.

RESPIRATORY ASSESSMENT OF THE VENTILATED PATIENT
The basis of any physiotherapy intervention is an accurate assessment of the patient's overall status. The principles of a respiratory assessment are set out in Chapter 2. This section will focus on the patient who is mechanically ventilated.

When assessing ventilated patients as opposed to those not ventilated there are fundamental differences which have to be addressed. Firstly, there is a vast, almost overwhelming, amount of objective data available. Patients are monitored continuously during their time on intensive care, with data being documented hourly. The most frequently collected information is listed in Table 6.8. Secondly, the sedated and ventilated patient will not be able to give you any subjective data or history. Thirdly, the patient's condition can change very rapidly. The following guide to the objective assessment of sedated and ventilated patients is based on asking a series of questions:

WHAT IS THE GENERAL CONDITION OF THE PATIENT?

Several critieria need to be taken into account when assessing the general condition of the patient. These include:
- Position of the patient: the cardiopulmonary assessment will establish if this is appropriate.
- Type of bed: does it allow for the patient to be therapeutically positioned, or does it hinder mobilisation?
- Site and type of all infusion lines, drainage tubes, monitoring equipment, surgical incisions and external fixators.
- Colour and condition of skin, e.g. cyanosed, flushed, sweating, presence of pressure sores, dry and flaking skin, peripheral or generalised oedema, finger clubbing.
- Core and peripheral temperatures: have heating or cooling devices being employed? Poor peripheral perfusion will decrease the accuracy of SO_2 monitoring.
- Nutritional status, i.e. obesity and malnutrition.

HOW MUCH VENTILATORY SUPPORT DOES THE PATIENT NEED?

It is important to decide the level of ventilatory support a patient needs. Criteria useful in deciding this include:
- Airway: endotracheal tube (oral or nasal), tracheostomy (i.e. fenestrated, allowing speech or unfenestrated) cuff (i.e. inflated, deflated or uncuffed). How long has this been employed? Is the patient likely to aspirate?
- Type of ventilator, i.e. volume or pressure cycled, high frequency jet ventilation, non-invasive.

- Ventilation setting, i.e. controlled ventilation, SIMV, with or without PEEP, continuous positive airway (CPAP) pressure, positive pressure support. Is the ventilatory support to the patient increasing or is the patient being weaned?
- Spontaneous and mechanical respiratory rate, V_T, minute volume, lung compliance, increasing or decreasing airway pressure, i.e. look at long-term trends and for sudden changes (Table 6.11).
- Percentage oxygen delivery, i.e. increasing or decreasing reliance, is pre-oxygenation needed before suction?
- Arterial blood gas analysis, i.e. the effectiveness of gas exchange. Is the patient improving, static, deteriorating?

IS ANY LUNG PATHOLOGY PRESENT AMENABLE TO PHYSIOTHERAPY TECHNIQUES?

Deciding whether lung disease is amenable to physiotherapy will depend on:
- Chest appearance, e.g. deformities, congenital or acquired; presence of incision sites and intercostal drains.
- Chest movement, i.e. is it symmetrical? Asymmetry may indicate pneumothorax, intubation of right bronchus or sputum plugging. During weaning, a high spontaneous respiratory rate, shallow depth, use of accessory muscles, indrawing of intercostals, paradoxical abdominal movement and asynchrony with the ventilator indicate fatigue or respiratory failure.
- Palpation: the position of the trachea indicates midline shift, percussion note, e.g. dull, resonant or hyperresonant, tactile fremitus indicating sputum.
- Auscultation, i.e. are breath sounds symmetrical, diminished, absent, increased? Added sounds include ventilator/tubing noise, crepitations, wheeze, cuff leak (usually adventitious squeak) and pleural rub.
- Sputum, i.e. quantity, colour, character, microbiology.
- Humidification: heat and moisture exchanger or heated water humidification, temperature of heated water humidification. Is the humidification adequate?
- Chest X-ray findings. N.B. X-ray findings may lag 24–48 hours behind clinical signs. A sudden change in

Table 6.11 The ventilated patient: causes of change in airway pressure.

The ventilated patient: causes of change in airway pressure		
	High airway pressure	**Low airway pressure**
Consistent or slow change	Fibrosis, Bronchospasm Pulmonary oedema	Pressure controlled ventilation
Sudden change	Coughing Fighting ventilator Pneumothorax Obstructed tubing	Leak in tubing

Characteristic cardiovascular signs					
	CVP	PAP	PCWP	BP	CO
Left ventricular failure			↑ >20	↓	↓
Right ventricular failure	↑				
Adult respiratory distress syndrome		↑	<18		
Hypervolaemia (overload)	↑			↑	
Hypovolaemia	↓			↓	
IPPV	↑	↑	↑		

Table 6.12 Characteristic cardiovascular signs.

respiratory signs warrants an immediate X-ray to confirm/exclude pneumothorax or acute atelectasis.

IS THE CARDIOVASCULAR SYSTEM LIKELY TO BE AFFECTED BY PHYSIOTHERAPY INTERVENTION?

It is important to decide whether any physiotherapy intervention will affect the cardiovascular system by considering the following criteria:

- The pre-set cardiovascular parameters set by the medical staff, e.g. keep systolic blood pressure below 150 mmHg, CVP at 8–12.
- Heart rate and rhythm from ECG—what are the prescribed anti-arrythmic drugs?
- Blood pressure, i.e. low, normal, high, wide fluctuations, requiring inotropic support or vasodilators to maintain blood pressure in stable limits. Adverse cardiovascular responses to previous intervention.
- Cardiac output studies, i.e. CVP, PCWP, pulmonary artery pressure, BP, CO (Table 6.12).

IS THE RENAL FUNCTION CONTRIBUTING TO RESPIRATORY PROBLEMS?

To determine whether renal function is contributing to respiratory problems, check:

- Fluid balance, i.e. cumulative balance, evidence of oedema or dehydration.
- Renal function tests.
- Type of dialysis.

IS THE PATIENT ABLE TO TAKE AN ACTIVE ROLE IN TREATMENT?

To determine whether a patient is able to take an active role in treatment, check:

- Consciousness level and ability to co-operate, i.e. is it increasing or decreasing?
- Pain management, i.e. is it adequate?
- The level of sedation, use of paralysing agents, e.g. are adverse reactions to suction due to inadequate sedation?
- Pupil size and reaction, i.e. response to stimuli.

- ICP and cerebral perfusion pressure, i.e. response to intervention.

ARE THERE ANY LIMITATIONS TO MOBILISATION?

The patient's level of mobility will depend on several factors:

- Degree of dependence, i.e. from needing assistance to totally paralysed and sedated.
- Decreased muscle strength or paralysis.
- Limitations to range of movement to any joints, especially thoracic spine, neck and shoulder girdle, tendo achilles, and finger joints in oedematous patients.
- Fixation of fractures and their stability. Possible spinal fracture, then log roll patient until cleared by medical staff.

ARE THERE ANY CONTRAINDICATIONS TO PHYSIOTHERAPY?

Several factors may preclude physiotherapy intervention. These include:

- Low or unstable blood pressure, i.e. systolic blood pressure <80–90 mmHg.
- High blood pressure, i.e. systolic blood pressure >180 mmHg. N.B. Following vascular surgery the limit may be lower, e.g. 120 mmHg.
- Raised ICP, i.e. >15, cerebral perfusion pressure <70 mmHg.
- Active treatment withdrawn, unless to make the patient comfortable.
- Patient or carers refuse treatment.

PHYSIOTHERAPY MANAGEMENT OF CRITICALLY ILL PATIENTS (FIGURE 6.9)

PRO-ACTIVE ROLE IN VENTILATED PATIENTS WITH PULMONARY PATHOLOGY

The role of the physiotherapist in the ICU in the treatment of respiratory problems is well established. The common pathologies amenable to physiotherapeutic techniques are

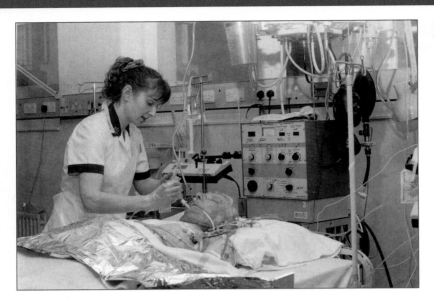

Figure 6.9 Physiotherapist treating an intensive care patient.

retained secretions, consolidation and acute/progressive atelectasis. The causes, recognition and treatment of these problems are outlined below.

Retained Secretions

Causes
The causes of retained secretions include infection, aspiration, inadequate humidification and patient immobility.

Signs
The signs of retained secretions can be determined by:
- Auscultation, e.g. coarse crackles, decreased breath sounds if combined with atelectasis.
- X-ray, i.e. sometimes patchy consolidation is present.
- Arterial blood gas analysis, i.e. deteriorating PaO_2 and SaO_2; $PaCO_2$ may increase.
- Ventilator, i.e. airway pressure may increase if secretions are very thick and copious or plugging bronchi.

Treatment
The sedated and ventilated patient is unable to make an active effort to remove excessive secretions, and therefore passive methods have to be employed. Percussion and manual vibrations on expiration are the traditional methods to facilitate sputum clearance. Adverse cardiovascular events during percussion have caused some researchers to advise against such use (Connors *et al.*, 1980; Hammon *et al.*, 1992; Jones *et al.*, 1992; Dean, 1994) when performed at the optimal 5–6 Hz. Slow one-handed percussion at 1 Hz has not been evaluated, but used appropriately by clinicians in North Staffordshire, rarely has adverse effects. A mechanical vibrator is well tolerated by patients with rib fractures and head injuries, although less efficient at mobilising secretions.

Regular position changes of sedated patients, and active movement of conscious patients, is highly effective in mobilising secretions and stimulating a cough reflex.

Thick and tenacious sputum may indicate inadequate humidification; therefore, institute heated humidification;

if it is already in use, check it is working correctly and the patient is not underhydrated. Nebulised 0.9% saline can be administered to raise the humidity before treatment.

Manual hyperinflation may be used for mobilising secretions. This technique is frequently contraindicated in critically ill patients, and should not be used routinely. Vibrations on expiration assist the peripheral clearance of secretions but do not affect central clearance (Bateman *et al.*, 1981). The conscious patient may find the procedure very distressing unless the hyperinflations are synchronised with his or her own respiratory cycle. Postural drainage positions may be utilised to enhance clearance, but as the abdominal contents force the diaphragm upwards, the ventilator cannot aerate the bases. The modified postural drainage positions for basal lung segments will be side lying and prone lying; it is not normally appropriate to head down tip. The active cycle of breathing technique (Pryor and Webber, 1992) can be taught to patients who are able to take spontaneous breaths.

Consolidation

Causes
Causes of consolidation include infection, persistent atelectasis, lung contusion, ARDS, pulmonary oedema and carcinoma.

Signs
The signs of consolidation can be determined by:
- Auscultation, i.e. of the area of bronchial breathing.
- Percussion, e.g. dull.
- X-ray, e.g. opacity of area involved with loss of border, air bronchogram in large area consolidation.

Treatment
Active treatment of unproductive pneumonic consolidation is limited to positioning to maximise V/Q matching. Infective consolidation will begin to resolve with antibiotics; resolution is indicated by a change in the type and/or quantity of

secretions and fine crackles on auscultation. Treatment can then be instituted to clear the sputum (see above).

Example

A 64-year-old male patient was admitted in respiratory failure with right lower and middle lobe pneumonia, and a history of COPD. Medical management included sedation and SIMV, FiO_2 40% with five of PEEP, 20 positive pressure support, supportive therapy and antibiotics. On auscultation, there were bronchial breath sounds throughout the right lung except for a small apical area; the left lung was intermittently wheezy. X-ray confirmed the consolidation. Scanty secretions were extracted by suction for 4 days. Bronchoscopy excluded obstruction and revealed only infective material. On the 5th day of ventilation, coarse crackles were audible on auscultation, tactile fremitus was present and copious yellow secretions had been suctioned by the nursing staff.

Treatment consisted of left side lying percussion and suction three times per day, with this position being preferred between treatments. X-ray examination confirmed complete resolution after 6 days of treatment. A 10 day slow wean from mechanical ventilation followed, and the patient was discharged from intensive care.

Atelectasis

Causes

Causes of atelectasis include:
- Acute lobar atelectasis, e.g. sputum plug, inhaled foreign body, intubation of right main bronchus.
- Progressive atelectasis, e.g. IPPV, abdominal distension, post-operative splinting, immobility, bronchial carcinoma.

Signs

The signs of atelectasis can be determined by:
- Auscultation, i.e. area of diminished or absent breath sounds.
- Chest movement, e.g. reduced over area.
- Acute lobar atelectasis.
- X-ray, i.e. tracheal shift to affected side and raised diaphragm on affected side (Figure 6.10).
- Arterial blood gas analysis, i.e. sudden deterioration in SaO_2 and PaO_2.
- Ventilator, i.e. sudden increase in airway pressure.

Treatment

Acute loss of breath sounds warrants an immediate X-ray to exclude pneumothorax or intubation of the right main bronchus.

Physiotherapy management of acute atelectasis requires positioning the atelectatic lobe uppermost, manual hyperinflation with vibrations and suction being most effective (Stiller *et al.*, 1990). The research evidence that sputum is affected by the instillation of normal saline is lacking. In the authors' experience 2–5 ml slowly trickled into the endotracheal tube while the affected lung is dependent can greatly assist clearance of sputum plugs. Following a successful treatment, check the humidification is adequate, leave instructions for continuing positioning, and suction to prevent recurrence (Figure 6.11).

If the cause is removed, progressive atelectasis can be treated by manual hyperinflation, which improves the lung compliance for up to 2 hours after treatment (Jones *et al.*, 1992). The dangers of this technique for the patient have to be weighed against the benefits, by the clinician.

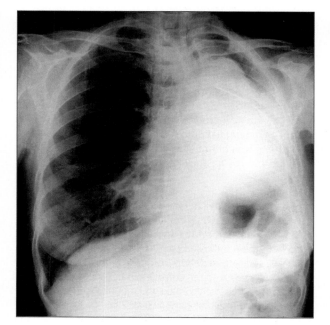

Figure 6.10 Chest X-ray showing collapse of left lung due to sputum plug.

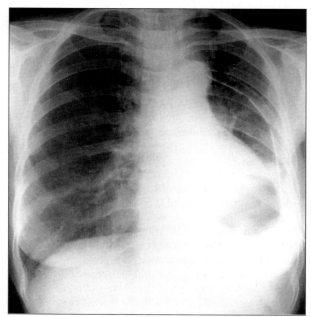

Figure 6.11 Chest X-ray showing the same lung as in Figure 6.10 after physiotherapy treatment.

Example

A 28-year-old male patient, comatose but self-ventilating via a tracheostomy tube following a head injury 3 weeks previously, had an acute episode of hypoxaemia (SaO_2 of 75%). Oxygen therapy initially at 100% gradually improved SaO_2 to normal limits. Chest X-ray showed a small mediastinal shift to the left, and a slightly raised left diaphragm. Medical staff assessed and diagnosed a pulmonary embolus. A subsequent V/Q scan showed reduced perfusion on the left side but totally absent ventilation. Nursing staff positioned the patient in right side lying but minimal secretions had been extracted. Physiotherapy was requested. Assessment noted an SaO_2 of 99% on 40% oxygen via a heated humidifier temperature of 34.5°C for the patient. Breathing was regular and not distressed (11/min). Chest expansion was reduced on the left side, and breath sounds were reduced on the same side.

Treatment consisted of left side lying and instillation of 5 ml of saline (0.9%); the patient was then turned to right side lying. Suction via a tracheostomy tube resulted in two large plugs of green mucus being extracted, followed by copious loose green secretions. The procedure was repeated producing copious secretions. After treatment, the oxygen requirement was reduced to 30%, and breath sounds and chest movement had increased on the left side. The temperature of the humidification was increased to 37°C for the patient. A bronchoscopy performed after physiotherapy treatment found no abnormality present. It was surmised that the perfusion defect was due to reflex hypoxic vasoconstriction in the left lung.

PRO-ACTIVE ROLE IN PATIENT MOBILISATION

The sedated and ventilated patient will succumb to the physiological effects of immobility, and the longer this period lasts the weaker the patient will be when weaning commences. Therefore, commence mobilisation when the patient is cardiovascularly and neurologically stable by routinely moving the limbs through their anatomical ranges. Patients nursed supine for long periods are prone to shortening of the tendo achilles. Stiffness in the neck and shoulders is particularly common in tracheostomy patients. Sit the patient up in bed for short periods to counter the effects of postural hypotension.

Positioning is a vital part of minimising the negative effects of immobilisation (Ross and Dean, 1989), but so long as all activity is passive, muscle wasting will occur.

Before active exercise can commence, the patient must be able to increase minute volume by taking spontaneous breaths, be cardiovascularly stable and have decreasing dependence on inotropic support. It is not necessary to wait until the patient is weaned from the ventilator before active exercise and even ambulation can begin. When the patient has been ventilated for hours rather than days, is fully conscious, pain free and co-operative, transfer him or her to a chair and ambulate as soon as practicable. The presence of intravenous lines is not a contraindication to mobilisation, but when many lines and tubes are present it may take several assistants to care for all the drip stands! If ambulation away from the bedside is limited by an underwater sealed drain on suction, exercises in standing or an exercise bike can be used instead.

The long-term ventilated patient can begin with simple exercises for the major muscle groups progressing from active-assisted to free movement and then resisted work. Initially, use low repetition rates, then gradually increase the rate and the resistance to increase endurance and strength (Sciaky, 1994), and encourage the patient to change his or her own position. The patient's relatives can be enlisted to help with these exercises. Prepare and involve the patient in the decision to sit out of bed for the first time. Following an acute life-threatening illness the patient will feel too weak and frightened to get out of bed. The severely debilitated person can be safely transferred using a mechanical hoist to minimise the work needed and prevent distress. Even if fully supported in a chair, the change of position and the perception of progress is very rewarding for patients, relatives and staff. The first adventure out of bed should be limited to 1 hour, building up gradually and always ensuring that fatigue is kept at bay. Frequently, the patient sitting out of bed for the first time in weeks will, on return to the bed, fall into the first non-drug-induced deep sleep.

Standing is much easier if it begins after independent sitting balance is achieved. Sitting on the side of the bed without support promotes the re-establishment of the normal balance mechanisms. Physiotherapists should take advice from their specialist colleagues in neurology before beginning this type of exercise with neurologically damaged patients. Standing a patient up for the first time after prolonged immobility will require three or more assistants—one therapist on either side of the patient and one other to take charge of the ventilator tubing and other lines. A patient with weak quadriceps and hip extensors (less than grade 3, Oxford scale) will require extra help to provide support. Postural hypotension may occur, and the patient should be returned quickly to bed. Falling blood pressure can be spotted if an indwelling arterial line is *in situ*, or by asking patients if they feel dizzy. Progress from standing to weight transference walking, then increase the distance and reduce the support.

Example

A 60-year-old female patient was admitted with sepsis from a leg wound, and ARF. Ventilation, CVVHD, and inotropic and antibiotic support for 3 weeks resolved the sepsis but kidney function indicated continuing failure. As the patient was weaned off sedation and the ventilatory support reduced, active exercises commenced. Tendo achilles (TA) stretching of the affected ankle was required. Sitting over the side of the bed for short periods over 2 days was followed by sitting out in a chair. While on a CPAP pressure of 5 cmH_2O and positive pressure support of 12 cmH_2O, standing and weight transference was practised. The following day the patient was extubated and later transferred to the HDU.

PRO-ACTIVE ROLE AFTER WEANING FROM VENTILATION

The period immediately after extubation is one where the physiotherapist can actively be involved in ensuring a smooth transition to full recovery. Common problems encountered by patients at this time are caused primarily by fatigue due to their generally poor condition.

Sputum Retention

Causes

Causes of sputum retention include:

- Inadequate cough, e.g. caused by weak muscles, poor co-ordination or reduced conscious level.
- Pain; patient will therefore resist expectorating the sputum to avoid discomfort.
- Inadequate humidification.
- Aspiration; a sluggish gag reflex.

Signs

See Table 6.13 for a list of the signs representative of retained sputum.

Treatment

Firstly, look at the reason why the patient is unable to expectorate. Check that the problem is pulmonary and not cardiac in cause (see Table 6.13). If sputum retention is due to fatigued muscles then put the patient into a position where he or she can cough most effectively with the minimum of energy expenditure. It is extremely difficult to expectorate when lying slumped in bed so if it is possible get the patient out of bed, the movement will assist sputum clearance. Pain is a common cause of sputum retention in the post-operative patient; the priority is to get analgesia prescribed and to give it immediately. Poor humidification resulting in tenacious secretions also requires early rectification; this can be identified by the patient being able to

perform an adequate cough or forced expiratory technique but being unable to clear the secretions.

The unconscious patient can be stimulated to cough by neurophysiological facilitation techniques which increase the rate and depth of breathing (Bethune, 1975).

When all other means have failed, suction using an airway or via the nasopharynx may be required; this procedure is contraindicated in some patients, and so a mini-tracheostomy will have to be inserted (Preston *et al.*, 1986) by a suitably trained doctor, ensuring suction is not traumatic.

Respiratory Distress

Causes

Causes of acute respiratory distress include:

- Chronic lung pathology.
- Fatigue.
- Bronchospasm.
- Neuromuscular dysfunction.

Signs

Signs of respiratory distress can be caused by:

- Respiratory problems, e.g. increasing tachypnoea and dyspnoea, and increased use of accessory muscles. Paradoxical breathing, recession of intercostal muscles and a tracheal tug may be evident.
- Cyanosis.
- Cardiovascular problems, e.g. hypertension and tachycardia.
- Neurological problems, e.g. decreased mental state.
- Increasing hypoxaemia, followed by increasing hypercarbia (shown by arterial blood gas analysis).

Treatment

Using positioning to allow breathing to take place by the minimum expenditure of energy is of primary importance. In bed the patient should be well supported and high side lying utilised. In a chair the patient should be either upright with arms supported on pillows, or forward lean sitting with arms resting on pillows on a bed-table.

Table 6.13 Differences between sputum retention and pulmonary oedema. (URT – upper respiratory tract; CVP – central venous pressure.)

Differences between sputum retention and pulmonary oedema		
Procedure	**Sputum retention**	**Pulmonary oedema**
Auscultation	Coarse crackles over URT	Dependent fine crackles
Temperature	Normal, or pyrexia if infection	Normal
Sputum	Purulent or mucoid	Frothy, white or pink
Chest X-ray	Normal, or lung collapse or consolidation	Engorged hilar, enlarged heart, pleural effusion
Fluid Balance	Normal	Retained fluid (+ve balance)
CVP	Normal	Raised
Orthopnoea	No	Yes

If positioning fails then mechanical support will be required. The hypoxaemic patient can be administered CPAP via a nose or face mask. A mouth piece can be used for periodic CPAP, and a 'T' piece if the patient has a tracheostomy or endotracheal tube. CPAP reduces the inspiratory work of breathing by increasing lung compliance. A reduction in work of breathing of 45% is achieved by CPAP at 10 cmH$_2$O, but the work increases above 20 cmH$_2$O (Gherini et al., 1979). As CPAP does not affect the V$_T$ it will not be appropriate to use it for cases where hypoventilation or hypercarbia are evident (Keilty and Bott, 1992).

When hypoxaemia and hypercarbia are present, intermittent positive pressure breathing (IPPB), nasal intermittent positive pressure ventilation (NIPPV) or BiPAP (both the latter have the facility to increase the tidal and minute volume) may be appropriate. The hyperventilation achieved will reduce the hypercarbia and correct hypoxia, without increasing the workload. The disadvantages of IPPB of inadequate flow rate, pressure controlled V$_T$, and lack of apnoea back-up have been remedied by NIPPV and BiPAP (Bott et al., 1992). No matter which profession, whether physician, anaesthetist, respiratory nurse or physiotherapist, applies, the mechanical aids will depend on the policy of the unit. If the patient fails to respond to non-invasive ventilation due to intolerance of the mask or extreme fatigue then the anaesthetists will need to re-intubate and ventilate the patient.

PHYSIOTHERAPIST IN AN ADVISORY ROLE

There are many situations on the ICU when physiotherapists can act in an advisory role; their assessment and problem solving expertise, skills learnt in other fields of physiotherapy, and clinical autonomy can all be used to benefit patients.

Not all patients admitted to the ICU will require physiotherapy intervention—assessment may indicate that there is no active lung pathology present, and therefore a prescriptive regimen of regular turning and suction is advised to maintain this status. ICU nursing staff are trained to perform this basic care, freeing valuable physiotherapy time for patients requiring pro-active intervention. Other patients may require a positioning regimen to prevent deterioration overnight, e.g. after a day of active treatment for atelectasis. Document the regimen you require so that each subsequent carer is aware of this.

An accurate chest assessment may signal a need to change the type of humidification. Interpreting the difference between scant and retained secretions will determine whether a heat and moisture exchanger or water bath humidifier is required. Experienced physiotherapists will recognise whether a change to the ventilatory mode is required, and when the optimal status has been achieved to commence weaning or to carry out extubation.

Physiotherapists are at an advantage on the ICU in bringing skills and knowledge from other areas of the profession. While the care is primarily respiratory, patients admitted to the general unit can have multiple and varied pathologies. The appropriate positioning of a neurological patient with increased tone can minimise stimulation of abnormal patterning. Advise on the proper handling of these patients will prevent a conflict of interest detrimental to recovery. Likewise, the management of fractured limbs either in plaster or after fixation is within the scope of practice, with the physiotherapist able to advise on care and detect any problems early.

There are some patients for whom physiotherapy would be detrimental, and other members of the multi-disciplinary team should be informed of this immediately; for example, if a patient with unstable blood pressure has a respiratory problem, the clearing of the chest should take second place to maintaining vital organ perfusion.

ROLE OF THE PHYSIOTHERAPIST IN PREVENTIVE CARE

The adverse effects of ventilation and immobilisation cannot be overcome by preventive care, but good care may minimise some of the difficulties. Patients admitted to the unit without lung pathology ideally would not acquire nosocomial pneumonia, which would hinder recovery. Therefore:

- Ensure all personnel pay scrupulous attention to their sterile technique of suction.
- Prescribe regular changes of position.

Avoiding the supine position is more difficult to achieve. Haemodynamically unstable patients will not tolerate changes in position, which can precipitate a fall in cardiac output of up to 25% (Winslow et al., 1990). Continuous lateral rotation beds have been used to attempt to overcome this problem, but some patients will not tolerate the gentlest movement. Maintaining muscle strength, joint movement and cardio-respiratory reserves by active exercise has been discussed above.

PHYSIOTHERAPY FOR SPECIFIC CONDITIONS

NEUROSURGICAL/HEAD INJURED PATIENTS
Acute Stage
These patients are frequently sedated, paralysed and hyperventilated for 24–48 hours to prevent hypoxia or hypercarbia causing secondary brain damage. The rule with these patients is minimal necessary handling. These patients will not normally be treated unless the parameters below are achieved and stable:

- Cerebral perfusion pressure = mean arterial pressure – ICP ≥70.
- ICP ≤15.

During the acute stage, the physiotherapist's assessment is required to identify any respiratory problems which may affect gas exchange. Aspiration of gastric contents at the time of injury is common, and if lack of treatment may affect gas exchange. No routine treatment should be administered during this phase, and suctioning should be kept to a minimum as it raises the ICP.

When treatment is indicated, request additional sedation to minimise its detrimental effects (Klein *et al.*, 1988). Very gently change the patient's position (harmonise with nursing procedures to keep the handling to a minimum). Keep the head in a midline position, raised 30° from the horizontal, and minimise flexing the hips to maintain the brain's venous drainage. Manual techniques to clear secretions can all potentially raise the ICP; a mechanical vibrator is less likely to have this effect than manual percussion, but vibrations are most likely to be detrimental (Garradd and Bullock, 1986). Manual hyperinflation is controversial, but if used it is essential to hyperventilate the patient to maintain a low carbon dioxide level.

Subacute Stage

As the sedatives are eliminated from the patient's body, the full extent of the neurological damage becomes apparent. Weaning from the ventilator can be problematic as the patient's central control systems may be damaged causing either hypo- or hyperventilation. Cough and/or gag reflexes may be absent. Apart from irreversible brain damage, chest infection is the largest killer of these patients, therefore constant attention to the respiratory system is needed. Sitting out of bed is advocated as early as possible, before full consciousness and, in some cases, before weaning from the ventilator to provide normal stimulus to the patient. Refer to neurological specialists for advice on ongoing management.

DRUG OVERDOSE

Patients having intentionally taken a drug overdose or having taken illegal substances are frequently seen in the ICU. Previously healthy individuals require assessing for possible aspiration of gastric contents. These patients are screened for toxic damage and weaned early. If neurological damage has occurred then treat under guidance from specialist colleagues.

UPPER ABDOMINAL SURGERY

Since the advent of shorter anaesthesia and better pain control, the majority of general surgery patients no longer require physiotherapy; a regimen of sitting out of bed on the first post-operative day and encouragement to mobilise by the nursing staff is normally adequate. Those patients with the risk factors of COPD, current smoking history, obesity or malnutrition, or musculoskeletal or neurological impairment may be nursed on an HDU post-operatively. Those seen on the ICU have undergone radical resection, or have had peri- or post-operative complications.

The spontaneously breathing patient needs adequate analgesia to promote the ability to deep breathe and cough effectively, without inducing drowsiness or decreased respiratory drive. Sputum retention and basal atelectasis are common problems. Close attention to fluid balance is needed as over- or underhydration are often the causes of problems; a CVP reading will confirm suspicions.

ABDOMINAL AORTIC ANEURYSM REPAIR

Patients who undergo repair of an abdominal aortic aneurysm (AAA) require close monitoring for 48 hours after surgery for signs of bleeding from the graft site, and hence are nursed. Encourage the patient to basal ventilate by positioning in side-lying and to practise deep breathing with an inspiratory hold. Teach the patient to support the wound when coughing and, if stable, mobilise after 48 hours.

These patients are often cardiovasculary unstable for many days after surgery, and therefore mobilisation will have to be deferred. Renal failure and lower limb ischaemia may complicate their recovery.

SEPTIC SHOCK

Septic shock is a complication of uncontrolled infection or ischaemia of the bowel. It is diagnosed by a Swann–Ganz catheter showing a very high cardiac output, profound peripheral vasodilation (systemic vascular resistance index <300) and hypotension. These highly cardiovascularly unstable patients often develop multi-organ failure. The benefit of physiotherapy is limited in the early stages, but if supportive treatment is effective then pro-active treatment will be required to reverse the effects of prolonged immobility.

ARDS

On auscultation these patients have harsh breath sounds and often interstitial crackles in the dependent lung areas. The X-ray will show a generally ground glass appearance with the costophrenic angles spared. The fibrotic lung changes are characterised by rising airway pressures and refractory hypoxaemia in ventilated patients of ARDS. Pressure controlled or jet ventilation reduce the risk of pneumothorax.

Secretions are often scant in these patients, and manual physiotherapeutic techniques inappropriate. Physiotherapeutic positioning in the prone position to maximise V/Q matching is indicated (Pappert *et al.*, 1994). A concurrent infection in some patients can be treated by manual hyperinflation while PEEP is maintained (Enright, 1992). The prognosis for these patients is poor but the survivors range from those who have full recovery of their respiratory function to those who have permanent lung damage.

COPD

Treatment should take account of the previous irreversible lung damage. These patients often have copious thick secretions, and physiotherapists should ensure the patient is optimally humidified. A heated water bath will have less irritant effect on sensitive airways, and will assist the removal of tenacious secretions. Manual hyperinflation is hazardous as the high pressures needed to inflate the lungs can result in barotrauma with emphysematous bullae being particularly vulnerable. Weaning is often slow as the patient's 'normal' hypoxic drive may have been lost by the use of high levels of oxygen. Mobilisation should take account of previous exercise tolerance. These patients will often not be invasively ventilated because of the irreversible lung damage and difficulty of weaning from IPPV.

ASTHMA

During an acute exacerbation of asthma, physiotherapy aims to reduce the work of breathing. Positioning in relaxed breathing stance, IPPB may be effective if initiated before the patient is fatigued. If in spite of these techniques the PCO_2 begins to rise, then IPPV is required with heated humidification to assist removal of sputum plugs. Acute bronchospasm indicated by high airway pressures and an expiratory wheeze will contraindicate manual techniques.

NEUROMUSCULAR DISORDERS

The disease pathology may determine the support required by these patients. When the inspiratory muscles are weak, positive pressure support is required. If ventilation is adequate but the expiratory muscles are affected, the patient's cough may be ineffective and a mini-tracheostomy is advised. Passive movements and splinting are essential for the paralysed limbs. Active exercise should not fatigue the patient with either the Guillian–Barré syndrome or myasthenia gravis.

Critical Illness Neuropathy

Some acutely ill patients suffer from critical illness neuropathy, which becomes apparent when difficulty is experienced during weaning. Characterized by low tone, this is a self-limiting syndrome with complete recovery taking from weeks to years. Treatment will depend on the extent and the severity of the neuropathy.

Spinal Injuries

Patients with spinal injuries cannot be moved in the normal way until the spine is stabilised. They must be log rolled in bed or nursed on a spinal bed. Treatment for concurrent respiratory problems will have to be adapted during this phase. Injury above T6 will leave abdominal muscle paralysis, and the patient will need to be assisted to cough. This is done by placing the heels of both hands together on the centre of the abdomen immediately below the rib cage and pressing in an upward and inward direction in synchrony with expiration. When mobilisation is allowed, begin by progressively lifting the head of the bed until the patient can sit erect without suffering postural hypotension. The patient is normally transferred to a specialised spinal unit as soon as medically stable, but until then exercise should concentrate on increasing the strength of spared muscle groups, and maintaining functional range of movement of the paralysed muscles can begin. High level tetraplegics can now survive with lifelong use of positive pressure support via a tracheostomy or by using a negative pressure cuirass.

BURNS/SMOKE INHALATION

The clinical picture may include elements of sputum retention, bronchospasm and pulmonary oedema. Continuous humidification is required and suction kept to a minimum with the gentlest pressure possible. Using manual techniques to assist sputum clearance will depend on the site and extent of external burns (Keilty, 1993).

PULMONARY OEDEMA

Production of copious frothy white secretions indicates that fluid has been forced into the alveoli. This has two causes:

- Cardiogenic, i.e. left ventricular failure causing increased pressure in the pulmonary vascular system.
- Non-cardiogenic, i.e. caused by hypervolaemia or shock.

The management by physiotherapists may include distinguishing pulmonary oedema from a problem of sputum retention (see Table 6.13). Treatment should consist of positioning the patient upright if the problem is cardiogenic. The patient should not be suctioned as this removes surfactant, causing atelectasis.

PHYSIOTHERAPY TREATMENT TECHNIQUES

SUCTION
General Points
Indications

Suction should be used for excessive bronchial secretions and sputum retention, when all other means to aid expectoration have failed or are not possible.

Adverse effects

The adverse effects of suction include:

- Patient distress.
- Hypoxia—use sealed unit catheters in patients with a high FiO_2 and/or high PEEP.
- Cardiovascular instability.
- Raised ICP.
- Introducing infection.
- Epithelial and submucosal damage.
- Pulmonary oedema and disordered blood clotting. N.B. Care should be taken to avoid these.
- Atelectasis (Branson et al., 1993).

Contraindications

Suction should not be used in patients:

- With acute head injury or after intracranial surgery, unless gas exchange is threatened.
- With severe bronchospasm.
- With a fracture to the base of the skull or cerebrospinal fluid leak; particularly naso/pharyngeal suction.
- Following oesophageal/high gastric surgery, or with tracheo/oesophageal fistulae, or high calcium in the gatrointestinal or respiratory tract—these patients need a mini-tracheostomy.

Pre-oxygenation

The following patients should be given 100% oxygen before suction:

- Those with acute head injuries or after intracranial surgery.
- Those cardiovascularly unstable.
- Those requiring FiO_2 >50%.
- Those with pulmonary pathology.
- Those with bradycardia due to vasovagal response.

The FiO_2 will have to be manually increased unless a modern ventilator with a 3 minute 100% pre-oxygenation mode is used. In COPD patients being weaned, pre-oxygenation at 10% above baseline level is advised. Some centres advise pre-oxygenation before all suction, but, this is not necessary for stable patients when the technique is performed quickly and with the minimum effective suction pressure.

Sterile technique
Recent evidence shows that no extra protection is gained by using sterile gloves (Rossof *et al.*, 1995) for each suction procedure or from using catheters more than once. The principal means of preventing cross-infection are for medical staff to wash their hands thoroughly between patients and to wear a new plastic apron before contact with each patient. The wearing of latex gloves is advised to protect the clinician from contact with body fluids. The physiotherapist should adhere to the policy of the hospital.

Technique via Endotracheal Tube and Tracheostomy Tube (Ventilated Patient)
When using the suction technique in a ventilated patient, the following procedure should be followed:
- Put on a clean plastic apron, a pair of latex gloves and goggles for your own and your patient's protection.
- Explain the procedure to the patient.
- Pre-oxygenate the patient if indicated.
- Select a catheter of less than half the diameter of the endotracheal tube:
    Size 10—endotracheal tube <7 mm diameter.
    Size 12.
    Size 14—very thick secretions and endotracheal tube >9 mm diameter.
- Use only suction catheters that have multiple tip holes.
- Attach the catheter to the suction source.
- Put a sterile glove on to your dominant hand. N.B. This glove should be used once only.
- Remove the catheter from its packaging; test that the suction pressure is 10–15 kPa, 70–100 mmHg maximum for adults (in the event of extremely thick secretions, up to 20 kPa, 150 mmHg, and review humidification).
- Let the patient know the procedure is to commence.
- Silence the ventilator alarm; detach the patient from the ventilator at the end of inspiration—you now have 10–15 seconds to perform the procedure.
- Introduce the catheter swiftly but gently into the endotracheal tube (a cough is normally stimulated), apply suction and withdraw the catheter smoothly.
- Reattach the patient to the ventilator.
- Reassure and reassess the patient.

Technique via Endotracheal Tube, Tracheostomy or Mini-tracheostomy (Spontaneously Breathing Patient)
This procedure is as above except that there will not be a ventilator alarm to silence.

N.B. The largest catheter that can be used with a mini-tracheostomy is size 10.

Technique via an Airway
When using a suction technique via an airway, the following procedure should be followed:
- Select an airway (size 3 for an average sized adult) and catheter.
- Prepare yourself and the patient as above. N.B. Clean latex gloves must be worn but sterile gloves are not indicated.
- Position the patient with the neck slightly extended and the head in line with the body.
- Insert the airway upside down and turn it over when half-way inside the mouth, and gently slide it into the oropharynx. N.B. Do not force the airway at any point as this will cause damage to the mouth and stimulate the gag reflex. When inserting the catheter into the airway, a cough will be stimulated.
- If you have difficulty passing the catheter ask the patient to take a deep breath and cough, or use neurophysiological techniques.

Technique for Naso/Pharyngeal Suction
The following technique is advised for naso/pharyngeal suction:
- Prepare yourself and the patient as above.
- Position the patient as for the airway technique.
- Cover the tip end of the catheter with lubricating jelly.
- Insert the catheter into the nose, pointing it slightly towards the midline and in a slightly downwards direction.
- Proceed as for the airway technique.

MANUAL HYPERINFLATION
General Points
Indications
Manual hyperinflation is used for:
- Re-inflation of atelectatic lung tissue.
- Mobilisation of large airways secretions.

Adverse effects
The adverse effects of manual hyperinflation include:
- Decreased cardiac output, cardiac arrhythmia.
- Increased ICP.
- Barotrauma.
- Patient distress (Paratz, 1992).

Contraindications
Manual hyperinflation should not be used in patients with:
- Cardiovascular instability, i.e. systolic blood pressure <80 or >180 mmHg.
- FiO_2 >80%.
- PEEP >5 cmH_2O without a PEEP valve.
- Peak airway pressure >40 cmH_2O in bronchospasm.
- Undrained pneumothorax.
- Emphysema.
- For 10 days following lung surgery including pneumonectomy and lobectomy.
- Patients on nitric oxide.

Technique

When using manual hyperinflation, the following procedure should be followed:

- Explain the procedure to the patient.
- Select a 2–3 litre bag depending on the size of patient; attach the manometer to the circuit.
- Turn the oxygen supply to 15 litres.
- Silence the ventilator alarm, and detach the patient from the ventilator.
- Allow six tidal breaths to assess compliance.
- To mobilise secretions, allow three hyperinflations to double baseline V_T using a slow inspiration and quick release expiration.
- To re-inflate the atelectatic lung, hyperinflate up to a pressure of 40 cmH$_2$O and hold (Rothen *et al.*, 1993).
- Allow six tidal breaths, and repeat if necessary.
- Return the patient to the ventilator.
- Reassess the patient.

For patients on high PEEP, use the ventilator sigh/hyperinflation mode, although this is less effective for mobilising secretions due to the lack of a quick release.

PRONE LYING

General Points

Indications

Prone lying is used in patients with ARDS, or when aspiration of gastric contents is likely.

Adverse effects

The adverse effects of prone lying include:

- Occlusion of the tracheostomy tube or central lines.
- Concern about being unable to return the patient to a supine position in the event of resuscitation being required. N.B. If preparation is adequate the procedure is quick and uneventful.

Technique

When placing a patient in the prone position:

- Explain the procedure to the patient.
- Place all equipment attached to the patient on one side of the patient (the ventilator side) or at the head of the bed if it is likely to become entangled.
- Switch off nasogastric feeding.
- Place the patient in a side lying position facing the ventilator (as far across the bed and away from it as possible), with lower arm under the body.
- Place pillows on the bed at chest and hip level (ensure the abdomen will be free hanging). A small pillow or towel is positioned for the head to rest on.
- Recheck that all lines are safe.
- Roll the patient on to the pillows.
- Recheck all lines and ventilator tubing.
- Check the patient is comfortable and stable.

ROLE OF THE DIETICIAN

The nutritional status of patients is usually the concern of more than one member of the multidisciplinary team, and many units will have formal nutrition teams with their own policies and procedure rules. Such teams can comprise dieticians, pharmacists, nutrition nurses, and a clinician with a special interest in nutrition, and together they will make and implement decisions which will meet the nutritional targets of the critically ill patient. However, specialist nutrition teams do not always exist, and in some units there may be close links with other healthcare professionals without a formal team. One thing is certain, however: that nutrition is seen as a fundamental need in people and can become an emotive subject, being regarded as a treatment or right for the critically ill. The right time to start feeding, if to start feeding, how much to feed and how this is to be done (enteral, i.e. via the gut, or parenteral via the bloodstream) are all considerations which need addressing throughout the patient's stay as nutrition therapy is not without its own risks.

PATIENT'S NUTRITIONAL REQUIREMENTS

How to feed the critically ill patient has been the subject of vigorous debate for many years, and in recent years there has been a gradual reduction in the calorie requirements recommended (Elia and Jebb, 1992). Until recently, the response to the severe wasting that occurs was to feed enormous amounts of calories and protein without understanding how the body responds to critical illness and its ability to cope with large infusions of nutrients.

Calories are generally derived from fat and carbohydrate, fat supplying 9 kcals/g and carbohydrate 4 kcals/g. Regimens supplying excessive quantities of either have been linked with abnormal liver function test results and hepatic steatosis. Excessive amounts of carbohydrate can elevate carbon dioxide production, and increase oxygen requirements and therefore ventilatory requirements, the respiratory quotient being elevated. Commercial enteral feeds exist that are intended as specialised nutrition for pulmonary patients; such feeds supply 1.5 kcals/ml (most enteral feeds supply 1 kcal/ml) and supply as much as 55% energy from fat, with some of this as medium chain triglyceride to aid absorption. Such feeds may have beneficial effects and help in the weaning of ventilator patients (Laaban, 1995). Many units will use a standard enteral feed using both fat and carbohydrate and ensure that overfeeding does not allow the respiratory quotient to rise unnecessarily. Excessive amounts of lipid may be deposited in the lung, and impair diffusion of gases. There is therefore much interest in the lowering of calorie targets in the acute hypercatabolic phase to 30–35 kcals/kg (Elia, 1995), which is very similar to the requirements of healthy adults. Some units are now very conscious of the metabolic effects of overfeeding and choose to aim on the lower side of recommendations, allowing for more intensive nutrition therapy in the recovery phase.

The metabolic consequences of nutrition in the patient with a critical illness must always be considered, and malnutrition should be prevented if at all possible. The successful outcome of patients with pulmonary failure often hinges on the use of appropriate and aggressive nutrition therapy (Pinard and Geller, 1995). Special consideration must also be given in the event of renal or hepatic complication with attention focusing on fluid volume available as well as tailoring regimens to meet specific vitamin, mineral and electrolyte requirements. Care must be taken to accurately assess the whole patient picture, accounting, in particular, for any other substrate infusions which could distort the total nutrition delivered. Dextrose infusions and peritoneal dialysate can contribute to the total carbohydrate load. Sedatives may be given in 10% lipid emulsions which when infused provide 1 kcal/ml, and can easily contribute significant calories when infusion rates over 24 hours are totalled.

Respiratory insufficiency and ventilator dependence can cause problems in the feeding of the critically ill patient. Malnutrition is prevalent in many of these patients and indeed may have been in existence before the onset of the precipitating acute illness. The need to feed must be met in order to try to normalise body function as much as possible, including the need to preserve diaphragmatic function.

METHODS OF FEEDING THE CRITICALLY ILL

The mechanical problems of introducing nutrition into such patients need addressing, as the vast majority will be unable to have their needs met without some form of nutritional support, namely, enteral feeding or parenteral feeding. Enteral nutrition is used in preference to parenteral for many reasons. It is more physiological, helping to minimise the effects of gut atrophy, and prevents the translocation of bacteria and toxins. We can offer a diet closer to the norm—diet is a complex medium and still not fully understood. It is difficult to replicate the ideal feeding solution, as we remain in a learning curve about what the ideal components are, although new interest has centred on such components as β-carotene, glutamine and others present in the diet but not in feeds (Elia, 1995). Enteral feeding is cheaper and generally much easier to implement, and is also associated with fewer complications. Parenteral feeding is used only when it is not possible to use the gut, and as such should be used much less frequently. The absence of bowel sounds is not in itself an indication for parenteral nutrition but must be taken into account along with a detailed history and current clinical picture. Indeed, many patients previously fed parenterally

can subsequently be managed with specialised elemental and peptide feeds, and with better controlled feeding pumps and systems.

Tube feeding into the oesophagus, using a hollow tube attached to a bladder, was used as long ago as 1598. In 1617, tetanus patients were fed via a silver tube inserted through the nostril into the nasopharynx. But it was some 30 years later that leather tubing was used, which could be passed into the stomach.

Today there is still a wide range of feeding tubes available. Ryles tubes, designed for gut aspiration, have been used for nasogastric feeding; however, they tend to be fairly rigid and require frequent replacement if the risk of oesophageal ulceration is to be minimised. The more commonly used tubes are the fine bore feeding ones, with diameters varying but generally 1–2 mm. These are most commonly made from PVC and polyurethane. PVC tubes are designed for short-term use and should be replaced after 7–10 days, while polyurethane tubes are designed for long-term use of 3–6 months, depending on the manufacturer. Most units will have policies relating to the insertion of enteral feeding tubes. Specialised tubes exist which are weighted and can be used to bypass the stomach or used in cases at risk of aspiration; however, the function of the gut in providing a gastric acid barrier to infection must not be overlooked.

Enteral feeding tubes can also be placed in the stomach as gastrostomy tubes, or the jejunum as a jejunostomy, when it is not possible to use the nasogastric route. Indeed, some users of long-term feeding have opted for gastrostomy placement to provide a less visible and more socially acceptable alternative, for example, in the treatment of malnutrition associated with cystic fibrosis, where overnight feeding via gastrostomy has proved beneficial. Gastrostomies have been placed surgically but endoscopic placement means that laparotomy and general anaesthetic are not required. Percutaneous endoscopic gastrostomy also has fewer complications and the endoscope is easier to remove.

Enteral feeding systems have become more advanced; for example, the feeding tube has a male luer lock which links to a female luer in the giving set, but because of the number of sets available it is essential to check compatibility. Fixing sets which are not compatible increase the chance of infection and of introducing pathogens into the feed, which is an ideal medium for growth. Many giving sets now allow the feed container to act as the feed reservoir, enabling the feed to be attached directly to the giving set, negating the need for decanting sterile feed into another reservoir, and limiting the opportunity for infection. Feeding pumps are not always essential. It is possible to gravity feed, counting the number of drops of feed per millilitre; however, when feeding the critically ill patient, accuracy is much more important in assessing the total volumes delivered. Many feeding pumps will deliver feed in

5 ml increments but where finer control is needed there are pumps available that deliver 1 ml increments; these are useful in the paediatric setting.

ENTERAL FEEDING

Enteral feeding solutions are now mostly commercially prepared. It is rare that food prepared in the hospital is used, as modular components are tailored to specific requirements, e.g. powder preparations which need careful calculation and preparation. Most enteral feeds are liquid, normally supplying 1 kcal/ml, and in 500 ml or 1 litre reservoirs. The feeds are sold as complete nutrition with a full range of the known requirements for vitamins and minerals. Calorie sources are from both fat and carbohydrate. Most feeds do not contain dietary fibre, but there are feeds available which have additional fibre. Energy dense feeds, giving 1.5 or 2 kcals/ml, may be requested if there is a need to restrict fluid; these feeds are administered cautiously at first as they tend to be hypertonic. Specialised feeds in the form of elemental or peptide feeds exist and are useful where there is severe digestive impairment, e.g. after total pancreatectomy, Crohn's disease, or if there has been some iatrogenic gut atrophy. Many disease-specific feeds are appearing; for example, those specialised for patients who are HIV positive. These feeds are generally more expensive and are still moderately new to the ranges.

The enteral feeding regimen will vary. Continuous 24 hour infusion, bolus feeding (e.g. 250 ml as eight separate feeds) or cyclic feeding (the feed is run continuously for a period then stopped to rest the gut before restarting) may be used. Cyclic feeding is thought to offer a more physiological method, especially in relation to the circadian effect on hormones. What is important is that records are kept of what is given so that calculations of feed can be made in relation to the feed prescription, as it is not unusual for patients to receive only half of their intended prescription due to stoppages. If a feed is stopped for any other treatment episode, this must be noted and the feed restarted as soon as possible. If the feed has been stopped for some while it may be prudent to hang fresh feed rather than one that has been left opened in ambient temperatures. If treatment requires physical handling or the need to cough, it may be necessary to alter the timing of feeds to ensure a more comfortable treatment session; good communication with the other team members can help here so that the patient receives the best available option.

The stopping of enteral feeding should be done as a planned approach, helping to ensure that the patient is able to have nutritional needs met. Transferring from enteral to oral nutrition is a vulnerable time and may require the need for additional sip feeds. If sip feeds are prescribed these should be encouraged by all the carers of the patient.

PARENTERAL FEEDING

When enteral feeding is not possible, parenteral feeding may be required, where a nutrient solution is passed directly into the bloodstream. This can be a peripheral feed or a central line feed. Generally, peripheral feeds are short term and tend to give fewer calories and less nitrogen in similar volumes. Most feeds are made up in large quantities and require no mixing at ward level, having been prepared by a pharmacy manufacturing service. The feeds have amino acid solutions to give nitrogen contents generally between 9 g and 14 g, although there are regimens which supply more (1 g nitrogen is the equivalent of 6.25 g protein). Most feeds also have dual energy sources as both a glucose solution and a fat solution. Water-soluble and fat-soluble vitamins are added together with trace elements, minerals, phosphate and electrolytes. The use of all additions needs to be carefully monitored. New preparations designed for use as a stop gap while tailored regimens are being prepared need care as these feeds are not designed for long-term use because they are not complete in vitamins and minerals. These feeds do not contain additional phosphate, other than that present as phospholipid. In the critically ill patient who has been receiving some glucose and is malnourished, the patient is likely to become phosphate depleted and re-feeding will exacerbate this. Hypophosphataemia can cause muscular fatigue (particularly of respiratory muscles) and poor oxygen uptake by haemoglobin, so phosphate levels should be monitored.

When parenteral nutrition is stopped there needs to be a planned approach, preferably tailoring off the parenteral feed while another form of feeding is established. This is usually done by decreasing the rate of the parenteral feed while introducing an enteral feed. This has many benefits, including the prevention of rebound hypoglycaemia.

RECOVERY

Once the patient has moved from the critical setting it is important to continue to monitor nutritional status and meet the nutrition targets set by the nutrition team or other appointed specialist. Patients continue to need help and encouragement, and during this phase of recovery they are very often exhausted and need time to come to terms with their acute illness. Ideally food and drink intake should be monitored until they consistently achieve their nutrition targets. Any further dietary interventions can be tackled as appropriate, if necessary on an out-patient basis. The prime in-patient priority remains the prevention or correction of any malnutrition.

OUTCOME OF INTENSIVE CARE

Scarce resources, cost restraints, an ever-growing number of candidates for ICU care, and a medically enlightened population has prompted the generation of 'outcome' research. The majority of ICUs in the UK can provide overall annual mortality figures, both for within the ICU and ultimate discharge statistics. Few can, however, provide detailed assessment of their patients months or years later. Short-term (6 months) survival is determined by severity of acute physiological disturbance, while quality of survival is limited by pre-morbid health status and physiological reserve (Bion, 1995). Quality of life is multidimensional and must include not only an individual's functional status, such as ability to self-care, which is relatively easy to document, but also the presence of psychological sequelae, which, without doubt, will impair an individual patient's ultimate outcome.

The development of psychological sequelae in conjunction with physical illness is being increasingly recognised as having an impact on length of hospital stay and functional outcome for an individual patient. Indeed, it has been suggested that psychological liaison teams in acute hospitals could produce significant financial savings by decreasing length of stay and improving outcome from physical illness (Le Gall, 1984).

The intensive care arena is not immune to psychological sequelae, indeed quite the opposite. The longer stay patients are most vulnerable but short stay does not protect. Auditory stimulation is intense and sleep deprivation occurs. During weaning from opiates there is 'heightening' of the patient's surroundings; perception is altered causing unpleasant dreams or nightmares where the patient is usually the victim. In an attempt to reduce the impact of this period of withdrawal of addictive drugs, it is our belief that if at all possible patients should be removed from the busiest, noisiest area of a unit, and placed in a calming environment (helped by appropriate decoration with pastel colours), where the noise level is less, a degree of day-time and night-time routine can be established, and it is more welcoming to family and friends. This sort of environment is less heavily invaded by technology and, hence, alarms, and the staff can begin the orientation of the patient back to 'normal' life. Televisions, radios, cassette recorders, large armchairs, simple unobtrusive pictures, large calendars and clocks populate the area and the lighting is subdued (wall lights) for night-time. This is still an intensive care area, as the patients have embarked on the process of weaning from ventilatory support. It may take several weeks to accomplish such weaning in long-stay patients due to the weakness they usually experience. Physiotherapists have a vital role in the progression of patients at this crossroad in their illness. Only patients who are well rested can actively participate at this all important time. Theoretically such a pleasant, peaceful, and yet 'intensive' environment (during the day-time) should produce fewer psychological sequelae, speed up the weaning process and hence have positive financial implications for a unit.

REFERENCES

Abraham E, Park YC, Covington P, Conrad SA, Schwartz M. Liposomal prostaglandin E1 in acute respiratory distress syndrome: A placebo-controlled, randomised, double-blind, multi-centre clinical trial. *Crit Care Med* 1996, **24:**10-15.

Aitkenhead AR. Analgesia and sedation in intensive care. *Brit J Anaes* 1989, **63:**196-206.

Ashbaugh DG, Bigelow DB, Petty TL, *et al*. Acute respiratory distress in adults. *Lancet* 1967, **12:**319-323.

Baker CF. Discomfort to environmental noise. Heart rate responses to SICU patients. *Crit Care Quart* 1992, **15(2):**75-90.

Ballard K, Cheeseman W, Ripiner R, Wells S. *Intens Crit Care Nurs* 1992, Mar; **8(1):**2-9.

Bateman JRM, Newman SP, Daunt KM, Sheahan NF, Pavia D, Clarke SW. Is cough as effective as chest physiotherapy in the removal of excessive tracheobronchial secretions? *Thorax* 1981, **36:**683-687.

Baum M, Benzer H, Putensen C. Biphasic positive airway pressure (BiPAP)–a new form of augmented ventilation. *Anaesthetist* 1989, **38:**452-458.

Bergbom-Endberg I, Haljamae H. The communication process in the ICU as perceived by the nursing staff. *Intens Crit Care Nurs* 1993, **9(1):**40-47.

Bethune DD. Neurophysiological facilitation of respiration in the unconscious adult patient. *Physiother Can* 1975, **27:**241-245.

Bion J. Rationing intensive care. *BMJ* 1995, **310:**682-683.

Bion JF. Audit and quality assurance in critical care. In: Dobb G, Bion JF, Burchardi H, Dellinger EP, eds. *Current topics in intensive care*. Philadelphia: WB Saunders; 1994.

Bion JF. Sedation and analgesia in the intensive care unit. *Hosp Update* 1988, **14:**1272-1286.

Bott J, Keilty SE, Noone L. Intermittent positive pressure breathing–a dying art? *Physiotherapy* 1992, **78:**656-660.

Braden BJ, Bergstrom N. Clinical utility of the Braden scale for predicting tissue sore risk. *Decubitus* 1988, **2(3):**34-38.

Branson RD, Campbell RS, Chatburn RL, Covington J. Endotracheal suctioning of mechanically ventilated adults and children with artificial airways. *Resp Care* 1993, **38:**500-503.

Choi SC, Nelson LD. Kinetic therapy in critically ill patients: combined results based on meta-analysis. *J Crit Care* 1992, **7:**57-62.

Connors AF, Hammon WE, Martin RH, Rogers RM. Chest physical therapy: the immediate effect on oxygenation in acutely ill patients. *Chest* 1980, **78:**559-564.

Crunden E. With the aid of an algorithm. *VFM Update* 1994, **12:**14-15.

Dean E. Oxygen transport: a physiologically based conceptual framework for the practice of cardiopulmonary physiotherapy. *Physiotherapy* 1994, **80:**347-355.

Department of Health. *Guidelines on admission to and discharge from intensive care and high dependency units*. London: NHS Executive, Department of Health; 1996.

Department of Health. *Pressure sores a key quality indicator*. London: Department of Health; 1993.

Department of Health. *The health of the nation*. London: HMSO; 1991.

Dinh-Xuan AT, Brunet F, Dhainaut JF. Inhaled nitric oxide: The light and shadow of a therapeutic breakthrough. In: Fink MP, Payen D, eds. *Update in intensive care and emergency medicine: Role of nitric oxide in sepsis and ARDS*. Berlin: Springer Verlag; 1995:**24:**414-425.

Elia M. Changing concepts of nutrient requirements in disease: implications for artificial nutritional support. *Lancet* 1995, **345:**1279-1284.

Elia M, Jebb SA. Changing concepts of energy requirements in critically ill patients. *Curr Med Lit Clin Nutr* 1992, **1:**35.

Enright S. Cardiorespiratory effects of chest physiotherapy. *Intens Care Britain* 1992, 118-123.

Fink MP, Helsmoortel CM, Stein KL, Lee PC, Cohn SM. The efficacy of an oscillating bed in the prevention of lower respiratory tract infection in critically ill victims of blunt trauma. *Chest* 1990, **97:**132-137.

Flanagan M. Pressure sore risk assessment scales. *J Wound Care* 1995, **2(3):**162-167.

Froese AB, Bryan AC. Effects of anaesthesia and paralysis on diaphragmatic mechanics in man. *Anaesthesiology* 1974, **41:**242-255.

Garradd J, Bullock M. The effect of respiratory therapy on ICP on ventilated neurological patients. *Aust J Physiotherapy* 1986, **32:**107-111.

Gauger PG, Pranikoff T, Schreiner RJ, Moler FW, Hirschl RB. Initial experience with partial liquid ventilation in paediatric patients with acute respiratory distress syndrome. *Crit Care Med* 1996, **24:**16-22.

6

REFERENCES

Gentilello L, Thompson DA, Tonneson AS. Effect of a rotating bed on the incidence of pulmonary complications in critically ill patients. *Crit Care Med* 1988, **16:**783-786.

Gherini S, Peters RM, Virgilio RW. Mechanical work on the lungs and work of breathing with positive end-expiratory pressure and CPAP. *Chest* 1979, **76:**251-257.

Gow GL. Influence of sedation regimens. *Brit J Intens Care* April, 1995.

Hammon WE, Connors AF, McCaffree DR. Cardiac arrhythmias during postural drainage and chest percussion of critically ill patients. *Chest* 1992, **102:**1836-1841.

Hardinge FM, Davies RJO, Stradling JR. Effects of short term high frequency negative pressure ventilation on gas exchange using the Hayek oscillator in normal subjects. *Thorax* 1995, **50:**44-49.

Inman KJ, Sibbald WJ, Rutledge FS, Clark B. Clinical utility and cost effectiveness of an air suspension bed in the prevention of pressure ulcers. *JAMA* 1993, **269(11):**39-43.

Jones AYM, Hutchinson RC, Oh TE. Effects of bagging and percussion on total static compliance of the respiratory system. *Physiotherapy* 1992, **78:**661-666.

Keilty SE. Inhalation burn injured patients and physiotherapy management. *Physiotherapy* 1993, **79:**87-90.

Keilty SE, Bott J. Continuous positive airways pressure. *Physiotherapy* 1992, **72:**90-92.

Kelley RE, Vibulsreth S, Bell I, Duncan RC. Evaluation of kinetic therapy in the prevention of complications of bed rest secondary to stroke. *Stroke* 1987, **18:**638-642.

Kirkpatrick AW, Meade MO, Stewart TE. Lung protective ventilatory strategies in ARDS. In: Vincent JL, ed. *1996 Yearbook of intensive care and emergency medicine.* Berlin: Springer-Verlag; 1996:398-410.

Klein P, Kemper M, Weissman C, Rosenbaum SH, Askanazi J, Hyman AI. Attenuation of the hemodynamic responses to chest physical therapy. *Chest* 1988, **93:**38-42.

Laaban JP. Nutritional support in patients with chronic respiratory failure undergoing surgery. *Ann Fr Anesth Reanim* 1995, **14(suppl. 2):**112-120.

Laing A. The applicability of a new sedation scale for intensive care. *Intens Crit Care Nurs* 1992, **8(3):**149-152.

Le Gall J, Loirat P, Alperovith A, *et al.* A simplified acute physiology score for ICU patients. *Crit Care Med* 1984, **12:**975-977.

Marshall JC, Cook DJ, Christou NV, Bernard GR, Sprung CL, Sibbald WJ. Multiple Organ Dysfunction Score: A reliable descriptor of a complex clinical outcome. *Crit Care Med* 1995, **10:**1638-1652.

McMurray TC. Propofol for sedation following cardiac surgery. *J Drug Develop* 1991, **4(3):**51-58.

Mitchell P. Intracranial hypertension: influence of nursing activities. *Nurs Clin N Am* 1986, **21(4):**563-576.

Mudler GD, Taro N, Seeley JE, Andrews K. A study of pressure ulcer response to low air loss beds vs conventional treatment. *J Geriatr Dermatol* 1994, **2:**87-91.

NHSME. *Junior doctors. The new deal.* London: NHS Management Executive; 1991.

Norton D, McLaren R, Exton-Smith AN. *An investigation of geriatric nursing problems in hospital.* London: Churchill Livingstone; 1962.

O'Dea K. Pressure reducing mattresses. *J Wound Care* 1995, **5(5):**207-211.

Oh TE. *Intensive care manual,* 3rd ed, Chapter 24. Sydney: Butterworths; 1990.

Pappert D, Rossaint R, Slama K, Gruning T, Falke KJ. Influence of positioning on ventilation-perfusion relationships in severe adult respiratory distress syndrome. *Chest* 1994, **106:**1511-1516.

Paratz J. Haemodynamic stability of the ventilated intensive care patient. *Aust Physiother* 1992, **38:**167-172.

Pennock BE, Cranshaw L, Maher T, Price T, Kaplan PD. Distressful events in the ICU as perceived by patients recovering from coronary bypass surgery. *Heart Lung* 1994, **23(4):**323-327.

Petros AJ, Fernando SSD, Shenoy VS, Al-Saady NM. The Hayek Oscillator. *Anaesthesia* 1995, **50:**601-606.

Pinard B, Geller E. Nutritional support during pulmonary failure. *Crit Care Clin* 1995, **11(3):**705-715.

Pingleton S. State of the art: complications of acute respiratory failure. *Am Rev Respir Dis* 1988, **137:**1463-1493.

Pryor JA, Webber BA. Physiotherapy for cystic fibrosis—which technique? *Physiotherapy* 1992, **72:**105-108.

Rappaport SH, Shpiner R, Yoshihara G, Wright J, Chang P, Abraham E. Randomised, prospective trial of pressure-limited versus volume-controlled ventilation in severe respiratory failure. *Crit Care Med* 1994, **22:**22-32.

Reeve W, Wallace P. A survey of sedation in intensive care. *Care Crit Ill* 1991, **7(6):**238-241.

Ross J, Dean E. Integrating physiological principles into the comprehensive management of cardiopulmonary dysfunction. *Phys Ther* 1989, **69:**255-259.

Rossof LJ, Borenstein M, Isenberg HD. Is hand washing really needed in an intensive care unit? *Crit Care Med* 1995, **23:**1211-1216.

Rothen HU, Sporre B, Engberg G, Wegenius G, Hedenstierna G. Re-expansion of atelectasis during general anaesthesia. *Brit J Anaes* 1993, **71:**788-795.

Rouby J-J. High frequency ventilation. In: Vincent J-L, ed. *Update in intensive care and emergency medicine.* Berlin: Springer Verlag; 1990:201-213.

Ryan DW. Low air loss therapy. *Care Crit Ill* 1995, **11(1):**5-6.

Ryan DW. The fluidised bed. 2. Burns, catabolism, nursing and medical care. Conference paper reprinted from *Intensive Care World,* 1990.

Sciaky AJ. Mobilising the intensive care patient: pathophysiology and treatment. *Phys Ther Pract* 1994, **3:**69-80.

Sim KM, Evans TW. Supporting the injured lung. *BMJ* 1993, **307:**1293-1294.

Stiller K, Geake T, Taylor J, Grant R, Hall B. Acute lobar atelectasis—a comparison of two chest physiotherapy regimes. *Chest* 1990, **98:**1336-1340.

Summer WR, Curry P, Haponik EF, Nelson S, Elston R. Continuous mechanical turning of intensive care unit patients shortens length of stay in some diagnostic-related groups, *J Crit Care* 1989, **4(1):**45-53.

Tapson VK, Fulkerson WJ. Infectious complications of mechanical ventilation. *Prob Resp Care* 1991, **4:**100-117.

UKCC. *The scope of professional practice.* London: United Kingdom Central Council; 1992.

Vinik HR, Kissin I. Sedation in the ICU. *Intens Care Med* 1991, **17:**20-23.

Waterlow J. A policy that protects: the Waterlow pressure sore prevention/treatment policy. *Prof Nurse* 1991, **6:**258-262.

Winslow EH, Clark AP, White KM, Tyler DO. Effects of a lateral turn on mixed venous oxygen saturation and heart rate in critically ill adults. *Heart Lung* 1990, **19:**557-561.

GENERAL READING

Allison A. High frequency jet ventilation—where are we now? *Care Crit Ill* 1994, **10(3):**122-124.

Bernard GR, Artigas A, Brigham KL, *et al.* Report of the American–European concensus conference on acute respiratory distress syndrome: Definitions, mechanisms, relevant outcomes, and clinical trial co-ordination. *Am J Resp Crit Care Med* 1994, **151:**818-824.

Castella X, Artigas A, Bion J, Kari A. A comparison of severity of illness scoring systems for intensive care unit patients: Results of a multi-centre, multinational study. *Crit Care Med* 1995, **8:**1327-1335.

Collier ME. Pressure-reducing mattresses. *J Wound Care* 1996, **5(5):**207-211.

Dolmage TE, Hayek Z, De Rosie JA, Goldstein RS. Effects of high frequency chest wall oscillation (HFCWO) at 1.5 Hz on gas exchange in normal lungs. *Am Rev Resp Dis* 1992, **145:**A528.

El-Baz N. High frequency ventilation for thoracic surgery. *Clin Anaes* 1987, **1:**99-105.

Ferrell BA, Osterweil D, Christenson PA. A randomised trial of low air loss beds for the treatment of pressure ulcers. *JAMA* 1993, **269:**494-497.

GENERAL READING

Hanson III CW, Marshall BE, Frasch HF, Marshall C. Causes of hypercarbia with oxygen therapy in patients with chronic obstructive pulmonary disease. *Crit Care Med* 1996, **1:**23-28.

House A, Farthing M, Peveler R. Psychological care of medical patients. *BMJ* 1995, **310:**1422-1423.

Jackson C, Webb AR. An evaluation of the heat and moisture exchange performance of four ventilator circuit filters. *Intens Care Med* 1992, **18:**264-268.

Knaus WA, Wagner DP, Draper EA. The APACHE III prognostic system. *Chest* 1991, **100:**1619-1636.

Knaus WA, Zimmerman JE, Wagner DP, *et al*. APACHE–Acute Physiology and Chronic Health Evaluation: A physiologically based classification system. *Crit Care Med* 1981, **9:**591-597.

Lemeshow S, Teres D, Pastides H, *et al*. A method for predicting survival and mortality of ICU patients using objectively derived weights. *Crit Care Med* 1985, **13:**519-525.

Martin C, Papazian L, Perrin G, Saux P, Gouin F. Preservation of humidity and heat of respiratory gases in patients with a minute ventilation greater than 10L/min. *Crit Care Med* 1994, **22:**1871-1876.

Milberg JA, Davis DR, Steinberg KP, *et al*. Improved survival of patients with acute repiratory distress syndrome (ARDS): 1983-1993. *JAMA* 1995, **273:**306-309.

Molloy AR, Edmondson SJ, Hinds CJ. High frequency jet ventilation in acute respiratory failure. *Br J Intens Care* 1992, **2:**126-131.

Preston IM, Matthews HR, Ready AR. Minitracheostomy. *Physiotherapy* 1986, **72:**494-496.

Rombeau JL, Caldwell FT. *Enteral and tube feeding*, 2nd ed. Philadelphia: WB Saunders; 1990.

Smith BE, Scott PV, Fischer HBJ. High frequency jet ventilation in intensive care–a review of 63 patients. *Anaesthesia* 1988, **43:**497-505.

Spiby J. Intensive care in the United Kingdom: report from the King's Fund panel. *Anaesthesia* 1989, **44:**428-431.

Thomas B. *Manual of dietetic practice*, 2nd ed. London: Blackwell Science; 1994.

7 K Jeyansingham, R Kanagasabay, G Morritt, B Smith, M Smith, T Treasure

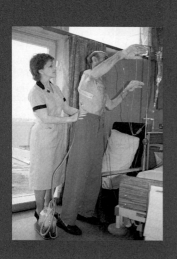

THE CARDIOTHORACIC UNIT

CHAPTER OUTLINE

- Surgery to the heart
- Investigations
- Coronary artery bypass surgery
- Complications from coronary artery bypass surgery
- Other forms of surgery for ischaemic heart disease
- Operations on the great vessels
- Other cardiac operations
- Pulmonary surgery
- Surgery to the oesophagus and stomach
- Post-operative pain control
- Physiotherapy in the cardiothoracic unit
- Physiotherapy and the cardiac patient
- Physiotherapy and thoracic surgery

INTRODUCTION

Within the lifetime of the present generation of surgeons, operations on the heart have gone from being regarded as difficult and dangerous to their present status as routine procedures. Just to give some historical context, it is worth remembering that the cardiopulmonary bypass, that is the 'heart–lung machine' used to support the patient's circulation during the majority of heart operations, was first used in the mid 1950s, and it was not until the mid 1960s that it was reasonably safe and reliable. Before that, cardiac surgery was limited to a relatively few procedures that could be performed in and around the heart without having to interfere with its function. These included 'closed' valvotomies on the mitral and pulmonary valves, and correction of some congenital abnormalities outside the heart, e.g. coarctation and persistent patent ductus arteriosus. Valve replacement surgery started in the early 1960s and coronary artery surgery in the late 1960s. These now are the bulk of the work performed in cardiac surgical units. To give some idea of the frequency of these operations,

about 100 patients per million of the population have a heart valve operation each year. The figure for coronary surgery varies from 500 to 1000 cases per million of the population in the developed world, with the USA having the highest operation rate. The organisation also differs from one country to another. The UK has fewer units, about 40 altogether, with each of the majority doing 500–900 coronary operations per year. There are many more units in the USA, in both relative and absolute terms, but each tends to deal with 200–300 cases per annum.

Cardiac surgery depends heavily on sophisticated technology and highly trained teams. This is one reason for the relatively large units in the UK where cost effectiveness has required that we work in reasonably large groups and use our teams and equipment as efficiently as possible. The heart lends itself to modern surgery remarkably well. Most of the problems are 'mechanical'. We can correct narrowed or leaking valves, restore more normal anatomy in congenital heart disease, and bypass blocked coronary arteries. As judged by mortality figures, cardiac sugery is remarkably safe and compares favourably with operations of similar magnitude in patients of similar age, undertaken on the lungs or abdominal organs. A simple explanation for this is that unrectified cardiac complications present the biggest hazard in the perioperative period for patients undergoing surgery for lung cancer, abdominal disease or hip replacement. Our patients, on the other hand, leave the operating theatre physiologically better equipped to survive than when they went in. Whatever the reason, there is no doubt that the risks are minimised by careful selection of patients and attention to detail at every stage.

SURGERY TO THE HEART

INCISIONS

The majority of cardiac operations are carried out through a median sternotomy (Figure 7.1). This involves cutting down onto the sternum, which is then sawn in two vertically. It is important to stay exactly in the midline at every stage to ensure no muscle is cut and instability of the chest is minimised. The two halves of the sternum are separated with a heavy spreader, to allow access to the heart, and they are re-opposed at the end of the operation with steel wires threaded through or around the sternum. These may be seen on the post-operative X-ray (some surgeons, however,

prefer sutures of synthetic polymer which are not radio-opaque). This incision allows good access to the heart and ascending aorta and heals soundly, usually allowing the patient to mobilise early with relatively little post-operative discomfort. However, something has to give when the two sternal edges are separated (sometimes quite widely) by 6 inches or more. The costal cartilage or the costochondral junctions may buckle, giving characteristic localised pain in the front of the chest. One or more ribs may fracture, giving pain laterally. Sometimes there is pain in the back which we believe is due to the strain put on the articulation between the ribs and the vertebrae.

An anterolateral thoracotomy is occasionally used for repair of atrial septal defect (ASD), particularly for cosmetic reasons in girls, because the median sternotomy scar is disfiguring and can become keloid. The skin incision is in the submammary fold. The serratus anterior muscle is partly cut and partly split and the chest is entered through the 5th intercostal space (Figure 7.2). Bilateral submammary incisions (Figure 7.3) are sometimes used for cosmetic reasons in young patients and also in cases where access to both pleural cavities is required, e.g. double-lung transplantation.

There is growing interest in the use of other types of incision for cardiac surgery, with the aim of reducing morbidity further. These include a small anterior thoracotomy, a paramedian incision through the costal cartilages, and incision for viewing the inside of the chest with an endoscope. These minimal access techniques are not as yet widespread.

SUPPORT AND PROTECTION OF THE ORGANS DURING SURGERY

The cardiopulmonary bypass machine is central to cardiac surgery. It temporarily replaces the function of the heart and lungs. The patient's blood is fully anticoagulated with intravenous heparin. Tubes are placed in the arterial and the venous sides of the heart. The desaturated, systemic venous blood is drained through a tube of up to 3 cm in diameter, into an oxygenator, and then pumped back into the arterial circulation through a cannula about 1 cm in diameter, in the ascending aorta. There are various modifications that can

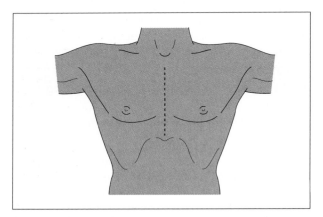

Figure 7.1 **Median sternotomy.**

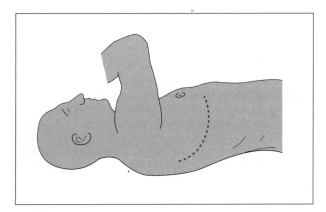

Figure 7.2 **Thoracotomy.**

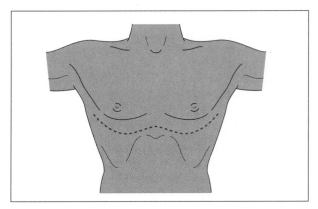

Figure 7.3 **Bilateral submammary incisions.**

be made to the circuit, e.g. cannulating the femoral vessels, but the essential principle of replacing the function of the heart and lungs is the same.

Cardiopulmonary bypass has become a very safe technique but once the blood is exposed to any surface other than vascular endothelium, changes take place including activation of the clotting cascades and a range of inflammatory processes. These have effects on all the organs of the body. Some degree of malfunction of the lungs, brain, kidney, liver and other organs and systems seems inescapable and occasionally there are severe consequences. There are good reasons to avoid bypass, or to use it for as little time as possible, but for most heart surgery it provides essential circulatory support while the heart is being operated on.

INVESTIGATIONS

Most patients come to the cardiac surgeon already investigated extensively, and the indications for surgery and the proposed operation are already worked out. The surgical team is nevertheless responsible for checking that the proposed operation is appropriate and that nothing important has been overlooked. It is not unusual for the specialist cardiologists to refer a patient for vein grafts who has already had the saphenous veins removed as part of a varicose vein operation or for peripheral vascular surgery, or in whom some important surgical complicating factor has been overlooked while concentrating on the heart.

Heart operations are sometimes performed in patients with no symptoms at all, to correct some abnormality which is known to put their life or future wellbeing at risk. In most cases, however, it is to relieve distressing symptoms and disability. Often, both motives apply. In every case, in the final run up to the operation, the following questions should be asked:
- Is the expected benefit great enough to justify the risk?
- Has anything been overlooked?
- Is the patient fully informed?

All the members of the team, i.e. nurses, physiotherapists, anaesthetists and junior doctors, see the patient and are entitled to take an intelligent and informed interest, and you can be sure that the patient will assume you know something about it. Patients often ask questions of younger, more junior, or ancillary staff and seek their support and reassurance.

SYMPTOMS
Angina Pectoris
Eighty per cent of all operations in adults are for coronary artery disease, and the characteristic symptom is angina. Angina describes a choking in the chest and although 'pain' is mentioned it is important to note that many patients do not spontaneously call it as such but use words like tightness, crushing, pressure or aching. The gesture of a hand placed firmly across the chest is more consistent than the words used to describe it. The aching feeling may spread into the left arm or to the jaw. Angina is typically brought on by exercise, relieved by rest, exacerbated in the cold, and is more likely to come on after a heavy meal. Sometimes it is precipitated by emotion, anxiety or stressful situations. In easy cases, particularly if the diagnosis has been confirmed by an angiogram, it is obvious, but the symptom has often been blamed on 'indigestion' and the descriptions vary widely from one case to another.

Breathlessness
The feeling of being out of breath accompanies so many illnesses that although it may point to a cardiac cause, there are many other explanations. Breathlessness on exertion is a feature of valvular heart disease and of left ventricular damage due to coronary artery disease, particularly from a previous myocardial infarction. More specific symptoms of heart failure include orthopnoea (breathlessness on lying flat) and paroxysmal nocturnal dyspnoea (PND; spasms of breathlessness occurring at night).

Other symptoms which are encountered much less commonly in patients awaiting surgery are palpitations (awareness of irregularity of the heart), cyanosis (bluish coloration due to desaturation of the circulating blood) and peripheral oedema and enlargement of the liver due to right-sided cardiac congestion.

SPECIFIC INVESTIGATIONS
Electrocardiogram at Rest and on Exercise
The 12 lead electrocardiograph producing an electrocardiogram (ECG), taken at rest, is a standard means of investigating the heart and tells the expert cardiologist a great deal about abnormal rhythms, the relative size of the different chambers, and the site and severity of an infarction, old or new. In those patients admitted for coronary artery surgery, we are often more interested in an exercise ECG (see Chapter 4).

An exercise ECG involves a continuous ECG recording during graded exercise during which time the test may be considered positive if the ECG shows ischaemic features. The test may also be aborted if the patient develops chest pain, breathlessness, arrhythmias or particularly if the blood pressure falls as this is a strong predictor of ischaemic heart disease. A positive exercise test may prompt further investigation by coronary angiography.

Cardiac Catheterisation
The process of threading fine tubes or 'catheters' through the arteries and veins into the heart to measure pressures, take samples, or to inject radiographic contrast material, is called cardiac catheterisation.

Coronary angiography was pioneered at the Cleveland Clinic, Ohio, USA, in the 1960s. It involves passing an arterial catheter through the femoral or brachial artery and directly cannulating the right and left coronary ostia, allowing contrast to be injected and coronary angiograms recorded with biplanar X-ray equipment. A left ventricular angiogram may also be performed, allowing an estimate of ventricular performance to be made. If there is suspicion of valvular heart disease, the aortic valve gradient can be directly measured, and similarly with a right heart catheter (inserted via a central vein), the pressures in the right heart, the gradient across the valves and the pressure in the pulmonary artery can be measured directly. After coronary angiography, patients have to lie flat for several hours to prevent haemorrhage from the arterial puncture site, and groin haematomas are not infrequently seen after this procedure. In less than 1% of cases, coronary angiography leads to acute coronary occlusion due to dissection or thrombosis, and this may necessitate emergency surgery. Patients are therefore warned of this possibility and blood is taken for potential cross-matching before the angiography.

Echocardiography and Doppler

Echocardiography is a valuable non-invasive tool in the investigation of cardiac disease. By means of reflected ultrasound waves a two-dimensional image of the heart can be displayed. The size of the cardiac chambers and the contractility can be seen, and by means of Doppler shift calculations, the velocity of the blood flowing across the valves can be measured; then by calculation an estimate of the pressure gradient can be made.

Post-operatively, echocardiography may be employed to investigate suspected cardiac tamponade in the surgical patient as well as to assess patients with poor ventricular function. Echocardiography may be combined with some means of putting stress on the heart, for example, either exercise or injection of a drug such as dobutamine, to bring out regional dysfunction of the left ventricular wall, which may correlate with ischaemia.

Nuclear Imaging Techniques

Thallium scanning

Thallium scanning requires an injected radiopharmaceutical which is taken up into functioning myocardium. A gamma camera is used to take images both at rest and with exercise to show areas of the heart deprived of blood supply by coronary atheroma. More prolonged studies are capable of demonstrating myocardium which is 'hibernating', that is non-functioning muscle which may recover if revascularised by surgery. Another use of nuclear imaging is to make the red cells radioactive and then take pictures over the precordium with the gamma camera. By taking repeated counts over the chest and 'gating' them to the cycle of the heart from the ECG, a picture of the volume of the heart in systole and diastole can be built up.

Positron emission tomography

Positron emission tomography (PET) is a sophisticated technique available in only a few centres. It may allow the metabolism of the heart to be examined. It is also useful in the investigation of hibernating myocardium and in research.

Computed tomography and magnetic resonance imaging

Cardiac computed tomography (CT) and magnetic resonance imaging (MRI) are not widely used in ischaemic heart disease, but may allow some structural detail to be assessed—including, with MRI, an assessment of vessel and graft patency—while MRI can provide impressive images of the great vessels. MRI has the advantage that, unlike conventional and CT angiography, it does not require a contrast injection to obtain images of the blood vessels. CT and MRI have an important role in the preoperative assessment of patients with diseases of the great vessels, e.g. aortic dissection and aneurysm.

Intravascular ultrasonography

The most direct method of assessing coronary atheroma is with intravascular ultrasonography (IVUS), where an ultrasound probe is passed directly inside a coronary artery at cardiac catheterisation. IVUS is currently a research tool, but may in the future allow more accurate assessment of coronary artery disease, including recurrent disease after surgery, and its treatment.

ISCHAEMIC HEART DISEASE

Ischaemic heart disease is one of the major causes of death in the Western world. For pathophysiology refer to Chapter 9.

CORONARY ARTERY BYPASS SURGERY

The first series of successful operations to bypass blocked coronary arteries was performed in the Cleveland Clinic in the late 1960s, and throughout the 1970s the operation became progressively safer. In the 1980s, the number of bypass operations performed increased world-wide. In the UK there are about 500 operations per million of the population each year, and in the USA the figure is about double. During the 1980s, many surgeons were able to report large series of patients with a mortality of 1–2%. The realistic mortality figures are now rather higher, at 3–5%, for many series because the operation is used in progressively older, more advanced and less stable cases.

All narrowed or blocked coronary arteries are bypassed with a combination of artery grafts, most commonly with left internal thoracic artery, which surgeons often call by its old name of internal mammary artery, or with long saphenous vein. When deciding which vessels to bypass, a reduction in diameter of 50% is considered critical (this is equivalent to a 75% reduction in area). This relieves angina in the large majority of patients and most operations are for symptomatic benefit.

FURTHER INDICATIONS

Coronary artery disease is very unpredictable. Many angina sufferers carry on for years, going through good and bad phases, but up to 5% die each year of myocardial infarction. We also try to identify these and recommend surgery to increase their chances of survival over a 5–15 year period. On the basis of large trials, it is known that patients most at risk of death are those with all three vessels critically narrowed, or with the left main stem coronary artery involved. This effect is even more pronounced if there is evidence of impaired left ventricular function on the angiogram, although these patients also have a slightly higher risk from surgery.

Recurrence of angina of some degree occurs in up to 20% of patients at 1 year, reaching 40% by 6 years. Results from coronary artery bypass grafting have been extensively surveyed. Operative mortality is around 2–3% for elective cases, while complete or substantial relief of angina can be achieved in more than 90% of cases. Left ventricular function is the most important predictor of long-term survival both before and after surgery. Most patients no longer have to take antianginal drugs, and prognosis is improved. Aspirin is advised for its antiplatelet action, and cardiac risk factors such as hypertension, smoking and cholesterol merit continued treatment. The operation is palliative in the sense that the underlying disease is still present, and 10–15% of patients may come back for a second operation after 10 years. The main causes of this are progression of the native coronary artery disease and graft atherosclerosis. At 10 years, 55–70% of saphenous vein grafts are narrowed or occluded compared with 3% of internal mammary arteries. This realisation has led to the increasing use of one or both internal mammary arteries (and in some cases other arterial conduits such as the inferior epigastric artery or the radial artery as free grafts, and the gastroepiploic artery on a pedicle brought up through the diaphragm); however, most patients will still require a number of vein grafts to achieve complete revascularisation; this is linked to survival and freedom from angina. Use of the left internal mammary artery to graft the left anterior descending coronary artery has been shown to reduce operative mortality and improve long-term survival and freedom from angina or the need for re-operation, but more extensive arterial revascularisation has yet to show clear benefit in long-term studies. In some cases, graft disease can be treated by angioplasty, but in others repeat operation is needed. The mortality from this is double that of first-time operations, and freedom from angina is less often achieved.

OVERALL MANAGEMENT OF ADMISSIONS

We try to arrange for as many patients as possible to attend a presurgery day, where they can learn more about the coronary artery bypass graft (CABG) procedure and may be able to visit the wards and Intensive Care Unit (ICU) where they will recover. Printed information is often distributed and we have a telephone helpline for both pre- and postoperative patients and families.

Most patients are admitted electively for CABG the day before surgery. Blood tests, blood cross-matching, chest X-ray and ECG are performed, and patients will be seen by the nursing, surgical, anaesthestic and physiotherapy staff for assessment. Before surgery, the chest and legs are shaved and these areas are also washed with an iodine antiseptic on the ward. In the operating theatre, central venous catheters, an arterial cannula, central and peripheral temperature probes and a urinary catheter are placed before surgery.

THE CORONARY BYPASS OPERATION

In the majority of coronary bypass operations (Figure 7.4), we use the heart–lung machine to support the circulation (see above). The coronary arteries are then grafted beyond the stenoses with reversed segments of long saphenous vein harvested from the leg. The proximal ends of these veins are anastomosed to the ascending aorta. One or both internal thoracic arteries may also be dissected off the chest wall and used as bypass grafts—the proximal end being left in continuity with the subclavian artery.

PROTECTING THE HEART MUSCLE

In order for the grafts to be sewn onto the heart, some method has to be employed to stop the heart beating. The two main techniques are known as 'cross-clamp/fibrillation'

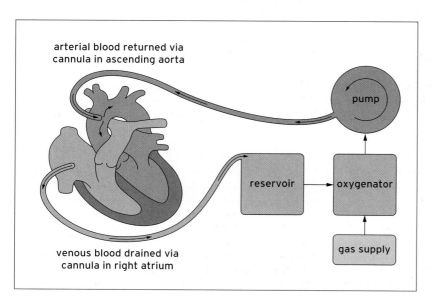

Figure 7.4 Diagram of the bypass circuit.

arterial blood returned via cannula in ascending aorta

pump

reservoir → oxygenator

gas supply

venous blood drained via cannula in right atrium

and 'cardioplegia'. In the former the heart is put into ventricular fibrillation by an electrical stimulator, and a clamp is placed across the aorta to prevent blood reaching the coronary arteries. The clamp allows the anastomosis to be made without blood spilling out of the coronary arteries and obscuring the view. During the period of aortic clamping, the heart is deprived of oxygen, but this is well tolerated for the short periods required for coronary anastomoses (5–15 minutes). After completion of the distal anastomosis, the clamp is released and the heart defibrillated and allowed to reperfuse while the proximal end of the vein is sewn to the aorta. This process is repeated a number of times until all the bypass grafts have been fashioned. This technique is often called 'Fast Track'.

If cardioplegia is used, a solution (usually cold) rich in potassium is infused into the aortic root between the aortic valve and the cross-clamp, thus perfusing the coronary arteries selectively. We use the commonest technique, i.e. very cold (<10°C) oxygenated blood, with a potassium content raised to 20 mM (normal, about 4 mM). This results in cardiac arrest, and since the metabolic requirements of the heart are much reduced in this state, the heart can tolerate longer periods of ischaemia than with ventricular fibrillation, allowing all the distal antastomoses to be made first. The cross-clamp is then removed, the heart perfused and the proximal anastomoses fashioned. Surface cooling of the heart with ice is also carried out with this technique and this can occasionally result in temporary post-operative palsy of the phrenic nerve leading to diaphragmatic paralysis. With either cardioplegia or fibrillation, the cardiopulmonary bypass circuit allows the heart to be arrested while the bypass machine sustains the circulation, perfusing the brain and other vital organs.

In some cases it is possible to perform CABG on the beating heart without cardiopulmonary bypass. This avoids the deleterious effects of heparinisation and bypass, but it is not yet clear whether these advantages outweigh the technical difficulties of operating without bypass, with the potential for graft failure due to anastomoses made under these more difficult conditions being of lower quality.

Once all the grafts are fashioned, the flow in the heart–lung machine is reduced and the heart takes over again. Protamine is given to reverse the heparin anticoagulant, and the chest is closed after any residual bleeding has been stopped. At the end of the operation, chest drains are placed around the heart and in the pleural cavities, if these have been opened, e.g. for dissection of a mammary artery. The drains will remain on continuous suction to prevent the accumulation of blood in the chest which would otherwise compress the heart leading to a reduction in venous return and a drop in cardiac output (cardiac tamponade).

Some patients will have temporary epicardial pacing wires attached to the surface of the heart and threaded out through the chest wall, to allow the heart to be paced externally. These wires may be located on the right atrium (conventionally these exit the chest on the right side) or the right ventricle (exiting the chest on the left side). In high risk patients, a monitoring line may be retained in the left atrium to allow direct measurements of left heart pressures and more accurate manipulation of fluids and inotropes, and this will also exit the front of the chest near the sternal wound.

Most patients go to the ICU for at least a few hours postoperatively, for monitoring of cardiac function and observation for bleeding or other adverse features. For routine cardiac surgery, however, this is a much simpler process than the care needed for multisystem failure in a general ICU. We aim to have our patients conscious and breathing spontaneously soon after operation but a planned period of ventilation for a few hours, or overnight, may be used, particularly in less stable patients. Many patients are vasoconstricted after bypass and it is common practice for a glyceryl trinitrate (GTN) infusion to be used to counter this. Most patients return to the general ward the day after surgery, and the chest drains and arterial line are removed at around this time. The central venous line and urinary catheter are removed the following day, and the patient is disconnected from cardiac monitoring and mobilised. Most patients are discharged home after 6 to 8 days. Regular analgesia is given throughout this time with oral analgesics usually being sufficient after the first 24 hours—most patients find that their pain is well controlled on this regimen. Many patients in fact find the leg wound more troublesome than the sternotomy.

COMPLICATIONS FROM CORONARY ARTERY BYPASS SURGERY

EARLY COMPLICATIONS
Haemorrhage
Bleeding is normal after coronary surgery due to the effects of heparin (which are largely, but not necessarily completely, reversed by protamine) and the damaging effects of the bypass circuit on platelet numbers and function. In addition, the patient may have been taking aspirin preoperatively for its protective effect, and due to this may still have impaired platelet function. For this reason, some surgeons stop aspirin 3 to 4 days pre-operatively. This bleeding should rapidly decrease in volume after the first hour, and prolonged or excessive bleeding may be due to either a coagulation defect or a surgical cause. If the bleeding persists once any coagulation defect has been corrected, the patient may need to go back to theatre for re-exploration. This is needed in about 3% of cases. Occasionally, patients will suffer catastrophic haemorrhage due to, for example, a tie coming off one of the venous side branches, or other surgical cause, and in these cases the patient's condition may have to be re-explored in the ICU.

Cardiac tamponade occurs when blood collects around the heart and is not adequately drained. It may occur after the initial excessive haemorrhage has apparently settled, and where, in fact, the drains have become blocked with blood clot. The blood compresses the heart leading to poor venous return to the heart and low cardiac output. The cardinal signs are hypotension with a rising central venous and/or left atrial pressure. Oliguria and acidosis commonly occur and chest X-ray or echocardiogram may be helpful to confirm the diagnosis. The treatment consists in surgical evacuation of the clot.

Arrhythmias

Atrial fibrillation is common after coronary surgery (in up to 30% of cases) generally occurs after the first 24 hours. Treatment consists in giving digoxin or other antiarrhythmics, although if the patient is still ventilated or seriously compromised electrical cardioversion may be preferable (see Chapter 9).

Low Cardiac Output

Low cardiac output is usually due to pre-existing or perioperative myocardial damage. The features are cool clammy peripheries, relatively low blood pressure, higher than normal atrial pressures and poor urinary output. Treatment includes ensuring adequate filling volume (guided by the central venous pressure), and correcting any rhythm disturbances, and then giving inotropic drugs. These drugs act by increasing the force of contraction of the heart. Inotropes commonly used are dobutamine, adrenaline, isoprenaline (which also increases heart rate) and dopamine (this is also used for its beneficial effect on renal blood flow).

A pulmonary artery flotation catheter (Swan–Ganz) is often used to measure the pressures in the pulmonary artery and, indirectly, the left atrium in order to allow an appropriate choice of inotropes (Figure 7.5). The Swan–Ganz catheter can also enable direct measurement of the cardiac output. If the cardiac output is low, and moderate doses of inotropes alone are insufficient, an intra-aortic balloon pump (IABP) may be used to provide further support. This is inserted via the femoral artery and sits in the descending aorta. It inflates in diastole and deflates in systole. This increases the blood pressure in the aorta during diastole, thereby increasing coronary artery perfusion (which mainly occurs during diastole), and by deflating in systole it reduces the work that the left

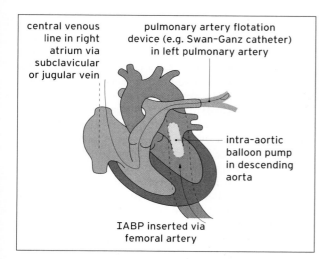

Figure 7.5 Diagram of relative positions of central venous line, pulmonary artery flotation catheter and intra-aortic balloon pump (IABP).

central venous line in right atrium via subclavicular or jugular vein

pulmonary artery flotation device (e.g. Swan-Ganz catheter) in left pulmonary artery

intra-aortic balloon pump in descending aorta

IABP inserted via femoral artery

ventricle has to perform in pumping blood. It is important to realise that an IABP does not actually pump blood as such and is more correctly referred to as a counterpulsation device.

Low urine output (oliguria) may reflect a low cardiac output state, and the first step is to treat the heart and circulation. Once the circulation is optimised, oliguria may respond to treatment with a diuretic, e.g. frusemide, which is often given to increase urine output and, in severe cases, may be given as an infusion to rescue the kidneys. Prolonged oliguria may lead to acute renal failure and this may require temporary renal support with a haemofiltration machine; the blood is taken from a large vein, filtered to remove waste products and excess water and then returned to the venous system.

Bypass Reactions

Cardiopulmonary bypass provokes an inflammatory reaction which in most patients is clinically unimportant. In a few cases, however, bypass may produce a severe reaction resulting in vasodilation and hypotension. It may also result in an acute lung injury with features similar to the adult respiratory distress syndrome (ARDS), i.e. diffuse lung shadowing on radiography and poor oxygenation without evidence of fluid overload.

Pneumothorax

Pneumothorax is occasionally seen in post-operative patients, requiring further chest drain insertion.

Hyperglycaemia

Hyperglycaemia, requiring insulin, is frequently seen in patients not known to be diabetic pre-operatively. A proportion of these will subsequently be shown to have either diabetes or impaired glucose tolerance, but many more will not need further treatment after the initial post-operative period.

Myocardial Infarction

Perioperative myocardial infarction occurs in 5% of patients, and carries an increased risk of death and long-term left ventricular impairment.

Cerebrovascular accident (CVA)

Cerebrovascular complications of CABG can be divided into major embolic stroke (1%) and more diffuse neurological dysfunction after surgery. The latter is usually transient although, depending on the sensitivity of the tests used, many patients show some evidence of this condition.

Atelectasis

This is common and is related to pain and immobility. Left-sided collapse is also common after internal mammary artery harvesting. Such cases generally respond to physiotherapy, and antibiotics are reserved for cases where sputum culture has identified an organism or where there are clear signs of infection, i.e. persisting purulent sputum, fever or raised white blood cell count. Occasionally, major lobar collapse will be caused by mucous plugging and require bronchoscopy.

Wound Infections

These may be superficial in which case local toilet and antibiotics will suffice, or may be deep sternal infections that could lead to mediastinitis. This is extremely serious and may need re-exploration and debridement. In some cases, irrigation of the mediastinum with antiseptics and even laying open of the sternum may be needed. Long-term non-healing of the sternum may ensue, requiring involvement of plastic surgeons to create muscle flaps for wound closure.

Pain and Immobility

The sternal wound generally heals well with little pain after the first few days. The leg wound may be more troublesome with a serous discharge, swelling and discomfort, but will usually settle with conservative measures.

OTHER FORMS OF SURGERY FOR ISCHAEMIC HEART DISEASE

There are several complications of ischaemic heart disease which may be amenable to surgical therapy. Infarction of the papillary muscles in the left ventricle may lead to mitral regurgitation. This may be effectively treated with mitral valve replacement, with or without CABG. Myocardial infarction may lead to development of a left ventricular aneurysm. This may compromise ventricular performance, act as a source of thrombus formation and subsequent embolism, and provoke cardiac arrhythmias. In this case, surgical resection may be advised. Myocardial infarction may also cause rupture of the ventricular septum and shunting of blood from left to right. If the shunt is large, this rapidly leads to heart failure and pulmonary oedema unless corrected, and emergency surgery may be indicated—the mortality from this condition remains high even with surgery. Rupture of the free wall of the ventricle may occur after myocardial infarction, and this is almost always fatal. In rare cases, the rupture is contained by thrombus and adherent pericardium and the patient may reach hospital alive. In such cases surgical repair may be possible.

SURGERY FOR HEART FAILURE

Cardiac transplantation is established as an effective treatment for patients with severe heart failure (see Chapter 11).

Cardiomyoplasty is an experimental technique whereby skeletal muscle is used to wrap the heart and is then stimulated by a pacemaker in order to provide additional contractility. Mechanical hearts can save a patient but their complications, expense and other implications are enormous.

VALVULAR HEART DISEASE

Surgery for valvular heart disease remains a major part of the workload of most centres, although the proportion of valve to coronary operations in the Western world has decreased over the past 30 years. In 1994, 5738 valve operations were performed in the UK, two-thirds of these being aortic valve replacements, mitral valve replacements or repairs constituting the majority of the remainder.

Normal heart valves cause no resistance to onward flow when open, and allow no backward flow when closed. If they are narrowed or 'stenosed' the chamber before the valve has to generate higher pressure. If they are 'regurgitant' the heart has to cope with an extra volume load.

Aortic stenosis is a result of congenital abnormality. Severe cases present in infancy and childhood. Mild degrees of abnormality, where two of the cusps have failed to separate properly, cause the valve to stiffen and calcify with time. This begins to cause trouble in the fifth or sixth decade of life. Sometimes a previously normal valve calcifies; such patients are seen in their 70s and 80s. Aortic stenosis is characteristically a disease of old age and many of our patients are over 70.

The left ventricular systolic pressure has to increase to maintain a normal arterial pressure beyond the valve. Typical symptoms are angina, dyspnoea on exertion and effort syncope. There may also be co-existing coronary artery disease, and a coronary angiogram is required before any valve surgery is contemplated. Surgery is usually advised once the gradient across the valve reaches 60 mmHg, or if there are signs of left ventricular failure, both to improve symptoms and reduce the chance of sudden death. Patients with severe aortic stenosis should avoid strenuous exercise (including exercise testing) as this may lead to sudden death.

Aortic regurgitation may occur with aortic stenosis or in isolation. It may be rheumatic, congenital or related to conditions such as endocarditis, hypertension, aortic dissection, Marfan's syndrome, ankylosing spondylitis, syphilis or Reiter's syndrome. Blood regurgitates across the leaky valve resulting in progressive volume overload and dilation of the left ventricle. This eventually leads to heart failure, and surgery is required once signs of ventricular enlargement or heart failure arise. Moderate aortic regurgitation may be effectively managed with drugs, e.g. venous vasodilators such as nifedipine.

Mitral stenosis is almost always rheumatic in origin. The left atrial pressure is elevated resulting in transmission of this pressure to the pulmonary circulation and ultimately to the right heart. This can then lead to right heart failure and peripheral oedema. A rapid rise in pulmonary-capillary pressure may lead to pulmonary vascular congestion and oedema. The long-term effects of mitral stenosis include progressive damage to the pulmonary vasculature resulting in pulmonary hypertension which may not resolve after surgery. Atrial fibrillation is common due to the enlargement of the atrium, and may result in thrombus formation and systemic embolism. Patients with mitral stenosis are also at risk of recurrent chest sepsis and pulmonary infarction and embolism. Mitral stenosis may present in pregnant women in whom the extra haemodynamic demands of pregnancy make their previously asymptomatic disorder show itself with dyspnoea. Treatment of mitral stenosis consists in medical stabilisation with digoxin, anticoagulation and diuretics and subsequent surgery. Closed or open mitral valvotomy may be performed or the valve may be replaced. A closed valvotomy is performed via a left anterior thoracotomy, and an expandable dilator is inserted through the valve via an invagination in the atrial appendage without the need for cardiopulmonary bypass. The operation is still widespread in India where rheumatic heart disease is still common and may give several decades of palliation before open replacement is necessary. There has been a resurgence of interest in mitral valvotomy with the development of catheter techniques allowing percutaneous balloon mitral valvotomy in suitable cases.

Mitral regurgitation may occur with rheumatic mitral stenosis or in isolation. Most cases that we see now are due to a form of degenerative disease called 'floppy' mitral valve disease. It may also be caused by endocarditis, papillary muscle rupture or ischaemia, connective tissue diseases, Marfan's syndrome or rupture of the chordae tendinae. Severe mitral regurgitation results in progressive enlargement of the left atrium and left ventricular failure. Treatment entails mitral valve repair if possible or otherwise replacement.

Tricuspid valve disease is usually secondary to heart failure and enlargement of the tricuspid valve ring. As such it may respond to medical treatment. Rheumatic tricuspid disease is rare and infrequently requires surgery, although valvotomy and valve replacement are occasionally performed. Tricuspid regurgitation secondary to mitral valve disease may respond to treatment of the latter although sometimes tricuspid valvuloplasty, i.e. sewing a ring around the tricuspid valve to prevent it becoming stretched and incompetent, is required.

Pulmonary stenosis is usually congenital and may be treated by valvotomy or replacement. Pulmonary regurgitation is usually secondary to pulmonary hypertension and responds to treatment of the latter.

VALVE TYPES

Valves may be mechanical, i.e. metal and plastic, or tissue. The latter include xenografts from animal tissue or homografts from human donors. Mechanical valves have the advantage of longevity although the patient is committed to long-term anticoagulation to prevent clots forming on the valve, and there is a 1–2% annual risk of serious complications involved, together with a higher risk of infection of the valve (endocarditis). Xenografts avoid the need for anticoagulation but do not have the same longevity, resulting in a need for re-operation of 5% at 10 years (this figure is somewhat higher when xenografts are used in younger patients). Overall, it is felt that elderly patients should receive xenografts and younger patients mechanical valves, provided they are suitable for anticoagulation, e.g. no active peptic ulcer disease, etc. Homografts prepared from human donors may combine the advantages of both groups and are being used particularly in young patients, although their long-term superiority over mechanical valves is yet to be proven. All valve recipients should be made aware of the risk of endocarditis, and counselled to take antibiotics when undergoing dental treatment or surgery. They should also be given an information card to carry with them.

Rarely, aortic or pulmonary stenosis may be caused by stenosis of the outflow tract from the ventricle rather than the valve itself (infundibular, or subvalvular stenosis). Supravalvular stenosis may also occur and in these cases resection of the appropriate stenosed tissue rather than replacement of the valve is the treatment of choice.

OPERATIONS ON THE GREAT VESSELS

AORTIC DISSECTION

This is a surgical emergency and arises when a tear in the intimal layer of the aorta allows blood to track between the intima and the media. This results in pain and may lead to occlusion of the arterial branches or rupture of the aorta. The dissection may track back into the aortic root leading to occlusion of the coronary arteries and myocardial infarction together with aortic valve incompetence. The condition is commonest in hypertensive patients aged 50–70, and there may be an underlying abnormality in the structure of the aortic wall. Aortic dissection is a major risk in Marfan's syndrome, where there is also aneurysmal dilation of the aorta. Aortic dissection can be divided into that which involves the ascending aorta (Stanford type A) and that which does not (type B). Type A dissections should be treated by urgent surgical replacement of the dissection (which may also require aortic valve replacement), although this carries a 25% mortality and a significant risk of paraplegia due to compromise of the blood supply to the spinal cord. Without surgery, mortality from type A dissection exceeds 90%. Type B dissections are generally treated medically with control of the blood pressure, usually using β-blockers, although rarely surgery may be indicated where major abdominal blood vessels are involved.

AORTIC TRANSECTION

This occurs after major trauma where sudden deceleration causes rupture of the aorta, usually at the level of the ligamentum arteriosus just beyond the left subclavian artery. The rupture may initially be confined by the intact adventitia, allowing the patient to reach hospital alive, but without urgent surgery the condition is usually fatal. Occasionally, patients survive such an injury without surgical intervention and may develop a calcified (false) aneurysm later in life.

PULMONARY EMBOLECTOMY

In cases of massive pulmonary embolism, the clot can obstruct the flow of blood from the right ventricle to such a degree that there is haemodynamic compromise. In such cases, pulmonary embolectomy, where the pulmonary artery is opened without the need for cardiopulmonary bypass, and where the clot is removed, may be life saving. Very few patients who are ill enough to merit this type of operation survive long enough for it to be feasible.

OTHER CARDIAC OPERATIONS

Atrial myxoma is a rare primary tumour of the heart which can present with symptoms of obstruction mimicking mitral stenosis, thromboembolism or non-specific systemic features such as fever, malaise and joint pains. It can be diagnosed by echocardiography, and treatment entails surgical excision.

Pericardectomy is the surgical removal of the pericardium and is indicated for constrictive pericarditis. This may be the result of previous tuberculous, viral or bacterial infection.

Ventricular tachycardia surgery is performed in patients with recurrent ventricular tachycardia despite anti-arrhythmic therapy. The underlying cause is usually ischaemic and these patients often need CABG as well. Electrical mapping of the heart both before and during surgery allows the electrically unstable myocardium to be identified (this is often around the scarred area where previous myocardial infarction has occurred) and resected. If surgical ablation cannot be performed, an implantable defibrillator may be inserted at a separate operation.

Insertion of permanent pacemaker systems is usually carried out by cardiologists. The pacemaker box is inserted in a pocket in the upper chest wall, the leads being fed into the heart via a great vein under X-ray guidance. Post-operatively, the pacing box will be checked and programmed for each individual patient.

The surgical management of congenital heart disease is discussed in Chapter 19.

PULMONARY SURGERY

INDICATIONS FOR SURGERY

Malignancy
The commonest indication for pulmonary resection is bronchial carcinoma, which accounts for about 90% of all resections, e.g. primary bronchial carcinoma, bronchial carcinoid and isolated secondaries from cancer of kidney.

Inflammatory
Lung resection is occasionally required for lung abscess, tuberculosis, bronchiectasis, aspergillosis and hydatid disease.

Trauma
Trauma, e.g. stab wounds and gunshot wounds to the chest.

Degenerative
Degenerative pulmonary disease, e.g. emphysema bullae.

Congenital
Congenital pulmonary conditions, e.g. arteriovenous fistula, lobar sequestration and lobar emphysema.

PULMONARY RESECTION
Patients with bronchogenic carcinoma usually present with cough, haemoptysis, shortness of breath and weight loss. They are first investigated by pulmonary physicians before referral for surgical resection.

Pre-operative Investigations
These investigations are designed to answer two questions: Can the carcinoma be removed? Is the patient fit for thoracotomy?

The patient usually presents with symptoms of cough, haemoptysis, shortness of breath (SOB) and stridor. Preoperative investigations of these patients will include:
- Chest X-ray, which usually shows a peripheral or central shadow.
- CT scan.
- Bronchoscopy and biopsy.
- Fine needle aspiration biospy (FNAB).
- Staging, e.g. mediastinoscopy, fibre bronchoscopy, and biopsy. This will decide whether the condition is operable. Treatment consists of either thoracotomy and radiotherapy or resection and chemotherapy.

BRONCHOSCOPY
This procedure can be carried out in two ways: fibreoptic flexible bronchoscopy, usually carried out by a chest physician on a conscious patient, under local anaesthesia; and rigid bronchoscopy, usually carried out by a chest surgeon, under general anaesthetic. The fibreoptic technique allows visualisation of the smaller bronchi; however, larger biopsies and better assessment of operability of central tumours can be obtained using the rigid bronchoscopic technique. The two methods are complementary and if necessary can be performed under the same anaesthetic.

INVESTIGATION/CT SCAN
CT scanning of the thorax and upper abdomen to include the adrenals is now a routine clinical work-up for patients with lung cancer. It is particularly useful for identifying metastatic deposits in the liver or adrenals. It will also detect enlarged mediastinal lymph nodes but cannot identify whether carcinoma is present in the lymph node. Therefore, if the CT scan demonstrates abnormally large mediastinal lymph nodes this should be confirmed by mediastinoscopy and biopsy.

INVESTIGATION/CHEST X-RAY
The cancer will appear as an area of shadowing. Posteroanterior and lateral films of the chest are necessary. The lateral film is useful in locating the position of the cancer whether in the upper or lower lobe.

MEDIASTINOSCOPY
This procedure is used to biopsy mediastinal lymph nodes related to the trachea which have been noted on CT scanning. It is useful both for diagnosis and as a staging procedure to plan treatment for the particular patient.

A small transverse incision is made 1 cm above the suprasternal notch, strap muscles are separated and the pretracheal fascia entered. Abnormal paratracheal and subcranial nodes can then be felt. A mediastinoscope is inserted and biopsies taken. It is impossible to reach all the lymph node stations, in particular the left-sided subaortic nodes;

in order to sample these nodes, a left anterior media-stinoscopy incision in the second intercostal space is made and a mediastinoscope introduced.

LUNG FUNCTION TESTS

Clinical assessment gives a good indication of the fitness of the patient to sustain lung resection; however, formal respiratory function tests are helpful and routinely performed. Forced expiratory volume in 1 second (FEV_1) and forced vital capacity (FVC) are recorded on a spirometer and compared with predicted values. If the FEV_1/FVC ratio is less than 40% of the predicted value or the arterial carbon dioxide level ($PaCO_2$) is greater than 5 kPa (40 mmHg) then operation is definitely contraindicated. In borderline cases, ventilation–perfusion scans are particularly helpful, allowing the surgeon to decide on whether the patient would tolerate pulmonary resection; for example, where normal lung is perfused but not ventilated and therefore shunting of deoxygenated blood from right to left occurs. Under these conditions removal of the abnormal lung can be expected actually to improve overall lung function.

OTHER INVESTIGATIONS

Occasionally, radionuclide scans of bone and liver are performed and ultrasound scans of the liver are screened for distant metastases. Some patients will also have coronary artery disease and will require full cardiological investigations.

Patients who have been found to have significant coronary stenosis sometimes undergo successful coronary bypass surgery before lung resection. In patients who have undergone recent myocardial infarction it may be necessary to postpone lung surgery for 6 weeks from the time of infarction.

INCISIONS IN THORACIC SURGERY

Most thoracic operations are performed through a posterolateral thoracotomy. This incision is made in line with the ribs under the scapula and divides the lower fibres of the trapezius, latissimus dorsi and serratus anterior muscles, and external and internal intercostal muscles. An anterolateral thoracotomy is occasionally performed for procedures such as closed mitral valvotomy or lung biopsy.

DRAINAGE OF THE CHEST

The purpose of drains in thoracic surgery is to remove fluid or air which collects within the pleural space. Drainage may be open or closed.

Closed Drainage

A tube with end and side holes is introduced into the thorax via an intercostal space. It is connected to a closed bottle via a transparent tube which ends under water. A second short tube left unconnected maintains atmospheric pressure within the bottle. This arrangement provides a simple one-way valve. If the short tube is connected to a suction apparatus, the air pressure within the bottle will be reduced below atmospheric. If sufficient suction is applied, the negative pressure which exists between the lung and the chest wall will be increased. Calibrations on the bottle allow easy measurement of blood loss in the post-operative patient.

On free drainage, the water level in the bottle will rise on inspiration and fall on expiration due to the change in intrathoracic pressure. If the fluid level ceases to swing this means that the lung is fully expanded or that the tube is blocked. If the drainage is connected to suction there should be no swing. The drainage bottle should be kept at a level lower than that of the patient's chest to prevent the siphoning of fluid back in to the pleural cavity. The drain should not be clamped except during difficult changes in the patient's position.

After pneumonectomy, intercostal drains are never connected to suction because of the danger of mediastinal shift. After other types of lung resection, usually two drains are present—one to drain the apex to accommodate unwanted air and the other contacting the base of the pleural space to remove fluid, typically blood after resection.

Open Drainage

A tube in the pleural cavity connects directly with air. This arrangement is safe only when the pleural cavity has become rigid and immovable. This is used to drain a chronic empyema where the infection is localised from the rest of the pleura by fibrosis. This method is very rarely used at the present time. If permanent drainage is necessary then a fenestration operation is performed to connect the interior of the pleural space directly with the skin surface allowing pus to drain out freely.

COMPLICATIONS OF LUNG SURGERY

Early (0–2 Weeks)

Local complications include haemorrhage, atelectasis/lobar collapse, wound infection, surgical emphysema, pleural effusion, empyema, bronchopleural fistula, and nerve damage (e.g. recurrent laryngeal, phrenic). General complications include ventilatory insufficiency, atrial fibrillation, myocardial infarction, pulmonary embolus/deep vein thrombosis and CVA.

Late (2 Weeks Onwards)

Local complications include thoracotomy wound pain, recurrence of carcinoma, chest wall deformity and restricted arm movements. General complications include distant spread of carcinoma.

Bronchopleural Fistula

A bronchopleural fistula implies breakdown in the bronchial stump, and it occurs any time post-operatively. If small, it may not be noticed until much later. It is recognised by dyspnoea, an irritating cough and possible expectoration of dark fluid. An associated empyema is inevitable. The patient should be sat up or turned to the side operated on to prevent spillover of infected fluid into the remaining lung. The pneumonectomy space should be drained promptly and the patient treated with antibiotics.

Recurrent Laryngeal Nerve Damage

Damage to the recurrent laryngeal nerve may occur during left pneumonectomy or left upper lobectomy due to its course around the arch of the aorta. Such damage seriously impairs the ability of the patient to cough, and the patient presents with a hoarse voice. If the damage is permanent, an injection of Teflon into the vocal cord can be performed by the ear, nose and throat surgeon. This can improve the symptoms by stiffening the vocal cord.

TYPES OF PULMONARY RESECTION

Pneumonectomy

The entire lung is removed. Operative mortality in the UK is around 7–10%, but for patients over 70 years of age 20% mortality can be expected. In a radical pneumonectomy, mediastinal lymph nodes and part of the chest wall may also be removed. The resulting cavity is reduced by lateral shift of the trachea and heart and upward shift of the diaphragm, and collection of fluid and fibrin. In addition, there is reduction of the intercostal spaces on the side operated on. Occasionally, much later, scoliosis develops.

Lobectomy

Any of the five lobes may be removed. On the right side, the middle and lower lobes are often removed together because of the common lymphatic drainage. If a tumour in the upper lobe protrudes into the main bronchus a segment of bronchus can be removed with the lobe, and the remaining lung and bronchus joined to the trachea. This is termed a sleeve resection.

Segmental Resection

A pulmonary segment is removed with its segmental artery and bronchus. This used to be indicated for tuberculosis but is now rarely performed.

Wedge Resection

This non-anatomical resection is used for excision of localised peripheral carcinomas in patients with reduced lung function, and for obtaining biopsies of lung using the automatic stapling device. This operation is commonly performed.

PNEUMOTHORAX

Details of pneumothorax are discussed in Chapter 12. Surgical management of recurring pneumothorax is highlighted below:

Pleurodesis

A chemical pleurisy is produced by the insertion of an irritant, e.g. tetracycline or iodised talc, into the pleural cavity.

Pleurectomy

Via a small posterior thoracotomy, the parietal pleura over the apex of the pleural space is removed leaving a raw surface to which the visceral pleura and lung will adhere. At the same time the area on the visceral pleura which is leaking air is stapled or oversewn. At present this procedure is generally carried out using video assisted thoracoscopic surgery.

EMPYEMA

This is a localised collection of pus in the pleural cavity. It may be associated with lung or subphrenic abscess or bronchopleural fistulae. Most empyemas these days arise after pneumonia.

Treatment

The aims of treatment are to abolish infection, obtain full lung expansion and prevent development of a rigid chest wall.

Early cases (acute)

These can be treated by pleural aspiration, oral antibiotics and physiotherapy, intercostal tube drainage, and video assisted thorascopic drainage.

Late cases (chronic)

These are more difficult to treat and will require thoracotomy and decortication of lung. The principle is to peel the thickened fibrotic layer of visceral pleura (cortex of the surface of the lung). This allows the lung to expand fully and adhere to the parietal pleura.

OPERATIONS ON THE CHEST WALL

Individual ribs or parts of a rib may be resected during excision of a neoplasm or for drainage of an empyema.

Fractured Ribs

This operation is performed only if the lungs are damaged. Pinning of the fractured rib is carried out in some centres. The rib ends are proximated and fixed with medullary pins.

Major Injuries

Injuries of the chest wall occur frequently in road traffic accidents. Multiple rib fractures may result in a flail chest. If a segment of the chest wall becomes detached (flail) paradoxical breathing occurs which seriously compromises ventilation. During inspiration, when intrathoracic pressure becomes more negative, the flail segment moves inwards while the remainder of the chest wall expands. During expiration, when intrathoracic pressure becomes less negative, the flail segment moves outwards. (Details of chest injuries are covered in Chapter 12.)

CONGENITAL DEFORMITIES

Pectus Carinatum (Pigeon Chest)

From this deformity the sternum projects forward and is held in a prominent position by the ribs and costal cartilages. The rectifying operation is performed mainly for cosmetic reasons. The prominent costal cartilages are removed and the sternum split horizontally and fixed in its new position with stainless steel wires.

Pectus Excavatum (Funnel Chest)

This deformity is probably caused by overgrowth of the lower costal cartilages and ribs, which is compensated for by depression of the lower end of the sternum, presumably due to pull of the diaphragm. Ventilatory and cardiac function may be impaired but the rectifying operation is performed usually for cosmetic reasons. The lower costal cartilages are resected on both sides and the sternum is split horizontally. The position is maintained by a metal bar, which is removed later. An alternative method is to place a pre-formed silastic prosthesis subcutaneously to improve the contour of the chest wall.

Thoracoplasty

This operation is now uncommon. It used to be performed in some cases of pulmonary tuberculosis before effective chemotherapy was available. An extensive resection of the ribs is performed, and as the chest wall loses this support it falls inwards and obliterates the pleural cavity and/or lung tissue. Infected pneumonectomy spaces are some-times closed in this manner. The first rib may or may not be removed.

Video Assisted Thoracic Surgery (VATS)

Recently, there has been a vogue to perform thoracic oper-ation using video assisted thoracoscopic techniques. All pulmonary resections and operations including lobec-tomy/pneumonectomy have been performed by VATS. The aftercare of these patients would be exactly as for patients who have undergone open surgery. The advantage of VATS is that small access incisions are made in the chest which result in minimal trauma and therefore reduced post-operative pain. This allows the patient to mobilise rapidly and be discharged early.

The commonest VATS procedures performed include:
- Apical pleurectomy and stapling of bullae.
- Wedge biopsy of lung.
- Pleural biopsy and talc pleurodesis.
- Pericardial window for pericardial effusion.

In VATS, the patients undergo standard general anaes-thesia for thoracic surgery. A double lumen endotracheal tube is inserted. In order to allow the lung on the opera-tion side to be collapsed, three to four 1 inch incisions are made in the chest wall for introduction of the telescope attached to the video camera and other instruments. At the end of the procedure, the lung is re-inflated and the intercostal drains inserted and connected to an under-water seal in the usual way. These drains will usually be connected to low pressure suction to facilitate lung expan-sion. The post-operative care of these patients is identical to that in patients undergoing open procedures.

SURGERY TO THE OESOPHAGUS AND STOMACH

This section covers the signs and symptoms of oesophageal and gastric abnormalities, and the investigations, diagnosis and treatment methods, in particular types of surgery. It is important to realise that because of the anatomical relation-ship between the organs and the respiratory system which derive congenitally from a common stem, and the anatomical relationship between other structures in the mediastinum,

neck and upper abdomen, it is not unusual to have patho-logical changes in neighbouring structures. This alone can determine whether a patient is a candidate for surgery or for more palliative care and radiotherapy. If, for example, a patient is diagnosed as having cancer of the oesophagus, and further investigations find secondary deposits in the liver, then the patient will probably be referred to the department of radiotherapy for treatment; the prognosis is not good.

ANATOMY

In its course in the neck, chest and abdomen, the oesophagus is subject to varying pressures. These begin with the positive pressure of the contiguous organs of the neck followed by the negative intrathoracic pressure and finally, in conjunction with the stomach, the positive intra-abdominal pressure. The oesophageal and stomach musculature, in common with the rest of the gastrointestinal tract, consists of an outer longitu-dinal and an inner circular layer. However, in the stomach there are also oblique fibres which are seen predominantly in the cardia and the vicinity of the fundus and lesser curves. Although the musculature of the gastrointestinal tract is essentially non-striated, the oesophagus at its cervical end consists of striated muscles almost entirely, while in the mid-dle third approximately 50% of the muscle is non-striated; in the lower third it is entirely smooth. The nerve supply derives from the autonomic system and the lymphatic drainage of the oesophagus and stomach is of considerable importance when considering the management of malignant disease by surgery or other modalities.

The various parameters of oesophageal and gastric pathophysiology lend themselves to investigations by sev-eral techniques, the most important of which are a detailed clinical history, radiological imaging of the two organs, endoscopy of the upper gastrointestinal tract, and oesophageal and gastric motility assessment combined with ambulatory pH measurement of the oesophagus. In addition to these measurements, transit of the upper gastrointestinal tract is also measured by radio-isotope studies while the secretory function of the stomach is estab-lished by total acid secretion.

Clearly, it is more cost effective and time saving if these investigations can be performed at one specialized diagnostic centre.

SIGNS AND SYMPTOMS

The common symptoms of oesophago-gastric disease include:
- Heartburn.
- Difficulty or incapability of swallowing, i.e. dysphagia.
- Regurgitation.
- Chest or epigastric pain.
- Cough induced by swallowing.

The rate of progression of the symptoms becomes signifi-cant where malignancy is concerned, as opposed to benign pathology, and also, if the symptoms occur later in life, the likelihood of malignancy is higher in contrast with develop-ing the symptoms in a younger age group. If the patient demonstrates motility disturbances as a 30-year-old, these must be regularly assessed as benign symptoms may lead to malignancy in later life. Dysphagia of malignant disease is very often rapidly progressive as opposed to dysphagia of benign pathology, for example, a stricture in the oesophagus or motility (peristalsis) disturbances.

INVESTIGATIONS

Radiological Tests

These involve the use of a radio-opaque substance such as barium or gastrograffin, performed as a barium swallow or meal; the former outlines the pharynx and oesophagus and the latter outlines the entire gastrointestinal tract to the duodenum. The barium is radio-opaque, the flow of the contrast being seen on an X-ray screen and any abnormalities demonstrated as obstruction to the flow. The motility of the oesophagus can also be assessed and a further more detailed study can demonstrate mucosal damage or inflammation caused by malignancy or acid regurgitation from the stomach.

Endoscopy

Here, a flexible fibreoptic scope is introduced into the pharynx via the patient's mouth while they are sedated. This allows a visual inspection of the pharynx, oesophagus, stomach and first part of the duodenum. In addition, the endoscopist can take samples of mucosa for pathology and identify any abnormalities in contractions of the oesopahagus, the presence of gastro-oesophageal reflux (GOR), any shortening of the oesophagus due to the presence of herniation of the stomach into the thorax, i.e. hiatus hernia, abnormalities of the different areas of the stomach, e.g. polyps, tumours, gastric ulcers, and with further introduction of the scope into the duodenum, duodenal ulcers and malignancy distal to the stomach within the limitations of the visual field of the oesophagoscope. If there is a need to investigate further along the gastrointestinal tract, then endoscopy may be performed rectally to identify the more distal structures.

Oesophageal Motility Studies and pH Levels

If the patient suffers from acid or bile regurgitation, this can be investigated by introducing a probe into the oesophagus and/or duodenum to measure the amount of acid produced, the efficiency of the motility of the oesophagus, particularly with eating or drinking, and evidence of acid in the oesophagus. Acid in the oesophagus tends to cause inflammation of the mucosa, known as oesophagitis.

To date, we have discussed the pathological changes that can occur with abnormalities. Now we turn to acquired lesions affecting the oesophagus or stomach.

Foreign Body Impaction

Here, the patient complains of an inability to swallow as the oesophagus has become occluded with a large bolus of food. This can be caused by dysmobility or an obstructive lesion or object, e.g. a small toy.

Removal of a foreign body is ideally carried out under a general anaesthetic using a rigid or a flexible fibreoptic scope.

Traumatic Perforation

Traumatic perforation often results from either a direct impact or a crush injury to the chest (see Chapter 12).

Spontaneous Rupture of the Oesophagus

The patient has a history of a motility disorder or has a violent episode of vomiting, and presents to casualty with surgical emphysema around the upper thorax, and chest pain. If treatment occurs soon after the insult, typically surgical repair of the rupture, then the prognosis is good with a 10% mortality rate. If, however, the patient is seen at a later stage there may be irreparable damage to the oesophagus and surgery will not be recommended—the mortality rate is high at approximately 80%.

Intrinsic Rupture of the Oesophagus

This occurs, for example, if the patient is undergoing an oesophagoscopy and, because of the 'friability' of the oesophagus, the scope causes a perforation.

PATHOPHYSIOLOGY

Tumours of the oesophagus are commonly squamous or adenocarcinomatous whereas tumours of the stomach are adenocarcinomatous with varying degrees of differentiation. Benign tumours of the oesophagus are predominantly those arising in the muscular and submucosal layers of the wall and, similarly, benign tumours of the stomach are either of muscular origin or arise from the submucosal fatty tissue. In addition to these tumours, lymphoma can be seen in both oesophageal and stomach wall, dependent on the diffuse nature of the manifestation. Peptic ulcer disease of the oesophagus, while it is secondary to GOR, may occur localised in the upper part of the oesophagus.

TREATMENT

The following conditions are the more common types seen by the thoracic surgeon and needing the aid of the physiotherapist.

Gastro-oesophageal Reflux (GOR)

Common symptoms of GOR are heartburn, acid reflux, oesophagitis and, sometimes, regurgitation. The majority of patients can be managed conservatively with medication such as antacid therapy and dietary advice to avoid food that produces the symptoms. If the patient has a hiatus hernia where the stomach enters the thorax through an enlarged hiatus of the diaphragm, then an operation to repair the diaphragmatic lesion may be performed through a thoracotomy and, depending on the mobility of the stomach, it may be pushed back through into the abdomen and the diaphragm repaired (Belsey's repair). In the event that the hernia is too difficult to repair, the stomach above the diaphragm is wrapped around the distal end of the oesophagus and sutured to form a pseudosphincter at the cardia, the junction between the stomach and the oesophagus. The procedure is called a fundoplication and a common surgical method is the Nissan fundoplication.

In recent years, video assisted endoscopic surgery has had a similar impact on simple procedures involving the oesophagus as in other branches of surgery. Thoracoscopic and laparoscopic procedures are currently used for the control of GOR. The more popular route is via a laparoscope whereby a total or partial fundoplication is performed through a minimum of five portholes, one of which carries a camera and another the instruments. Despite this innovation, the long-term results of laparoscopic and thoracoscopic antireflux procedures are not adequately documented and circumspection about such operations is needed.

Open techniques have been widely documented over the past few years and the success of repair ranges from 85% to 95%.

Malignant Tumours

The treatment of malignant tumours of the oesophagus and stomach needs a multimodality approach but the only treatment method with any success rate is resection. This involves surgical removal of the segment containing the tumour and an adequate margin of tissue to ensure removal of all the tumour cells. Lymph node involvement means a poor result and often surgery is for palliation of symptoms. Regardless, the results from surgery are more successful than, for example, chemo- or radiotherapy, laser or stenting of the occluded oesophagus.

SURGICAL APPROACHES TO THE STOMACH AND OESOPHAGUS

Apart from keyhole and endoscopic access to the oesophagus and stomach, open access for surgery on these organs is achieved by cervical, thoracic and abdominal incisions. One or more of these may be employed in any one operation.

The Cervical Incision

The cervical incision in the neck is essentially for access to the cervical oesophagus and pharynx and this is performed either as an oblique incision along the anterior border of the sternomastoid or as a transverse incision along one of the skin crease lines centred at the sixth cervical vertebral level. This allows access to the oesophagus as well as the cricopharyngeal area without too much difficulty.

The Thoracic Incision

For lower oesophageal tumours, the thoracic incision involves a thoracotomy through the left seventh intercostal space, and for tumours of the mid or entire oesophagus, through a right thoracotomy incision at the fifth intercostal space. A thoracolaparotomy is indicated if the tumour extends into the stomach from the distal end of the oesophagus or if the lesion is gastric; however, big incisions cause post-operative complications because of damage to the musculature and pain. This is when the services of the physiotherapist are needed to prevent atelectasis and encourage mobilisation (see physiotherapy section).

In recent years, multiple incisions of the chest have been replaced by an upper midline laparotomy, permitting complete access to the entire length of the stomach and duodenum as well as the lower aspect of the oesophagus. A trans-hiatal incision allows access to the lower two thirds of the oesophagus and is achieved by increasing or enlarging the anatomical hiatus. Trans-hiatal oesophagectomy is becoming increasingly more popular with general surgeons although thoracic surgeons still employ the thoracic approach.

During the operation, elective collapse of the lung on the side of the incision is established by use of the double lumen intubation tube allowing ventilation of a single lung during mobilisation and operation of the transthoracic part of the oesophagus. After the procedure, the anaesthetist can re-ventilate the deflated lung and the surgeon introduces intercostal drains to help re-inflate the lung and to drain any post-operative blood.

In some units, the patient is ventilated post-operatively, but with advances in anaesthesia, good post-operative pain control (see below) and the help of the physiotherapy team, the risks attached to major surgery are fewer and the patient's stay in hospital is reduced.

COMPLICATIONS

The complications after oesophagectomy or gastrectomy are covered later in this chapter.

POST-OPERATIVE PAIN CONTROL

Pain following thoracic and upper abdominal surgery can be very severe, as the operations involve extensive incisions and manipulation of organs. In both types of operation, the skin incision involves cutting a large number of cutaneous nerves and several muscles are either incised or retracted. The pressure of drains post-operatively also contributes to the problems.

Pain may also be conducted via the vagus and phrenic nerves and, in thoracic surgery, even from the shoulder joint via cervical nerves C5–C7. The sympathetic nervous system is also involved, conducting pain from the viscera, although this mechanism is poorly understood at present.

Many of these considerations also apply to cardiac operations and, in addition, pain may arise from enlarging the sternotomy, resulting in damage to the ribs and costochondral junctions. However, the midline incision is surprisingly less painful than after thoracotomy. In fact, most patients undergoing CABGs complain more about the discomfort in their legs from which the saphenous vein grafts have been taken.

POST-OPERATIVE RESPIRATORY FUNCTION

Apart from the humanitarian aspect of relieving a patient's suffering, the provision of adequate post-operative pain relief in cardiothoracic and upper abdominal surgery can have a significant effect on respiratory morbidity.

Major changes in lung volumes, mechanics and gas exchange occur after such surgery, with a reduction in total lung volume, FRC and residual volume. This results in an increased proportion of the resting tidal respiration taking place below the closing volume and thus ventilation/perfusion mismatching with shunting. Compliance is decreased and the work of breathing is increased.

Although the extent and duration of these changes is proportional to the extent of the surgical procedure, they will also be influenced by the ability of patients to deep breathe, cough and co-operate with their physiotherapist. Pain results in shallow tidal volumes and the absence of deep breathing, leading to underventilation and gradual collapse of alveoli. Inability to clear secretions may lead to plugging of bronchioles or even major airways, which further increases the shunting. Infection of such atelectatic areas results in pneumonia.

The results of these changes and the efficacy of post-operative analgesia can be assessed and compared by the use of chest X-rays, spirometry, arterial blood–gas analysis and pulse oximetry. It has been shown that patients receiving good pain relief will have better lung function tests, less X-ray evidence of atelectasis and a lower incidence of hypoxaemic episodes.

DRUGS AND OTHER MODALITIES

The drugs and techniques available for the prevention and treatment of post-operative pain include opiate analgesics, non-steroidal anti-inflammatory drugs (NSAIDs), regional local anaesthesia, transcutaneous electric nerve stimulation (TENS) and acupuncture.

The severity of post-operative pain after cardiothoracic or upper abdominal surgery means that adequate analgesia usually cannot be provided using a single drug or technique, without incurring serious side effects. However, relief can be achieved using a combination of them and each anaesthetist or surgeon will, from experience, have devised a suitable regimen. The exact details will vary from one practitioner to another but the results can be equally as good.

Special considerations apply to cardiac surgery patients and, for this reason, the techniques are described with details of how they relate to thoracic and upper abdominal surgery. This is followed by a description of those techniques applicable to cardiac surgery.

SYSTEMIC OPIATE ANALGESICS

Although opiates are powerful analgesics, they can have a deleterious effect on the respiratory system. Opiates can depress the respiratory centres, causing desensitisation to the stimulating effects of hypercarbia and hypoxia, and also inhibit coughing and deep breaths. In addition, they cause sedation which, if excessive, can decrease the ability of the patients to co-operate with their physiotherapist. The appropriate use of opiate analgesia aims to achieve a balance between pain relief and avoiding side effects. This therapeutic range is small and there is also a considerable variation in response from one patient to another. Therefore, the traditional method of intramuscular injections of opiates is poorly suited to the control of post-operative pain, and the best way to use these drugs systemically is to titrate small doses intravenously until a satisfactory

response is obtained. A development of this approach is the use of patient controlled analgesia (PCA) in which the patient can self-administer, via a specialized pump, a preset intravenous dose of opiate. The practitioner who programmes the pump can select the dose to be given at each demand and the interval between doses during which the pump will not respond to a patient demand (the 'lock-out' time). The most commonly used drugs are morphine and fentanyl.

Intravenous opiates should not be administered by a syringe pump at a constant rate. Such a method will not respond to varying pain levels and the drug may accumulate, leading to oversedation and respiratory arrest. Respiratory depression has also been reported with PCA and the use of the method does not obviate the need for careful observation of the patient.

TRANSDERMAL OPIATES

An interesting development in analgesia is the formulation of a fentanyl patch for transdermal administration. The first license has been granted for its use in chronic pain but it may be extended to acute pain. There are some potential problems, such as variable absorption, slow build-up in blood levels and continuing absorption after the patch has been removed. It is not possible to predict whether this mode of use will find a place in the prevention or treatment of post-operative pain.

NON-STEROIDAL ANTI-INFLAMMATORY DRUGS (NSAIDs)

A wide variety of NSAIDs have been used to reduce pain in patients after thoracic and abdominal surgery. Although they are not powerful enough alone to prevent or control such pain, they can reduce the amount of opiate which is required. They have also been used to good effect in combination with intercostal nerve blocks in patients after thoracic surgery.

NSAIDs can be given as a premedication, or intraoperatively or post-operatively, and are formulated so that a choice can be made regarding the route of delivery, i.e. oral, rectal, intravenous or intramuscular. Success has been reported using several NSAIDs so the choice of agent is probably not important.

The NSAIDs are not without their potential problems, including gastrointestinal bleeding, acute reversible renal dysfunction and bleeding associated with platelet dysfunction. The effects are unlikely to cause significant clinical problems with short-term use and none have been recorded in published studies, although these have excluded patients with known peptic ulceration or renal disease.

REGIONAL LOCAL ANAESTHETIC TECHNIQUES

Intercostal Nerve Block

Each intercostal nerve can be blocked by a separate injection of 3–5 ml of local anaesthetic, and it is possible to block nerves from T2 to T12. To be effective, the lateral cutaneous branch needs to be blocked, which requires the injection to be given at the midaxillary line. If used at thoracotomy, the block can be performed by the surgeon. It is important to remember to block the nerves supplying the site of a chest drain as well as the line of incision.

The duration of analgesia is limited by the type of local anaesthetic, but even at best is only 4–8 hours. Repeating the block at intervals is difficult practically and is uncomfortable for the patient. Attempts have been made to provide a more prolonged period of pain relief by the use of catheters which may be introduced percutaneously into the intercostal space. The use of both intermittent boluses and continuous infusions of local anaesthetic has been reported, with better results being achieved by the continuous method.

Intercostal nerve block carries a risk of pneumothorax. This is not a problem following thoracotomy if a chest drain has been inserted, but is of concern in upper abdominal surgery, particularly if a midline incision would require a number of blocks bilaterally.

In addition, there is a risk that large total volumes of local anaesthetic injected close to the neurovascular bundle will lead to rapid absorption, high plasma concentrations and toxicity. The addition of adrenaline will reduce peak plasma concentrations but the systemic effect of the adrenaline will then have to be taken into account.

Extrapleural Analgesia

Extrapleural analgesia is an extension of the intercostal space catheter technique, and is used in thoracotomy patients. At operation, a packet of parietal pleura is formed by retracting it medially from the posterior wound edge, a catheter is then inserted percutaneously and the pleura attached to the wound edge. The procedure adds only 10–20 minutes to the operation.

An extrapleural technique creates a more extensive block than an intercostal nerve block because the local anaesthetic enters the paravertebral space (PVS; see below) and spreads into adjacent spaces. Although a sympathetic block would also be expected, studies have not demonstrated that this occurs.

The results of the extrapleural technique have been very impressive in terms of both pain relief and improvement of respiratory function. It is a relatively safe procedure and worth the extra surgical time.

Cryoanalgesia

When nerves are exposed to extreme cold, long-lasting but reversible analgesia can be produced . A cryoprobe uses a high-pressure gas which is allowed to expand rapidly within the tip of the probe. This produces cooling (the Joule–Thompson principle) down to temperatures of –20 to –60°C. This technique has been applied to intercostal nerves during thoracotomy.

In the 1980s, cryoanalgesia became popular as it was thought to be without serious side effects. However, its use can cause paresis of intercostal and abdominal muscles with reduction in effective coughing. In addition, the time to recovery of normal nerve sensation is unpredictable and nerve damage may actually be permanent. Anaesthesia of the breast and nipple can be distressing,

especially in young women, and problems with breast-feeding reflexes have been reported. Cryoanalgesia can also produce the formation of neuromata and long-lasting neuralgia. Consequently, it has fallen out of favour and is little used now.

Intrapleural Analgesia

In 1990, the injection of local anaesthesia intrapleurally, i.e. between the visceral and parietal pleura, was shown to produce pain relief after cholecystectomy and renal surgery. The technique was then applied to patients undergoing thoracotomy using catheters inserted by the surgeon before closing the chest.

The mode of action of intrapleural local anaesthetics is not well understood. It may consist in diffusion through the pleura to the intercostal nerves or into the PVS.

The local anaesthetic may be diluted by blood, rapidly absorbed from injured pleura and lung tissue or lost from chest drains. Although some studies have shown lower pain scores in patients receiving intrapleural analgesia, the reduction of opiate consumption has not been significant.

It is possible that future work may determine better regimens in terms of how many catheters are needed, what concentration of local anaesthetic is required, what size dose to use and the best way to administer it.

Paravertebral Block

The PVS is the area the spinal nerves enter as they leave the intervertebral foramen. The nerve divides into the anterior and posterior rami during its passage through the PVS, and the sympathetic chain also lies within it. Injection of local anaesthetic into the PVS can produce motor, sensory and sympathetic nerve blockade.

There is no direct communication between one PVS and another but injected local anaesthetic can spread via the loose connective tissue, and in only 10% of cases does the block remain confined to the PVS into which the injection is given. The local anaesthetic also spreads into the epidural space and a unilateral injection can even spread bilaterally over a wide area. Usually, however, the block remains more localised and the reduced sympathetic block leads to a lower risk of hypotension, bradycardia and urinary retention when compared with epidural blockade.

Both a single shot injection and the placement of catheters into the PVS are possible. Complications can arise from the accidental puncture of the dura and pleura, and catheters can also be misplaced into the cerebrospinal fluid (CSF) or epidural space, or intrapleurally.

Epidural Block Anaesthetic

Epidural block anaesthetic can produce excellent analgesia both intra- and post-operatively. When performed at the lumbar level, a large volume has to be injected to extend the block to the required segments. This can cause an unacceptable sympathetic block with severe hypertension, urinary retention and unwanted motor block of the lower limbs, resulting in reduced mobility and the risk of pressure sores. Systemic toxicity may also be a problem.

By using a thoracic epidural technique, the level of block can be confined to the required segments. The insertion is technically more difficult to carry out because the epidural space is narrower and there is risk of damage to the spinal cord at this level. The angle of thoracic vertebral spinous processes also makes a midline approach difficult, although this can be overcome using a lateral technique. In addition, a sympathetic block at this level can produce significant cardiovascular effects and these may limit the use of thoracic epidurals in elderly patients.

Epidural Opiates

The discovery of spinal opioid receptors led workers to develop pain relief regimens involving the injection of opiates directly into the epidural space or intrathecally (see below). It was hoped that this would offer great advantages over other routes of administration, including a more localised effect, no nausea, no sedation and no respiratory depression. Unfortunately, this has proved not to be the case. Epidural opiates can still produce respiratory depression and the great danger is that this can occur many hours after administration. Nausea, vomiting and sedation also remain possible side effects, and some patients also develop urinary retention and pruritus which affects the face and groin area.

Opiates delivered into the epidural space work by first diffusing into the CSF and binding with the receptors in the spinal cord. An effect may also be produced by systemic absorption, although this varies with the type of drug used. Some drugs, e.g. fentanyl, have an affinity for fat (lipophilic) and can pass readily across membranes to produce significant blood levels, whereas others, e.g. morphine, do not have an affinity for fat (lipophobic) and therefore do not cross membranes so easily, resulting in very low blood levels.

The approaches to the epidural space and problems with them are discussed under epidural block anaesthetics (above). The situation with regard to epidural opiates is even more difficult and depends on the type of drug used. A lypophobic drug, e.g. morphine, will spread widely, and a lumbar injection of a small dose will produce excellent analgesia. The effect is long-lasting (24 hours) and, therefore, a single injection is all that is required but continuing spread may lead to respiratory depression many hours later. If a lipophilic drug, e.g. fentanyl, is chosen then the effect is more localised and the route of choice would then be the thoracic level. The effect is much shorter and either repeated boluses, a continuous infusion or even a PCA device may need to be used. However, because significant blood levels are produced, comparable degrees of analgesia can be produced by an intravenous infusion of fentanyl, and it may be thought that the added risks of performing a thoracic epidural are not justified.

Intrathecal Opiates

Opiates can be injected directly into the CSF (a 'spinal' anaesthetic), which eliminates the need for the drug to pass across the dura. The dose of opiate can therefore be considerably reduced and the speed of onset of analgesia is rapid. However, the technique is currently available only as a single dose administration and the duration of action is, therefore, limited. As morphine is long acting it is therefore the drug most commonly used but is associated with greater speed of action and respiratory depression. Once the analgesia wears off, parental opiates will be required, which reduces the advantage of using the intrathecal route in the first place.

Combined Thoracic Epidural Local Anaesthetic and Opiates

Local anaesthetic agents and opiates have been given together using the thoracic epidural route. The aim of this technique is to be able to decrease the dose of both and provide good analgesia while reducing the dose-related adverse effects of either agent alone.

Some good results have been obtained. However, the optimum combination dose regimens and the derived benefits have not yet been determined.

Nitrous Oxide

An inhaled mixture of 50% nitrous oxide in oxygen (Entonox) produces a level of analgesia very approximately equal to 10 mg morphine. It is usually delivered from a cylinder via a demand valve, with the patient self-administering using a face mask. The effect is short-lasting and can be used post-operatively to provide additional analgesia during physiotherapy.

TRANSCUTANEOUS ELECTRICAL NERVE STIMULATION (TENS)

TENS has been developed as a result of the formulation of the gate theory of pain. This postulates that the stimulation of large nerve fibres closes a physiological 'gate', preventing pain information, carried in smaller nerve fibres, from passing into the nerve tracts in the spinal cord. The stimulation may also cause the release of naturally occurring chemicals which have an opiate-like effect. The only side effects are local skin sensitivity to the pads which are applied and the possibility that there may be interference with implanted cardiac pacemakers.

Originally used in chronic pain conditions, the technique has been applied to patients post-operatively. The reports of its use have been very variable, with some workers having claimed good analgesia with improved respiratory function but others not.

ACUPUNCTURE

The traditional Chinese therapy of acupuncture has been used for analgesic effects. It is another technique which may act by releasing naturally occurring opiates. Its use in Western countries is extremely limited but may find a place as a technique free of side effects which can be used as an adjunct to other methods.

CARDIAC SURGERY

As noted previously, the intensity of pain suffered after cardiac surgery is less than after thoracic or upper abdominal surgery. In addition, the pain from leg incisions means a systemic regimen is usually required.

The use of spinal or epidural techniques is contraindicated by the use of fully anticoagulating doses of heparin and the risk of persisting coagulation defects post-operatively.

The most frequent method of analgesia is the use of opiate infusions while the patient remains ventilated. During the weaning from mechanical ventilation, PCA can be substituted as the patient regains consciousness and is able to use the control device.

Once the coagulation state is satisfactory, epidural analgesia can be considered but is seldom used. Useful adjunctional analgesia can be provided by NSAIDs given by the most convenient route, although most practitioners would also wait until they were satisfied that there was no coagulation or renal impairment before using these drugs.

The use of TENS is thought to be ineffective after cardiac surgery.

Pre-emptive Analgesia

It has been suggested that providing analgesia before the surgical incision, reduces the pain experienced post-operatively. This is thought to act by decreasing the sensitisation of the CNS which may otherwise occur.

Pre-incisional local anaesthetic infiltration, epidural fentanyl, intercostal nerve block and systemic opiates have been found to have a small but significant effect. Further work may clarify the situation and lead to a definite recommendation for the timing of the administration of analgesia.

Chronic Post-thoracotomy Pain

The incidence of long-term chronic pain following thoracotomy deserves special mention. The problem is being increasingly recognised although, as yet, most studies have been retrospective. Chronic post-thoracotomy pain (CPP) does not present as a single, definable entity and the nature and severity of the pain varies considerably and may be dull, burning, stabbing, painful numbness or hyperanaesthesia. The duration also varies but CPP is usually classed as chronic if it persists for more than 6 months and is not related to the pathology of the underlying disease.

The reported incidence of chronic post-thoracotomy pain ranges from 44% to 67% and the symptoms are usually mild. However, a small number (approximately 5%) of all patients have pain of such severity that they require help from chronic pain clinics. Severe chronic pain is not easily treated.

The cause of the condition is not known. It is suggested that patients who experience severe pain and have a high analgesia requirement in the first 48 hours post-operatively are more likely to develop chronic pain. Factors which may play a part are the surgical technique, efficacy of post-operative analgesia and patient psychology. Cryoanalgesia is associated with long-term neuralgia but chronic pain also develops in patients in whom this technique has not been used.

PHYSIOTHERAPY IN THE CARDIOTHORACIC UNIT

In this section, the physiotherapeutic treatment of the various conditions will be dealt with separately. The routines for cardiac and thoracic patients do not vary a great deal but the need to understand the operative procedures and the post-operative care and complications is important. If there are any specific problems in theatre or the operation varies from the norm, then this must be highlighted by the surgeon, as some physiotherapy techniques may cause harm to the patient (examples of these are given below). Physiotherapy involving patients after cardiac surgery is well documented, particularly with CABG surgery (Dull and Dull, 1983; Stock, et al., 1984; Jenkins et al., 1989, 1994) but there is not much literature on physiotherapy and valve surgery and less still on those patients who undergo thoracotomy, in particular oesophageal and stomach surgery. Patients in the last two groups are far more pront to develop respiratory complications and are more at risk of pulmonary embolus and chest infections. They are also less inclined to mobilise initially post-operatively, mainly because of the number of drips and drains they have and their general condition. By virtue of the pathology, many patients undergoing oesophagectomies and gastrectomies are malnourished and thin, with poor muscle bulk, and are physically incapable of demanding exercise. For such patients 'little and often' is the best approach. The medical care of all the main groups of conditions has been discussed earlier with their respective pathologies, and so this section will cover the role of the physiotherapist and how the nursing staff tend to cater for basic physiotherapy under the education of the physiotherapy team.

PHYSIOTHERAPY AND THE CARDIAC PATIENT

Coronary artery surgery is now considered routine in the cardiothoracic unit, and the turnover rate of this group of patients is high. In Stoke on Trent, 15 to 18 patients are operated on per week and yet this unit is not large. The majority of patients have an overnight stay in the ICU, not necessarily ventilated, and return to the ward the next day. They will then spend between 5 and 7 days in hospital and return to see the surgeon at approximately 4 to 6 weeks after discharge. In most units, cardiac rehabilitation starts at 6 to 8 weeks after discharge but we have found great benefits with beginning rehabilitation at 1 week after discharge as the in-patients are already involved in formal exercise on the wards or in the physiotherapy gymnasium at 4 days post-operatively. The benefits are discussed later.

The role of the physiotherapist in the cardiac unit is:
- To assess the patient's respiratory status both before and after surgery.
- To address any chest problems arising and to advise the patient and nursing staff on positioning in bed and breathing techniques.

- To initiate the mobilising of the patient and assess the progress on a daily basis, and to advise the nurses on the distances the patient is managing to negotiate and therefore also to encourage the patient to mobilise independently.
- To introduce exercise as a daily routine and encourage the patient and spouse to enjoy activity as their norm.
- To address any problems arising after discharge with the cardiac rehabilitation. Typically, the problems are musculoskeletal as a result of the sternotomy or removal of the internal mammary artery for grafting, or leg wound pain as a result of the saphenous vein graft.

Coronary artery surgery is split into two groups—those that are fast track and those that are routine. The differences in theatre procedure have been discussed earlier, and from the physiotherapy aspect, the fast-track group tend to be a day ahead of the routine group. We tend to mobilise fast-track patients on the first day post-operatively whereas the routine patients are mobilised on the second day post-operatively. The fast-track patient is typically discharged at day 5 post-operatively and the routine patient at day 7 post-operatively.

PHYSIOTHERAPY ROUTINE

To keep the format as clear as possible, the physiotherapist's role is described from the day before surgery to day 7 post-operatively.

Pre-operative

In some units, the physiotherapists will see the in-patients the day before surgery to discuss their role in the patient's management and to emphasise the importance of deep breathing, the use of incentive spirometry (Dull and Dull, 1983; Stock *et al.*, 1984), if employed, and early mobilisation. The depth of explanation will depend on the mental state of the patient. If patients are extremely anxious about the operation and do not want to know the details, then it is enough to assess their chest and to say that the physiotherapist will help them to mobilise after surgery and ensure that they can clear their chest of any sputum. Covering more detail serves only to confuse and intimidate the patient and the likelihood is that they will not remember much detail anyway. If, however, the patient wants to know more, then the role of the physiotherapist can be discussed further. Some units have out-patient clinics where pre-operative explanation of the surgery, including physiotherapy and any blood sampling or ECGs, is catered for well before admission, and the patient is less anxious and able to take in the information. Clearly, this depends on the budget of the hospital and the resources available to set up such a system.

Operation Day

As a rule, there is no physiotherapy input unless there is a respiratory complication intra-operatively or immediately post-operatively. Typically, patients will be supine and ventilated, or at least still intubated, until they have stabilised and warmed up. The nursing staff will then sit patients up upon waking and will encourage deep breathing. Once airway and

blood gas analysis has been maintained, the extubation can be considered. This will occur any time between an hour of returning from surgery to overnight. Again, fast-track cardiac patients will be extubated at the early stage; in fact, often they are not ventilated. Patients who are known to be high risk pre-operatively because of poor left ventricular function or problems in theatre, may be less stable as their underlying pathology requires them to have inotropic support, anti-anginal therapy, a balloon pump or temporary pacemaker. Cardiac function, in particular that of the left ventricle, will be known and, therefore, the risks attached to the surgery. The patient will also be informed by the medical team of the risks of surgery, and therefore the physiotherapist's approach before the operation must respect the patient's situation.

Day 1 Post-operatively

The patient is seen by the physiotherapist first thing in the morning. If the surgery was routine, then the patient will be awake and oriented, on occasion still intubated and sitting up in bed. The role of the physiotherapist is to assess the respiratory status, in particular post-operative atelectasis (Wilcox *et al.*, 1988; Vargas *et al.*, 1993) and sputum retention, and to encourage the patient to deep breathe and/or use the incentive spirometer, e.g. Triflo 2. The physiotherapist will assess the need for further humidification. Saline nebulisers are useful and nebulisers such as the Inspiron, and steam inhalation. At this stage, the need to ease expectoration and deep breathing is important so any method to facilitate these is employed.

There is a percentage of early lower lobe atelectasis after cardiac surgery (Wilcox *et al.*, 1988; Vargas *et al.*, 1993) and the position for optimum expansion with least discomfort is forward sitting, preferably with elbow support. This can be achieved by having the patients place their elbows on either their bent knees or on a table. The patient is supported by the physiotherapist from behind (Figure 7.6), and the physiotherapist's hands are placed over the patient's lower lobes; in this position, the patient can also hold the incentive spirometer with both hands. Fixing the shoulder girdle in this manner enables expansion of the lower lobes with minimal sternal wound pain, and the physiotherapist can encourage assisted basal expansion with his or her hands. Expectoration is eased by sternal wound support in forward sitting. The patient is encouraged to use the spirometer on the hour until mobile.

The physiotherapist will assess the patient twice daily unless further input is required. Blood gas analysis or pulse oximetry will determine the patient's respiratory status, and early physiotherapy intervention prevents the possibility of chest infection and further atelectasis. The nurses are advised about the positioning of the patient in bed through the night and, in particular, if there is an element of persistent atelectasis or consolidation, they will encourage the use of the spirometer and deep breathing.

Day 2 Post-operatively

The major complaint at this stage is lack of sleep and a sore posterior. The patient will have been turned from side to side during the night or kept upright, and with hourly observations will have had little sleep. Often at this stage patients are less compliant and the last person they want to see is the physiotherapist. Here, gentle persuasion and encouragement are required with the reminder of the importance of chest physiotherapy. As a rule, once patients are out of bed, they can begin to mobilise. If the drains are still *in situ* and attached to wall suction, patients can be stood up and encouraged to mobilise on the spot or within the confines of the suction tubing. A good policy is to assess the chest and encourage an active cycle of breathing techniques when patients first sit out and then mobilise before lunch. We tend to mobilise the patient to 30 m for the first walk and then in the afternoon to 60 m. Often more than one physiotherapist or one qualified member of staff and a helper are needed to mobilise the patient as there may still be drips and drains *in situ* (Figure 7.7).

Day 3 Post-operatively

The emphasis at this stage is increased mobilisation. As a rule, the patient's chest is clinically clear and he or she will have started to mobilise independently. Rid of drips and drains, the patient is still encouraged to use the incentive spirometer but the physiotherapist is more involved in the exercise. Now the patient will be managing to climb a flight of stairs and the mobilising will have increased. Dizziness is the common sign of overdoing things and therefore it is prudent to warn the patient of this before starting exercise, and during the activity question casually, for example, 'How is your head feeling?' If the dizziness persists, take the patient's pulse and sit him or her down. A common situation post-operatively is to develop atrial fibrillation, and the clinical signs for this are a fast, irregular heart rhythm, palpitations and dizziness. Low blood pressure also causes dizziness and therefore it is a good idea to check the observation charts and cardiovascular status before mobilising, especially if the patient has required inotropic support and/or has had low blood pressure in the immediate past. If the patient is still on oxygen therapy and has a tendency to be hypoxaemic, then the mobilising can occur but with the patient on oxygen via a mobile oxygen cylinder. The use of pulse oximetry during exercise is recommended if the patient is oxygen dependent.

Day 4 to Discharge

By now, there is talk of discharge, and the preparation of the patient for coping at home is underway. The nursing

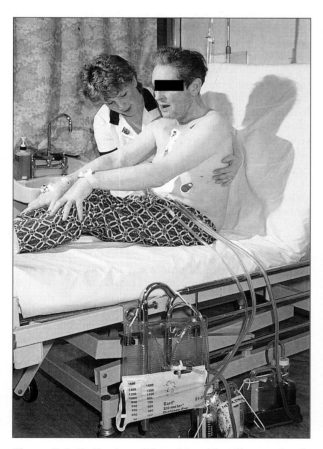

Figure 7.6 Patient positioned to aid optimum chest expansion with minimum discomfort on the first day post-operatively.

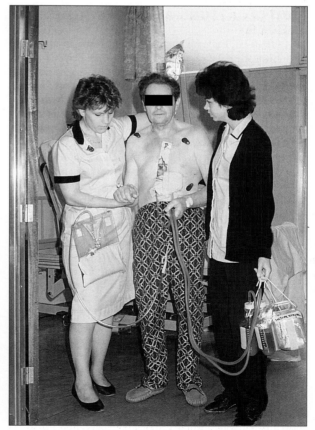

Figure 7.7 Physiotherapists mobilising patient with drains.

staff will give advice on medication, wound care, counselling agents and support groups. One of the biggest support groups nationally is the British Cardiac Patient's Group (formally known as the Zipper Club) whose members are ex-cardiac surgery patients. They offer a social forum and the wealth of their personal experience. If a formal counselling service is required then the patient has contact numbers. The psychological effects of any major surgery need to be addressed and access to the professional groups is important. The physiotherapy input is increased to involve formal gymnasium sessions with the use of stationary bikes, steps, light weights, press-ups against the wall and sitting to standing. We have found that equilateral arm exercise does not cause any sternal wound discomfort; in fact, there is a reduced number of musculoskeletal problems arising as a result of immobility, in particular in patients who generally suffer from conditions such as cervical spondylosis and osteoarthritis of the spine or shoulders. Exercise which involves opposing arm movement tends to put a strain on the sternum and so the patient is recommended to avoid activities that will aggravate this, e.g. dusting with one hand, ironing, carrying a heavy carrier bag or bucket. Unilateral activity can be considered at approximately 8 weeks after discharge.

COMPLICATIONS AFTER CARDIAC SURGERY

As mentioned, the investigations before surgery will have established the risk factor attached to the operation. The common problems arising from the surgery reflect the state of the patient's myocardium and therefore the cardiac output. If the patient has hypertrophy of the muscle or ischaemic changes, then treatment methods may be of little use as they often rely on reasonable contractility of the cardiac muscle. If the cardiac output improves with inotropic support, for example, then the myocardium is of a fair calibre. Patients requiring drug support and/or the balloon pump are in effect unstable, despite a reasonable blood pressure. For example, if a patient needs adrenaline and noradrenaline to maintain a systolic pressure of 120 mmHg, then he or she is still unstable, and where the physiotherapy is concerned, the patient's blood pressure may drop when altering their position in bed and so any physiotherapy techniques must be performed in the supine position. As mentioned, the physiotherapist must assess the overall patient condition before treating the chest, as the patient's stability is the priority and the chest complaint can be addressed when the patient's condition allows. If the patient is severely hypoxaemic due to pulmonary status and the reason is lobar atelectasis, for example, it is worth discussing with the surgeon the risks attached to treating the chest condition as in this situation a contribution to the poor cardiac output may be poor oxygenation of the myocardium. The balloon pump is not a contraindication to physiotherapy but the reason it is *in situ* is because of poor coronary artery perfusion and impaired cardiac output. Turning the patient is hazardous due to the risks attached to flexing the groin where the pump is inserted, e.g. femoral artery infarct. It is best to turn the

patient and ensure the hip is extended at all times. As the patient becomes more stable, the drug dependence lessens and physiotherapy can start but always refer to the patient's blood pressure to confirm that the treatment is not affecting the cardiac output. Once the patient is sitting out of bed, again check medication and blood pressure to establish if the patient can mobilise without dropping the cardiac output. If there is some doubt refer to the patient's surgeon.

There is an incidence of patients needing temporary pacing after cardiac surgery, in particular in mitral and aortic valve replacement. There are no contraindications to physiotherapy but if the patient has a fixed, set heart rate, e.g. 80 beats/min, then any exercise that would require a faster rate, e.g. climbing two flights of stairs, is not recommended and the patient would become fatigued and dizzy. Once the patient's own underlying rhythm is evident, more exercise will be possible. Patients needing a permanent pacemaker can resume normal exercise the day after the insertion of the device once its functioning is checked.

RESPIRATORY COMPLICATIONS AFTER CARDIAC SURGERY

The unstable cardiac patient may develop respiratory problems as a result of being supine for a long time. Typically, the patient is ventilated and the presentation is atelectasis of the lower lobes and further consolidation, then infection of the dependent lobe. Sputum retention can be avoided by maintaining adequate humidification and regular suctioning. Atelectasis in this scenario is a result of poor ventilation of the lower lobes with selective ventilation of the most compliant areas of the lungs in the supine position, i.e. the upper lobes. As soon as the patient can be turned, routine physiotherapy may take place with percussion, bag squeezing and vibrations. Again, refer to the contraindications to bag squeezing before treating the patient using this procedure (see Chapter 6).

In the extubated patient, sputum retention may become an issue if the patient does not have an effective cough, therefore nasopharyngeal or oral suction or, the use of a mini-tracheostomy tube for ease of access into the trachea, may be required. The long-term ventilated patient needs rehabilitation and more intense physiotherapy, similarly to the patient recovering from an episode on the general ICU.

A less common problem after cardiac surgery is a cerebrovascular accident . The patient returns from theatre with a paralysis. If the cause is an air embolus, then the recovery rate is high and often within days the patient regains use of the affected side. If the cause is an infarct due to poor cardiac output intra-operatively and poor perfusion to the brain, then the clinical presentation is that of a serious stroke and the patient will require major rehabilitation. The physiotherapy is impeded by the patient's cardiac condition and also the sternal wound pain. The imbalance of muscle tone around the shoulder girdle, sternum and trunk causes unequal forces about the chest wall and so the patient suffers increased pain, and the risk of chest wall instability is evident if manhandled. Physiotherapy starts as soon as the patient is cardiovascularly stable, and the emphasis on correct positioning in bed and in sitting is communicated to the nursing staff who are made aware of the problems arising in cardiac patients with paralysis and the need for specialist positioning.

CARDIAC REHABILITATION OF THE OUT-PATIENT

Most units nationally offer a rehabilitation service for post-operative cardiac patients. This can join up with the myocardial infarct service and/or the transplant service. The range of facilities covers exercise, relaxation, diet advice, psychological support, family support, drug and pain control and a chance to meet patients who have also had cardiac surgery. Depending on the unit, the rehabilitation can begin between 2 and 8 weeks post-operatively. The exercise prescription and the amount of monitoring will also vary. Some units employ the services of exercise physiologists to assess the exercise tolerance of the patients formally, and often there is a team approach that includes a cardiac nurse and doctor. Obviously this depends on funding of the service and so it is not unusual to find the physiotherapy department offering the entire package.

Exercise is known to be beneficial to cardiac patients and the success rate is high with patients returning to work and enjoying a healthy lifestyle. They are encouraged to join a local gymnasium after they are discharged from the rehabilitation group, or at least to continue with regular exercise for the rest of their lives. The best approach is to offer a finite time attached to the hospital as there is a risk of allowing the patient to become too reliant on the service. We tend to have patients on the programme for 6 weeks and their fitness levels are assessed at weeks 2, 4 and 6. They then return to the gymnasium at 3-monthly intervals for reassessment until 1 year post-operatively.

The prescription of exercise depends on the unit, and as a whole there is a combination of cardiovascular, mobility and muscle strengthening exercises. A common patient perception chart is the Borg Scale, established in 1985, and this gives an accurate measurement of the patient's perceived exertion. The patient refers to the chart during exercise and works at progressively higher levels, with the ultimate aim of a heart rate of less than 130 beats/min.

The rating of perceived exertion is performed on a scale comprised of 15 category points. The scores include:

6   No exertion at all.
7   Extremely light.
8
9   Very light.
10
11   Light.
12
13   Somewhat hard.
14
15   Hard.
16
17   Very hard.
18
19   Extremely hard.
20   Maximal exertion.

Patients are then encouraged to use the scale when they exercise at home or at their local gymnasium.

PHYSIOTHERAPY AND THORACIC SURGERY

Post-operative thoracic surgery can be very painful, and depending on the extent of the resection and the state of the lungs prior to surgery, the potential risk of chest infection is high. Many patients requiring lung resection have underlying chronic lung disease and therefore poor lung compliance. This impedes the re-inflation of the remaining lobes, and the patient's chest drain is often on suction for quite a while post-operatively. The patient's underlying lung condition may present with the production of sputum on a daily basis and with the effects of anaesthesia and the handling of the lung intra-operatively, the pain associated with the thoracotomy incision and general tiredness post-operatively. The physiotherapist therefore has a task on his or her hands.

Patients undergoing oesophageal or gastric surgery are often thin and malnourished; this is because they present with difficulty in swallowing since the cancer is occluding the oesophagus and, sometimes, by the time they come to the ward for surgery, they can swallow fluids only. Physiotherapy for lung resection and oesophageal resection will be dealt with separately.

PULMONARY SURGERY

The reason for the patient's admission and the pre-operative investigations will give an indication of the post-operative situation. Details of the patient's condition are covered in the section on lung resection (p.128) but those of most interest to the physiotherapist include:

- Lung cancer as a result of heavy smoking. The patient will probably have chronic bronchitis or emphysema, or, at least, a productive cough.
- Ruptured bulla with emphysema. Lung compliance will be affected and therefore lung expansion impeded.
- Persistent pleural effusion as a result of an empyema. Both lung and chest wall compliance will be affected.
- Failed pleuradesis requiring pleurectomy in the persistent pneumothorax scenario.
- Ruptured bronchus with bronchopleural fistula in the lung resection patient or chest trauma patient with lung contusion.

These are examples of problematic situations where the lung is stiff or there is reduced chest wall compliance and where the difficulty in re-expanding the lung is evident. The problems occur if the lung remains deflated for any length of time, e.g. lung tissue infection and consolidation are present. If the patient is an elective admission, he or she will have had lung function tests before surgery which confirm the lung pathology, and therefore the anticipation of post-operative complications. The physiotherapist will know this and will have assessed the patient before surgery with the emphasis on the ability to cough effectively and exercise tolerance. A very simple test is the matchstick test whereby the patient holds a lighted matchstick and tries to blow it out. If the patient can, then they will have enough elastic recoil in the lungs to cough. If not, the patient may be a candidate for a mini-tracheostomy. Be careful to adhere to the hospital's health and safety regulations when dealing with lighted matches!

In lung resection, the patient will have one or two intercostal drains *in situ* to remove unwanted air and/or blood from the hemithorax. Assessment of the drains will tell whether there is an existing pneumothorax and the extent of the bleeding post-operatively. If the remaining lobes have expanded into the space where the affected lobe used to be, then the column of fluid in the drain will minimally rise with inspiration and fall to its original level with expiration. If the patient has poor lung compliance but the lung has expanded, then the swing is accentuated. If the lung has not re-inflated, then there will be bubbling on expiration and coughing and, worse still, bubbling with minimal effort, suggesting a bronchopleural fistula. A bubbling drain is normally attached to a wall suction unit with between 3 and 5 kPa of suction to increase the negative pressure in the thorax and so aid expansion. If there is no swing then either the lung has fully expanded or the drain is blocked.

PHYSIOTHERAPY AND THE LUNG RESECTION PATIENT

All physiotherapy relies on good pain control post-operatively but more so in the thoracotomy patient. The anatomy of the muscles incised causes reduced intercostal movement on the operated side, reduced lung volume, often impaired lung and chest wall compliance, uncomfortable chest drains and, together with pain, a high incidence of chest infection. The role of the physiotherapist is:

- To assess the patient before surgery and to familiarise him- or herself with the lung condition.
- To teach the patient the active cycle of breathing techniques and the use of incentive spirometry, if employed. Also, to demonstrate wound support for the aid of coughing.
- To encourage expansion of the dependent lung and to prevent development of complications with the other lung post-operatively. The pneumonectomy patient is especially vulnerable if the remaining lung becomes infected.
- To encourage early mobilisation, i.e. first day post-operatively.
- To assess chest drains.
- To encourage arm elevation on the affected side.
- To improve stamina by introducing early formal exercise and the use of stairs, thereby increasing lung function.
- To reassure the patient and family of the benefits of exercise.
- To introduce the patient to an out-patient service and pulmonary rehabilitation where available.

PRE-OPERATIVE PHYSIOTHERAPY

Having read the medical notes and seen the lung function tests, the physiotherapist will have an idea of the state of the patient's lung condition. Formal assessment of the lungs with auscultation, chest expansion, adequacy of cough and the ability to huff will establish whether the patient will be able to expectorate adequately post-operatively and, also, what medication the patient needs, e.g. bronchodilators. The use of the matchstick test is a good indication of the patient's lung compliance. The patient will be informed of the exercise routine and of the need to elevate the arm on the side of the incision, to prevent frozen shoulder through reluctance to move the arm because of pain.

POST-OPERATIVE CARE

Patient compliance comes with adequate reassurance and direction from physiotherapists as to their role in management post-operatively. To attempt to treat patients when they are in pain serves only to intimidate them and lose their confidence in the individual providing the treatment. Clearly, if a patient has had the maximum analgesia allowed and is still in pain, then the situation needs to be reviewed.

As a rule, the patient stays in hospital for 7 to 10 days, and if the chest drains are not on suction, then the exercise regimen follows the routine of the fast-track cardiac patient. If the patient is confined to the bed space then the use of an exercise bike, steps, and exercise in sitting and standing, with general arm exercise, is beneficial and aids the prevention of complications such as pulmonary embolism, deep vein thrombosis and chest infection. The out-patient service will be discussed in conjunction with oesophageal surgery.

Day of Operation

The patient will return from theatre in the side lying, operated side uppermost or high sitting position. Note that in the pneumonectomy patient, side lying with the operated side uppermost promotes the risk of bronchial stump breakdown and the problems attached to aspiration of the hemithorax contents into the unoperated lung. The optimum position of the chest drain in the hemithorax depends on its function. As a rule, the patient is drowsy but co-operative and can manage to cough. The analgesia is taking affect and so this is a good time to assess the chest and ask the patient to take some deep breaths. Coughing will establish whether there is an air leak—assess the chest drain and therefore whether the drain needs to go onto suction. The chest X-ray immediately post-operatively will confirm the position of the chest drain in the hemithorax and whether a pneumothorax exists or whether the remaining lobes have expanded into the space remaining. The blood loss through the drain is measured hourly by the nurse in charge of the patient, major loss of blood suggesting a leaking vessel, with the patient returning to theatre. With pneumonectomies, some surgeons place intercostal chest drains in the operated cavity to reduce the risks of mediastinal shift and to establish equal intrathoracic pressure, whereas other surgeons prefer to leave the space with no chest drain, stating that the problems with cavity infection potentially caused by a foreign body outweigh the risks of mediastinal shift.

Patients are mobilised on the second day post-operatively and their exercise regimen increases. As mentioned, arm elevation is encouraged, to prevent shoulder girdle problems (Figure 7.8).

On discharge, patients are encouraged to walk at least 1 mile a day, building the distance up over 4 weeks, and at 6 weeks post-operatively they will be invited to the rehabilitation class if one is available.

OESOPHAGEAL AND GASTRIC SURGERY

As mentioned, patients undergoing oesophageal and/or gastric surgery are often very ill. Post-operatively there may be two or three intercostal drains *in situ*, a central venous line and a nasogastric tube, and the patients are monitored quite strictly. The incision may be an extended thoracolaparotomy depending on the site of the cancer.

By nature of the surgery and to visualise the oesophagus in theatre, the patient's lung will be electively deflated, or at least the lower lobe, if the lesion is in the lower third of the oesophagus. In upper oesophageal lesions, the patient will have an additional neck incision where the oesophagus is brought to the surface to sew the anastomosis of the healthy cut ends of the oesophagus.

Post-operatively, the patient remains nil by mouth until a radio-opaque swallow, typically gastrograffin, confirms there is no leak around the anastomosis. Then the patient starts to drink limited clear fluids for a day or so, followed by free fluids followed by a non-solid diet of mashed potatoes or

semolina, for example, and then a normal diet. Often the patient finds difficulty in eating foods that are difficult to digest, e.g. steak, or foods that become pulpy once chewed, e.g. peanuts, and for weeks after surgery the need to experiment with food is highlighted. The patient typically complains of feeling full, having eaten little, and so the common regimen is to eat five small meals a day.

After surgery, anatomically the stomach is partially or completely in the thorax (Figure 7.9) and, depending on the side of the incision, there will be an element of either right or left lower lobe collapse. It is the role of the physiotherapist to re-inflate the lung around the stomach, and the mobilisation follows the same regimen as for the fast-track cardiac patient depending on the cardiovascular state of the patient.

Complications

Leaking anastomosis

If the anastomosis breaks down, as confirmed by the gastrograffin swallow, the patient stays nil by mouth and hopefully the lesion eventually heals, but now there is a risk of pleural space infection as any substance ingested enters the pleural space via the leak. Returning to theatre is a hazardous procedure and is best avoided.

Chest infection

Any patient who has undergone major surgery for cancer is in effect immunosuppressed and prone to infection. If such a patient is thin and malnourished, the likelihood of developing infection is increased further. If a patient develops atelectasis as a result of oesophageal or gastric surgery, this is serious and the deterioration in the patient is rapid.

If a patient has sputum retention, there is a risk of disturbing the anastomosis in the high oesophageal or the pharyngo-oesophageal resection if oral or nasopharyngeal suction is attempted, especially if the physiotherapist is

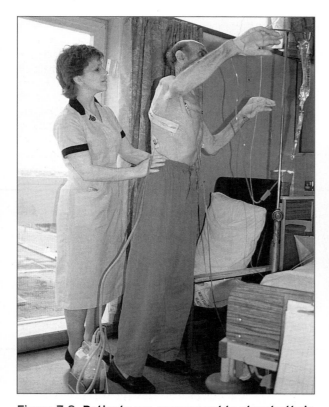

Figure 7.8 Patients are encouraged to elevate their arms on the second day post-operatively to prevent shoulder girdle problems.

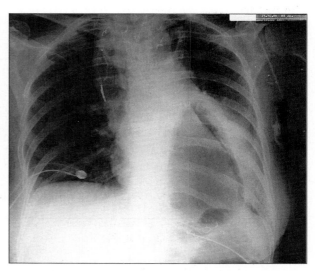

Figure 7.9 Post-operative chest X-ray of subtotal oesophagectomy. Early atelectasis of left lower lobe is present.

inexperienced, and so mini-tracheostomy is the preferential early choice of treatment.

As a whole, in the uncomplicated post-operative resection, the patient remains in hospital for 1 to 2 weeks and is fully mobile having also climbed stairs and exercised formally on the ward. The patient will be eating a reasonable diet and, depending on location, will have access to out-patient physiotherapy to increase stamina.

Some areas offer a local oesophageal surgery support group but these are few and far between. Most patients have to fend for themselves with the advice from the hospital and their recovery is slow.

Encouraging exercise helps patients' self-esteem and improves their appetite, but eating as a whole is arduous and not really a pleasure.

OUT-PATIENT REHABILITATION FOR THE THORACIC PATIENT

With the establishment of pulmonary rehabilitation in many districts, lung resection patients can be accessed (see Chapter 10). We have found that thoracic patients benefit from gentle exercise at 6 weeks post-operatively. A retrospective audit carried out on six oesophagectomies and 12 lung resections showed that exercise in a gymnasium at 2 weeks post-operatively, the same as for the cardiac group, made the oesophagectomy group totally exhausted and the few calories

they were taking in were used up in the exercise, the lung resection group also being depleted. Bringing the patient back for gymnasium sessions at 6 to 8 weeks post-operatively has been successful and the patients can start training with light weights for their arms, redressing the situation of incised back muscle groups such as latissimus dorsi and serratus anterior. The patients tend to stay in the rehabilitation class for 6 weeks and are then encouraged to join their local gymnasium.

CONCLUSION

The cardiothoracic unit caters for a wide spectrum of pathology and is one of the few units where virtually all the patients require physiotherapy.

The advisory role of the physiotherapist is evident: to increase the nurses' input for routine physiotherapy, releasing the specialist to concentrate the workload on the more needy situations.

Recognition of high risk patients is paramount and therefore the capacity to prioritise is important.

There is little literature on physiotherapy and the thoracic patient but local audits have shown that an out-patient service is of great benefit, and that in-patients benefit from early physiotherapy intervention, reducing the number of serious chest complications.

REFERENCES

Dull JL, Dull WL. Are maximum inspiratory breathing exercises or incentive spirometry better than early mobilisation after cardiopulmonary bypass? *Phys Ther* 1983, **63:**655-659.

Jenkins SC, Soutar SA, Loukota JM, Johnson LC, Moxham J. Physiotherapy after coronary artery surgery: are breathing exercises necessary? *Thorax* 1989, **44:**634-639.

Jenkins S, Akinlube Y, Corry G, Johnson L. Physiotherapy management following coronary artery surgery. *Physiother Theory Prac* 1994, **10:**3-8.

Stock MC, Downs JB, Cooper RB, *et al*. Comparison of continuous positive airway pressure, incentive spirometry and conservative therapy after cardiac surgery. *Crit Care Med* 1984, **12:**969-972.

Vargas FS, Culkier A, Terra-Fihlo M, Hueh W, Teixeira LR, Light RW. Influence of atelectasis on pulmonary function after C.A.B.G. *Chest* 1993, **104:**434-437.

Wilcox P, Baile EM, Hards J, *et al*. Phrenic nerve function and its relationship to atelectasis after C.A.B.G. surgery. *Chest* 1988, **93:**693-698.

GENERAL READING

Alferi A, Khotler MN. Non cardiac complications of open heart surgery. *American Heart Journal* 1990, **119:**149-158. Euroston, Spencer. *Gibbons surgery of the chest*, 5th ed. Philadelphia: WB Saunders.

Gothard JWW. *Anaesthesia for thoracic surgery*. London: Blackwell Science; 1993.

Gravelee GP, Rauch RL. *Pain management in cardiac surgery*. Philadelphia: JB Lippincott; 1993.

Kalan, Starr, Wewin. *Manual of cardiac surgery*. Springer-Verlag.

Kaplan JA. *Cardiac anaesthesia*. Philadelphia: WB Saunders; 1993.

Kaplan JA. *Thoracic anaesthesia*. New York: Churchill Livingstone; 1991.

Morris PJ, Malt RA. *Oxford textbook of surgery*. Oxford: Oxford University Press; 1994.

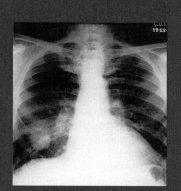

8

M Conway & F Macbeth

LUNG CANCER AND OTHER THORACIC TUMOURS

CHAPTER OUTLINE

- **Tumours**
- **Investigations**
- **Radiotherapy**
- **Chemotherapy**
- **Lung rejection**

- **Role of physiotherapy**
- **Assessment**
- **Respiratory problems**
- **Neurological problems**
- **Psychological problems**

INTRODUCTION

The aim of this chapter is to introduce the reader to common cancers of the thorax and to explain treatment modalities, including physiotherapy and the role of the physiotherapist when dealing with the cancer patient. The approach of the physiotherapist with cancer patients is different from that in other areas of medicine because often there is a time factor as the patient has not long to live, and so the aim of the physiotherapy is to improve the patient's quality of life and not to follow an orthodox treatment plan often adopted in other areas of medicine. The patient's comfort is paramount and the least stress encountered by the patient the better. Often the relatives are more involved in the care of the patient at home and are taught basic physiotherapy techniques such as good positioning in bed, gentle chest physiotherapy aids to mobility and adequate humidification if applicable.

This chapter describes tumours, their pathology and progression, and the role of chemotherapy, radiotherapy and surgery, and, finally, physiotherapy.

TUMOURS

Tumours can grow in any body tissue, and consist of clones of cells whose growth has become disordered and, to some extent, out of normal control. Tumours are either benign or malignant.

Benign tumours tend to grow slowly, do not invade into adjacent normal tissues, and never spread through the blood or lymphatics. They can cause problems if they grow in a relatively confined space or when they obstruct important ducts or tubes.

Malignant (or cancerous) tumours have two important characteristics:
- Invasive growth into surrounding tissues.
- The ability of individual cells to spread either through the lymphatics or the bloodstream to other places in the body—the process known as metastasis.

The commonest malignant tumours arise from epithelial tissues and are known as carcinomas. Those starting in connective tissues, i.e. cartilage, bone, muscle and fibrous tissues, and in lymph nodes are known as sarcomas and lymphomas, respectively, and are rarer.

LUNG CANCER
Epidemiology
In the UK, lung cancer is the commonest cancer in men and the second commonest in women. Overall about 45 000 people currently are diagnosed each year and about 40 000 die from the disease. It is therefore a major health problem.

Aetiology
It has been well known since the research of Doll and Hill on British doctors published in 1976 that tobacco smoking (especially cigarettes) is a major risk factor for developing lung cancer. Lung cancer was rare before 1900 and since then its increasing incidence has followed the increase in cigarette smoking in both men and women

with a time lag of about 20 years. Recently, there has been an encouraging decrease in the incidence in men as smoking habits change, but the rate is still increasing in women. At the moment more than 90% of lung cancers in the UK occur in people who are or have been smokers. It is probable that 'passive' smoking can also cause lung cancer.

There are other environmental agents which are associated with lung cancer (Table 8.1). Radon, a radioactive gas which is released from some minerals, e.g. granite, and is detectable in some buildings, can cause lung cancer in people who are heavily exposed to it, e.g. uranium miners, but its contribution in the UK is uncertain and probably small. Asbestos, which is the major cause of mesothelioma (see below), is thought to be a 'co-carcinogen' with smoking.

Pathology

Lung cancer arises from the epithelial tissues that line the bronchial tree and alveoli, and so is also referred to as 'bronchial carcinoma'. It most commonly occurs in the major airways beyond the trachea (main and lobar

Causes of lung cancer
Cigarette smoking
'Passive' smoking
Pipe and cigar smoking (some evidence)
Asbestos exposure (co-carcinogen with cigarette smoking)
Radon gas
Nickel
Chromium
Polyvinyl chloride
Other air pollutants (smoke, car exhausts) (some evidence)

Table 8.1 Causes of lung cancer.

bronchi), but a variety known as bronchoalveolar carcinoma, with a characteristic clinical course, seems to start in the distal airways and alveoli.

The main histological types of lung cancer are listed in Table 8.2. The most important clinical distinction to be made is between small cell carcinoma and the rest (referred to collectively as 'non-small cell' carcinoma). This is because small cell lung cancer (SCLC) has a distinct biological behaviour: it grows quickly, spreads early and is very sensitive to anticancer chemotherapy. The other varieties may be localised at the time of diagnosis and are all managed in much the same way (see later).

Lung cancer first spreads by local growth into, along and around the airway. It can then grow into nearby structures such as the pleura, chest wall, mediastinum, brachial plexus and heart.

A key feature of a malignant tumour is that cells can break away from the primary tumour, lodge in other tissues, and grow to form secondary tumours or 'metastases'. Lung cancers, especially SCLC, tend to metastasise early and the majority of patients have metastases, either clinically obvious or occult, at the time of diagnosis.

Lung cancers can spread through lymphatics to the draining peribronchial lymph nodes and from there to the mediastinal and supraclavicular fossa nodes. They can also metastasise to other parts of the body through the bloodstream, and any organ may be affected. The commonest sites of these 'systemic' metastases are shown in Table 8.3.

Symptoms and Signs

Because of its very variable clinical course and its ability to spread throughout the body, lung cancer can cause a wide variety of symptoms and signs. These can be divided into local problems in the chest, problems due to metastatic spread, and other systemic effects not directly due to metastases. The clinical problems due to growth and spread within the chest are summarised in Table 8.4 and those due to metastases in Table 8.3.

The commonest presenting picture is of a middle-aged or elderly smoker with a significant change in chest symptoms, such as haemoptysis, and increasingly troublesome cough, a sudden increase in breathlessness or an unre-

Table 8.2 Histological types of lung cancer.

Histological types of lung cancer (percentages vary in different series because of different histological criteria)	
Type	Percentage of cases
Squamous carcinoma	30-50
Adenocarcinoma	15-20
Large cell anaplastic carcinoma	10-20
Small cell anaplastic carcinoma	15-20

solving chest infection. If a patient having chest physiotherapy for another reason admits to any of these symptoms, it must be brought to the attention of medical staff.

INVESTIGATIONS

A variety of different tests are used in the management of patients with lung cancer, both to establish the initial diagnosis and to determine the extent of tumour spread. These are summarised in Table 8.5.

Treatment

The treatment of lung cancer depends on the pathological type and extent of disease at diagnosis.

Non-small Cell Lung Cancer
Surgery

Surgery is the best treatment for non-small cell lung cancer (NSCLC), but unfortunately this is possible for only about 10% of patients. The rest are unsuitable either because of other medical problems, e.g. chronic obstructive pulmonary

Common sites of systemic metastases	
Site	**Common symptoms and signs**
Bones	Pain, pathological fracture, hypercalcaemia
Liver	Pain, anorexia, nausea, jaundice
Brain	Headache, ataxia, hemiparesis
Lung	Breathlessness, pleural effusion
Adrenal glands	Pain, lump (adrenal failure rarely seen)
Skin	Skin lumps

Table 8.3 Common sites of systemic metastases.

Local chest problems (from growth of primary tumour or lymph node metastases)	
Pathological problem	**Clinical problem**
Narrowing of trachea or main bronchus	Breathlessness, stridor
Blockage of bronchus	Cough, breathlessness, lung/lobe collapse, infection
Ulceration in bronchus or trachea	Cough, haemoptysis, increased sputum
Growth into pleura	Pain, pleural effusion
Growth into chest wall	Pain, lump, rib fracture
Growth into mediastinum	Pain
Growth around/into oesophagus	Difficulty swallowing
Growth around/into heart	Pericardial effusion, cardiac dysrhythmia, sudden death
Obstruction of superior vena cava Growth into root of neck (Pancoast tumour)	Swollen face/arms, headache Shoulder/arm pain, paraesthesiae/numbness/weakness in hand/arm, swollen arm, Horner's syndrome
Growth into spine	Back pain, vertebral collapse, spinal cord compression

Table 8.4 Local chest problems.

disease (COPD) or ischaemic heart disease, or because the tumour has already spread to the mediastinal lymph nodes or beyond at the time of diagnosis. The usual operations are lobectomy or pneumonectomy, depending on the size and position of the tumour, but very occasionally a small wedge resection is carried out on patients with small peripheral tumours whose lung function does not allow a larger procedure (see Chapter 7).

Radiotherapy

Radiotherapy can be useful. A few patients with small tumours, who cannot have surgery because of other medical problems or local involvement of mediastinal structures, can be treated with high dose, 'radical', radiotherapy with a significant chance of cure. Radical radiotherapy is a complex procedure that usually involves daily treatment for 4 to 6 weeks.

Most patients can be treated with low dose radiotherapy for palliation only, i.e. relief of symptoms. Patients with cough, haemoptysis and chest pain have a good chance of an improvement in their symptoms after radiotherapy, which can, in this situation, be given in a short course of only one or two treatments. Breathlessness sometimes does not improve after radiotherapy, because a collapsed lung or lobe may not re-expand, or because of severe underlying COPD.

Radiotherapy to the chest can cause side effects. General tiredness is common and nausea and vomiting is usual. Soreness with swallowing due to radiation oesophagitis occurs about 2 weeks after the start of radiotherapy, and usually settles quite quickly after the end of treatment. Occasional patients may have severe, prolonged problems after radical radiotherapy, especially if given after chemotherapy, and may need special dietary supplements or even tube feeding for a while.

Chemotherapy

Chemotherapy has an increasing but still largely experimental place in the management of patients with non-small cell lung cancer. Combinations of drugs such as cisplatin, ifosfamide, etoposide and vincristine may produce tumour responses in 30–50% of selected patients with advanced disease. They can also produce a small but significant improvement in the length of survival, but may be toxic. There are a range of new drugs (such as the taxanes and gemcitabine) which are promising but not yet fully tested. It seems likely that in the future more patients with cancer will receive chemotherapy.

Small Cell Lung Cancer (SCLC)

SCLC is a tumour that grows quickly and has a tendency to spread early. Most patients have metastases at the time of diagnosis, though these may not be picked up on the usual screening tests. The patient's prognosis can be predicted not only by the extent of tumour but also by general fitness ('performance status') and weight loss.

Investigations for patients with lung cancer		
Purpose	**Test**	**Comments**
To make the diagnosis	Chest X-ray	Essential screening test for patients with suspicious symptoms
	Sputum cytology	Useful if patients too ill for bronchoscopy
	Bronchoscopy	Essential test for patients with suspicious symptoms on X-ray
	Mediastinoscopy or mediastinotomy	If bronchoscopy negative
	Needle biopsy of lung mass	If bronchoscopy negative
	Lymph node biopsy	
	Biopsy of metastasis	
To look for tumour spread	Liver function tests	
	Computerised tomography (CT) of chest and upper abdomen	Only for patients fit for surgery or radical radiotherapy
	Mediastinoscopy	Only for patients fit for surgery
	Liver ultrasound	If local pain or abnormal blood tests
	Bone scan	If bone pain or abnormal blood tests
	Brain CT scan	If clinical suspicion of brain metastases

Table 8.5 investigations for patients with lung cancer.

Chemotherapy

Chemotherapy is the best initial treatment. SCLC is very responsive to a wide variety of drugs, but those most commonly used are doxorubicin, cisplatin, carboplatin, etoposide and cyclophosphamide. However, very few patients are cured by chemotherapy because the tumour, even after responding well initially, tends to return and develop drug resistance.

A few very fit patients can be treated with high dose chemotherapy and, if they respond well, radical radiotherapy. Most patients are treated less intensively with palliative intent, and the difficulty is balancing the potential benefit from getting a good tumour response with the risk of toxicity.

Radiotherapy

Radiotherapy is useful for the palliative treatment of patients whose disease relapses and spreads, but is also part of the intensive treatment of a few patients who may be cured. These patients receive high dose radiotherapy to the chest and also to the brain to prevent metastases.

Outcome

Overall, the outcome from lung cancer is very poor with only 5% of patients surviving 5 years. The majority of patients with NSCLC have only a 20% chance of living 1 year and a 5–10% of living 2 years. However, a patient with NSCLC who has successful surgery, has a 30–50% chance of 5 year survival.

Even with optimal chemotherapy the prognosis of patients with SCLC is poor. Of the 'good' prognosis patients treated intensively only 20–30% will live 2 years and 10–15% to 3 years. Recurrence of the tumour after 3 years is, however, uncommon.

MALIGNANT MESOTHELIOMA

Malignant mesothelioma is a relatively uncommon tumour. It arises from the pleural lining of the lung and occasionally from the peritoneal lining of the abdomen. There is convincing evidence that it is related to exposure to and inhalation of asbestos fibres, although the time interval between exposure and the appearance of the tumour can be very long, up to 50 or 60 years. Most patients have a history of asbestos exposure in their work, e.g. boiler makers, ship builders and building workers, but some patients were exposed in their homes from nearby asbestos processing plants. A few patients give no clear occupational or domestic exposure and there are fears that widespread low level environmental contamination by asbestos may lead to a continuing increase in incidence.

The tumour grows in a characteristic manner, spreading first through the pleural cavity, encasing the lung, and then into the adjacent tissues. Although metastases (brain, liver and bone are frequent sites) are quite common, they are rarely apparent until late in the course of the disease.

Patients usually present either with breathlessness due to a pleural effusion or with chest pain due to invasion of the parietal pleura and chest wall, sometimes producing an obvious lump on the chest wall.

Treatment is unsatisfactory. Only a very few patients are suitable for surgery and the tumour does not respond well to either chemotherapy or radiotherapy. The emphasis has to be on controlling the pleural effusion and the pain.

OESOPHAGEAL CARCINOMA

This is described in Chapter 7.

CARCINOID TUMOUR

This uncommon tumour is usually benign and arises from specific cells of neural (nerve) origin in the walls of bronchi. It is not known to be associated with tobacco smoking and tends to occur in younger patients.

Carcinoids tend to grow as a small polyp in the lumen of the bronchus without invading widely, and cause problems only when they become large enough to obstruct the airway, or when they bleed. They are frequently discovered only coincidentally when the patient has a chest X-ray. The histological appearances are usually typical.

Treatment consists of surgical resection, which is almost always curative. Very occasionally these tumours can metastasise to local lymph nodes or the liver. A patient with liver metastases may develop the carcinoid syndrome with episodes of flushing and diarrhoea. There is no satisfactory treatment for metastatic carcinoid but the tumour tends to grow very slowly and the patient may survive for a number of years.

OTHER TUMOURS

The commonest tumours in the chest other than lung cancer are metastatic tumours from other sites. Almost all tumours can spread to the lung but the commonest are breast cancer and bowel cancer. Sarcomas typically spread to the lung as the first site of metastasis and, if solitary, may occasionally be resected.

A number of other more unusual tumours can occur in the chest and mediastinum (Table 8.6). They can present in a variety of ways depending on the site but may cause pain, dysphagia, breathlessness or superior vena cava obstruction.

Rarer chest tumours
Lymphomas
Germ cell tumours (teratoma and seminoma)
Thymoma (benign and malignant)
Soft tissue sarcoma
Bone tumours (osteo- and Ewing's sarcoma)

Table 8.6 Rarer chest tumours.

ROLE OF PHYSIOTHERAPY

Physiotherapy has an important place in the assessment, management and rehabilitation of patients with lung cancer. Its role in the surgical patient with cancer is discussed in Chapter 7.

Patients with lung cancer may have a variety of symptoms all of which may be helped by appropriate physiotherapy along with standard medical management. The most important problems that physiotherapy can help with are respiratory or neurological.

ASSESSMENT

Patients with lung cancer may be referred for physiotherapy at any stage of their illness, and a full assessment should always be carried out including:
- Respiratory function.
- Neurological function.
- Mobility.
- Functional ability.
- Emotional state.

Information should be obtained on:
- The anatomical site and extent of the tumour.
- Any previous treatment.
- The intended treatment.

All of these may affect the interpretation of the assessment and the effectiveness of any planned treatment. For example, physiotherapy techniques will have only a limited effect on dyspnoea caused by lung resection or post-irradiation pulmonary fibrosis.

RESPIRATORY PROBLEMS

DYSPNOEA

Patients with lung cancer may be breathless for a number of reasons, the commonest listed in Table 8.7. Awareness of these possibilities and a clear diagnosis are essential in order to treat the patient effectively.

Breathlessness, especially when associated with anxiety, can cause some patients to become restless and therefore increase their energy expenditure and oxygen consumption. So a vicious circle is induced and the fear of exertion may lead to further inactivity. These patients may be helped by training in breathing awareness and control, combined with relaxation therapy.

OXYGEN THERAPY

Most patients with lung cancer who are breathless at rest are hypoxic, and it has been shown that supplementary oxygen reduces dyspnoea. In patients with moderate to severe dyspnoea the use of oxygen may also help maintain mobility, function and independence. However, as many of these patients will also have underlying chronic obstructive airways disease and, perhaps, carbon dioxide retention, it is important to be cautious about the oxygen concentration. Lightweight portable oxygen equipment is of particular benefit for frail patients.

HUMIDIFICATION THERAPY

Dehydration of the periciliary layer increases sputum viscosity, decreases cilial activity and makes expectoration difficult. Patients with lung cancer often have particular problems with excessive secretions and sputum retention, and so humidification is an important adjunct to chest physiotherapy.

Table 8.7 Major causes of breathlessness in patients with lung cancer.

Major causes of breathlessness in patients with lung cancer	
Respiratory	
Tumour-related	Narrowing of trachea or main bronchus
	Lobe/lung collapse
	Lobe/lung consolidation
	Diffuse lung infiltration
	Lung metastases
	Pleural effusion
	Pleural thickening
Treatment-related	Lobectomy/pneumonectomy
	Post-radiotherapy fibrosis
	Chemotherapy-induced fibrosis
Other chronic obstructive pulmonary disease	Asthma
Cardiovascular	Pericardial effusion
	Pulmonary embolus
	Heart failure
Other	Anaemia
	Anxiety

Sterile heated humidifiers are most commonly used. Because of the risk of thermal injury and bacterial colonization, it is essential that they are serviced and sterilised regularly, and used correctly.

INHALATION THERAPY

Inhalation therapy may be helpful, and a variety of drugs can be administered by the physiotherapist in conjunction with chest clearance techniques. There are three main considerations:
- The purpose of inhalation.
- Mode of delivery.
- Positioning and breathing techniques.

The types of drug that can be used, their purpose and precautions are summarised in Table 8.8. It should be noted that not all of these are well validated and they should all be used with caution.

The inhaled drugs can be given either in dry powder form, through metered dose inhalers, or in solution through a nebuliser. Patients should sit upright with a relaxed posture and using abdominal breathing. They should take a deep breath in and hold it for as long as possible to allow adequate distribution of the inhaled drug to the periphery of the lung. If a particular part of the lung is a problem, the patient may be positioned to allow maximum ventilation to the affected area.

RETENTION OF SECRETIONS

Excessive bronchial secretions can contribute to airways obstruction in patients with lung cancer, particularly in bronchi that are narrowed by tumour. Bleeding from the tumour may result in patients coughing up blood (haemoptysis). This usually consists only of small amounts, which, though alarming to the patient, does not increase the bronchial obstruction. Occasionally, however, heavy bleeding may result in clots forming in the airways which may be more difficult to shift. There are a number of physiotherapy techniques which may help clear retained secretions:-

a) Thoracic Expansion Exercises

The patient is encouraged to take in some deep breaths followed by quiet, unforced expiration. This results in an increase in lung volume, promotes collateral ventilation flow, enables air to get behind bronchial secretions, and assists in mobilizing secretions up the bronchial tree. In some patients a 3 or 4 second breathhold will increase the effect.

Expansion exercises may be combined with careful chest shaking vibrations followed by breathing control techniques. These percussions can be helpful in some patients but not all. It has been suggested that percussion may decrease the force expiratory volume in one second (FEV_1) and oxygenation, but it has been shown that there is no detrimental effect on oxygen saturation when thoracic expansion exercises are accompanied by short periods of chest percussions.

Particular care should be taken with patients known to have bone metastases, especially in the ribs, because of the risk of causing a pathological fracture. Also many patients in the terminal stages of their disease are thin and emaciated or have chest wall pain, both of which might make percussion uncomfortable.

Drugs and solutions that may be used for inhalation therapy		
Drug	**Purpose**	**Precautions**
Bronchodilators, e.g. salbutamol	Improve dyspnoea and sputum clearance in patients with reversible airway obstruction	Overdose may produce tachycardia, tremor etc.
Corticosteroids, e.g. beclometasone	Reduce inflammation and mucosal swelling	Patients may develop oropharyngeal thrush
Mucolytics, e.g. isotonic saline	Reduce sputum viscosity and aid clearance	
Antibiotics	The clinical benefits are questionable	
Hypertonic saline	May help get specimens for sputum cytology	
Local anaesthetic, e.g. lignocaine	Treatment of intractable cough	Care with eating and drinking—reduced cough reflex
Opiates, e.g. morphine	Treatment of breathlessness	Overdose may produce respiratory depression

Table 8.8 **Drugs and solutions that may be used for inhalation therapy.**

b) Breathing Control

Patients should be encouraged to use normal gentle breathing at tidal volume, using the lower chest with relaxation of the upper chest and shoulders (previously termed 'diaphragmatic'). This allows them to rest after the exertion of coughing.

c) Forced Expiratory Technique

This can be used to help the patient mobilise secretions. It consists of one or two huffs combined with breathing control. If huffing is continued down to a low lung volume, this will help to mobilise and clear secretions from more peripheral sites. When secretions reach the larger, more proximal airways they are cleared by a huff or a cough at higher lung volumes. This technique can be used in any position, according to the individual's requirements, and studies have shown that there is no effect on hypoxaemia.

d) Autogenic Drainage

This is a method of controlled breathing in which patients adjust the rate, location and depth of respiration. The aim of treatment is to achieve the best possible air flow throughout the bronchi and therefore to increase the clearance of mucus. Patients have to be very co-operative, and so this technique is not suitable for everyone. A modified approach can sometimes be used with emphasis on self-treatment once patients have learnt the correct technique.

NEUROLOGICAL PROBLEMS

Many patients with lung cancer develop neurological problems which may result in impaired mobility and independence, particularly in the terminal stage of their illness.

The commonest problems are listed in Table 8.9. Sometimes the problems may improve after treatment with radiotherapy, corticosteroids or chemotherapy.

The physiotherapist has a clear role in assessing patients during and after therapy, and in rehabilitation. Rehabilitation should be aimed at achieving the best physical function within the restrictions of time and of the patient's wishes. This should involve careful consideration of the patient's possible prognosis and realistic physical goals. It is important to consider the patient's safety when deciding on the most appropriate aids and level of rehabilitation, especially when a fall could result in a pathological fracture in a patient with bone metastases.

Carers should be taught correct positioning, passive or active assisted movements and transfer techniques. It is important to remember that a wheelchair might improve the quality of life for patient, family and carers not only when disability is severe but also when it is only modest.

Proximal myopathy can be a particular problem in patients on high dose or long-term steroid therapy. Reducing the steroid dose combined with an appropriate exercise programme may lead to improvement. In addition, functional aids, such as a raised toilet seat or a high chair, may be appropriate.

PSYCHOLOGICAL PROBLEMS

Patients with lung cancer may experience a number of emotional and psychological problems including anxiety, fear, hostility, denial and depression. All of these may in turn produce symptoms of dyspnoea and panic. Techniques for breathing awareness, breathing control and relaxation, and the correct positioning of the patient in a bed or chair, can all be helpful and reassuring. It is also important to train carers in the best way to help patients through acute attacks of dyspnoea.

PAIN

Many, but not all, patients with lung cancer experience pain at some time during their illness. This may be caused

Major neurological problems in patients with lung cancer	
Symptom/signs	Likely cause
Hemiparesis or hemiplegia	Brain metastasis
Cerebellar ataxia	Brain metastasis
Paraparesis or paraplegia	Spinal cord compression
Proximal myopathy	Corticosteroids
Arm/hand weakness	Tumour invasion of brachial plexus
Painful movement	Bone metastases
Peripheral neuropathy	Chemotherapy, 'non-metastatic' effect

Table 8.9 Major neurological problems in patients with lung cancer.

by tumour invasion into soft tissues, nerves or bone, either at the primary site or from metastases, and is best treated by antitumour therapy or appropriate analgesics.

Neurogenic pain can cause particular problems. It may result from tumour infiltration into nerves or nerve roots, e.g. into the brachial plexus from an upper lobe tumour, or following thoracotomy. Transcutaneous electrical nerve stimulation may be helpful in relieving the discomfort, particularly when used in conjunction with drugs such as tricyclic antidepressants.

GENERAL READING

Association of Chartered Physiotherapists. *Oncology and palliative care: Guidelines for good practice*. London: Chartered Society of Physiotherapy; 1993.

Macbeth FR, Milroy RM, Steward WP. *Lung cancer: a practical guide to management*. London: Harwood Academic; 1996.

Michie J. An introduction to lung cancer. *Physiotherapy* 1994, **80(12):**844-847.

Saunders C, Sykes N. *The management of terminal malignant disease*. London: Edward Arnold; 1993.

Shia B, Vlad G. Rehabilitation of the lung cancer patient. In: McGarvey C, ed. *Physical therapy for the cancer patient*. New York: Churchill Livingstone; 1990.

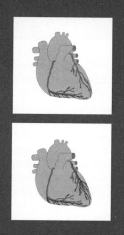

9 S Brean & R Carroll

THE CORONARY CARE UNIT

CHAPTER OUTLINE

- **Coronary artery disease**
- **Angina**
- **Unstable angina**
- **Myocardial infarction**
- **Haemodynamics**

- **Long-term treatment and prognostication**
- **Physiotherapy after myocardial infarction**

THE CORONARY CARE UNIT

The concept of the Coronary Care Unit (CCU) dates back to the early 1960s, and since then the typical unit has undergone tremendous change. Although the principles of care remain the same, focusing on early recognition and prompt intervention in the treatment of potentially life-threatening complications, the equipment and techniques available are evolving at a rapid pace.

The vast majority of patients entering the CCU have coronary artery disease causing an acute coronary syndrome, such as myocardial infarction or unstable angina with pain at rest. A smaller proportion may have life-threatening disturbances of heart rhythm or severe heart failure requiring intravenous therapy, or need temporary stabilisation before emergency surgery.

The duration of admission to a CCU is highly variable, but usually coincides with the time the patient is most likely to be vulnerable to complication. For example, the first 24 to 48 hours of an acute myocardial infarction will be spent in the CCU, and thereafter the patient will be transferred to an adjoining, specialised cardiac medical ward. Staffing levels are high and usually in the order of one nurse to 1.5 patients.

The management of unstable patients is progressively more invasive, both in terms of gathering diagnostic or haemodynamic data and in terms of interventional treatment.

CORONARY ARTERY DISEASE

INCIDENCE

Coronary artery disease is the biggest single killer of adults in the developed world. It is responsible for 160 000 deaths annually in the UK and accounts for 40–50% of all deaths in the developed world.

PATHOPHYSIOLOGY

Cholesterol in the blood is transported in the form of complex structures called lipoproteins. Dietary cholesterol is incorporated into lipoprotein complexes in the liver, which allow it to be transported in the blood in an aqueous miscible phase. The key lipoprotein involved in the generation of atheroma in humans seems to be low density lipoprotein (LDL). Various stressors such as cigarette smoke, dietary oxidants, etc., cause oxidation of the LDL complex, and in this activated state it penetrates the endothelium and into the arterial wall. The arrival of these oxidised LDL complexes stimulates rapid migration of immunologically active cells from the blood and hyperplasia of vascular wall smooth muscle cells. The immunological cells avidly take up the cholesterol and other lipids from the LDL complex and form foam cells. As this process continues, the coalescing cells form the young atheromatous plaque and the process perpetuates itself forming larger and larger plaques and eventually causing stenotic coronary lesions.

RISK FACTORS FOR CORONARY DISEASE

A number of independent factors have been identified that predispose the individual to coronary artery disease. Some are hereditary and as such cannot be modified. Others such as cigarette smoking are environmental and can be modified (Table 9.1). Collectively they are known as risk factors.

ANGINA

PATHOPHYSIOLOGY

The myocardium is highly metabolically active, and depends normally on aerobic generation of adenosine triphosphate (ATP) and other high energy phosphate compounds for muscle contraction and relaxation. It has a high resting demand for oxygen, which seems to be its limiting metabolic substrate. This is reflected by the almost complete extraction of available oxygen from the coronary arterial blood. Unlike in skeletal muscle, which can increase its oxygen supply by increasing the arteriovenous oxygen difference, i.e. oxygen extraction, myocardial oxygen supply can be increased only by raising the coronary artery blood flow.

In the healthy adult heart, when heart rate increases as a result of exercise coronary blood flow increases by as much as fourfold, due mainly to coronary artery vasodilation and due partially to an increase in the perfusion pressure, i.e. a slight increase in systemic blood pressure. This coronary artery vasodilation is thought to be mediated by products of metabolism such as ATP breakdown products or by a drop in pH, or more likely by modulation by nitric oxide.

In the heart with diseased coronary arteries, two processes act to limit this increase in blood flow and oxygen delivery. Firstly, the accumulation of atheromatous plaque causes physical obstruction in the coronary vessel, and greatly decreases flow downstream. Secondly, and perhaps more importantly, the process of atherosclerosis itself causes a dramatic decrease in the degree of vasodilation in response to the usual stimuli. The net result is a heart which cannot meet the increased requirement for oxygen to maintain aerobic metabolism; a switch to anaerobic metabolism occurs with a consequent accumulation of metabolites such as lactate. These metabolic changes cause the stimulation of various chemical messengers such as bradykinin and adenosine which activate receptors in the coronary vessels and myocardium and cause pain—usually experienced as angina.

CLINICAL FEATURES

The onset of angina is usually a steady process. Typically, the patient will become aware of a central retrosternal crushing dull sensation related to exertion, and worsened by emotion or stress. This is often associated with a sensation of breathlessness or sweating. The pain may often radiate to the neck, jaw or left arm. If the patient stops and rests, the sensation abates over a matter of minutes. As the disease process continues, the level of activity that provokes angina inexorably decreases.

DIAGNOSIS

The diagnosis of angina is usually obvious if the features are typical in a patient with multiple risk factors. However, if doubt remains, the usual action is to perform a treadmill exercise test with continuous electrocardiogram (ECG) monitoring. If the patient is unable to perform a treadmill test, due to concomitant chest disease for example, either nuclear isotope imaging or dobutamine stress echocardiography can be used.

Coronary Arteriography

This is often described as the gold standard of diagnosis. In this procedure, the femoral artery is punctured and a flexible sheath placed *in situ*. Through this sheath, catheters can be guided under fluoroscopic imaging into the left ventricle and selectively into the coronary arteries. Injections of radiopaque contrast then outline the coronary anatomy giving detailed information about coronary stenosis morphology and severity.

MEDICAL TREATMENT

For a detailed discussion of cardiac drugs, see Chapter 5.

Oxygen is the limiting substrate in myocardial metabolism. It is often a useful concept then to understand angina as a mismatch of oxygen (or high energy phosphate) supply and utilisation. To redress this balance, agents may either enhance coronary oxygen delivery equivalent to supply or decrease myocardial energy utilization equivalent to demand.

β-Blockers

β-Blockers form the mainstay of treatment. Their action predominantly consists in decreasing heart rate and blood pressure, particularly during activity, and decreasing myocardial oxygen utilization. As a result of slowing the

Common risk factors for coronary artery disease
Cigarette smoking
Male sex
Hypercholesterolaemia
Hypertension
Family history of ischaemic heart disease
Diabetes mellitus
Central obesity
Sedentary lifestyle
Hyperfibrinoginaemia

Table 9.1 Common risk factors for coronary artery disease.

heart rate (bradycardia) they also prolong diastole and augment coronary blood flow.

Nitrates

Nitrates act primarily by vasodilation, and hence decrease ventricular wall stress and myocardial oxygen utilisation. They also cause a small degree of coronary artery vasodilation but this is not their primary mode of action.

Calcium Channel Blockers

Most patients will be maintained on a combination of β-blocker and nitrate; however, there are a significant number of patients in whom β-blockers are either contraindicated or who simply cannot tolerate the agents. These patients may be treated with a calcium channel blocker, preferably with some slowing effect on heart rate, e.g. diltiazem, in combination with a nitrate.

Potassium Channel Openers

This relatively novel group of agents, including nicorandil in the UK, have excellent antianginal properties but function in a dissimilar way from the usual antianginal agents described above. They also have the exciting potential to directly protect the myocardium from ischaemic insult, and allow greater survival of myocytes in the face of coronary occlusion and reperfusion.

INTERVENTION
Coronary Angioplasty

If, at diagnostic coronary arteriography, a lesion or lesions are identified that are amenable to coronary angioplasty, then using a modified coronary catheter of a wider bore, a thin (0.014 inch diameter) guide wire can be manipulated across the lesion and beyond into a stable position. Over this wire, a special angioplasty catheter can be positioned. When in position at the midpoint of the lesion, the balloon can be deployed and inflated to a pressure of many atmospheres. As the balloon inflates, it causes stretching and splitting of the plaque with consequent restoration of the lumen. Many complications can arise with this procedure, for example, dissection of the plaque and consequent acute closure of the vessel. Recently, devices known as coronary stents have entered widespread usage. These are thin metal coils of varying design but with the common principle that stent deployment via the balloon angioplasty catheter causes the stent to assume its predetermined shape, bracing its struts against the vessel wall and thus maintaining lumen patency. An important caveat of stent utilization is that, in the UK, to prevent thrombosis on the stent matrix, the patient must undergo aggressive anticoagulation with warfarin, but more effective regimens using the platelet inhibitor ticlopidine will, at the time of writing, soon become adopted globally.

One of the main limitations of coronary angioplasty is the development of restenosis, where, following the trauma to the vessel wall, there is a massive proliferation of vessel wall cells, causing re-narrowing of the lumen, and recurrence of symptoms.

SURGERY

Surgery for coronary disease is discussed in Chapter 7.

UNSTABLE ANGINA

There are many definitions of what constitutes unstable angina, but the three most useful considerations are the new development of angina symptoms during activity, the development of angina at decreasing levels of activity, i.e. more easily provoked angina (sometimes referred to as crescendo angina), and the development of anginal pain at rest. As you might appreciate, there is a spectrum of disease ranging from stable, exertional angina at high workload on the one hand, through angina at rest to the development of myocardial infarction at the other extreme. Unstable angina and myocardial infarction are often collectively referred to as the acute coronary syndromes.

PATHOPHYSIOLOGY

The critical feature of acute coronary syndromes is a sudden and definite change in the activity and number of immunologically active cells in a plaque. There is a simultaneous change in the morphology of the plaque and the thrombogenicity of the plaque surface. This sequence of events is known as plaque activation. There are many postulated triggers for this mechanism but none has been clearly confirmed. Amazingly, television violence has recently been implicated.

CRESCENDO ANGINA

In crescendo angina, the patient may well have had reproducible angina for many years, upon walking from the house to the local newsagent, for example. Then over the period of a week or a few weeks the patient finds that progressively less activity is sufficient to provoke angina, and this is often reflected in an increased usage of sublingual glyceryl trinitrate (GTN). The situation may often stabilise or even revert to the patient's previous level of activity. Commonly, with intensified medical treatment, the patient may stabilise. However, there is a distinct subgroup of patients who proceed to have angina at lesser and lesser exertion until they develop pain at rest.

REST PAIN

Rest pain may be the final point of the patient with crescendo-type unstable angina, or may arise *de novo*. It is a medical emergency, as a large number of these patients will go on to develop myocardial infarction if treatment is not aggressive enough.

MEDICAL THERAPY

The patient should be admitted to the CCU or a dedicated Cardiology Unit. In the first instance, the patient should be on strict bed rest, have continuous ECG monitoring and daily 12 lead ECG, and cardiac enzyme estimation. Intravenous access is established and the patient commenced on infusions of heparin and nitrate. At the same time, the patient's oral treatment should be rationalised; the patient must be fully treated with β-blocker unless there are definite contraindications, and co-administration of a calcium channel blocker should begin if symptoms are not fully resolved.

When the patient responds and rest pain is abolished, the next step is weaning off the nitrate infusion, and replacement of this with an oral preparation. We prefer the early use of a buccal GTN preparation such as suscard buccal, and then replacement with a sustained release preparation such as isosorbide mononitrate durules (Imdur). During this interval the patient is gradually and progressively mobilised with careful observation for the recrudescence of pain.

If the patient's symptoms are refractory to this medical 'triple therapy', coronary arteriography is proceeded to, with a view to angioplasty if amenable lesions are identified, and surgery of the lesions is unsuitable.

MYOCARDIAL INFARCTION

Myocardial infarction is the most common reason for admission to the CCU.

PATHOPHYSIOLOGY

One of the main complications of atheromatous plaque is a tendency, under certain circumstances, to become immunologically activated. The exact mechanism of this activation is unclear, and currently the subject of much research, but it leads to the chemotaxis of many immunologically active cells such as macrophages, polymorphs and lymphocytes. This in turn is intimately associated with change in plaque morphology and, most importantly, platelet activation and thrombus formation. The thrombus becoming occlusive is one of the reasons for the close interrelation between unstable angina and myocardial infarction, i.e. severe narrowing or even intermittent occlusion of the coronary vessel may cause unstable angina, whereas complete and persistent occlusion causes myocardial infarction.

When the myocardium is deprived of its blood supply, a number of changes occur very rapidly. Within eight or so heart beats the usual aerobic metabolism of the myocardium changes to anaerobic pathways with the resultant accumulation of metabolites such as lactate, and a marked decrease in intracellular pH, i.e. an intracellular acidosis. As this process continues there are more marked derangements in intracellular metabolism, and eventually irreversible release of intracellular calcium from the sarcoplasmic reticulum signals irreversible cell necrosis and myocyte death.

Under certain circumstances, in the setting of reperfusion for example (see below), myocytes may be significantly damaged, but blood supply is restored before irreversible cell death. In this situation, myocytes are alive and provided with all the metabolic substrate they need, but the intracellular mechanisms for cell contraction are impaired, and hence functionally inactive. This is usually a temporary phenomenon, and full recovery occurs in a matter of hours to days. Affected myocardium is said to be 'stunned'.

After myocyte death the area of infarction is invaded by numerous polymorphs, fibroblasts and tissue macrophages. These progressively phagocytose the dead myocytes and replace them with a variable amount of collagen matrix in among which may be a small number of surviving myocytes. This is then manifest as scar tissue.

CLINICAL FEATURES

In myocardial infarction, the patient usually develops characteristic cardiac pain, which is identical in nature to anginal pain but constant and unrelieved by rest or nitrates. It is frequently associated with marked autonomic upset such as sweating, nausea and vomiting, and occasionally by a sense of impending death (angor animi).

In certain groups of patients, e.g. the elderly or people with diabetes, such characteristic features may be attenuated or even absent, and a high index of clinical suspicion is essential for correct diagnosis and treatment.

Examination usually finds a cold, clammy, sweating patient, but may be remarkably normal if no complications have arisen.

DIAGNOSIS

In combination with the clinical features, diagnosis is usually confirmed with specific ECG changes or changes in the profiles of blood cardiac enzymes.

ECG Changes

In myocardial infarction, there are a variety of specific changes in the leads directed at the surface of the myocardium undergoing ischaemia. Initially there is inversion of the T waves in the leads followed shortly by elevation of the S–T segment and shortly the loss of the R wave and development of deep Q waves. These changes are not invariable, and varying degrees thereof may co-exist depending on the nature and extent of the infarction.

The ECG is not used only to diagnose myocardial infarction, but also to locate the site of myocardial damage, bearing in mind that the different ECG leads evaluate different surfaces of the heart. See Chapter 4 for typical examples of the ECG in myocardial infarction.

Blood Analysis

The second common diagnostic technique is the analysis of the patient's plasma for the presence of 'cardiac enzymes'. These are actually cytosolic enzymes from the myocyte, and during ischaemia they leak from the myocyte into the plasma. The two most commonly measured cardiac enzymes are creatine kinase (CK) and aspartate transaminase (AST). Unfortunately, these enzyme systems co-exist in other organ systems such as skeletal muscle and liver. If diagnostic doubt persists, then further assays can be performed on the same serum sample to calculate ratios of iso-enzymes and hence determine the tissue of origin. It is usual to accept a rise in the blood concentration by 2.5-fold as significant.

More recent efforts have focused on 'near patient' diagnosis with bedside blood or urine analysis for markers of myocyte injury such as troponin T.

TREATMENT
First Aid
If possible, small doses of an opiate such as diamorphine should be administered as this is analgesic, anxiolytic and vasodilatory. At the same time, an antiemetic such as maxolon should be administered.

ADMISSION TO THE CCU

TREATMENT
Immediate
The critical concept behind treatment of myocardial infarction is the restoration of blood flow down the occluded coronary vessel as soon as possible. To achieve this, a group of agents known as thrombolytics have been developed. The most commonly used of these is streptokinase and recombinant tissue plasminogen activator (rtPA). These agents share a similar mode of action, which is the degradation of fibrin to its smaller breakdown products and thus disruption of the thrombus matrix and restoration of blood flow (thrombolysis). International, large scale trials have demonstrated significant reductions in mortality by the co-administration of these two thrombolytic agents; the effect of aspirin appears to be additive.

The benefit of restoring blood flow down the occluded vessel (reperfusion) is greater protection of the left ventricular myocardium (myocardial salvage), which translates into better preservation of left ventricular function—the most important determinant of survival and symptomatic status.

The agents are administered by intravenous infusion, and the ECG repeated at a predetermined time interval after administration to identify markers of restoration of blood flow. If there is no evidence of reperfusion at this time then either a further attempt at thrombolysis or an alternative strategy of reperfusion should be undertaken such as coronary angioplasty (see page 157).

At the same time other measures will need to be undertaken as explained below.

β-Blockers should be administered by cautious intravenous injection under the guidance of continuous ECG monitoring. These decrease myocardial oxygen uptake and have a remarkable effect on the patient's pain but also decrease the risks of cardiac rupture and dysrhythmia (see below).

THE FIRST 3 DAYS AND BEYOND
Angiotensin Converting Enzyme (ACE) Inhibitors
In humans, maintenance of blood pressure is governed by a complex interactive system of neurohumoral control. One of the most common manifestations of dysfunction of this system is hypertension. More importantly, in acute myocardial infarction, especially in the presence of extensive damage to the left ventricle or overt left ventricular failure, there is intense activation of the neurohumoral system with elevation of systemic blood pressure, increased left ventricular wall stress and consequently adverse remodelling of the infarcted area.

Over the past decade a group of agents called angiotensin converting enzyme (ACE) inhibitors have become available for clinical use. These agents bind to and irreversibly block the enzyme which catalyses the conversion of angiotensin I (an inactive peptide) to the active compound, angiotensin II, a potent vasoconstrictor. This occurs not only on a systemic basis but also at the tissue level where local renin–angiotensin–aldosterone activity modulates cell growth and division.

Recent evidence from a number of large scale clinical trials has shown that early treatment of patients with extensive damage to the left ventricle improves survival in both the short and long term. One practical approach is to identify those with evidence of pulmonary congestion (either clinically or on chest X-ray) or extensive anterior infarction on the ECG, and start them on ACE inhibitor on or around the third day after infarction.

β-Blockers
There is evidence that the early use of intravenous followed by oral β-blockers improves survival in patients following myocardial infarction. This is particularly apparent in anterior myocardial infarction. However, these data are from the so-called pre-thrombolytic era, i.e. before the widespread use of thrombolysis in myocardial infarction, and may not be applicable to current clinical practice. It is our practice to continue patients on β-blockers for at least 3 months after anterior infarction.

Aspirin
There is extensive evidence that low dose aspirin, continued long term, has a beneficial effect on survival. Following myocardial infarction, patients should remain on aspirin indefinitely.

Lipid Lowering Agents
There has been great interest lately in the use of two classes of agents, namely statins (HMG CoA reductase inhibitors) and fibrates. In patients with elevated plasma lipids or even with 'normal' cholesterol levels following myocardial infarction, early and sustained treatment with a statin, e.g. simvastatin, reduces the likelihood of further ischaemic events such as heart attack or unstable angina.

The effect is more complex and stronger than is likely to be due to the lowering of cholesterol levels alone, and may reflect alteration in the balance of intercellular transmitter synthesis from cholesterol by the sterol pathway.

COMPLICATIONS OF MYOCARDIAL INFARCTION

DYSRHYTHMIA: CARDIAC ARREST
Diagnosis and Management
Diagnosis of cardiac arrest is confirmed by the presence of patient collapse and absence of a palpable central pulse. There are well established protocols for the delivery of both basic and advanced life support. The current European Resuscitation Council guidelines appear in the *British*

National Formulary and on the walls of most CCUs. The vast majority of hospitals now train all personnel in basic life support, and all medical personnel in advanced life support.

OTHER RHYTHM DISTURBANCES: TACHYDYSRHYTHMIA

During the initial phase, and especially during the reperfusion phase, of thrombolysis, the development of dysrythmia is commonplace. The most common tachyarrhythmic disturbances are shown in Table 9.2. There is considerable difference of opinion on the management of tachydysrhythmia, but the key feature would appear to be the presence or absence of haemodynamic compromise as a result of the dysrhythmia.

If the patient has haemodynamic compromise (see below), then urgent action is indicated. Almost invariably this takes the form of synchronised direct current (DC) cardioversion by the use of a defibrillator.

The paddles of the defibrillator are placed in contact with the patient's chest via two conductive gel pads. The defibrillator is charged to a high potential in the order of tens of thousands of volts, and then discharged, synchronised with the upstroke of the R wave on the ECG. A pulse of electrical energy lasting only a few milliseconds but of 200–400 J energy passes through the chest and myocardium. The idea is that the magnitude of the pulse is sufficient to depolarise the entire myocardium and allow re-emergence of the highest order pacemaker, usually the sino-atrial (SA) node (see Chapter 4). This should restore normal sinus rhythm.

If the patient is haemodynamically stable, then a variety of pharmacological treatments are available.

If the patient becomes unstable, with dropping blood pressure, poor perfusion or pulmonary congestion, then the treatment of choice is DC countershock, synchronised with the upstroke of the ECG R wave.

In all situations it is imperative to search for any aggravating or precipitating factors, especially hypokalaemia, hypoxia or acidosis.

BRADYDYSRHYTHMIA

This is a situation where the effective heart rate is too slow to maintain adequate cardiac output. There are two main causes:

Sinus Bradycardia

This is usually due to excessive vagal stimulation in the setting of myocardial infarction, but can occasionally be due to occlusion of blood supply to the SA node. It is often transient and almost invariably responds to intravenous injection of atropine 600 µg. It may also be iatrogenic, for example, due to β-blockade or diltiazem administration. Treatment is indicated only if the patient is symptomatic or has haemodynamic compromise.

Heart Block

Prolongation of the P–R interval is not uncommon in inferior myocardial infarction, and is almost invariably of no consequence. In the setting of inferior myocardial infarction, second degree and third degree (complete) heart block is frequently transient and well tolerated. It can be treated with atropine as above. If the rhythm disturbance is persistent or causes compromise, a temporary pacing wire should be inserted.

Common dysrhythmias			
Dysrhythmia	**First-line**	**Second-Line**	**Comments**
Occasional ventricular premature complexes	None	β-blocker if symptomatic	
Self-terminating runs of ventricular tachycardia	None	β-blocker	Usually occur in setting of reperfusion and self-limiting
Sustained ventricular tachycardia	Lignocaine IV or β-blocker IV	Amiodarone IV	Again usually during reperfusion
Paroxysmal atrial fibrillation	β-blocker	Amiodarone	
Sustained atrial fibrillation (usually reverts spontaneously)	Verapamil, diltiazem, β-blocker	Digoxin	
Narrow complex/re-entry tachycardia ('SVT')	Adenosine	β-blocker/amiodarone	Adenosine is ultra short-acting agent and terminates a large percentage effectively

Table 9.2 Common dysrhythmias.

In the setting of anterior myocardial infarction, second or third degree heart block is a grave feature, signifying extensive myocardial damage, and the decision to site a temporary pacing wire is usually taken prophylactically.

Temporary Cardiac Pacemaker

The pacemaker is attached to a wire threaded through the superior vena cava in a similar route to that of the central venous line. The wire is then fed through the tricuspid valve and becomes attached to the wall of the right ventricle. The pulse generator is then attached.

The pulse generator has two essential circuits, one for the detection of spontaneous cardiac electrical activity and one for the generation of an electrical pulse capable of stimulating the myocardium. When the generator is operated, it monitors the electrode tip for any evidence of electrical activity, i.e. the QRS complex on the surface ECG. If there is no spontaneous electrical activity after a predetermined time, usually in the order of 900 ms, the second circuit delivers a brief low energy electrical pulse to the pacing wire tip. The duration, energy and interval of the pulse are variable but there must be sufficient energy and duration to 'capture' the myocardium and hence cause effective cardiac contraction.

Usually, after a period of hours to days, spontaneous electrical conduction returns and the pacing generator can be turned down and the pacing wire removed.

More recently, many defibrillators have been designed with a high energy external pacemaker facility. Here two large electrodes are attached to the front and back of the thorax. The heart can be stimulated via high current flow but if the patient is conscious then this is extremely uncomfortable and should be used as an emergency holding measure only until a transvenous pacing wire can be positioned.

HAEMODYNAMICS

PULMONARY CONGESTION (OEDEMA)

Pathophysiology

The pulmonary capillaries are extremely permeable to most small molecules, including water. Normally there is a well controlled balance between forces causing and preventing the passage of water from the pulmonary capillary space into the pulmonary interstium and alveolar spaces. On the one hand, there is the hydrostatic pressure within the capillary which tends to cause the movement of water out of the capillary and into the interstitium. This is usually counteracted by a combination of opposing forces of the oncotic (or colloid osmotic) pressure, caused by the osmotic effect of plasma proteins in the capillary, and the lower hydrostatic pressure in the interstitium.

In the setting of myocardial infarction there may be transient or permanent left ventricular damage. This may manifest in two ways: the first, and most common, is diastolic dysfunction. Here the end diastolic pressure of the left ventricle is greatly raised due to over-filling (mediated through autonomic reflex mechanisms) and failure of the ventricle to eject a normal volume of blood with each contraction. This elevation of pressure is translated directly into an increase in pulmonary venous pressure and then pulmonary arterial pressure. When the pressure reaches a critical value, the outward forces acting in the capillary overcome the inward acting forces and fluid begins to leak out of the pulmonary capillaries and into the interstitium. As the pressure increases, more fluid leaks and pulmonary compliance drops dramatically, i.e. the lungs become much stiffer. Gas exchange across the alveolar membrane is steadily impaired, and as oxygen is much less soluble in water than is carbon dioxide, the patient becomes progressively more hypoxic with a low or normal PCO_2. Eventually, free fluid leaks into the alveolar spaces (pulmonary oedema) and gas exchange is gravely impaired.

Clinical Features

The first feature is usually a sensation of breathlessness. The patient then becomes progressively more tachypnoeic and agitated, remains upright, and cannot lie flat. On examination, initially the lung bases display fine mid-inspiratory crackles, but as the pulmonary oedema worsens the crackles may progress to involve the whole of both lungs. The chest X-ray shows characteristic features (see Chapter 3) and the patient becomes progressively more desaturated and hypoxic on arterial blood gas analysis.

Treatment

The first action is to sit the patient upright and administer as high a concentration of oxygen as possible by mask (unless there is definite evidence of concomitant structural lung disease). The aim of treatment is to decrease the pressure in the pulmonary vasculature and hence decrease and reverse the leakage of fluid into the pulmonary interstitium. This is achieved by decreasing the pressure loading of the left ventricle. Three agents achieve this. Firstly, diamorphine, given slowly in a dose of 2.5–5 mg intravenously not only is a vasodilator, but has a great anxiolytic effect. Secondly, nitrates, often in the form of GTN given by intravenous infusion, are potent vasodilators. Finally, the loop diuretic frusemide, given by slow intravenous push in a dose of 40–80 mg, has some vasodilating properties.

At the same time, specific causes for the pulmonary oedema must be sought, especially dysrhythmia.

After the initial treatment, the patient will usually be started on a regular oral loop diuretic. Recent trials have shown that in the group of patients who develop pulmonary oedema during their in-patient episode, there is a great survival benefit in treatment with ACE inhibitor drugs (see page 159).

CARDIOGENIC SHOCK

The second manifestation of left ventricular damage is cardiogenic shock.

Pathophysiology

Cardiac pump function is extremely dependent on the effective delivery of oxygen and metabolic substrates by coronary blood flow. Coronary blood flow in itself is highly dependent on perfusion pressure, i.e. the driving force of blood pressure difference between the aorta and the coronary sinus. In the healthy human, about two thirds of coronary blood flow occurs during diastole, when the myocardium is relaxed. However, in patients with atheroma, the aorta and coronary vessels are much less compliant, i.e. stiffer, and coronary blood flow is much more pressure dependent, needing a good systolic blood pressure to be maintained. If there has been extensive damage of the myocardium to the left ventricle with either death of the muscle or stunning or a mixture of both, the left ventricle cannot pump efficiently to maintain adequate systolic blood pressure. Therefore coronary blood flow falls and delivery of metabolic substrates and oxygen to the remaining viable myocardium is decreased. When this happens, the remaining myocardium becomes ischaemic, contracts less well, and cardiac pump function is further impaired.

This initiates a vicious cycle, with a drop in systolic pressure causing worse perfusion so causing worse pump function so causing a further drop in systolic pressure, and so on.

Cardiogenic shock may often co-exist with pulmonary oedema. At the same time, there is hypoperfusion of other vital organs, particularly the kidneys and brain. Unless treated aggressively, it is rapidly fatal.

Clinical Features

The patient usually has a large anterior myocardial infarction. Cardiogenic shock may be the presenting feature of the myocardial infarction, but it can occur at any time. Initially the blood pressure begins to fall. The peripheries become poorly perfused and the patient becomes 'shut down' as intense sympathetic nervous system activation causes profound skin vessel constriction to try and maintain the falling blood pressure. Urine output tails off and the patient becomes obtunded or confused. This may co-exist with any of the features of pulmonary congestion. The patient develops a systemic acidosis, and dysrhythmia may supervene, in which setting it is almost invariably fatal.

Treatment

The key aim of treatment is to restore coronary blood flow and thus restore cardiac pump function and blood pressure. This can be achieved in two ways; the most effective is the restoration of coronary blood flow directly either by thrombolysis or by direct angioplasty.

The second and more frequently used way is the use of pharmacological techniques to restore blood pressure. In the setting of cardiogenic shock, an accurate picture of the patient's haemodynamic status is needed and this is usually obtained by the insertion of a pulmonary artery balloon flotation catheter (commonly a Swan–Ganz catheter).

Agents such as dobutamine, adrenaline and enoximone are administered by intravenous infusion at various doses, based on the patient's body weight. These act either directly on receptors on the myocardium or by affecting the intracellular signalling pathways. The overall common effect is to enhance cardiac pump function by increasing stroke volume and, to a lesser extent, heart rate. Unfortunately, this is usually at the expense of increased myocardial oxygen demand.

In order to improve kidney function, a low dose infusion of dopamine is often administered, the idea being that it acts at a low dose as a selective renal artery vasodilator; however, evidence for its effect is contentious.

More recently, and particularly as a holding measure while waiting for emergency coronary angioplasty in the emergency setting of myocardial infarction, the use of intra-aortic balloon pumping is becoming more widespread (see Chapter 7).

Any compounding factors such as dysrhythmia must be treated aggressively.

SPECIAL CONSIDERATIONS

Mitral Valve Rupture

Mitral valve rupture may occur in the setting of acute myocardial infarction or several days after the patient is making an apparently good recovery. It is usually seen in the setting of inferior myocardial infarction. The mitral valve leaflets are anchored to the left ventricular papillary muscles. If these muscles are damaged by infarction, the chordae tendinae may break off and allow free prolapse of a mitral valve leaflet. This in turn causes torrential regurgitation of blood into the left atrium with consequent severe pulmonary oedema and a low cardiac output state.

The diagnosis is usually clinically obvious with the appearance of a new murmur of mitral regurgitation, and severe pulmonary congestion. The chest X-ray confirms frank pulmonary oedema. If doubt remains, diagnosis can be confirmed by trans-thoracic or trans-oesophageal echocardiography, or by Swan–Ganz catheterization.

Treatment consists of emergency surgical repair of the mitral valve apparatus, as medical treatment is ineffective other than as a temporary holding measure.

Ventricular Septal Defect

Similarly, if the interventricular septum has been infarcted, it can become disrupted and develop either a single small defect or multiple defects of varying size (so-called Swiss cheese defects). This allows flow of left ventricular blood into the relatively low pressure right ventricle. Consequently there is a massive drop in effective cardiac output to the systemic circulation, and if the defect is large enough, cardiogenic shock supervenes. Clinically, if the defect is significant, there is brisk deterioration in the patient's condition and a harsh systolic murmur develops. Once again balloon pumping can be used as a holding measure, but the definitive treatment consists of surgical repair.

Pericardial Tamponade

Pericardial tamponade is an uncommon and extremely dangerous situation. Normally, the parietal and visceral pericardia are separated by a potential space. In certain circumstances fluid can accumulate in this potential space. If sufficient fluid accumulates, the limited space will not allow an increase in pressure to be accommodated, and this pressure is transmitted to the right atrium and right ventricle. This inhibits cardiac filling and hence cardiac output.

The clinical features are of a patient with low blood pressure, small volume pulse, pulsus paradoxus (both pulse volume and blood pressure drop significantly on inspiration) and often engorged neck veins. The chest X-ray shows a featureless, globular cardiac silhouette.

Treatment consists of the insertion of a fine bore needle, under ECG guidance, from the xiphisternum into the pericardial space, and aspiration of the fluid. Usually, aspiration of even a small volume is sufficient to restore cardiac output.

MONITORING

In the presence of haemodynamic instability, and especially cardiogenic shock, invasive measurement of blood pressures and cardiac output is highly desirable. This is done at the bedside in most CCUs.

The insertion of a Swan–Ganz catheter is beneficial to establish the damage and/or function of the left side of the heart. It also allows measurement of right atrial, right ventricular and pulmonary artery pressures, and approximation of left atrial pressures.

Incorporated near to the tip in modern Swan–Ganz catheters is a tiny thermistor capable of changing its electrical resistance proportional to the temperature of its environment. If a given volume of cold saline of a known temperature is then injected into the proximal port of the catheter, the thermistor will measure the rate of temperature drop in the pulmonary artery as the bolus of cold fluid goes past. These data can be incorporated into an algorithm to determine cardiac output.

Armed with these indices, the doses of inotropes, vasodilators and volume infusions can be accurately calculated, and their effects measured and titrated to the patient's response.

BALLOON PUMPING

Details of the function of the balloon pump are described in Chapter 7. After insertion of the device, the results on blood pressure, perfusion and cardiac performance can be extremely dramatic; and they may well be life saving in the time interval spent waiting to perform angioplasty.

MASSIVE HAEMORRHAGE

In the setting of myocardial infarction treated by thrombolysis, it is not uncommon to have minor bleeding from venepuncture sites. However, a small percentage of patients will develop significant bleeding from, for example, peptic ulcer. Treatment is standard resuscitation with colloids and blood transfusion, but specific agents such as tranexamic acid can be administered, along with fresh frozen plasma (rich in depleted clotting factors) and platelet concentrates.

PERICARDITIS AND THE DRESSLER SYNDROME

Following myocardial infarction, there is considerable inflammation and immunological activity at the site of the healing infarction; fibrin is deposited at the infarct site and on the adjacent pericardium. Patients commonly develop pericarditis a few days after the infarct, and this is manifest by a localised, almost pleuritic pain in the praecordium that is worse lying flat and better sitting forward. Clinically, a rub may be heard over the site, sounding like the creak of sailing ships in harbour. Treatment consists of non-steroidal anti-inflammatory drugs such as indomethacin. Unfortunately, there is evidence to suggest that these agents also cause myocardial scar thinning and adverse remodelling of the left ventricle.

A small subgroup of these patients go on to develop a constellation of pericarditis, pericardial or pleural effusion fever and oligoarthritis. This is known as Dressler syndrome and may require systemic steroids for its control, but the majority of patients settle with symptomatic treatment only.

LONG-TERM TREATMENT AND PROGNOSTICATION

The aims of long-term management of myocardial infarction are to return the patient to as active a functional capacity as possible and to prevent the development of long-term complications. In order to best identify which patients are likely to gain benefit from the limited resources of, for example, surgical revascularization, or to identify which patients are at risk of complications such as sudden cardiac death or heart failure, intense research activity into different strategies of assessment is underway. Commonly used techniques are exercise treadmill testing and ambulatory ECG. Alternative techniques are isotope stress scanning, dobutamine stress echocardiography, or, a more recent development, positron emission tomography.

Whatever method of stressing the heart or imaging modality is employed, the underlying principles are the same. An area of dead myocardium will not function at all and shows as a wall motion abnormality or 'defect' on the imaging system. An area of myocardium supplied by a coronary vessel with a significant stenosis may function near normally in the resting state but will manifest abnormal function on imaging or changes on the related surface ECG as it is stressed. An area of stunned or hibernating myocardium will gain function as the stress is increased to a certain level but will then begin to differ from the surrounding normal myocardium.

These techniques can be used to target those who have poor ventricular function or extensive coronary artery disease remote to their original myocardial infarction site. In combination with clinical assessment, resources can be targeted at those most at risk, hence most likely to gain benefit.

RISK FACTOR MODIFICATION

Of the many interdependent risk factors for coronary artery disease, several are open to modification. There is currently great interest in four key areas—stopping smoking, blood pressure control, increasing physical activity, and aggressive 'normalization' of blood lipids. Recent large scale trials have confirmed laboratory based experiments on the stabilization of active coronary plaques and improvement in survival in patients with abnormal and 'normal' lipids using the HMG CoA reductase inhibitor drugs or 'statins'.

OTHER CONDITIONS FOUND ON ENTERING THE CCU

Valvular disease, cardiomyopathy and septal defects are covered in Chapters 7 and 11. The symptoms of cardiac failure and the medical support required are described above. Clearly, the majority of patients entering the CCU have ischaemic heart disease and, hence, the emphasis of this chapter.

Many centres have integrated post-infarction rehabilitation programmes run by dedicated dietitians, nurses and physiotherapists.

PHYSIOTHERAPY AFTER MYOCARDIAL INFARCTION

Cardiac rehabilitation is defined as 'the sum of activities required to influence favourably the underlying cause of disease, as well as the best possible physical, mental and social conditions, so that they [patients] may, by their own efforts, preserve or resume, when lost, a normal place as soon as possible in the community. Rehabilitation cannot be regarded as an isolated form of therapy but must be integrated with the whole treatment of which it forms only one facet' (World Health Organisation, 1993).

The physiotherapist's role in the rehabilitation of a patient after myocardial infarction is as part of a co-ordinated multidisciplinary team effort , involving physician or cardiologist, nurse specialist, physiotherapist, occupational therapist, dietitian and pharmacist. The ultimate goal of the team is to return the patient to his or her normal physical and psychological status, through reassurance, education and secondary prevention.

As a rapidly developing service, more randomised trials are necessary to establish guidelines for good practise and effective rehabilitation. In order to consolidate information, the British Association of Cardiac Rehabilitation (BACR) was established in 1992, and in 1995 the World Council for Cardiac Rehabilitation was founded to promote international communication.

In the guidelines laid down by the BACR (Coats *et al.*, 1995), it is suggested that treatment of the patient should cover four phases:
- The in-patient stay.
- The immediate post-discharge period.
- The intermediate post-discharge period.
- Long-term maintenance.

PHASE I: IN-PATIENT STAY

Heart attacks are a devastating experience for patients who have previously considered themselves to be fit, and therefore considerable reassurance and guidance is required. The physiotherapist's involvement should begin as soon as possible after the cardiac event. The primary aim is to encourage a positive attitude and emphasise that the aim of the post-infarction care is to return the patient to a normal and active lifestyle.

Information must be accurate, prompt and non-conflicting. Verbal information should be backed up with written information which the patient may refer to, and should be clear, precise and well presented. Studies have shown that high levels of distress and anxiety have been related to a lack of information and that inappropriate assumptions may hinder the whole rehabilitation process (Lewin *et al.*, 1992). It should not be forgotten that the spouse and immediate family will also need advice, reassurance and support.

On admission to hospital, the patient is usually nursed on the CCU, where the ECG can be continuously monitored for potential dysrythmias. Provided patients remain stable for 48 hours they may then be moved to the medical ward for the rest of their hospital stay.

The physiotherapist is predominantly concerned with the physical aspects of recovery, to counteract the deconditioning effects of bed rest and to encourage a return to a normal and active lifestyle.

While the patient is sedentary, it is essential that breathing and circulatory exercises are taught to prevent complications such as a chest infection or deep vein thrombosis. After 48 hours, the physiotherapist encourages the patient to gradually increase activities through supervised exercise and gentle mobilization. The patient is advised gradually to increase the frequency and distance of walks before climbing the stairs in preparation for discharge.

However, although a structured format should be followed, each patient will progress at his or her own pace, dependent on the size and site of the infarct, age and other medical conditions. The usual length of stay in hospital is between 5 and 7 days; however, in some cases it may be longer. A typical programme is summarised in Table 9.3.

Before discharge, the patient must feel confident to cope at home. Occasionally a referral may be made to the occupational therapists for assessment, especially if the patient is elderly, infirm or living alone. If living alone, it is recommended a patient stays with friends or family for the first couple of weeks to reduce anxieties and allow time to gain confidence in his or her condition. Instructions regarding recovery once at home are summarised in Table 9.4.

These instructions are intended as a guideline only as it is important to stress that each patient is an individual, and that patients will progress at different rates.

In general, patients should be advised that activities should be restricted for approximately 6 weeks to allow time for a strong scar to form over the repaired heart muscle. For this reason it is advisable to begin activities gently and build up gradually, resting where necessary. Before 6 weeks, all strenuous activities must be avoided, especially involving work above shoulder height.

The patient must be warned never to work through any chest pain, as this is a warning sign that the myocardium is being starved of oxygen. The patient must rest, and once the pain has subsided may resume the activity. If the pain does not disappear within a couple of minutes, GTN must be taken.

It is the responsibility of the whole multidisciplinary team to ensure that the patient receives and understands all the information regarding his or her condition and recovery before discharge. It may be the job of the physiotherapist or cardiac liaison worker to conscript the patient on to the out-patient rehabilitation programme.

PHASE II: IMMEDIATELY POST-DISCHARGE

Previously at this stage patients received little input from the healthcare team. However, this phase has since been recognised as a time where patients and their families may require further support, counselling, education and encouragement. In many trusts, this role is now performed by a coronary liaison worker, a position equally suitable for physiotherapist or nurse.

HOME VISIT

The liaison worker will meet the patient in hospital and follow up with a home visit, the timing of which may vary between 2 days to 2 weeks post-discharge. By visiting the patient in his or her own surroundings, the psychological and physical recovery may be assessed. Thus any problems encountered may be referred to the appropriate place of management at an earlier stage.

EDUCATION PROGRAMME

Patients are encouraged to attend out-patient educational sessions, aimed at continuing health promotion and secondary prevention. Motivation to comply with advice has been limited to an understanding of the illness and a need for risk factor assessment (Oldridge, 1991).

Topics included are how the heart and arteries work, the disease process, medication, risk factor assessment and management, introduction to stress and relaxation, dietary advice and return to work, and the importance of exercise.

Daily treatment programme	
On Coronary Care Unit Stage 0	On bed rest: ECG monitored via telemetry Rehabilitation advice booklet given Explanation on MI and plan for in-patient stay Respiratory assessment Breathing: circulatory and bed maintenance exercises
On medical ward Stage 1	May sit out Exercise as stage 0 plus: Alternate knee bends (5 each hour) Alternate straight leg raise (5 each hour) Alternate arm raise (5 each hour)
Stage 2	Exercise as stage 0 + 1 plus Sitting to standing (5 each hour) May walk one way to the toilet and around bed area
Stage 3	Walk to and from the toilet and around the ward more frequently
Stage 4	Increase the frequency and distance of walks Climb the stairs supervised Discharge advice given
Stage 5	Increase the frequency and distance of walks Climb the stairs unsupervised Enrol on cardiac rehabilitation programme

Table 9.3 Daily treatment programme.

As the topics involve expertise in several areas the whole multidisciplinary team should be involved.

Group interaction is psychologically important to the patient as it reduces the feeling of isolation. Through interaction with others in a similar predicament, confidence may be restored and hence a return to normal enhanced.

FORMAL EXERCISE TESTING

Exercise tolerance testing has been considered to be mandatory before the commencement of an exercise programme. It may be performed safely as early as 3 days after the cardiac event (Miller and Borer, 1988) or any time up to 6 weeks. Maximal or symptom-limited exercise tests provide therapeutic and diagnostic information which aids decisions regarding further evaluation and intervention (see Table 9.4).

The Bruce Protocol (Bruce et al., 1973) is commonly used. This is a progressive, incremental test using the treadmill to a maximal or symptom-limited effort.

It is essential for the physician performing the test to communicate with the co-ordinator of the rehabilitation programme as to the suitability of the patient to exercise. A copy of the exercise test result is useful.

PHASE III: INTERMEDIATE POST-DISCHARGE

This phase is often thought of as the 'exercise phase'. Historically, supervised graduated exercise has been the central component to the cardiac rehabilitation programme and therefore is predominantly run by physiotherapists.

Out-patient programmes vary widely from centre to centre, but typically begin within 3 weeks of the cardiac event. Programmes are often run in the hospital physiotherapy department, but may be held in community health centres or leisure centres. Although a low rate of cardiac complications has been reported, all staff should be trained and updated regularly in advanced cardiopulmonary resuscitation.

PHYSIOLOGICAL EFFECTS OF EXERCISE

Physical improvements with exercise training are due to peripheral adaptations through more efficient extraction and metabolisation of oxygen by skeletal muscle. High intensity training has also demonstrated central cardiovascular adaptations of myocardial hypertrophy and dilation of the heart chambers and, consequently, increase of stroke volume, ejection fraction, myocardial contractility

Progression of activities on discharge	
Week 1	Take things slowly. Dress yourself each day. Concentrate on sedentary interests, e.g. reading or listening to music. Avoid getting over tired or tense. Walk up to 0.5 miles.
Week 2	Begin light household activities, e.g. dusting, preparing simple meals and tending to household plants. Rest when necessary.
Week 3	Increase household activities, i.e. ironing, washing up. Begin gardening, i.e. light cutting, weeding and hoeing. Begin light social activities, i.e. visiting friends, going for a meal, going to the cinema or theatre. Begin out-patient rehabilitation programme.
Week 4	Increase household activities to include washing by machine and making beds. Increase walking to 1.5 miles. Begin driving (inform insurance company).
Week 5	Increase activities to include cleaning, mopping floors and light shopping. Increase walking to 2 miles.
Week 6	Become more active. Vacuum clean in stages. Gardening may now include light digging, raking and mowing. Return to work for light occupations (up to 4 months for manual work). Increase walking 2-3 miles. Resume active hobbies such as cycling, bowling, swimming and hiking.

Table 9.4 **Progression of activities on discharge.**

and left ventricular wall thickness. It has been reported that patients who have trained for more than a year have shown improved stroke volume (Horgan *et al.*, 1992). Exercise training ultimately improves functional work capacity by reducing metabolic and circulatory demand during activity.

BENEFITS OF EXERCISE

The benefits of exercise include:

- Improved exercise tolerance and general physical fitness. VO_2 peak improvements have been reported of 10–55% in post-myocardial infarction patients after 3 to 6 months of exercise training (Coats *et al.*, 1995).
- Raised anginal thresholds through lower myocardial oxygen demands, resulting from peripheral and central adaptations of exercise training.
- Improved lipid profile through a greater production of cardioprotective high density lipoproteins (Hartung *et al.*, 1990).
- Greater glucose tolerance in patients with diabetes.
- Lower resting heart rates and blood pressure.
- Improved psychological function through a greater sense of wellbeing, improved confidence, and reduction in anxiety and depression (Oldridge *et al.*, 1993).
- Socioeconomic gains due to improved return to work rates (Levin *et al.*, 1991), a reduction in hospital admission rates (Hartung et al., 1990), and a reduction in the need for antianginal and antihypertensive drugs.

TYPE OF EXERCISE

Aerobic (endurance) exercise forms the core component of the exercise programme. Activities which promote the greatest cardiovascular protection involve regular and rhythmical use of large muscle mass. Hence, walking, cycling and stepping are ideal activities by allowing vasodilation of large muscle mass which lowers peripheral resistance and subsequently opposes a rise in blood pressure which would otherwise occur.

Exercises to involve both the upper and lower limb are included to meet the everyday and/or occupational requirements of the patient, and to promote an all over body training effect. As arm exercises have been shown to cause a greater stress on the heart (Astrand and Rodahl, 1996), the intensity of the arm exercise should be lower than that of the leg exercise. Variation of exercise will minimise overuse and encourage motivation.

In the past, isometric exercise, which maximises strength, was considered to be contra-indicated in patients with cardiac disease due to left ventricular pressure increases and dysrhythmia provocation. However, it has since been demonstrated that strength training is safe, provided that workloads are low and repetitions high (Vonder *et al.*, 1994). Circuit interval training is commonly used; suitable exercises are identified in Table 9.5.

FREQUENCY AND DURATION OF EXERCISE

As the metabolic benefits of exercise are short-lived, it is necessary for the patient to exercise regularly to achieve maximum benefit. It has been recommended that patients should exercise three times a week for 20 to 30 minutes per session. The majority of programmes run 2 to 3 times a week, but for optimal effect patients are advised to exercise at home between attendances. As a high cardiac output must be sustained, the duration of exercise should be between 20 and 30 minutes, excluding warm up and cool down.

INTENSITY OF EXERCISE

Submaximal workloads are used to train the cardiac patient, and are compensated for by a greater duration of activity. Exercise intensities of 60–80% VO_2 max (equivalent to 70–85% maximal heart rate) are used. Higher intensities may provoke cardiac complications such as ischaemia and dysrhythmia without additional aerobic benefit.

PROGRESSION OF EXERCISE

All exercises are pursued on an individual basis. Continual monitoring allows the supervisor to assess when the patient is ready to increase his or her level of activity. Pulse palpation identifies whether the training heart rate (about 75% maximal heart rate) is being achieved. For patients on β-blockers, i.e. atenolol, which act by lowering the heart rate, the Borg Scale of perceived exertion (Borg, 1992) is used to determine the level at which the patient is working. The Borg Scale is a 10 point scale of at what level the patient feels he or she is working on during activities, ranging from 1 (extremely light) to 10 (maximum), points 4–6 (moderate to hard) being the optimal range at which to work. Only when the training heart rate is not being met, or the rate of perceived exertion is low, are the exercises increased. Safe progression is achieved by increasing the frequency and duration before increasing the workload.

Suitable exercises for interval training
Stride jumps
Trunk curls
Bench stepping
Bench dips
Exercise bicycle–progressive resistance
Marching
Sit to stand
Skipping
Half squats
Gentle jogging
Arm swinging–with or without light arm weights
Wall press-ups

Table 9.5 **Suitable exercises for interval training.**

WARM UP AND COOL DOWN EXERCISES

The warm up is an essential prerequisite to the exercise programme as it prepares the body for the ensuing activity. It should include:

- Mobility exercises to improve joint range, i.e. shoulder circles and hip and knee swinging.
- Static stretch of muscle groups, i.e. quadriceps, hamstring stretch. Each stretch must be maintained for approximately 10 seconds.
- Dynamic activities to raise the heart rate, i.e. marching and walking.

Ideally the warm up should raise the heart rate to within 20 beats of the training heart rate. For cardiac patients an effective warm up of 10 to 15 minutes duration has been shown to increase the anginal threshold.

Following the exercise circuit, an active cool down of 5 to 10 minutes duration is performed to prevent blood pooling and post-exercise hypotension. A gradual decline in activity guards against post-activity dysrhythmia evoked from higher plasma catecholamine levels.

CONTRAINDICATIONS TO EXERCISE

Exercise should not be considered in patients with:
- Severe aortic stenosis.
- Active myocarditis.
- Exercise-induced dysrhythmia.
- Unstable angina.
- Severe orthopaedic disability.
- Uncontrolled hypertension (160/100 mmHg) or above.
- Uncontrolled diabetes.
- Acute left ventricular failure.
- Overt psychoses.
- Left ventricular aneurysm.
- Bilateral bundle branch block.

PRECAUTIONS TO CARDIAC REHABILITATION

Cardiac rehabilitation should be considered carefully in patients with:
- Gross obesity.
- Chronic chest conditions.
- Transient ischaemic attacks (TIAs).
- Intermittent claudication.
- Poor ejection fraction.
- Heart failure.

STRUCTURE OF THE EXERCISE PROGRAMME

An initial assessment is performed on an individual basis to gain relevant information about the patient and his or her condition. A resting ECG and blood pressure recording are taken for future reference.

Ideally, a submaximal exercise test is performed on the exercise bicycle or treadmill to ascertain the appropriate starting point of exercise, and to detect any potential risks. If all is satisfactory, warm up exercises are taught and general advice is given.

Often the rehabilitation programme is the first contact with healthcare professionals that the patient has received since his or her discharge from hospital. Therefore both patient and relatives are encouraged to ask questions relating to the condition in order to allay possible anxieties regarding recovery.

Subsequent visits are as a group session with each patient performing his or her own individual level of exercise, and progressing at his or her own rate. The structure of the assessment and exercise session is summarised in Table 9.6.

PHASE IV: LONG-TERM MAINTENANCE

It is becoming increasingly recognised that the way forward in the treatment of cardiac patients is through secondary prevention and long-term maintenance (Sivers, 1996). Until a few years ago, cardiac rehabilitation offered only a short-term solution by accelerating the return to normal following a cardiac event. Oldridge (1991) highlighted the fact that approximately 50% of patients who began the rehabilitation programme failed to continue their lifestyle modifications within 6 to 12 months. It is only through habitual modifications over several months or years that a reduction in the progression of the disease is likely to occur.

Through a close liaison with the primary healthcare team, long-term maintenance is possible. Risk factor clinics are being established to monitor lipid profiles, blood pressure, smoking habits, medication and weight control. Some healthcare trusts have initiated long-term follow-up of patients in their own homes to provide on-going support, monitoring and education. Furthermore, cardiac support groups are growing following a network initiated through the British Heart Foundation.

CONCLUSION

Until the late 1960s, cardiac rehabilitation was identified fundamentally with the physiotherapist and physical training. More recently, research has shown that exercise should form only one component in a comprehensive long-term approach to the disease process. Rehabilitation procedures must include risk factor modification, education and changes in lifestyle, monitored over a long period of time. Through effective health awareness in the community and the ripple effect of health promotion through families, greater awareness and earlier modification of risk factors may be established.

Coronary heart disease has been identified as a great economic burden to the NHS (Horgan et al., 1992). Comprehensive cardiac rehabilitation programmes are now being recognised as a means to reduce healthcare costs, achieved through lower hospital admissions, the need for fewer antianginal and antihypertensive drugs and a higher return to work rate, and are therefore seen as a justifiable use of healthcare resources. *The Health of the Nation* document has begun to address this issue through secondary prevention, aiming to reduce by 40% coronary heart disease mortality in under 65 year olds by the year 2000. As a direct consequence, recent years have seen a boom in the provision of cardiac rehabilitation programmes which otherwise would have been slow to develop, despite having been established for over 25 years.

Cardiac rehabilitation remains very diverse; the programme may vary from trust to trust and from one country to another. Although the importance of exercise programmes has been established (Oldridge et al., 1988; O'Connor et al., 1989), more audit, evaluation and randomised trials are necessary to establish guidelines of good practise, effective evaluation and demonstration of long-term benefit (Sivers, 1996).

Table 9.6 Structure of the exercise programme.

Structure of the exercise programme	
Session 1 **Assessment**	One to one General advice Relevant patient history and condition since discharge Risk stratification ECG trace, and blood pressure Submaximal Bruce Protocol—important for devising appropriate exercise programme and detecting potential risks Warm up exercises taught
Other sessions **Twice weekly** **for 6-8 weeks**	Group session Resting heart rate and blood pressure Warm up 10-15 minutes Circuit interval training 20-45 minutes, monitoring via pulse and Borg scale Post-exercise blood pressure and pulse Cool down 5-10 minutes Relaxation Education and advice

9

REFERENCES

Astrand PO, Rodahl K. *Textbook of work physiology, physical basis of exercise*, 3rd ed. New York: McGraw-Hill; 1996.

Borg G. Psychophysical bases of perceived exertion. *Med Sci Sports Exerc* 1992, **14(5):**377-381.

Bruce RA, Kusumi F, Hosmer D. Maximal oxygen intake and nomographic assessment of functional aerobic impairment in cardiovascular disease. *Am Heart J* 1973, **85:**546-562.

Coats A, McGee H, Syokes H, Thompson D. *BACR guidelines for cardiac rehabilitation*. London: Blackwell Science; 1995.

Hartung GH, Foreyt JP, Reeves RS, *et al.* Effect of alcohol dose on plasma lipoprotein subfractions and lipolytic enzyme activity in active and inactive men. *Metabolism* 1990 **39:**81-86.

HorganJ, Bethell H, Carson P, *et al.* Working party report on cardiac rehabilitation. *Br Heart J* 1992, **67:**412-418.

Levin LA, Perk J, Kedback B. Cardial Rehabilitation - a cost analysis. *J of Int Medi* 1991, **230:**427-434.

Lewin B, Robertson I, Lay EL, *et al.* Effects of self-help post myocardial infarction rehabilitation on psychological adjustment and use of health services. *Lancet* 1992, **339:**1036-1040.

Miller DM, Borer JS. Exercise testing early after myocardial infarction: Combined experience of random trials. *JAMA* 1988, **260:**945-950.

Moghissi K. *Essentials of thoracic and cardiac surgery*. London: William Heineman Medical Books.

O'Connor T, Buring J, Yusuf S, *et al.* An overview of randomised trials of rehabilitation with exercise after myocardial infarction. *Circulatia* 1989, **80:**234-244.

Oldridge N. Compliance with cardiac rehabilitation services. *J Cardiopul Rehab* 1991, **111:**115-127.

Oldridge NB, Guyatt G, Fischer M, Rimm A. Cardiac rehabilitation after myocardial infarction: Combined experience of randomised trials. *JAMA* 1988, **260:**945-950.

Sivers F. *Evidence based strategies for secondary prevention of coronary heart disease*. United Kingdom, Merck Sharp and Dohme; 1996.

Vonder LB, Franklin BA, Wrisley D, Ruberfive M. Acute cardiovascular responses to nautilus exercise in cardiac patients: implications for exercise training. *Ann Sports Med* 1994, **2:**165-169.

GENERAL READING

Braunwald E. *Heart disease, A textbook of cardiovascular medicine*, 5th ed. 1996 WB Saunders & Co. Pennsylvania.

Caine N, Harrison S, Sharples L, Wallwork J. Prospective study of quality of life before and after coronary artery bypass grafting. *BMJ* 1991, **302:**511-516.

Huang D, Ades P, Weaver S. Cardiac rehospitalizations and costs are reduced following cardiac rehabilitation. *J Cardiopul Rehab* 1990, **10.**

Kehl P. A retrospective look at the effects of cardiac rehabilitation—post myocardial infarction. *Physiotherapy* 1991, **77(2).**

Kellerman J. Long term comprehensive care and tasks of cardiac rehabilitation (Editorial). *Euro Heart J* 1993, **11(14):**1441-1444.

Laure C, Miliani R. Cardiac rehabilitation and health care reform (Editorial). *Chest* 1995, **107(S):**1189-1190.

Oldridge N, Furlong W, Feeny D, *et al.* Economic evaluation of cardiac rehabilitation soon after myocardial infarction. *Am J Cardiol* 1993, **72:**154-161.

Opie LH, Lionel K, Phil D. *Drugs for the heart*. *Pennsylvania:* WB Saunders & Co; 1997.

Oldridge NB, Guyatt G, Jones, *et al.* Effects on quality of life with comprehensive rehabilitation after acute myocardial infarction. *Am J Cardiol* 1991, **67:**1084-1089.

Royal College of Physicians Report. *Medical aspects of exercise: Benefits and risks*. London: Royal College of Physicians; 1991.

Wheatley. *Coronary artery disease, valvular disease. Lecture notes of cardiology*. Ceatumm, Bull and Braimdridge. Oxford: Blackwell Science.

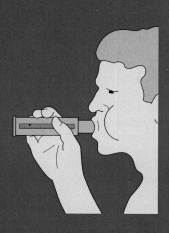

10 MB Allen, CFA Pantin & S Singh

THE MEDICAL UNIT

CHAPTER OUTLINE

- Asthma
- Acute severe asthma
- Chronic bronchitis and emphysema
- Bronchiectasis
- Tuberculosis
- Pneumonia
- Pneumonia in the immunocompromised patient
- Obstructive sleep apnoea

- Hyperventilation syndrome
- Pleural effusion
- Lung abscess
- Pulmonary embolus
- Interstitial lung diseases
- Occupational lung diseases
- Pulmonary rehabilitation
- Setting up a rehabilitation programme

THE MEDICAL ASSESSMENT UNIT

This chapter will describe common medical chest conditions seen by physiotherapists. Some of the conditions covered may not benefit from hands-on physiotherapy, but there is a high likelihood that the clinician will encounter patients with, for example, sarcoidosis and, because of the underlying pathology, may be able to advise or offer general exercise in an attempt to improve the patient's wellbeing.

The current emphasis on physiotherapy management of chronic respiratory disease is moving away from traditional chest physiotherapy techniques of postural drainage, percussion and vibrations, towards pulmonary rehabilitation. While there is still a place for techniques to enhance sputum clearance, e.g. during an acute exacerbation, the physiotherapist will predominately provide the patients and their carers with advice on positioning, humidification, bronchodilation assessment and methods to increase exercise tolerance. Patients with lung disease need to be encouraged to assess their own condition and put into practice methods to improve their general health. General exercise should be applied both in the ward and at home.

In many acute hospitals, the trauma patients are admitted through an accident and emergency department, whereas the medical patients are brought to a Medical Assessment Unit (MAU). The role of the MAU is to stabilise patients and to admit them if necessary.

ASTHMA

DESCRIPTION

No one has been able to define asthma satisfactorily, although the disease can be described. The British Thoracic Society (BTS) description states:

'Asthma is a common and chronic inflammatory condition of the airways whose cause is not completely understood. As a result of inflammation the airways are hyper-responsive and they narrow easily in response to a wide range of stimuli. This may result in coughing, wheezing, chest tightness and shortness of breath; these symptoms are often worse at night. Narrowing of the airway is usually reversible, but in some patients with

chronic asthma the inflammation may lead to irreversible obstruction of airflow.

Characteristic pathological features include the presence in the airway of inflammatory cells, plasma exudation, oedema, hypertrophy of smooth muscle, mucus plugging and shedding of epithelium. The changes will be present even in patients with mild asthma when they have few symptoms.'

Thus asthma is a chronic inflammatory disease of the airway; however, the diagnosis has to be made clinically and by measurement of the flow of air through the narrowed airway. Variation in the narrowing clinches the diagnosis.

AETIOLOGY AND EPIDEMIOLOGY

Asthma has a genetic component, running in families. This tendency is inherited separately from the tendency to atopy, the allergy which is shown by positive skin prick tests to common environmental allergens such as one in the faeces of the house dust mite, others in the fur of the cat, dog and other animals, or another in grass pollens. Atopic families show a high incidence of hay fever, rhinitis, flexural eczema and asthma. The inheritance of either or both of these genetic tendencies raises the probability of an individual developing asthma. Thus, a person, usually a child, may develop atopic (childhood, extrinsic) asthma where airway narrowing is triggered by exposure to one of the common environmental allergens (Table 10.1). Others may develop non-atopic (adult-onset, intrinsic) asthma where only non-specific events, such as viral infections, cold, exercise or stress may trigger an asthma attack. Such non-specific events can also trigger an attack in an atopic asthmatic.

Inheriting a genetic tendency to either asthma and/or atopy does not mean a person will inevitably develop asthma however. There must be an environmental inducer of the first attack. Contrariwise, a person with no genetic tendency may develop asthma, if the environmental inducer is in high concentration, such as in some occupations, e.g. bleach in hairdressing, colophony in soldering, animal urine in laboratories. The exposure to environmental chemicals and pollutions is blamed for the current increase in the prevalence of asthma, but conclusive evidence for this claim is still lacking. In the UK an estimated 10% of children and 5% of adults are affected. The peak onset occurs between the ages of 5 and 10 years with a male to female ratio of 1.5 to 1. However, the asthma in up to 70% of affected children remits by the age of 20 years, although it is possible that it will return in later life.

Evidence is growing that avoidance of allergens by the mother in late pregnancy and by the baby in its first year can reduce the risk of the baby in an atopic family developing asthma.

CLINICAL FEATURES

The classic symptoms of wheeze, breathlessness, chest tightness and cough typically show considerable temporal variation, often being worse at night or in the early morning. The severity can vary from mild with wheeze after running, to constant and severe, dominating the patient's lifestyle. This severity can vary during the same person's life. Thus, a patient may complain of episodic asthma with sudden onset of a feeling of tightness in the chest with breathlessness and wheeze. Expiration becomes prolonged with a short, gasping inspiration. Polyphonic wheeze may be heard over the chest, often without the use of a stethoscope. Patients may know the triggers which cause these attacks, which are often short-lived, with recovery as patients remove themselves from the stimuli and use a bronchodilator inhaler. However, such an attack may be prolonged into an acute severe asthma attack. The same patient may later develop chronic severe asthma with persistent wheeze and breathlessness. Cough productive of mucoid sputum is often a major symptom, and may turn purulent in episodes of respiratory infection.

Non-atopic asthma usually starts later in life, even into the 60s and 70s. It is often chronic and rarely remits. Precipitating factors are non-atopic and skin tests negative (see Table 10.1).

In children under 5 years of age, wheezing cannot confidently be regarded as equivalent to asthma. It is common with minor respiratory infections and acute bronchiolitis. Non-asthmatic wheeziness will usually resolve as the child grows. Often, the experience of a paediatric respiratory physician is needed to make the diagnosis in infancy. Features suggestive of asthma are that the wheeze and/or cough is episodic, nocturnal, seasonal or exertional; the child is atopic with a positive family history.

COMPLICATIONS

Asthma is a chronic disease and may lead to retarded growth rate in children. thoracic cage deformity, recurrent bronchial infection, fixed airways obstruction and chronic respiratory failure.

Chronic colonization of the lungs with the aspergillus fungi may lead to the development of allergic bronchopulmonary aspergillosis (see page 188). Acute severe asthma increases the risk of pneumothorax, and may lead to respiratory arrest and death.

INVESTIGATIONS

An objective diagnosis of asthma depends on demonstrating a variable degree (>15%) of airflow obstruction. The peak flow meter, being inexpensive, is widely used to measure the patient's maximum peak expiratory flow (PEF) to determine the degree of obstruction.

In patients with a low PEF at time of test, a bronchodilator reversibility test or steroid test may be used. In the first, the PEF is measured; the patient inhales the bronchodilator, and the PEF measurement is repeated after 5–10 minutes. In the second, the patient monitors PEF morning and evening for at least a week; oral prednisolone is given for 3 days in children and up for to 3 weeks in adults continuing to monitor PEF. In both tests an improvement in PEF of at least 15% indicates reversible airflow obstruction, suggesting asthma.

In patients with a normal PEF at time of test, diurnal variation or exercise test may be used. In the first, the patient monitors PEF morning and evening for 2 weeks. If there is at least a 15% variation in PEF between mornings and evenings, asthma is indicated. In the second, PEF is measured if the patient exercises vigorously for 5–6 minutes. The PEF is recorded every 5 minutes after exercise for 15 minutes. After vigorous exercise, over 80% of asthmatics will show a fall in PEF of at least 15% within 10 minutes of the cessation of exercise.

Dynamic spirometry can be used to demonstrate airflow obstruction and bronchodilator reversibility. Airway hyper-responsiveness can be measured by the histamine challenge test, but this is restricted to very difficult cases and research.

Skin tests for common environmental allergens assess the atopic status of the patient, and give a guide to which allergens to avoid, e.g. cat hairs. Eosinophils may be raised in the blood or sputum of asthmatics, but are rarely checked for today.

TREATMENT

Management aims to find the minimum level of treatment to suppress symptoms and enable the patient to lead a normal life. The patient is encouraged to take responsibility for day-to-day management, with verbal or written advice from the professional and regular review.

AVOIDANCE

β-blocker drugs, used for hypertension and glaucoma, cause bronchospasm and must be avoided. Patients must not smoke. The patient needs to avoid any known triggers if possible (see Table 10.1). However, suppression of house dust mite, or avoidance of grass pollen, for example, can be difficult. It is preferable to adjust drug treatment to cover exposure to day-to-day triggers such as exercise and cold air, because avoidance can impose inappropriate restrictions on lifestyle.

DRUG THERAPY

There are two main types of drug treatment for asthma, classified 'Preventers' and 'Relievers'. Inhaled therapy is preferable to minimize side effects.

Preventers include anti-inflammatory drugs to suppress the underlying inflammation and 'prevent' airways obstruction, such as the inhaled steroids (beclomethasone, budesonide and fluticasone), sodium cromoglycate (Intal) and nedocromil sodium (Tilade). These drugs are given regularly, and even to mild cases, as inflammation is found in the airways of the mildest asthmatics. Prednisolone, a corticosteroid, may be needed as an oral 'preventer'.

Relievers include drugs that reduce bronchospasm. Unlike 'preventers', they are effective only in relieving existing bronchospasm and exercise induced asthma. These drugs include short-acting β_2-agonists such as salbutamol and terbutaline, long-acting β_2-agonists such as salmeterol, formoterol and bambuterol, and anticholinergics such as ipratropium and oral theophyllines.

'A combination of an inhaled "preventer", usually a corticosteroid, to treat the underlying inflammatory pathogenesis and inhaled short acting β_2-agonist to treat symptom breakthrough, can provide an effective, safe and logical approach to asthma therapy' (BTS Guidelines).

Table 10.1 Triggers causing asthma attacks.

Triggers causing asthma attacks		
Specific Atopic allergens (skin tests positive)	House dust mite Animal moulds Grass pollen Tree pollen	

Occupational allergies	**Source**
	Isocyanates
	Flour/grain/hay
	Soldering flux (colophony)
	Laboratory animals
	Wood dusts (African teak,
	    Western red cedar)
	Glues, resins
		Uses
		Paint spraying
		Milling, malting, baking
		Welding, soldering
		Laboratory animal work
		Saw milling,
		    woodworking
		Curing of epoxy resin

Non-specific	Viral infection Fumes, sprays, smokes Exercise, cold air Perfume Stress-related issues Drugs, e.g. β-blockers and non-steroidal anti-inflammatory drugs	

This philosophy is central to the first approach used in national and international guidelines to the use of drugs in asthma treatment with increasing doses of preventer and reliever as the asthma worsens, together with reduction as asthma severity wanes. In chronic severe asthma, the first step suggests the use of oral prednisolone, kept to the lowest level, which controls the symptoms to minimise side effects (if possible below 15 mg).

ACUTE SEVERE ASTHMA (STATUS ASTHMATICUS)

Acute severe asthma, severe wheezing and breathlessness lasting more than 24 hours and not responding to normal medication can occur in even the best controlled asthma patient. The severity of an attack of acute severe asthma is often underestimated by patients, their relatives and carers, and can be fatal. Potentially life-threatening features include the patient being unable to complete sentences in one breath, unable to get up from chair or bed, respiratory rate greater than 25/min (>40 in children, >60 in infants) and tachycardia greater than 110 beats/minute (>140 in children). The patient may even have a silent chest on auscultation, feeble respiratory effort, cyanosis and disturbance of consciousness. PEF shows a drop, often predicting an attack days before symptoms occur; a patient's best PEF below 50% is a danger sign.

TREATMENT

If a patient is alerted early to a worsening of his or her asthma by noticing a worsening of symptoms and reduction in PEF, then an increase in inhaled steroids or a course of oral prednisolone at home may abort the exacerbation.

Acute severe asthma is treated in hospital by high concentrations of oxygen, high doses of inhaled β_2-agonists and high doses of systemic steroids, either prednisolone by mouth or hydrocortisone by intravenous injection. Physiotherapy as an adjunct to drug therapy can be helpful. If the asthma attack does not respond, nebulised ipratropium and/or intravenous theophylline or β_2-agonist may be tried. Rarely, tracheal intubation and mechanical ventilation is needed, sometimes with bronchial lavage.

CHRONIC BRONCHITIS AND EMPHYSEMA (COPD)

DEFINITION

This disease is known by a variety of names, including chronic bronchitis and emphysema, chronic obstructive airways disease (COAD), chronic obstructive lung disease (COLD), and non-reversible obstructive airways disease (NROAD). The term that has gained widespread acceptance is chronic obstructive pulmonary disease (COPD). COPD is characterised by the presence of bronchitis and/or emphysema associated with airflow obstruction; the airflow obstruction may be accompanied by airways hyperreactivity and may be partially reversible. Chronic bronchitis is epidemiologically defined as cough and sputum for 3 months of each year occurring over 2 consecutive years, while emphysema is a pathological diagnosis. The airflow obstruction, best measured as forced expiratory volume in the first 1 second (FEV_1), is the important factor as this relates to mortality.

EPIDEMIOLOGY

The prevalence and impact of COPD within a community is difficult to determine because of different methods of recording the diagnosis, variable use of pulmonary function to confirm the airflow obstruction and considering chronic asthmatics in the same group. Information from 1982–3 suggests that 14% of sickness from work in men was of respiratory nature, 56% of which was due to COPD and only 9% asthma. For women 11% of certified incapacity was of a respiratory origin of which 24% was due to COPD. Mortality from COPD is high, with an estimated rate of 48 per 10 000 in men and 18.8 per 10 000 in women. There is a three-fold variation throughout the UK with the industrialised North having the highest rates. The prognosis is much worse if patients develop fluid retention, with only a 30% survival rate over 5 years.

PATHOLOGY

The pathological changes in the lungs of patients with COPD can be considered as three entities: chronic bronchitis, emphysema and small airways disease. The cough and sputum production found in chronic bronchitis are due to increased numbers of mucous glands and are not related to airflow obstruction. Emphysema is a pathological definition of permanent enlargement of air spaces distal to the terminal bronchioles accompanied by the destruction of alveolar walls without fibrosis. This enlargement and destruction has several effects but the important ones are a change in alveolar surface area and relationships with the capillary network around the alveoli, making gas exchange less efficient. There is also loss of the surrounding supportive tissue of the small airways and it is likely that this, in conjunction with changes in bronchiole muscle tone, produces the small airways disease and airflow obstruction.

With progressive loss of alveolar tissue, patients become hypoxaemic initially at exercise and then at rest (PaO_2 less than 8 kPa). This can produce a variety of effects, with pulmonary hypertension, fluid retention and heart failure (cor pulmonale) being the most important.

AETIOLOGY

The above changes are due to smoking, especially of cigarettes. Environmental air pollution and passive smoking are far less important. There is a close relationship between the amount smoked and the chances of developing COPD; however, only around 20% of people who smoke actually develop the progressive airflow obstruction. Many smokers will have cough and sputum due to the increased mucous production but this improves markedly if they stop smoking.

The proposed mechanism of emphysema development is an imbalance between the protease enzymes within the alveoli and the antiproteases present in the blood. Cigarette smoking produces an influx of white cells into the lungs and also stimulates production of more protease, leading to a protease–anti-protease imbalance and lung damage. Very rarely (about 0.03% of the population) there is a deficiency of the blood antiproteases, predominately alpha 1 antitrypsin. Such individuals develop emphysema much more readily and often present with symptoms in their early 40s.

CLINICAL FEATURES

COPD is a disease which occurs in the middle-aged and elderly and may present to healthcare workers in several ways, including recurrent chest infections, progressive breathlessness and fluid retention of cor pulmonale. In the past patients were divided into two polarised groups. The so-called pink puffers are extremely breathless on minimal exercise, have a hyperinflated chest on examination and use the accessory muscles of respiration, fixing their arms, and breathe with pursed lips in an attempt to maintain pressure within their airways. The arterial blood gases on such patients often show only mild hypoxaemia due to the marked ventilatory effort. In contrast the so-called blue bloaters are often cyanosed, make little ventilatory effort, rarely complain of breathlessness and may have features of heart failure at presentation. The blood gases show marked hypoxaemia with an elevated carbon dioxide tension, but due to compensatory long-term renal retention of bicarbonate they are not acidotic. However, most patients fall between the two polarised types.

INVESTIGATIONS

By definition patients with COPD will have impairment of expiratory flow, best measured by spirometry and not peak flow. This can be used to classify the disease as mild (<60% predicted), moderate (40–59% predicted) or severe (<40% predicted). If detailed lung function tests are performed increased lung volumes are often noted together with a reduced gas transfer, reflecting a reduction in the number of functional alveolar units. Blood gases should be performed to identify the severity of the hypoxaemia and decide if oxygen therapy is required. In patients with heart failure an ECG and a biochemical profile should be requested and all patients should have a full blood count to see if there is an increase in the number of red cells (polycythaemia). This is a response to the hypoxaemia and if present the patient should be considered for venesection (blood volume reduction), as the benefits of the increased oxygen-carrying capacity of the additional red cells is offset by the reduced tissue perfusion from the increased blood viscosity.

A chest X-ray is important, not for confirming the diagnosis of COPD but to exclude other reasons for the presentation. Heart failure may be confirmed by an enlarged heart, interstitial shadowing and pleural effusions. Pneumonia may produce increasing symptoms, but, more importantly, lung carcinoma, which is much more common in the smoking population and thus may explain why an individual has deteriorated. Computerised tomography (CT) of the thorax is needed only if specific pulmonary surgery is being considered. In patients with a familial history or premature COPD the alpha 1 protease inhibitor levels should be checked as this may allow screening of individuals and allow targeting for smoking cessation advice.

DIFFERENTIAL DIAGNOSIS

There are few conditions associated with sputum production, progressive breathlessness and airflow obstruction, but bronchiectasis and asthma are the important ones to consider. As the management of asthma is different it is important to confirm the diagnosis of COPD. The characteristic feature of asthma is variability in both symptoms and degree of airflow obstruction. Diagnosis should be ascertained from symptom questioning and examination of patients' twice-daily peak flow measurements to see if there is any inherent variability of the airflow obstruction. A formal trial of oral steroids for 2 weeks is an additional method of examining for a reversible 'asthmatic' disease. Determining reversibility of airflow obstruction to standard and high dose bronchodilators should also be performed as a guide to therapy; some patients with COPD may have a significant response to bronchodilators but not to steroids.

TREATMENT

This may be considered under three headings:
- Stop the progressive decline in lung function: *smoking cessation.*
- Relieve the hypoxaemia: *long-term oxygen therapy.*
- *Symptom control.*

Smoking Cessation

The underlying decline in lung function is the factor which leads to death and the only method to prevent the decline is smoking cessation. It is important that the patient is advised to stop smoking at every encounter with healthcare professionals as, once the idea is accepted, the chances of stopping increase. There are a variety of different ways of achieving smoking cessation but it appears that stopping acutely, with appropriate support and advice, is the best method. A gradual reduction in the amount smoked often fails to lead to permanent cessation. In individuals who smoke excessively both nicotine replacement patches and chewing gum can play a role.

Long-Term Oxygen Therapy

The loss of alveolar units and gas exchange leads to hypoxaemia, pulmonary hypertension and, ultimately, cor pulmonale. Use of low flow oxygen corrects the hypoxaemia and limits the rise in pulmonary artery pressure and development of cor pulmonale. In selected patients (Department of Health criteria PaO_2 less than 7.3 kPa, $PaCO_2$ greater than 6 kPa, FEV_1 less than 1.5 litres) low flow oxygen for a minimum of 15 hours per day was associated with a 5 to 10 year increase in survival. Unfortunately if patients continue to smoke, oxygen therapy produces no benefit.

Long-term oxygen therapy is a large commitment for the patient, especially as it is associated with little symptom improvement. The oxygen is most efficiently delivered by a concentrator rather than oxygen cylinders and the oxygen is then piped to areas where patients spend most of their time, usually the bedroom and sitting room, although large lengths of tubing do allow patients freedom of movement. The concentrator is serviced on a regular basis and the amount of time used recorded to allow reimbursement of electricity costs to the patient.

Symptom Control

Regular inhaled bronchodilators play a major role in the relief of breathlessness even though most patients show little objective improvement in pulmonary function following use. The anticholinergic drugs appear to have a greater role than in asthma and have an additional benefit when used in conjunction with β-agonists. If there is a significant element of reversible airflow obstruction inhaled steroids should be used, although their role in patients with COPD without an asthmatic component is not yet clear and results from large trials are awaited. Oral theophyllines produce benefit for some patients, especially in improving exercise tolerance. In those patients not affected severely enough to require long-term oxygen therapy but who have marked breathlessness after exercise, supplemental oxygen via cylinders may produce more rapid relief of breathlessness. More portable forms of oxygen therapy such as liquid oxygen are not available on prescription in the UK at present.

To prevent infections, influenza and pneumococcal vaccination should be administered and for some patients the GP may provide a supply of antibiotics for home use to allow prompt treatment of any exacerbations. To improve patients' ability to feel in control of their illness and increase their exercise tolerance the patients should be considered for pulmonary rehabilitation. Such programmes encompass the important aspects of nutrition, education, appropriate use of prescribed therapy and advice on available benefits; see Pulmonary Rehabilitation.

For a few patients surgical interventions may be considered. If there is a large air-containing cyst (bullae) which is compressing the surrounding lung, excision can be considered. Young and middle-aged patients (less than 60 years of age) who remain symptomatic despite the above management should be considered for lung transplantation. Single lung transplant allows best use of the limited number of organs with a low operative morbidity. The role of excising lung tissue to allow the chest to regain its normal shape and improve mechanical function (lung volume reduction surgery) appears beneficial but is not yet established in the UK.

COMPLICATIONS

Several complications of COPD are recognised and include unexplained weight loss, rupture of an emphysematous sack to produce a pneumothorax, development of heart failure (cor pulmonale) and ventilatory failure. The latter is a common problem in patients with severe disease during infective exacerbations. Treatment is aimed at improving gas exchange by controlled oxygen therapy, clearing bronchial secretions, ensuring maximal bronchodilation and treating the underlying infection. If patients fail to improve, nasal intermittent positive pressure ventilation (NIPPV), with oxygen supplementation if necessary, allows patients to be managed without the need for endotracheal intubation and its associated problems.

BRONCHIECTASIS

DEFINITION

Ectasis is Latin for 'widened'. Bronchiectasis describes lungs where some or all of the bronchi are widened and damaged. It results from failure of airway protection, including mucociliary clearance and the inflammatory response. Thus bronchiectatic lungs can be a manifestation of many disease processes.

EPIDEMIOLOGY

The incidence of new cases of bronchiectasis in the UK is very low, the commonest causes of new cases being congenital, e.g. primary ciliary dyskinesia and cystic fibrosis. The estimated prevalence in the UK is 1–2 in 1000. It is more common in developing countries.

PATHOLOGY

The pathology following the initial breakdown of airways protection is due to poor clearance of mucus, through either loss of cilia or failure of the inflammatory response. This leads to infection with further damage to the bronchial walls, with the normal ciliated columnar epithelium changing to cuboid form with fewer or no cilia. Thus a vicious cycle can be set up. In addition, in severe cases, the bronchial arteries within the walls of the bronchi become dilated with anastomoses to the pulmonary circulation, giving a tendency to haemoptysis.

IMPAIRED CLEARANCE
Primary Ciliary Dyskinesia (PCD)

Cilia in normals beat in one direction only. In the bronchi and trachea, this is towards the larynx, thus clearing the lungs of mucus and inhaled debris. In PCD, the cilia are defective and do not beat in unison, so the mucus is not cleared from the lungs. Ciliated movement of embryonic cells is thought to direct the placing of the organs, with the heart and spleen placed on the right, and the liver on the left side. Therefore, a patient with PCD has a random (50%) chance of his or her organs being either on the left or right side. If on the unusual side, e.g. heart on the right (dextrocardia) the patient has situs inversus as part of his or her PCD—Kartegener's syndrome. As the tails of sperm have a similar structure to cilia, affected males are sterile.

Bronchial Obstruction

If a bronchus is obstructed for any length of time, local mucociliary clearance breaks down, causing localised bronchiectasis. The obstruction may be a foreign body, or an enlarged lymph node, e.g. a tubercular or congenital narrowing.

Cystic Fibrosis

The viscid mucus jams the clearance mechanisms, stopping the cilia beating.

INFLAMMATION

Congenital Breakdown of the Immune System

Children with immune system deficits, e.g. panhypogammaglobulinaemia, develop bronchiectasis. Patients with inadequate numbers of lymph drainage vessels (primary lymphoedema) may be unable to clear the debris after a chest infection, leading to bronchiectasis, and sometimes pleural effusions. Inadequate lymph drainage may also lead to thickened yellow nails—yellow nail syndrome.

Acquired

After severe inflammation from any cause, the lung may heal with minor or major bronchiectatic areas. This was very common in the pre-antibiotic era, but is rare now. Specific examples are, post-pneumonia, often viral, e.g. whooping cough, allergic bronchopulmonary aspergillosis or fibrotic or granulomatous lung disease, or following immunodeficiency in association with leukaemias and lymphomas.

Bronchiectasis is more likely in patients with rheumatoid arthritis, ulcerative colitis, vasculitis and connective tissue disorders. Male infertility often accompanies bronchiectasis (e.g. in PCD and cystic fibrosis).

CLINICAL FEATURES

These range from non-existent in those with only a small area of lung involved to extensive in those with widespread bronchiectasis. Cough, often with sputum, is the common symptom. The sputum may be purulent and large volume. Episodic fever or malaise, pleuritic pain, or night sweats related to intercurrent infection may occur. As ciliated respiratory epithelium extends into the sinuses and nasal passages, many patients suffer from nasal discharge and chronic sinusitis. Dyspnoea is felt if enough lung is affected. On examination, signs range from none through a few crackles to clubbing, halitosis, weight loss, tachypnoea, sputum which is often purulent, hyperinflation of the chest and coarse crackles on auscultation.

Complications can include infective exacerbations, pneumothorax, respiratory failure, cor pulmonale, emphysema, amyloidosis, and haemoptyosis. Chest pain, usually pleuritic, may be associated with an area of bronchiectasis. Metastatic spread of infection is now rare; brain abscess was the classic complication. Some patients may develop an arthropathy, either rheumatoid arthritis or non-specific related in intensity to the infective activity of the disease.

The prognosis of bronchiectasis depends on the severity of the disease.

INVESTIGATIONS

Sputum cultures are regularly taken, often with the help of the physiotherapist, to check for the presence of the bacteria, *Staphylococcus aureus*, *Haemophilus influenzae*, *Pseudomonas* species (especially *P. aeruginosa*) and *Bordetella cepacia*, and to exclude active tuberculosis.

Chest X-rays show hyperinflation, tramlines, crowded lung markings and ring shadows. A high resolution CT scan will delinate the extent of disease. Sinus X-rays may show associated mucosal thickening and fluid levels.

Respiratory function tests (see Chapter 2) show any defect, which may be obstructive or mixed.

Tests for the cause of the bronchiectasis include serum immunoglobulins, aspergillus skin and precipitin tests, nasal mucociliary clearance and tests for cystic fibrosis.

TREATMENT

The aim of treatment is to minimise lung damage by limiting pulmonary infection and increasing clearance of pulmonary secretions. Firstly, any underlying cause needs treatment, e.g. removal of foreign body, treatment of active tuberculosis, replacement of immunoglobulins for panhypogammaglobulinaemia. The patient must keep as fit as possible. Minor degrees of bronchiectasis may need no further treatment.

Physiotherapy is the main form of non-pharmacological treatment.

Antibiotics are given for infective exacerbations, in some cases at regular intervals. Drug choice is based on sputum culture. Courses should last 2–3 weeks with high doses of the drug. For patients colonised with *Pseudomonas* species, nebulised antibiotics, e.g. colomycin, are often given daily to suppress the bacteria.

Bronchodilators and inhaled steroids are used for patients with demonstrable airflow obstruction.

If the sputum contains DNA from the many disintegrating cells (usually neutrophils) seen in inflammation, the nebulised enzyme DNAase which chops up the DNA is effective in liquefying viscid sputum. This treatment is used mainly in cystic fibrosis sufferers.

Haemoptyosis is treated with bed rest and antibiotics. Selective bronchial embolisation, intubation and balloon tamponade, or local resection of bleeding segment of lung may be needed in severe cases. Respiratory failure and pneumothorax are treated as usual. Surgery may be required to remove severe locally diseased lung or even the whole lung in a transplant.

TUBERCULOSIS

DEFINITION

Tuberculosis is active infection with the bacterium *Mycobacterium tuberculosis*. It is a legal requirement that the details of patients with tuberculosis are passed to the consultant in communicable diseases in the Department of Public Health. There are many different types of mycobacteria and it is only the disease caused by *M. tuberculosis* that is tuberculosis proper, infections with other species, e.g. *M. kansasii*, *M. malmoense*, *M. avium-intracellulare*, produce atypical tuberculosis. Such affected patients are not infectious to other individuals and their details do not need to be passed to the public health authorities. Human tuberculosis can affect any tissue but the lungs are the most common site and only pulmonary tuberculosis will be considered further.

EPIDEMIOLOGY

World-wide, the incidence of tuberculosis is rising, such that approximately one third of the world's population has been infected. In places where there is co-existent HIV infection, which reduces immunity, tuberculosis is much more prevalent and associated with a high mortality.

In the UK there has been a gradual decline in tuberculosis since the 1860s due to improved public health measures, better nutrition, sanitation and housing. However, over recent years this gradual decline has ceased, while in many Westernised countries there has been an actual increase in tuberculosis. The reasons for this increase are multifactorial and relate to increasing poverty, immigration and an older population. Infection with HIV is not the explanation in the UK as the two diseases coexist in around only 2% of notifications.

PATHOLOGY

Although many healthcare workers and individuals have been exposed to and infected with *M. tuberculosis* few develop active infection as their own body defences destroy or wall off the infection. If vaccinated with BCG at school (or at birth in high risk groups) the chances of developing active disease are further reduced, BCG producing an approximate 75% protection.

When pulmonary infection does occur it may be of two types: primary and post-primary. Primary tuberculosis is active disease on first exposure to the bacteria and usually presents with constitutional symptoms and an abnormal chest radiograph. This is often hilar/mediastinal lymphadenopathy or a pleural effusion which contains many lymphocytes but few bacteria. In post-primary disease the area of infection which the body defences have walled off becomes active again, damaging the lung, which liquefies to produce multiple cavities. This is associated with cough, haemoptysis and constitutional symptoms. The reasons why this walled-off disease becomes active again may be due to changes in immunity which occur with increasing age, use of immunosuppressive drugs or infection with HIV, although there is often no obvious cause.

In post-primary tuberculosis the bacteria may be identified on examination of a sputum smear by use of special stains. With the commonly used Ziehl–Neelsen technique sputum is stained and then attempted to be removed with acid and alcohol. Mycobacteria, by virtue of their fatty cell wall, hold on to the stain, hence they are both alcohol- and acid-fast bacilli (AAFB). Culture of the sputum sample will allow identification of whether the mycobacteria is an atypical or *M. tuberculosis*. It is important to know if patients with suspected tuberculosis have bacilli in sputum or only on culture. If the latter they are effectively non-infectious, but the presence of AAFB on smear means patients may pass on infection to their contacts.

CLINICAL FEATURES

Patients with post-primary active disease may have no symptoms (and thus spread infection freely), but complain of respiratory problems and/or non-specific constitutional symptoms such as weight loss, malaise and night sweats. The respiratory symptoms are usually persistent cough (over 3 weeks), productive of small quantities of clear sputum; but if cavities have developed the sputum volume may increase with associated haemoptysis. If tuberculous infection occurs elsewhere presentation will be related to that organ together with the above constitutional symptoms, e.g. haematuria in renal tuberculosis. Examination usually reveals a low grade pyrexia with few signs in the chest.

INVESTIGATIONS

Examination of sputum is essential. If AAFB are found on direct examination, i.e. smear positive, the patient is infectious. In those individuals where AAFB are not found on direct inspection but only after the sputum has been cultured, i.e., smear negative, culture positive disease, there is minimal chance of spreading infection. New molecular medicine techniques are being developed which may allow more rapid diagnosis but at present these are still experimental.

In any patient who has a new cough for more than 3 weeks it is good practice to obtain a chest X-ray. In healed tuberculosis there may only be scarring while in active disease there is often a fluffy infiltrate predominantly in the upper zones, possibly with cavities. Blood tests may show only non-specific markers of chronic infection such as an elevated erythrocyte sedimentation rate (ESR), low serum albumin and a chronic anaemia. It is unusual for a patient to have active pulmonary tuberculosis and a normal chest X-ray and blood.

If tuberculosis is suspected but not identified on smear or culture, bronchoscopy should be considered. This allows direct inspection of the airways to ensure that there is no obstructing lesion and allows bronchial washings to be examined for AAFB. In individuals with an unproductive cough samples may be obtained by induced sputum. In this technique the patient breathes an aerosol of hypertonic saline which encourages a productive cough. However, caution is needed as there may be wide dispersion of acid-fast bacilli, increasing the risk of infection to others.

DIFFERENTIAL DIAGNOSIS

The frequency of constitutional symptoms and cough as a presenting complaint means that tuberculosis has a wide differential diagnosis. It should always be considered, especially in the presence of an abnormal radiograph, and sputum samples should be sent for smear and culture.

TREATMENT

The management of pulmonary tuberculosis can be considered under two headings: patient treatment and contact tracing.

Patient Treatment

With modern antibiotic chemotherapy using three drugs (rifampicin, isoniazid and pyrazinamide) patients are non-infectious within 2 weeks of treatment, even though they may still expectorate sputum containing AAFB. If resistance to one of the above drugs is possible, perhaps as a result of previous antituberculosis therapy, a fourth drug, ethambutol, should be added. Patients take these three (or four) drugs for approximately 2 months until the results of cultures can confirm the bacteria is *M. tuberculosis* and its antibiotic sensitivity patterns. Treatment is then modified so the patient takes only two drugs to which the bacteria are sensitive, for a further 4 months, i.e. 6 months' treatment in total. Pyridoxine is usually given to prevent any side effects which may occur with isoniazid.

If resistant bacteria are identified treatment should be modified according to the resistance pattern and may need to be continued longer. Regular monitoring of liver function tests is required and patients should be informed to seek medical advice if they become jaundiced or develop a rash. Rifampicin produces an orange/red discoloration of urine and patients should be informed of this and also that soft contact lenses may be stained. In addition, rifampicin makes the oral contraceptive pill less effective and supplementary contraception should be used.

Contact Tracing

The aim of contact tracing is twofold: firstly, to find the source of the infection (i.e. is there a close associate who has infected the patient?); and secondly, to determine whether the patient has infected others. Smear negative, culture positive disease and non-pulmonary disease are essentially non-infectious so few, if any, contacts will need to be examined. For smear positive disease all close contacts should be screened, and if a high proportion of these contacts also have tuberculosis fewer close contacts will also need screening— the classic 'ripple in the pond' concept, in other words.

Screening revolves around testing the individual's immunity to tuberculosis by Heaf testing and chest radiographs. To perform the Heaf test a small amount of tuberculous protein is inoculated under the skin and the reaction read after 7 days. This reaction can be graded from no reaction, zero, to strongly positive, grade 4. Depending upon age, previous BCG administration and Heaf grade, contacts can be offered further BCG, chest X-ray follow-up at regular intervals for 1 year or a short course of rifampicin and isoniazid for 3 months to prevent any latent infection from developing (chemoprophylaxis).

PNEUMONIA

DEFINITION
Pneumonia is infection of the lung parenchyma.

EPIDEMIOLOGY
Pneumonia is a common problem, despite the use of antibiotics, accounting for approximately one million deaths per year and 10% of hospital admissions to medical wards and is ten times more common than any other infectious cause of death. In the elderly, pneumonia occurs more frequently with a greater mortality.

AETIOLOGY/PATHOLOGY
Pneumonia can be sub-divided in a variety of ways: typical or atypical; on the basis of the causative agent; or community or hospital acquired. All of these have their advantages and problems. There is no clinical difference between typical and atypical pneumonia and in many patients no causative agent can be identified. It therefore appears that the best method of classifying pneumonia is whether the infection is acquired at home—community acquired pneumonia, or in hospital—hospital or nosocomial pneumonia. As the infecting agents tend to be different this definition may be used to consider the choice of antimicrobial agent before results of sputum or blood cultures are available. Other important diagnoses to consider are tuberculosis and pneumonia occurring in immunocompromised patients.

In community acquired pneumonia the commonest cause is *Streptococcus pneumonia*, accounting for 70% of cases. Depending upon the season, the year, history of travel and exposure to birds, other infective agents need to be considered. *Mycoplasma pneumonia* occurs in 4- to 6-yearly cycles while *Staphylococcal pneumonia* may follow infection with the influenza virus (which may also cause pneumonia itself).

Patients with hospital acquired pneumonia develop features after being in hospital for 24 hours or longer and the infective agents are often Gram-negative bacteria such as *Escherichia coli* or *Klebsiella* species. Mortality from nosocomial pneumonia may be over 30% and this infection is an important cause of prolonged hospital stay. A common reason for its development is aspiration of upper airway contents, predisposed to if swallowing is impaired, e.g. following a stroke, nasogastric intubation or after heavy sedation. Aspiration pneumonia can also occur in the community, e.g. following an alcoholic 'binge' or other causes of impaired consciousness.

The infective process takes place by colonisation of one or more lung segments followed by capillary leak to allow a white cell infiltrate.

This produces a solid and heavy lung which ceases to function for gas exchange. In the absence of effective antibiotic therapy there is an infective 'crisis' after about 10 days where at either the individual may die from overwhelming infection or the process resolves. With modern antibacterial agents death is usually secondary to organ failure from sepsis and hypotension. For patients who develop respiratory failure mechanical ventilation may be necessary, sometimes for several weeks.

CLINICAL FEATURES
Patients may present with a variety of symptoms and signs depending on the organism and speed of onset. With pneumococcal pneumonia malaise, dry cough, pleuritic pain and high pyrexia with rigors can occur within a few hours. Over the course of a few days the cough often becomes productive of green sputum which may contain blood, the so-called rusty sputum. All patient groups, but especially the elderly, may present with features of generalised sepsis, e.g.

headache, diarrhoea, confusion and collapse. With effective antibiotic therapy patients feel better and the pyrexia resolves in a few days but it may take several weeks before they return to normal. Resolution of the chest X-ray is much slower than clinical recovery. Pneumonia due to other organisms, e.g. *Mycoplasma*, *Legionella* and *Chlamydia*, usually has a more insidious onset over the course of a few weeks. It is important in the history to enquire about activities and events which may predispose to pneumonia. Around 50% of *Legionella* pneumonia is acquired abroad, while exposure to parrots or budgies may explain the development of psittacosis, pneumonia due to *Chlamydia psittaci*. Other risk factors, e.g. smoking, poor nutrition, and the immune status of the individual need to be considered.

On examination the patient may be pyrexial, hot and flushed with hypotension and a tachycardia. Some impairment of conscious level is not uncommon. In the respiratory system patients are often tachypnoeic with dullness to percussion over the affected area and increased high pitched breath sounds (bronchial breathing) noted on auscultation. Localised crackles may be heard at the outset or within a few days as the consolidation resolves; however, some patients have few or no physical signs.

INVESTIGATIONS

These may be considered under several headings:

- Confirm the diagnosis. Chest X-ray will show localised or widespread consolidation while the C-reactive protein and white blood cell count may be elevated to suggest infection.
- Assess the severity. Several investigations suggest a worse prognosis. These include a low serum albumin, high blood urea, raised (over 30×10^9) or low (less than 4×10^9) white blood cells, bacteria identified on the blood cultures and arterial hypoxaemia.
- Determine causative agent. Blood and sputum cultures should be undertaken, although sputum cultures may be negative despite being purulent if the patient has received antibiotics. Serology (including a convalescent sample to look for a fourfold rise in titres) should be performed for viruses and other agents, e.g. *Legionella* and *Mycoplasma*. Bronchoscopy or needle aspiration of the chest may be required to determine the underlying infected agent in patients who are deteriorating.

DIFFERENTIAL DIAGNOSIS

There are many causes for patchy consolidation on chest X-rays including lung cancer, pulmonary infarction, pulmonary oedema and, less commonly, vasculits. With the history, examination and simple investigations a diagnosis of pneumonia can be made. Although the causative agent is unknown, antibiotic therapy should be started immediately, before microbiological results are available. This is good practice as delay in starting treatment may lead to death or prolonged hospital stay. Further investigations to determine if there is an alternative diagnosis can continue while the antibiotics are being given.

TREATMENT

This can be considered under two headings: supportive and specific. Maintenance of fluid balance, correcting hypoxaemia with high flow oxygen, non-steroidal anti-inflammatory agents for pleuritic pain, paracetamol for its anti-pyretic action and bed rest are all important aspects of care.

Antibiotics should be given immediately with a choice of agent(s), reflecting what the underlying causative organism may be. Oral therapy is sufficient unless the individual is ill, nauseated or vomiting. For mild community acquired pneumonia amoxycillin with erythromycin is sufficient: if the patient is ill a third generation cephalosporin, e.g. cefotaxime or cefuroxime, should be used in place of the amoxycillin. For hospital acquired pneumonia one of the cephlosporins should be used, possibly with the addition of an aminoglycoside, e.g. gentamycin. If infection with *Staphylococcus aureus* is considered, flucloxacillin should be added; if aspiration is thought likely, amoxycillin plus metronidazole should be used. Treatment should be for a minimum of 5 days and may need to be prolonged in severe pneumonia.

Although most infections resolve, some patients progress to develop a pleural effusion (parapneumonic effusion), which should be aspirated, an empyema (pus in the pleural cavity), lung abscess or, if severely ill, multi-organ failure. It is important to ensure the chest X-ray returns to normal by a follow-up film after 6 weeks. If the chest X-ray has not improved in the elderly it should be repeated after a further 6 weeks. In young patients (and in the elderly if suspected) the delayed resolution may be due to an underlying bronchial carcinoma and fibre-optic bronchoscopy should be performed. In an attempt to prevent pneumonia it is important that the elderly, those with chronic lung disease or those with other debilitating illnesses receive the annual influenza vaccine. Pneumococcal vaccination should also be given to those thought to be at risk of pneumonia.

PNEUMONIA IN THE IMMUNOCOMPROMISED PATIENT

DEFINITION

Impaired host defences, which may be of different types, e.g. reduced levels of circulating immunoglobulins and impaired ciliary activity, predispose an individual to an increased risk of infection. World-wide the commonest problem is loss of cell mediated immunity due to infection with the HIV virus. In the Western world immunosuppressive drug therapy to prevent rejection of transplanted organs and cancer chemotherapy are additional factors. In such patients infections may be due to both the common organisms and agents which do not normally cause problems in those with intact immune systems, the so-called opportunistic infections.

EPIDEMIOLOGY

World-wide the incidence of HIV is rising through heterosexual transmission while in the UK most patients acquire HIV infection as a result of a homosexual relationship or the sharing of needles amongst intravenous drug abusers.

The suspected epidemic of HIV which was forecast fortunately has not occurred in the UK, the rate of new cases being stable.

AETIOLOGY/PATHOLOGY

Infection with the HIV virus produces a steady decline in the numbers of 'helper' T cell lymphocytes (measured as the CD4 group). As levels of these cells fall risk of infection increases, initially for the usual agents then for opportunistic organisms which include cytomegalovirus, disseminated fungal infections and atypical tuberculosis. The commonest opportunistic organism, accounting for around 75% of opportunistic infections, is the presumed protozoan *Pneumocystis carinii*. Infection with these agents is one criterion for a patient with HIV infection moving into the classification of having the acquired immune deficiency syndrome (AIDS).

CLINICAL FEATURES

Patients may present in a variety of ways. For *Pneumocystis* pneumonia the history is of progressive breathlessness over a few weeks usually associated with an unproductive cough. On examination there may be features of AIDS such as weight loss, and the cherry red skin lesions of Kaposi's sarcoma. *Pneumocystis* pneumonia tends to produce few signs with tachypnoea being present on mild exercise or at rest with occasional crackles on ausculation, though often the chest is clear. If the patient is not known to be immunosuppressed the diagnosis of an opportunistic infection may not be considered unless a careful history of at-risk behaviour is taken.

INVESTIGATIONS

The principles of management are similar to those of pneumonia in immunocompetent individuals. However, as there may be more than one organism producing the pneumonia a greater attempt should be made to identify the causative agent to ensure effective therapy. For those patients who are thought to be immunocompromised but unaware of their HIV status an HIV test should be performed after obtaining the patient's consent and ensuring that counselling can be provided. The number of CD4 helper cells will give an indication of how immunocompromised the patient is, a figure below 200×10^6 making infection with opportunistic organisms more likely.

In *P. carinii* pneumonia the chest X-ray may be normal or show a haze around the hilar regions. Patients are often hypoxaemic at rest or on minimal exercise and this can be a useful investigation in breathless patients. A fall in saturation below 90% during mild exercise in a patient who is immunocompromised and complaining of breathlessness suggests underlying early *Pneumocystis* infection. Sputum should be examined for standard bacteria as well as *Pneumocystis*, if necessary using induced sputum. This should be undertaken in a single room, ideally with negative pressure ventilation to ensure there is not dissemination of an aerosol of other bacteria, especially tuberculosis, to other immunocompromised patients.

If the diagnosis is thought to be *Pneumocystis* pneumonia many institutions start treatment and observe progress. If the patient continues to deteriorate or there is no improvement after 5–7 days an alternative or additional diagnosis should be considered. Acute deterioration may be due to a pneumothorax, which is more common in *Pneumocystis* infection. Further samples are best obtained by fibre-optic bronchoscopy with washings of the airway secretions and broncho-alveolar lavage, where 200 ml or more of saline in separate aliquots are injected into a particular bronchus and aspirated to obtain alveolar samples. Less commonly alveolar tissue may be sampled by transbronchial biopsy, although this is more hazardous and is associated with bleeding.

DIFFERENTIAL DIAGNOSIS

There are many potential pathogens which can produce pneumonia in an immunocompromised patient; taking the appropriate samples and observing response to therapy should enable a diagnosis to be made. However, there are many other causes of breathlessness and an abnormal chest X-ray, for example Kaposi's sarcoma and lymphoma, highlighting the importance of confirming the diagnosis.

TREATMENT

Similar supportive therapy described in the treatment of pneumonia should be used together with specific therapy. High dose co-trimoxazole for 14 days is effective, but around 40% of patients develop side effects. If hypoxaemia is present, high dose steroids should be given as they improve survival. If the patient is found to be HIV positive and has developed an opportunistic infection, i.e. he or she has now developed clinical AIDS, anti-retroviral therapy to limit progression of the HIV infection should be started. Once *P. carinii* pneumonia has occurred the patient has an increased risk of further infection with a worse prognosis so secondary prophylaxis with low dose oral co-trimoxazole or nebulised pentamidine should be commenced. In a patient noted to be immunocompromised (CD4 count below 200×10^6) but who has not developed *P. carinii* pneumonia, primary prophylaxis should be given.

The mortality from the first attack of *Pneumocystis* pneumonia is less than 10% but rises with subsequent attacks. As the AIDS progresses, other opportunistic infections, especially disseminated atypical tuberculosis, may cause problems.

OBSTRUCTIVE SLEEP APNOEA

DEFINITION

Apnoea is defined as cessation of air flow for an arbitrary minimum of 10 seconds, while hypopnoea is a reduction in air flow for a similar period. The events may be obstructive in nature when there is absent or diminished air flow with normal or increased ventilatory efforts. Alternatively, and less commonly, there may be cessation of ventilatory effort, i.e. central apnoea. The obstructive sleep apnoea–hypopnoea syndrome is a symptom complex which includes loud snoring and excessive day-time sleepiness, this being due to the rousal associated with the recurrent episodes of sleep disordered breathing. Periods of apnoea and hypopnoea may occur without symptoms, especially in the elderly; the number of episodes of apnoea and hypopnoea per hour (apnoea/hypopnoea index) necessary to have symptoms varies—Below five per hour is accepted as normal.

EPIDEMIOLOGY

As sleep apnoea can be confirmed only with detailed and expensive studies there have been few good epidemiological studies. In North America the incidence of obstructive sleep apnoea syndrome requiring treatment is approximately 2% of adult females and 4% of adult males. In the UK the figure is probably less than 1% of the adult population. Around 90% of patients with sleep apnoea are males, who normally present in their 4th decade. They usually seek medical advice because their partner finds the excessive day-time sleepiness, changes in personality and years of loud snoring intolerable. Sleep disordered breathing produces not only considerable morbidity but also increased mortality, with the deaths being due to cardiovascular factors and stroke. The excessive day-time sleepiness is associated with an increase in road traffic accidents, often fatal.

PATHOLOGY

Sleep apnoea and hypopnoea are caused by recurrent collapse of the upper airway during sleep. There is a gradation in the size of the upper airway, being smaller in patients with sleep apnoea than in simple snorers and in turn in normal individuals. With sleep onset there is a reduction in muscle tone, which allows the unsupported pharyngeal walls to narrow or collapse. In an effort to overcome this occlusion the patient makes increased efforts to breathe, which produce turbulent air flow and vibration of the tissues, the noise of snoring. The period of hypopnoea or apnoea may last well over a minute before being terminated by a temporary awakening from sleep, i.e. a rousal. During this rousal the airway returns to its awake size and ventilation is restored or temporarily increased for a few breaths before the individual returns to sleep. The cycle is repeated several hundred times per night. At the time of the rousal, which the patient is usually unaware of or when he or she may experience a choking sensation, there is a loud snore or grunt and limb movements.

CLINICAL FEATURES

The clinical features of sleep apnoea can be anticipated from the above pathological account. Patients complain of excessive day-time sleepiness due to the sleep fragmentation and disruption of normal sleep architecture. Loud snoring is due to vibration of tissues and the grunt and excessive movements constitute the arousal. Patients may complain of a dry mouth, morning headache or 'muzzy' feeling, as if they have been drinking alcohol excessively.

On examination about 70% of individuals are obese and often they will have a small oropharyngeal cavity with a thick set neck and a large collar size. Hypertension is present in many patients so it is essential to measure blood pressure. Sleep apnoea is more common in conditions which narrow the upper airway size, so acromegaly, hypothyroidism and abnormalities of the facial bones or tonsillar enlargement should be considered.

INVESTIGATIONS

Although the loud snoring, excessive day-time sleepiness and witnessed apnoeas are suggestive of the diagnosis further investigations are required for confirmation. Information on the impact of some of the symptoms may be collected by diaries or questionnaires, with the Epworth questionnaire, a simple self-administered series of questions relating to when patients fall asleep, being the most helpful in confirming the excessive day-time sleepiness.

To determine if episodes of apnoea or hypopnoea are occurring and their nature, measurement of thoraco-abdominal movement and air flow is needed. A microphone is also helpful to document the presence and magnitude of snoring. To assess the physiological impact of disordered breathing oximetry allows documentation of desaturation and an ECG can identify heart rate variation and cardiac dysrhythmia. If there is doubt over the diagnosis, simultaneous recording of an electroencephalogram (EEG), eye movements (electro-oculogram, EOG) and muscle tone at the chin (electromyogram EMG) will allow sleep to be divided into its specific stages and the frequency and nature of arousals to be documented, together with their relationship to episodes of disordered breathing.

DIFFERENTIAL DIAGNOSIS

There are several other causes of excessive day-time sleepiness, which include narcolepsy—a tendency for the brain to switch suddenly and unexpectedly into dreaming sleep—snoring, which itself may fragment sleep, and excessive leg movements during sleep. As obstructive sleep apnoea is common, multiple diagnoses should be considered if a full sleep study has not been used to confirm the diagnosis and/or initial treatment has failed.

TREATMENT

General measures should include stopping evening or night-time alcohol intake and/or sedatives/hypnotics as these not only allow the upper airway collapse to occur more readily but limit the arousal response. Weight loss is difficult to achieve and many patients have tried this before presentation. There is no simple and effective drug therapy for sleep apnoea. Surgery to enlarge the upper airway, e.g. uvulopalatopharyngoplasty (excision of the uvula, soft palate, tonsils and redundant upper airway tissue), may be helpful in simple snoring but it is not a treatment for obstructive sleep apnoea. Other surgical procedures can be considered if there is an abnormal jaw shape.

The most effective therapy is continuous positive airways pressure (CPAP). Via a nasal mask strapped to the face, air is blown into the upper airway. Provided the pressure is set correctly CPAP acts as a pneumatic splint holding the airway open. Although CPAP is strange and unpleasant for normal individuals patients with excessive day-time sleepiness due to sleep apnoea tolerate it remarkably well. With the abolition of apnoeas and hypopnoeas sleep patterns return to normal and the excessive day-time sleepiness rapidly improves. Although inconvienient the long-term compliance is good because of the benefits noticed by most patients.

The role for other mechanical devices to alter jaw position, e.g. mandibular splints, is being evaluated but initial work suggests that they may be effective in mild sleep apnoea.

HYPERVENTILATION SYNDROME

DEFINITION

The term hyperventilation syndrome was used in 1938 to describe patients with anxiety and hypocapnia. There remains considerable confusion about hyperventilation syndrome: is it associated with panic disorders or a disease in its own right; where disproportionate breathlessness ends and hyperventilation syndrome begins is unclear. A physiological definition of hyperventilation is taken as breathing in excess of metabolic needs, which produces a reduction in arterial carbon dioxide tension and subsequent alkalosis. The hyperventilation syndrome can be considered as a constellation of symptoms in association with hyperventilation.

EPIDEMIOLOGY

With the uncertainty over the diagnostic criteria it is difficult to determine the true incidence of hyperventilation syndrome. However, it has been estimated that 5–10% of patients attending a general medical out-patients department have hyperventilation syndrome. In patients with respiratory diseases and those attending psychiatric clinics the incidence is probably greater.

PATHOLOGY

Hyperventilation lowers the arterial carbon dioxide tension and is associated with a variety of different effects which can be considered as:
- Vascular changes. Cerebral and cardiac changes may contribute to the symptoms of light-headedness, dizziness, feeling of impending doom, chest pain and palpitations.
- Increased work of breathing. This leads to breathlessness and may lead to tachycardia, fuelling the anxiety.
- Neuromuscular excitability. The changes in distribution of calcium ions due to the alkalosis produce limb and especially mouth paraesthesia together with tetany.

In normal individuals an equivalent fall in carbon dioxide tension occasionally produces symptoms, suggesting that there may be an additional factor as to why patients with hyperventilation syndrome complain of symptoms. Whether this lies in an inherent difference in the sensitivity to carbon dioxide tension or due to a different cerebral perception of the effects is unclear.

CLINICAL FEATURES

With this wide variety of symptoms patients may present to their general practitioner with many complaints and be referred to different medical departments. Unfortunately, the diagnosis of hyperventilation syndrome is not always established and such a failure may produce more anxiety, which can make the syndrome worse. For example, a patient may be referred to a cardiologist with chest pain, initial investigations will be normal so the patient may proceed to further tests which have a definite morbidity, e.g. coronary angiography. Alternatively, patients may receive long-term medication which is either increased or repetitively changed because it is ineffective, again a problem which fuels anxiety.

Clues to the diagnosis may be elicited from the history. Breathlessness and chest pain may occur at rest or under certain circumstances and be less troublesome during exercise. Sometimes patients will admit to feeling anxious or worried prior to an attack. Apart from an increased respiratory rate there will be little to find on examination, although a full medical history and clinical examination should be undertaken to exclude other diagnoses.

INVESTIGATIONS

These can be considered under two headings, one to ensure there is no other diagnosis and a second to confirm that the problem is due to hyperventilation syndrome. The history will suggest if and what further investigations are necessary. For example if the patient presents with chest pain it may be necessary to do an exercise ECG, while if features of neuromuscular excitability are predominant it is important to ensure that the clinical chemistry, including the calcium and magnesium, are normal.

To confirm the diagnosis it is often possible to precipitate the patient's symptoms by asking him or her to hyperventilate at rest. It is not usually necessary to check the arterial carbon dioxide tension although this may be helpful for a few patients to confirm that hypocapnia has occurred. Under such circumstances the patients will also have a respiratory alkalosis as confirmed by a high pH. In those few patients with chronic hyperventilation syndrome, symptoms may develop after only a few deep breaths. Arterial blood gas analysis in these patients when stable usually shows low normal arterial carbon dioxide tension and a low bicarbonate.

DIFFERENTIAL DIAGNOSIS

Depending upon the method of presentation there may be a wide variety of differential diagnoses. Unfortunately, patients with obstructive airways disease have an increased incidence of hyperventilation syndrome and it may be difficult to differentiate what is causing the symptoms, especially as hyperventilation itself may produce bronchoconstriction. Patients presenting acutely, especially to Accident and Emergency departments, should not be labelled as suffering from hyperventilation syndrome until other causes of acute breathlessness have been excluded.

TREATMENT

Many patients are often anxious about their symptoms, especially if they experience chest pain, so a detailed and sympathetically taken history is an important aspect of management. Once the diagnosis is confirmed by the simple hyperventilation test the patient may be reassured that there is no serious underlying disease. Often this reassurance, together with the demonstration that they can produce the symptoms at any time, is sufficient for many patients. For some individuals, however, further support is required: during acute attacks re-breathing through a paper bag is sufficient to correct the low arterial carbon dioxide tension, limit the alkalosis and thus prevent or treat symptoms. A better method, however, is to prevent attacks by breathing re-training and the physiotherapist can play a great role in such advice. By using abdominal muscles to breathe and slowing the rate of breathing under conditions which often precipitate an attack the patient may be put in control of his or her problem with a good outcome.

For the few patients that have considerable psychiatric problems associated with hyperventilation syndrome general advice about relaxation therapy may be helpful and involvement of a psychiatrist or clinical psychologist should be sought. Care is needed if drug therapy is thought necessary to modify the anxiety state as some drugs, e.g. benzodiazepines, may depress ventilatory drive and be difficult to withdraw from at a later date.

PLEURAL EFFUSION

DEFINITION

A pleural effusion occurs when fluid collects in the pleural space. It is a complication of many diseases, and is divided into transudates and exudates (Table 10.2). A transudate is when the fluid collects due to pressure from surrounding fluid-logged tissues; the cause is usually obvious clinically and treatment with diuretics provides resolution. An exudate is caused by a local problem and needs local treatment.

CLINICAL FEATURES

If the effusion is small, no symptoms or signs occur. If larger, breathlessness, chest pain and positional discomfort or pain may occur together with features of the underlying disease. The signs may include decreased movement of affected side, dull percussion note and absent breath sounds.

A chest X-ray will show the extent of the effusion and any underlying disease. Aspiration of fluid and biopsy of the pleura are used to help diagnose the cause.

TREATMENT

The aim is to achieve resolution of the pleural effusion without residual fibrosis. The treatment is of the underlying disease and drainage of the effusion either by aspiration through a needle and a three-way tap or by inserting a chest drain linked to an underwater seal.

If a thick pleural rind persists, surgical removal may be required. Occasionally, chemical pleurodesis, the obliteration of the pleural space by the insertion of a chemical, e.g.

tetracycline, is required to stop recurrence, for example, in a malignant effusion.

LUNG ABSCESS

DEFINITION

A lung abscess is a cavitated infected necrotic lesion within the lung parenchyma.

PATHOLOGY AND AETIOLOGY

Infection with necrosis of the surrounding lung can occur for several reasons. An area of pneumonia can liquefy to produce an abscess, especially that caused by *Klebsiella* species or *Staphylococcus aureus*, while bronchial obstruction from a foreign body or underlying carcinoma can limit drainage and encourage abscess formation. Aspiration of gastric/upper airway contents, especially during sedation or after an alcoholic 'binge', may present as a lung abscess. Less common are bloodborne spread of infection, as seen in drug abusers, bacterial endocarditis affecting the right heart and *S. aureus* septicaemia. Less common causes are spread from below the diaphragm, penetrating injuries and infection of a sterile pulmonary infarct following pulmonary embolism.

Causes of pleural effusion
Transudates
i) Pulmonary oedema
Left heart failure
Constrictive pericarditis
ii) Low blood protein
Nephrotic syndrome
Hepatic cirrhosis
Exudates
i) Infections
Viral pleurisy
Bacterial pneumonia
Tuberculosis
Empyema
ii) Secondary malignancy
e.g. lung, stomach, breast
iii) Leukaemia
iv) Lymphoma
v) Primary pleural malignancy (mesothelioma)
vi) Pulmonary infarction
vii) Collagen vascular disorders
Rheumatoid arthritis

Table 10.2 Causes of pleural effusion.

CLINICAL FEATURES

Depending upon the speed of onset, patients may be acutely unwell or complain of constitutional symptoms such as weight loss and malaise. Usually the abscess will communicate with the bronchus so patients complain of cough productive of foul-tasting sputum, often associated with haemoptysis which is admixed with the sputum.

On examination clubbing may be obvious but this can occur from both the infection and an underlying carcinoma. The chest may be dull to percussion while breath sounds on auscultation may be diminished, harsh or blowing, depending upon the location and the pleural reaction. Rarely the infection can spread via the pulmonary veins into the systemic circulation with a risk of disseminated infection, cerebral abscess being the most commonly described.

INVESTIGATIONS

Chest X-ray will usually show a thick walled irregular cavity with an air/fluid level, though it may be difficult to differentiate from a collection of pus in the pleural cavity (empyema). If the diagnosis is uncertain imaging using ultrasound or CT may be performed to determine the anatomical appearances. Basic blood investigations would usually show a raised white count, high ESR and possible anaemia. If there is a suspicion of an underlying bronchial carcinoma, especially in a smoker, bronchoscopy should be undertaken.

Identification of the organism and antibiotic sensitivities allows a rational choice of therapy. Sputum samples are usually sufficient but more invasive methods may need to be considered.

DIFFERENTIAL DIAGNOSIS

The other conditions which need to be considered in the differential diagnosis are those which produce cavitation on the chest radiograph. Beyond those listed above, carcinoma, usually of squamous cell type, tuberculosis and vasculitis, e.g. Wegener's granulomatosis, are the important ones on a large list.

TREATMENT

The two principles of treating a lung abscess are to promote drainage of the infected material and to sterilise the cavity with antibiotics, the choice of which will depend upon bacteriology results. Often the patients will identify what position is associated with drainage and this should be encouraged by physiotherapy and nursing staff. If adequate drainage cannot be achieved and the size of the cavity is unaltered despite antibiotics a drainage procedure may need to be considered, either through the bronchial tree or via the skin; rarely, surgical removal of the affected segment needs to be performed.

Most cavities will close with the above therapy although the chest X-ray changes may persist for some time and not fully resolve. Clinical response, e.g. weight gain and return of appetite, are better markers of progress.

Occasionally the abscess cavity may fail to close and subsequently be colonised by fungi, forming an aspergilloma.

PULMONARY EMBOLUS

DEFINITION

Venous thrombosis, a clot, can form in any vein (see Chapter 13), encouraged by venous stasis, trauma to the veins or increased blood clotting (Table 10.3). If a piece of thrombus is dislodged from a systemic vein, generally 10 days after its initial formation, it will impact in the pulmonary arterial circulation. The impacted thrombus is called a pulmonary embolus.

EPIDEMIOLOGY

Over 90% of pulmonary emboli are thrown off from thrombi in the deep veins of the lower extremities and pelvis. A few may arise in the right atrium when a clot forms in association with atrial fibrillation or from a mural (wall) thrombus in a damaged area of the right ventricle following myocardial infarction. At postmortem, pulmonary embolism has been found in 9–26% of all patients.

CLINICAL FEATURES

Pulmonary embolism presents in many ways depending on the extent of the obstruction of the pulmonary arterial tree, the time during which the obstruction accumulates and whether there is pre-existing heart or lung disease. Pleuritic chest pain, dyspnoea and haemoptysis indicate acute minor pulmonary embolus. Acute onset of dyspnoea, faintness or collapse and central chest pain may indicate massive pulmonary embolus. Gradual onset of the symptoms may occur.

DIFFERENTIAL DIAGNOSIS

Pulmonary embolus is common and can be confused with many other diagnoses, e.g. pneumonia, cardiac failure and myocardial infarction. The lung distal to the obstructed artery may necrose, causing a pulmonary infarction, giving perhaps a pleural rub, fever and pleural effusion. The diagnosis may be made by pulmonary angiogram or CT scan of the thorax, where injected contrast shows up the clot. Ventilation/perfusion scanning is often used where one radioactive labelled substance is injected showing lack of perfusion of the pulmonary arteries in the area of the clot and where another is inhaled showing whether the airways are still open.

TREATMENT

A massive pulmonary embolus will need emergency resuscitation and treatment with clot-dissolving thrombolytic drugs, usually streptokinase, or surgical removal of the clot (embolectomy). Prevention is vital. In patients at risk (e.g. during and after surgery, when immobile), early mobilisation, pneumatic calf compression and graduated compression stockings are used. Heparin is injected to cover high risk periods.

INTERSTITIAL LUNG DISEASE

DEFINITION
Interstitial lung disease is characterised by an inflammatory exudate of the alveolar wall, with a tendency to fibrosis.

EPIDEMIOLOGY
It occurs mainly in patients aged between 50 and 70 years with a prevalence estimated at 2–5 per 100 000 population. Over 60% of the patients die from the lung disease, most within 5 years of diagnosis.

PATHOLOGY
The major disease in this group is cryptogenic fibrosing alveolitis (CFA). Its cause is unknown (cryptogenic). CFA may be associated with connective tissue disease of unknown cause, e.g. systemic sclerosis, systemic lupus erythematosis, rheumatoid arthritis and polymyositis. There are very rare diseases such as histiocytosis X and lympholeiomyomatosis, which also affect the lung parenchyma with similar clinical features. Certain drugs, e.g. bleomycin, methotrexate and amiodarone, can cause a similar disease.

CLINICAL FEATURES
The symptoms are usually a progressive breathlessness and a dry unproductive irritating cough. The patient develops clubbing of the fingers, and fine inspiratory crackles are heard initially at the lung bases on auscultation. Patients will develop cor pulmonale and respiratory failure.

Chest X-ray shows small lung fields, irregular nodular or recticulonodular opacities, and later signs of cor pulmonale (pulmonary artery enlargement and cardiomegaly).

High resolution CT scan is very sensitive in detecting CFA, showing a subpleural rind of increased density. Pulmonary function tests show a restrictive ventilatory defect, with low lung volumes, decreased lung compliance and reduced carbon monoxide transfer. Lung biopsy will show the typical pathological picture.

TREATMENT
The aim is to prevent deterioration of lung function, to relieve symptoms and to give supportive care if treatment fails. Drug treatment is unproven. Corticosteroids and an immunosuppressant, cyclophosphamide, are used to slow progress of the disease, but they often have side effects. Supportive therapy, such as supplemental oxygen, diuretics for cor pulmonale and opiates for the suppression of cough and breathlessness, will probably become necessary. Response to treatment is monitored by changes in clinical features, the chest X-ray and pulmonary function tests. Patients may be offered a lung transplant.

Risk factors for venous thrombosis
I) Venous stasis
Immobility
Bed rest
Obesity
i) Compression of calf muscles
Surgery
Bed rest
Long journeys
ii) Low venous flow
Cardiac failure
iii) Pregnancy due to compression of inferior vena cava
II) Trauma to veins
Indwelling venous catheter
III) Hypercoagulability
Oral contraceptive pill
Inherited
Antithrombin deficiency
Protein C deficiency

Table 10.3 **Risk factors for venous thrombosis.**

OCCUPATIONAL LUNG DISEASES

PNEUMOCONIOSES

Definition

The pneumoconioses are fibrogenic lung diseases caused by the inhalation of small particles (diameter <3.5 mm). Any particles of greater than a diameter of 3.5 mm will be eliminated by the mucociliary escalator or by turbulent air flow above the larynx.

Pathology

Coal workers' pneumoconiosis develops after prolonged exposure to coal dust. The incidence in the UK among miners is falling due to efficient dust extraction. Coal dust deposited around the alveoli and respiratory bronchioles provokes a cellular response with development of nodular fibrosis. Later, this causes atrophy of the bronchiolar wall and dilation of the respiratory bronchioles, producing focal centrilobular emphysema.

Clinical Features

The clinical features of fibrogenic lung disease are similar for each type of dust. Dependent on the severity, they range from nil through increasing breathlessness to cor pulmonale and respiratory failure. In simple pneumoconiosis, the chest X-ray characteristically shows small rounded or irregular opacities (2–10 mm in diameter) in the lung fields. If the miner is non-smoking, simple pneumoconiosis often produces no symptoms and only a mild decrease in lung function.

The coal dust deposits and focal emphysema may coalesce into dense black fibrotic masses, occurring most commonly in the upper lobes. This is called complicated pneumoconiosis or progressive massive fibrosis (PMF). Shortness of breath, significant impairment of pulmonary function and cor pulmonale now develop.

Silicosis

Silicon dioxide in crystalline form (quartz, cristobalite and tridymite) provokes severe fibrosis. The crystals set up an inflammatory response leading to fibrotic nodules. The onset of the disease may be rapid if the silica exposure is very high, leading to breathlessness in a few months, and then progressing on to death—from acute silicosis. More commonly, the level of exposure leads to a more gradual development of fibrotic nodules, which may coalesce to form large masses. The onset of progressive disease may occur many years after the initial exposure. The chest X-ray shows hilar gland enlargement with later calcification in the periphery and diffuse nodule shadowing, which may coalesce into larger masses.

Asbestosis

Asbestos describes a number of fire resistant naturally occurring fibrous mineral silicates. The asbestos fibres with a diameter of <1 mm and length of usually less than 50 mm can penetrate to the lung periphery and stimulate severe fibrosis, especially in the lower lobes. All forms of asbestos are fibrogenic, although crocidilite (blue) and chrysotile (white) have been regarded as more dangerous than amosite and anthophyllte. Asbestos has been used in insulation, textiles, asbestos cement products, brake linings and ship building and repair. Builders cut up asbestos sheets. The aim of legislation in the UK is to substitute other materials for asbestos.

The interval between exposure to asbestos and development of any problems is commonly 20 years or longer. The patient usually presents with insidious onset of shortness of breath. Clubbing of the fingers and fine inspiratory crackles at the bases occur. Chest X-ray changes begin as scattered opacities, usually irregular and small, between 2 and 4 mm in diameter, with less often a diffuse haziness. Honeycomb or ring shadows may occur in more advanced disease. Most changes are in the lower zones. Respiratory function tests show some changes as in CFA.

Asbestos exposure can also lead to the development of pleural plaques, which may calcify. These do not usually cause symptoms. There is an increased risk of lung cancer and of the pleural and peritoneal primary tumour, mesothelioma.

OTHER PNEUMOCONIOSES

Problems with fibrogenic and other lung diseases have been reported after inhalation of many materials, for example, talc, mixed mineral dusts (e.g. slate and china clay), hard metal and beryllium.

EXTRINSIC ALLERGIC ALVEOLITIS

Definition

Extrinsic allergic alveolitis (EAA), or hypersenstivity pneumonitis, is a specific immunological response to the inhalation of various organic dusts (Table 10.4).

Clinical Features

The clinical features depend on the amount of exposure and the individual's response. Acute allergic alveolitis typically follows exposure to a highly concentrated dust source. For example, several hours after exposure to a pigeon loft, a bird fancier develops 'flu'-like symptoms and breathlessness with sometimes inspiratory crackles over the lungs. These will settle unless he is further exposed within approximately 1 week. The chest X-ray may show a generalised haziness, sometimes with nodules, although it may be normal. Lung function shows reduction in lung volumes and gas transfer.

Acute allergic alveolitis becomes chronic when irreversible pulmonary fibrosis develops, perhaps after repeated short high exposures or one low-level long exposure. The breathlessness becomes chronic and again inspiratory crackles are heard. The diagnosis is based on identifying a source of antigen, forming a clinical picture and finding antibodies to the antigen in the serum. Occasionally, lung biopsy is required.

Treatment

Treatment consists of avoiding the source of antigen, e.g. the pigeons. Corticosteroids may hasten recovery.

SARCOIDOSIS

Definition

Sarcoidosis is a multi-system disease of unknown cause. It can, therefore, only be described.

Epidemiology

Sarcoidosis usually occurs in the 20–40 age group, with an incidence estimated at 10–20 per 100 000 in the UK. It is more prevalent in black populations where it tends to be chronic with higher risk of non-pulmonary manifestations.

Pathology

The appearance of the tissue on histological examination allows the most confident diagnosis, with the appearance in all of the affected organs containing non-caseating epithelioid cell granulomata, and focal, closely packed collections of macrophages and epithelioid cells, which often fuse to form multinucleate giant cells. The commonest organ involved is the lung. The chest X-ray is graded as follows: stage 1, 50% of cases show bilateral hilar lymphadenopathy only; stage 2 (25%), bilateral hilar lymphadenopathy and peripheral pulmonary infiltration plus paratracheal nodes enlarged in some cases; and stage 3 (15%), parenchymal infiltration only. Ten per cent may have a normal chest X-ray (stage 0). Pulmonary function tests range from normal to significant physiological dysfunction.

The involvement of other organs may lead to, for example, peripheral neuropathy, cranial nerve palsies, space occupying lesions, congestive cardiac failure and dysrhythmia, hypercalcaemia, enlarged parotid and lacrimal glands and chronic uveitis.

Treatment

Treatment is not needed in many patients as symptoms are mild and 70% of patients remit spontaneously. Corticosteroids can suppress the manifestations of acute sarcoidosis. However, it is unproven whether they prevent development of irreversible pulmonary fibrosis in those patients with progressive lung disease. Immunosuppressant drugs have been used in some cases with unproven success.

The pulmonary fibrosis can be complicated by upper zone bullous disease, aspergillomas, with recurrent infection and haemoptyses.

ASPERGILLOSIS

Aspergillus is a genus of ubiquitous fungi, which may be associated with a variety of pulmonary diseases and can be considered under the following headings:

- Allergic reactions.
- Simple colonisation: aspergilloma.
- Direct invasion: invasive aspergillosis.

Each behaves as a separate disease entity and will be considered as such.

ALLERGIC REACTIONS

Asthma

The features of asthma have already been described. Many asthmatic patients will show a positive skin prick test to *Aspergillus* species, especially *A. fumigatus*. Inhalation of the spores in these sensitive patients produces an attack of asthma; however, such patients should be managed as being atopic and treated with the usual therapy.

Allergic Bronchopulmonary Aspergillosis

In this disease, which almost always occurs in asthmatic patients, there is a marked inflammatory response in the proximal airways to the *Aspergillus* fungus. This has two effects. Firstly, the production of thick mucus leading to bronchial obstruction and subsequent collapse of the affected lung segment; and secondly, damage to the bronchial walls, producing bronchiectasis.

Clinical features

Allergic bronchopulmonary aspergillosis usually occurs in adults with asthma and is particularly common in cystic fibrosis. Patients may present with their asthma being difficult to control, fever, cough or with an abnormal chest radiograph. Bronchiectasis is the commonest cause of their ongoing symptoms.

Causes of extrinsic allergic alveolitis	
Antigen dust source	**Disease**
Mouldy hay, straw, etc.	Farmer's lung
Avian excreta and bloom, especially from budgerigars, pigeons	Bird fancier's lung
Contamination of air conditioning	Ventilation pneumonitis
Spores released by mushrooms	Mushroom worker's lung

Table 10.4 **Causes of extrinsic allergic alveolitis.**

Investigations

Diagnosis is usually made by the asthmatic history, fleeting shadows on chest X-ray, blood eosinophilia, positive precipitin (IgG) and reaginic (IgE) antibodies against the fungus. In established bronchiectasis the chest X-ray usually shows chronic changes, especially in the upper lobes, confimed by CT of the thorax.

Treatment

The fungus cannot be erradicated so management revolves around optimal control of the underlying asthma and bronchiectasis. Suppression of the host response to the fungus is best achieved by oral steroids but the relative risks need to be balanced against long-term use. Even with inhaled and low dose oral steroids patients may still develop new pulmonary infiltrates. These should be treated promptly with high doses of oral steroids in the hope of limiting further airway damage.

Extrinsic allergic alveolitis

This reaction has a rare association with *Aspergillus* species.

Simple Colonisation: Aspergilloma

In some individuals with areas of damaged lung, e.g. old tuberculous cavities, inhalation of fungal spores may be followed by their active growth. If there is normal host immunity the fungal mycelium is contained within the cavity but mixed with inflammatory cells to produce a fungal ball — an aspergilloma. Patients may present with periodic haemoptysis, expectoration of dark brownish material, or debris from the fungal ball or by chance on a chest radiograph.

No treatment is required unless the condition is associated with recurrent or brisk haemoptysis. Unfortunately there is no effective anti-fungal therapy and surgical removal may be considered, although this is often difficult due to poor pulmonary reserve and the underlying adherent pleura making resection hazardous. Occlusion of the artery by embolisation may eliminate or reduce the frequency of haemoptysis.

Direct Invasion: Invasive Aspergillosis

Aspergillus fungi may directly invade and destroy the lung, sometimes spreading in the blood to other organs. Such reactions are found in those individuals who are immunocompromised. The chest X-ray may show infiltrates with cavitation, which progress rapidly, thus the diagnosis often being made at autopsy. If the disease is suspected, treatment with systemic anti-fungal agents should commence early.

PULMONARY REHABILITATION

Major changes are occurring with respect to the physiotherapy treatment of chronic lung conditions in hospital and in the community.

The conventional hands-on approach with percussion, postural drainage and vibrations for all patients with chest complaints is being replaced by increased exercise, adequate bronchodilator therapy where applicable, assessment of the tenacity of secretions and therefore the need for humidification, and patients' education in the management of their own conditions.

Pulmonary rehabilitation occurs to some extent in all hospitals and formal out-patient groups are developing nationally. The success of the exercise is discussed below.

Chronic obstructive pulmonary disease (COPD) resulting from a combination of airways disease and emphysema presents a major burden to the National Health Service. In 1992 there were 26 033 deaths attributed to COPD, chronic bronchitis or emphysema, amounting to 6.4% of all male deaths and 3.9% of female deaths in England and Wales. In a recent survey of all medical and geriatric admissions to a UK health region 25% were with a respiratory disease and over half of these with COPD (Pearson *et al.*, 1994). The conventional medical treatment for this group of patients is aimed firstly at halting the progression of the disease (most obviously by stopping smoking), followed by optimising their pharmaceutical management, which may include correcting abnormal pathophysiology (for example, oxygen therapy). Only at this stage would it be appropriate to consider rehabilitation.

COPD is a progressive disease categorised by a insidious decline in FEV. The American Thoracic Society guidelines describe severe COPD as having an FEV_1 of less than 40% predicted, moderate COPD having an FEV_1 of between 40 and 60% predicted and an individual with mild COPD presenting with an FEV_1 of less than 80% predicted but more than 60%. The majority of patients with mild COPD are not known to their GP. It is not until patients have moderate to severe COPD that they present to their GP, commonly with breathlessness on exertion in the initial stages. Sadly the immediate impact of declining lung function is not obvious to the individual and it is not until lung function has been significantly and irretrievably disrupted that a functional limitation is noticed. This situation is further compounded by the creeping breathlessness and loss of physical performance which in turn leads to social isolation, immobility, loss of physical fitness and possibly depression. The individual unwittingly becomes trapped within this vicious circle of inactivity until fundamental activities such as bathing and walking around the home become a major undertaking, with crippling from severe dyspnoea. Pulmonary rehabilitation attempts to break this cycle of inactivity by providing a coherent package of education and exercise. Until quite recently pulmonary rehabilitation programmes have not been a popular treatment option for individuals with COPD in the UK, unlike in the United States and parts of Europe, where they have been utilised enthusiastically for a number of years. There are two possible explanations for this disparity. Firstly, there has been a paucity of research based evidence proving the benefit of this mode of treatment. Only recently have the results of randomised control trials been published and taken seriously (Goldstein *et al.*, 1994). The second reason relates to the shift of power within the health service. At present we are within an evolving organisation where the consumer of resources appears to have greater influence over budget allocation. What should not be overlooked is that a form of pulmonary rehabilitation has long been provided within the health service by the doctors, nurses, physiotherapists etc. passing on advice and practical tips. What we are now experiencing is a surge of enthusiasm for a more coherent approach to patient care provided by a multidisciplinary team. One of the most recent definitions for pulmonary rehabilitation was devised in the USA (Fishman, 1994). In essence rehabilitation is concerned with lessening the impact of disabling conditions. It is a complex process usually involving several professional groups. The key purposes of rehabilitation have been summarised by Young (1996) as being:

- Realisation potential.
- Re-enablement.
- Resettlement.
- Role fulfilment.
- Readjustment.

Pulmonary rehabilitation begins with the assumption that the underlying condition cannot be improved upon by any alteration in the pharmaceutical management of the patient at that time. Of course this does not mean that each patient considered for a course of rehabilitation will be on maximal therapy (e.g. supplemental oxygen and nebulised bronchodilators), but medication will be optimal for his or her particular stage of the disease.

SETTING UP A REHABILITATION PROGRAMME

The most fundamental consideration prior to setting up a programme is the local prevalence of COPD and the level of access available to diseased individuals via either consultant physician or direct GP referral must be established. Rehabilitation has to date been out-patient based, predominantly within a hospital setting. Alternatives to this, particularly in a rural setting, may be a series of satellite groups in community halls, or even home-based programmes. The effectiveness of the latter has recently been documented (Wijkstra et al., 1995). Regardless of the environment the principles of rehabilitation remain constant, offering a package of exercise training, disease education and psychosocial support. Once an adequate number of patients and a venue have been secured other aspects need to be considered. Service costs are frequently uppermost and areas to consider include:

- Equipment costs (including cycle ergometers, treadmills, pulse oximeter, ambulatory oxygen dispenser, heart rate monitors, stop watches, spirometer, etc.).
- Resuscitation equipment and nebulisers.
- Staff costs (principal co-ordinator, physiotherapists, nurses, dietitians, occupational therapists, etc.).
- Transport costs (of ambulances, hospital cars).

- Secretarial support.
- Stationery costs.

The overall cost of a pulmonary rehabilitation service depends upon the type of service offered. An in-patient programme as offered in the United States is inevitably expensive but short-term out-patient rehabilitation as offered in the UK need not be too costly. From our own experience we estimate the cost of a 7 week out-patient programme to be approximately £420 per patient, which could be set against the cost of just one brief hospital admission.

The precise structure and contents of the rehabilitation programme require careful discussion within a multidisciplinary framework. Areas to consider include:

- The frequency of sessions.
- The duration of each session and of the course.
- The components (type of exercise training and programme of disease education).
- Contributors to the programme.

The process of rehabilitation usually includes an element of exercise followed by a period of disease education. There are generally 2 or 3 weekly sessions, each lasting for between one and a half and 3 hours. The duration of the course is approximately 6 to 8 weeks. The exercise component will be discussed in more detail later in this chapter. The educational component of the programme includes contributions from the following members of the team:

- Contributor: topic.
- Doctor: anatomy, physiology and pathology.
- Physiotherapist: breathing control, chest clearance techniques, relaxation.
- Nurse: coping skills, smoking cessation.
- Occupational therapist: time management, conservation of energy, sexual relations.
- Dietitian: healthy diet.
- Psychologist: coping strategies, relationships, role changes.
- Technician: devices, oxygen, travel.
- Pharmacist: drugs and medication.
- Social worker: benefits and entitlements; agency.
- Self-help group member: role of self-help groups. (e.g. Breathe easy group)

Most of the educational sessions tend to be informal discussions or practical sessions, the relaxation sessions being particularly important. The dissemination of information is supported by a series of leaflets etc., designed by each professional group. The written information can be collated at the time of discharge in the form of a discharge folder containing advice from all professional and voluntary groups and used for future reference. The inclusion of smoking cessation classes at this stage can be controversial. By the time most people have become disabled by their lung disease they have already given up smoking.

PATIENT SELECTION

Patient selection is one of the most important considerations when starting a rehabilitation programme. The success of the programme can be prejudiced by inappropriate selection criteria. Not surprisingly a variety of opinions exist to identify the optimal client group to target for rehabilitation. Traditionally patients recruited for a course of rehabilitation are those with established COPD. However, it would appear from recent data (Ambrisino and Foglio, 1996) that all categories of patients can benefit from a course of rehabilitation. Therefore the most severely affected patients, using long-term domiciliary oxygen and nebulised bronchodilators, may well improve as a consequence of rehabilitation. However, what should not be overlooked is the importance of certain fundamental considerations such as patient motivation and travel difficulties.

The insidious loss of 'fitness' results in the individual adopting a less physically demanding lifestyle and in being trapped in a vicious circle of inactivity, breathlessness, depression and social isolation, until such time as the most basic activities become too demanding and are avoided. For example, in the early stages of the disease an individual may avoid social gatherings or leisure activities, but as the disease progresses even climbing the stairs may impose an enormous challenge and so is avoided. In the later stages of the disease the individual may avoid leaving the house altogether and find bathing and grooming very difficult. It is the aim of rehabilitation to reverse these trends.

The team accepting the referral for pulmonary rehabilitation needs to make two assumptions. These should be fulfilled but they require careful and precise information backup.

Firstly the team assumes that the individual has been thoroughly assessed and managed by the referring consultant/GP to such a degree that no further gains can be achieved by additional pharmaceutical intervention.

Secondly, that the decreased physical fitness and associated dyspnoea are related to a respiratory pathology and not for example as a consequence of other pathologies. Patients that are particularly difficult to rehabilitate within the context of a pulmonary rehabilitation course are those with other co-existing pathologies. For example, if the patient has both COPD and osteoarthritis careful attention needs to be paid to the exact limit of exercise. As indicated above, recently there have been reports demonstrating that other categories of patients can be treated effectively within a pulmonary rehabilitation setting. Perhaps one of the more exciting developments is the inclusion of a pulmonary rehabilitation programme in the pre-operative work-up of patients considered for lung volume reduction surgery (LVRS). LVRS attempts to utilise surgery to remove lung tissue to relieve dyspnoea by improving the mechanics of the respiratory system. This technique is reserved for those patients that have predominately emphysema with a large degree of hyperinflation (Cooper et al., 1995). This is a recent surgical development in the UK. The aim of rehabilitation is to optimise the individual's level of fitness and understandably there may be a place for post-operative rehabilitation as well. It would appear that the USA has defined precisely the level of achievement anticipated as a consequence of rehabilitation. In the UK we remain unclear if an absolute threshold or an individually calibrated target is most appropriate.

Overall there are few patients with a diagnosis of COPD that would not benefit from either component of a pulmonary rehabilitation course. However, a few exceptions need to be recognised. A formal selection procedure is therefore important. The identification of poorly motivated patients is critical. If recruited these patients may be the most likely not to attend regularly and/or not to adhere to lifestyle changes suggested throughout the rehabilitation programme. [Adherence is generally defined as 'the degree to which patient behaviour coincides with the clinical recommendations of the health care providers' (Rand, 1990).] Inclusion of these patients can have a demotivating effect on the rest of the group as well as constitute a recurrent source of frustration for the rehabilitation team. Other cases that need careful consideration prior to inclusion to a group are individuals with travel difficulties and/or work difficulties (either difficulties with time off for attendance, or requiring an 'out of hours' programme). In inner city areas with a substantial immigrant population, problems with language may be overcome by the use of an interpreter (either an official or a relative). Hearing problems are usually easily resolved. A barrier less easily overcome is an unstable psychiatric history; the inclusion of a patient with such a history on a pulmonary rehabilitation programme warrants very careful consideration, unless stabilisation measures are implemented. The final consideration must be directed towards the inclusion of current smokers onto the programme. Some centres may argue that the inclusion of current smokers onto a rehabilitation programme is inappropriate, until the latter can demonstrate a reasonable period of abstention. Furthermore, it could be suggested that if an individual with COPD is unwilling to stop smoking he or she is unlikely to be someone prepared to make the lifestyle exchanges proposed by members of the healthcare team, including a commitment to regular exercise.

PATIENT ASSESSMENT

An assessment before rehabilitation is vital to quantify the patient's capabilities and aspirations. Assessment is also important to judge the progress of the individual and consequently the success of the programme. The assessment usually concentrates on the determination of the extent of impairment, disability and handicap.

DEFINITIONS
Impairment,'any loss or abnormality of psychological, physiological or anatomical structure or function'.

10

Disability, 'any restriction or loss of activity in a manner, or within the range considered normal for a human being'. **Handicap**, 'disadvantage for a given individual, resulting from an impairment or a disability, that limits or prevents the fulfilment of a role that is normal (depending on age, sex, social and cultural factors)' (World Health Organisation, 1980).

Despite appearing relatively rigorous definitions they are subject to a range of interpretations. The definitions used in this chapter are for practical application to the area of pulmonary rehabilitation. It would be impossible to suggest for example that measures of disability measure disability exclusively, and similarly measures of handicap may measure in part levels of disability.

IMPAIRMENT

Typically, in COPD, impairment is judged by the disturbance in lung function. Commonly an FEV_1 (forced expiratory volume in 1 second) or FVC (forced vital capacity) is used in the rehabilitation setting. Despite being a useful prognostic indicator the measurement of lung volumes is not especially useful to those involved in rehabilitation. It is important to recognise that these measures do not change as a result of rehabilitation, but are commonly measured to categorise the type of patient (as judged by the American Thoracic Society, 1986) being referred to the service.

DISABILITY

A practical measure of disability should reflect a reduction in functional capacity. Exercise tests are used to quantify this objectively. An exercise test in the setting of a rehabilitation service is important for a number of reasons. Lung function values (e.g. FEV_1 and FVC) that are measures of impairment do not relate well to a patient's functional capacity. Most studies reveal a poor relationship between the two (McGavin et al., 1976; Swinburn et al., 1985). Therefore exercise tests are employed to evaluate more precisely a patient's level of disability and capacity to perform day to day activities. In terms of pulmonary rehabilitation an exercise test is not only useful to quantify the individual's exercise tolerance but also is important as an indicator of change. Rehabilitation, not surprisingly, has no effect upon lung function (Simpson et al., 1992). Furthermore, an exercise test is important prior to entry onto a rehabilitation programme to indicate the limitations to exercise, e.g. respiratory, peripheral or cardiovascular. If the individual fails to continue with an exercise test because of breathlessness it is likely that the respiratory system is the limitation to continued exercise. Alternatively, if the patient stops because of general fatigue it is likely that he or she is 'deconditioned' and will respond to exercise training. If, however, the test is aborted because of cardiovascular reasons, leg pain, intermittent claudication, angina, etc., it is unlikely that the patient will respond to exercise training within the context of pulmonary rehabilitation. It is vitally important to make this distinction. Patients presenting with a co-existing history of osteoarthritis, angina, etc., are not uncommon, but this may *not* be a limiting factor to exercise. Occasionally, it may not be clear to the observer why the patient terminated the exercise test prematurely. It may

simply be that the individual was frightened of becoming severely breathless and so avoided provoking this sensation.

The measure of disability in lung disease can be assessed in either the field or the laboratory. Perhaps the former is more familiar to physiotherapists. Laboratory assessment requires the patients to perform a treadmill or cycle ergometer test with detailed gas analysis measurements requiring the patient to wear breathing apparatus (either a face mask or mouthpiece and nose clips). Not least because of the expense (both equipment and technical support), this type of testing is not widely used as part of the rehabilitation service. Field exercise tests, such as the 6 and 12 minute walking test (McGavin et al., 1976; Butland et al., 1982), were developed as a cheap, simple but effective alternative to laboratory based assessment of disability. Walking ability is the most frequent mode of testing. The 6 or 12 minute tests were the first field walking tests specifically designed to assess patients with COPD. These tests are self-paced tests, i.e. the patient selects the speed that will allow him or her to walk as far as possible in the time allowed. The individual can vary his or her speed and indeed stop to rest within the time of the test. The total distance covered along with some estimation of the time taken to rest is recorded. Not surprisingly the administration of these tests is haphazard and difficult to standardise. The results can be further influenced by motivation of the individual and by encouragement and pacing by the operator. Furthermore, the tests' simplicity limits the information which can be obtained from them about the physiological and symptomatic changes that are occurring during exercise. More recently the shuttle walking test has been developed as a standardised field exercise test (Singh et al., 1992, 1994) that is both reliable and valid. The shuttle walking test is an incremental, externally paced exercise test that stresses the patient to a symptom limited maximum. Briefly, the test requires the individual to walk around a 10 m course, defined by two marker cones. The speed of walking is dictated by signals played from a tape cassette and increases every minute, until the patient is either too breathless to continue or cannot maintain the required speed. Because the speed of walking is externally controlled the influence of the operator and/or encouragement is dampened. At the end of the test the number of 10 m lengths completed can be converted to a total distance or else recorded as the number of completed levels (i.e. each minute at a particular speed). Into this measure of distance, measures of dyspnoea, exertion, oximetry and heart rate can be incorporated. However, a more specific diagnosis can be made with only laboratory testing.

The performance of a laboratory based exercise test provides the most accurate measure of $VO_{2\,max}$ (see Chapter 1 for details). In patients with respiratory disorders the oxygen consumption is limited because of abnormalities associated with the respiratory system. Consequently the maximal VO_2 that a patient attains is often described as the symptom limited $VO_{2\,max}$ or $VO_{2\,peak}$. A $VO_{2\,max}$ is traditionally defined as the point at which, despite an increase in the gradient/speed of the treadmill there is no accompanying increase in oxygen uptake (less than 150 ml O_2/min), i.e. a plateau effect. This point is seldom achieved in patients with COPD. For patients with COPD the limitation to exercise is due to the inability of the lungs to meet the demand for increasing ventilation. In healthy trained subjects the limit to continued exercise is the cardiovascular system, more specifically the stroke volume. It should be remembered that these individuals do not always stop exercising because of limits imposed by their respiratory system; alternative reasons include peripheral muscle fatigue, poor co-ordination (particularly important for a cycle ergometer test) and poor motivation. This is discussed in more detail below.

The measurement of oxygen saturation is important at rest and during an exercise test to identify those individuals requiring supplemental oxygen. Pulmonary rehabilitation does not exclude those individual requiring long-term oxygen therapy or those using short bursts of oxygen for symptomatic relief. The dilemma associated with oxygen prescription within the context of pulmonary rehabilitation is, at what level of desaturation supplemental oxygen is thought necessary. Although there are at the time of writing no strict guidelines there is a consensus of opinion suggesting that any drop of 4% below 90% saturation requires intervention. It should be noted that levels of desaturation alter with the mode of exercise. This has been highlighted in studies (Spence et al., 1993; Cockcroft et al., 1985) examining the response to both endurance and incremental tests, as well as corridor walking test and cycle ergometry. It is important to use a saturation monitor during exercise testing not only for reasons of safety, but also to monitor oxygen levels during the exercise classes when the exercise regimen may provoke a different response to that observed during the exercise test. At present supplemental oxygen can be provided in cylinders small enough to allow the patient to carry them whilst exercising.

Recently it has been proposed that the endurance test may be a more sensitive measure of improvements in exercise tolerance as a result of exercise training. This relates to the nature of the limitation in this group of patients. If the limit to exercise is truly a failure of the respiratory system to sustain the levels of ventilation required then rehabilitation will not alter those parameters and it is likely that improvements in maximal exercise will be minimal. In the laboratory endurance testing is straightforward, but in the field it is inevitably less precise where a step test or a walking test can be used. A constant rate step test would be easier to calibrate than a walking test. Recently a field endurance walk was described. The subject was instructed to walk as far as possible (at a pace as though late for an appointment) and to stop when unable to go any further (Davidson et al., 1988). Maintenance of a constant prescribed speed of walking is obviously difficult without a treadmill.

As stated above, the measurement of dyspnoea can enhance the information acquired from a field exercise test. Resting measures also give a useful baseline against which to judge any exercise induced change. Patients can present with a variety of responses post-exercise; for example, individuals may have a heightened perception of their breathlessness, downgrade their level of breathlessness or change very little from their resting level. During an exercise test the two most commonly used scales are the Borg Breathlessness Score (Borg, 1982) and a simple visual analogue score (VAS). The VAS requires individuals to mark along a 10 cm line the intensity of their symptoms, with either end of the line used to identify 'nothing at all' and 'maximal'. While the patient is at rest there is a small selection of other more functional scales that can be used. These ask the patient to identify what level he or she can function at before becoming breathless. It is important to take a measure of perceived breathlessness, as one of the proven benefits of rehabilitation is the reduction of shortness of breath on exercise (Reardon et al., 1994).

Limitations to Exercise in Patients with COPD

Pulmonary limitations have been discussed earlier with reference to impaired lung function and also the mechanical disadvantage of a flattened diaphragm and chest wall restrictions.

Cardiovascular factors appear to be relatively insignificant in limiting performance, and low maximal heart rates are consistently documented (Nery et al., 1983). Patients do however present with an upwards shift of the VO_2/heart rate slope, i.e. at a comparable VO_2 (oxygen consumption) a patient with COPD will have a higher heart rate. From personal experience it is rare for a patient to achieve 85% of his or her predicted maximal heart rate, and breathlessness and/or fatigue present prematurely.

Recently additional factors have been identified as co-existing ischaemic heart disease (most patients with COPD are old and have smoked) and pulmonary hypertension (associated with structural abnormalities of the lung, compounded by hypoxic vasoconstriction) (Wagner, 1992). It has also been documented that right ventricular function is decreased in this group of patients (Matthay et al., 1992), but its contribution to exercise cessation is unclear.

The perception of breathlessness is unique to each patient. The sensation is strongly influenced by the individual's psychological state at the time of assessment. Awareness of dyspnoea may itself limit exercise independent of any mechanical/physiological mechanisms. Altose (1985) proposes a variety of signals that may be responsible for mediating the sensation of breathlessness including chemoreceptors in the blood and brain, mechanoreceptors in the thorax and outgoing CNS respiratory motor commands.

HANDICAP

The degree of handicap imposed by an individual's disease is generally believed to be reflected in measures of quality of life. The term quality of life has recently been described as '...an individual's perception of their position in life in the context of the culture and the value system in which they live and in relation to their goals, expectations, standards and concerns. It has a broad ranging concept affected in a complex way by a person's physical health, psychological state, level of independence, social relationships, and their relationship to salient features of their environment' (World Health Organisation, 1993). The quality of an individual's life is understandably multi-factorial, and may include issues relating to financial position, social/leisure activities, family and religion. The use of quality of life and, in particular, health related quality of life instruments, is becoming increasing popular within the rehabilitation setting. It is believed that the use of these measures may allow the identification of more subtle beneficial changes that occur as a consequence of rehabilitation. Health related quality of life is an attempt to judge how the patient is affected both physically and psychologically by his or her respiratory disease and it is believed to reflect the level of handicap. Questionnaires are frequently employed as the mode of investigation. These can indicate the impact that the patient's breathlessness and other manifestations of respiratory disorders have upon his or her daily life. Questionnaires were developed to aid the overall evaluation of patient's psychological, emotional and functional status and to reveal any hidden links between directly measured pathophysiological parameters and a patient's quality of life. The questionnaires used to measure quality of life can be categorised as either general or disease specific. Examples of the former include the Sickness Impact Profile (SIP) (Bergner *et al.*, 1981) and the short form -36 (SF36) (Ware and Sherbourne, 1992). Disease specific questionnaires can be used, allowing the investigation of specific issues pertinent to an individual with COPD. Perhaps most obviously health related quality of life measures would focus upon the impact that dyspnoea has upon patients' lives.

The St George's Respiratory Questionnaire (SGRQ) has recently been introduced to assess both COPD and asthma patients (Jones *et al.*, 1992). It is proposed that this test is more standardised than previous questionnaires, and it consists of 76 items divided into three sections (symptoms, activity and impacts). The questionnaire, it is reported, correlates well with other reference values and also relates to more general measures of health, e.g. The Sickness Impact Profile (Bergner *et al.*, 1981).

The Breathing Problems questionnaire (Hyland *et al.*, 1994) is, like the St George's, a self-completed questionnaire. It directs questions to the functional limitations and the emotional impact caused by the symptoms of chronic respiratory disease. It has 33 items and is simple for the patient to complete in 10–15 minutes.

EXERCISE FOR PATIENTS WITH COPD

As healthy individuals involved in the provision of a pulmonary rehabilitation service we frequently assume that the ability to exercise is important to an individual's well being and as an extension of this process that the improvement in exercise tolerance is automatically beneficial to an individual's quality of life. This is quite clearly not so. The relationship between exercise tolerance and quality of life may be reasonably strong in a cross-sectional comparison at the time of the initial assessment but the changes generated in both dimensions do not appear to be strongly related. Therefore it would appear that the ability to exercise is just one component of perceived quality of life.

There are several different strategies that can be adopted to train patients with COPD. These can be broadly categorised as:
- Aerobic training.
- Peripheral muscle training.
- Upper limb training.
- Respiratory muscle training.

AEROBIC TRAINING

This approach attempts to optimise cardiovascular fitness, firstly by improving the efficiency of the heart by increasing stroke volume and secondly by improving oxygen extraction at the level of the exercising muscle. Typically an aerobic regimen would involve cycling, swimming or walking. Physiologically this training method remains controversial. We are unsure if patients with COPD are able to achieve a training level commensurate with a physiological training effect. This suggestion hinges upon the difficulty we frequently experience in measuring a lactate threshold. Exercise prescription can be based either on the results of a laboratory based exercise test or on a field exercise test where some estimation of maximal capacity is secured. From either exercise test there are a combination of parameters that can be used to prescribe exercise ($VO_{2\,peak}$, heart rate and lactate threshold). The training load can be further secured by matching peak performance with the response to the Borg Breathlessness Score or VAS. To obtain a physiological training effect in healthy individuals a course of approximately 6 weeks is recommended (American College of Sports Medicine, 1991). This is mirrored in training programmes for patients with COPD. Commonly a course is 6–8 weeks in duration and held twice a week; in addition, exercise sessions should be repeated at home, each ideally lasting 20–30 minutes. The intensity of exercise for a healthy population is commonly at 50–60% of maximal oxygen uptake. This coincides with the anaerobic threshold. The required intensity for patients with COPD remains unclear and it has been suggested that these individuals cannot train at the required intensity to provoke an aerobic training response. Casaburi and colleagues (1991) were able to demonstrate the anticipated response in a group of patients with mild to moderate disease. Punzal and colleagues (1993) suggested that in patients with COPD it may be possible to train at a much higher percentage of the measured $VO_{2\,peak}$.

PERIPHERAL MUSCLE TRAINING

As an alternative to whole body exercise, specific muscle training can be employed. This is an option for those individuals who become too breathless to participate in aerobic training. Killian *et al.* (1992) demonstrated that patients with COPD frequently terminate exercise because of peripheral muscle fatigue. It is this skeletal muscle fatigue that is directly addressed with specific muscle training. Simpson *et al.* (1992) employed weightlifting as a means of training with successful results in patients with COPD. The study reported an increase in arm and leg strength, an increased endurance time and an improvement in quality of life, as measured by the CRDQ. However, the system is likely to be more costly to set up (equipment costs, e.g. multi-gym) and support.

UPPER LIMB TRAINING

Patients with COPD frequently rely on the stability of their shoulder girdle to compensate for hyperinflation of their chest and the mechanical disadvantage that this imposes. Consequently when these individuals perform upper limb activities disproportionate breathlessness results. Upper limb exercise can include cycle ergometer, weightlifting and unsupported exercises. The result of this type of training is very specific with an increase in endurance and strength for arm activities. There is little transference of effect to improved whole body exercise.

RESPIRATORY MUSCLE TRAINING

The respiratory muscles are the only skeletal muscles required to contract regularly for the maintenance of life. In patients with COPD the functioning of these muscles is inadequate. There is disruption of the load applied (increased airways resistance), and a reduction in the force they are able to generate (hyperinflation, malnutrition and fatigue). Most patients attending rehabilitation will be on optimal medication and it is unlikely that the 'load' can be reduced. The principles underpinning respiratory muscle training are an increase in the efficiency of the respiratory muscles, improved co-ordination of all the muscles of respiration and a decrease of the respiratory frequency. There have been several attempts to measure the benefits, but to date these reports have had varying success (Belman and Shadmehr, 1988).

PROVEN BENEFITS OF REHABILITATION

There are several studies examining the benefit of rehabilitation in this group of patients (Goldstein *et al.*, 1994; Wijkstra *et al.*, 1995; Ries *et al.*, 1995). Most of the studies reported offer something quite different to the rehabilitation offered in the UK. Nevertheless they offer an established, successful framework by which we can develop programmes suitable to the health service in the UK. Although older studies examined benefits only in terms of increased exercise tolerance it is now common to examine the effects of rehabilitation upon changes of exercise tolerance and quality of life. Exercise tolerance can be measured by a vast spectrum of tests as described above. Most studies document an improvement in maximal oxygen consumption, walking distance or endurance time. The latter may reflect more accurately any changes in domestic activity that rehabilitation can provoke. Amongst healthcare professionals there is a widespread belief that an improved ability to exercise inevitably leads to an improved quality of life; although these parameters do improve after rehabilitation these changes may not be linked. Not surprisingly there are many components to both quality of life (including financial, social and leisure) and health related quality of life (role function, emotional and physical function) and the ability to exercise is just one

component of the latter. Other areas of interest include a reduced rate of hospital admissions. Such information was documented by Haas and Cardon (1969); which sources reported decreased admissions following a course of rehabilitation. It would therefore appear that pulmonary rehabilitation is of benefit not only in the short term but also in the longer term with financial benefits included.

THE ROLE OF THE PHYSIOTHERAPIST

The physiotherapist with an interest in chest diseases has witnessed several important changes over the last few years, two such being the proliferation of non-invasive positive pressure ventilation techniques and the resurgence of interest in pulmonary rehabilitation. With the additional pressures that these developments bring, many physiotherapists have been forced to redefine their role. The aim of physiotherapy is to maximise an individual's quality of life, achieved by teaching the individual or his or her carer the optimal therapeutic approaches. This aim is fulfilled largely by the shift in healthcare towards self-care supported by a large element of education. In the treatment of chronic respiratory disease the aims of treatment for the physiotherapist include:

- Reduction of fear and anxiety.
- Reduction of breathlessness and the work of breathing.
- Improved efficiency of breathing.
- Mobilising and aiding expectoration of secretions (Bott and Moran, 1996).

The active cycle of breathing techniques (Webber and Pryor, 1993) and autogenic drainage (David, 1991) are techniques that allow the patient to mobilise and clear excessive bronchial secretions independent of any external assistance, whether therapist, partner or equipment. If necessary other techniques can be added to assist in the achievement of the treatment's aims. The aims of pulmonary rehabilitation are reflected in the aims of conventional physiotherapy; the only difference lies in the progression from individual to group treatment. In addition, therapists may be required to implement exercise training regimens.

Overall the principles of physiotherapy treatments remain constant but with a shift of emphasis towards self-management and taking individual responsibility. The varied role of the physiotherapist sits comfortably in the pulmonary rehabilitation framework. For example, the physiotherapist may be responsible for the overall organisation of the service *and* operate as the service co-ordinator; alternatively, he or she may supervise the exercise sessions as well as taking part in the lecture programme.

CONCLUSION

Pulmonary rehabilitation is presently enjoying a resurgence within the British and European healthcare service. This expanding service for patients with chronic respiratory disease relies heavily upon the skills of physiotherapists within a multidisciplinary framework. It is an exciting development for both the patient and the physiotherapist.

REFERENCES

Altose DM. Assessment and management of breathlessness. *Chest* 1985, **88:**77s-83s.

Ambrisino N, Foglio K. Selection criteria for pulmonary rehabilitation. *Resp Med* 1996, **90:**317-322.

American College of Sports Medicine. *Guidelines for exercise testing and prescription*, 4th ed. Pennsylvania: Lea & Febiger; 1991.

American Thoracic Society. Evaluation of impairment/disability secondary to respiratory disorders. *Am Rev Resp Dis* 1986, **133:**1205-1209.

Belman MJ, Shadmehr. Targeted resistive ventilatory muscle training in chronic obstructive pulmonary disease. *J Appl Physio* 1988, **65:**2726-2735.

Bergner M, Bobbitt RA, Carter WB, Gilson BS. The sickness impact file: development and final revision of a health status measure. *Med Care* 1981, **19:**787-806.

Borg GAV. Psychophysical bases of perceived exertion. *Med Sci Sport* 1982, **14:**377-381.

Bott J, Moran F. Physiotherapy and NIPPV. In: Simonds AK , ed. *Non-invasive respiratory support*. London: Chapman & Hall; 1996:133-142.

Butland RJA, Pang J, Gross ER, Woodcock AA, Geddes DM. Two-, six- and twelve-minute walking tests in respiratory disease. *BMJ* 1982, **284:**1607-1608.

Casaburi R, Patessio A, Ioli F, Zanaboni *et al*. Reduction in exercise lactic acidosis and ventilation as a result of exercise training in patients with chronic lung disease. *Am Rev Resp Dis* 1991, **143:**9-18.

Cockcroft AE, Beaumont A, Adams L, Guz A. Arterial desaturation during treadmill and bicycle exercise in patients with chronic obstructive pulmonary disease. *Clin Sci* 1985, **68:**327-332.

Cooper JD, Trulock EP, Triantafillou AN, *et al*. Bilateral pneumectomy (volume reduction) for chronic obstructive pulmonary disease. *J Thorac Cardiovasc Surg* 1995, **109:**106-119.

David, A. Autogenic drainage – the German approach. In: Pryor JA, ed. *International perspectives in physical therapy*. 7: Respiratory care. Edinburgh: Churchill Livingstone; 1991:65-178.

Davidson AC, Leach R, George RJD, Geddes DM. Supplemental oxygen and exercise ability in chronic obstructive airways disease. *Thorax* 1988, **43:**965-971.

Fishman AP. Pulmonary rehabilitation research. *Am J Resp Crit Care Med* 1994, **149:**825-833.

Goldstein RS, Gort EH, Stubbing D, Avendano MA, Guyatt GH. Randomised controlled trial of respiratory rehabilitation. *Lancet* 1994, **334:**1394-1397.

Haas A, Cardon H. Rehabilitation in chronic obstructive pulmonary disease; a five year study of 252 patients. *Med Clin North Am* 1969, **53:**593-607.

Hyland M, Bott J, Singh SJ, Kenyon CAP. Development and validation of a patient-completed questionnaire for assessing quality of life in patients with chronic obstructive pulmonary disease. *Quality of Life Res* 1994, **3:**245-256.

Jones PW, Quirk FH, Baveystock CM, Littlejohns P. A self completed measure of health status for chronic airflow limitation. The St Georges Respiratory Questionnaire. *Am Rev Resp Dis* 1992, **142:**1321-1327.

Killian J, LeBlanc P, Martin DH, Summers E, *et al*. Exercise capacity and ventilatory, circulatory, and symptom limitation in patients with chronic airflow limitation. *Am Rev Resp Dis* 1992, **146:**935-940.

Matthay RA, Arroliga AC, Wiedermann HP, Schulman DS, *et al*. Right ventricular function at rest and during exercise in chronic obstructive pulmonary disease. *Chest* 1992, **(suppl 101):**255s-262s.

McGavin CR, Gupta SP, McHardy GJR. Twelve-minute walking test for assessing disability in chronic bronchitis. *BMJ* 1976, **1:**822-823.

Nery LE, Wasserman K, French W, Oren A, Davis JA. Contrasting cardiovascular and respiratory responses to exercise in mitral valve and chronic obstructive pulmonary diseases. *Chest* 1983, **83:**446-453.

Pearson MG, Littler J, Davies PDO. An analysis of medical workload by speciality and diagnosis in Mersey – evidence of a specialist to patient mismatch. *J Roy Coll Phys* 1994, **28:**230-234.

Punzal PA, Reis AL, Kaplan RM, Prewitt LM. Maximum intensity exercise training in patients with chronic obstructive pulmonary disease. *Chest* 1993, **100:**618-623.

Rand CS. Issues in the measurement of adherence. In: Shumaker SA, Schron EB, Ockene JK, eds. *The handbook of health behaviour change*. Springer Publishing Company; 1990:102-110.

Reardon J, Awad E, Normandin E, Vale F, Clark B, ZuWallack RL. The effect of comprehensive outpatient pulmonary rehabilitation on dyspnea. *Chest* 1994, **105:**1046-1052.

Ries AL, Kaplan RM, Limberg TM, Prewitt LA. Effects of pulmonary rehabilitation on physiologic and psychosocial outcomes in patients with chronic obstructive pulmonary disease. *Ann Intern Med* 1995, **122:**823-832.

Simpson K, Killian K, McCartney N, Stubbing DG, *et al*. Randomised controlled trial of weight lifting in patients with chronic airflow limitation. *Thorax* 1992, **47:**70-75.

Singh SJ, Morgan MDL, Hardman AE, Rowe C, Bardsley PA. Comparison of oxygen uptake during a conventional treadmill test and the shuttle walking test in chronic airflow limitation. *Eur Respir J* 1994, **7:**2016-2020.

Singh SJ, Morgan MDL, Scott SC, Walters D, Hardman AE. The development of the shuttle walking test of disability in patients with chronic airways obstruction. *Thorax* 1992, **47:**1019-1024.

Spence DPS, Hay JG, Carter J, Pearson MG, Calverley PMA. Oxygen desaturation and breathlessness during corridor walking in chronic obstructive pulmonary disease: effect of oxitropium bromide. *Thorax* 1993, **48:**1145-1150.

Swinburn CR, Wakefield JM, Jones PW. Performance, ventilation and oxygen consumption in three different types of exercise tests in patients with chronic obstructive lung disease. *Thorax* 1985, **40:**581-586.

Wagner PD. Ventilation-perfusion matching during exercise. Chest 1992, **101:**192s-198s.

Ware JE, Sherbourne CD. The MOS 36-item short form health survey (SF-36). *Med Care* 1992, **30:**473-483.

Webber BA, Pryor JA. Physiotherapy skills: techniques and adjuncts. In: BA JA Pryor, Webber, eds. *Physiotherapy for respiratory and cardiac problems*. Edinburgh: Churchill Livingstone; 1993:113-171.

WHOQOL Group. *Measuring quality of life: The development of the World Health Organization quality of life instrument (WHOQOL)*. Geneva: WHO; 1993.

Wijkstra PJ, Ten Vergert EM, Van Alten AR, *et al*. Long term benefits of rehabilitation at home on quality of life and exercise tolerance in patients with chronic obstructive pulmonary disease. *Thorax* 1995, **50:**824-828.

World Health Organization. *International classification of impairments, disabilities and handicaps*. Geneva:WHO; 1980.

Young J. Rehabilitation and older people. *BMJ* 1996, **313:**677-681.

GENERAL READING

Astrand PO, Rodahl K. *Textbook of work physiology*, 3rd ed. New York: McGraw-Hill; 1986.

Belman MJ, Kendregan BA. Exercise training fails to increase skeletal muscle enzymes in patients with chronic obstructive pulmonary disease. *Am Rev Resp Dis* 1981, **123:**256-261.

Calverley P. Ventilatory control and dyspnoea. In: Calverley P, Pride N, eds. *Chronic obstructive pulmonary disease*. London: Chapman & Hall; 1995:205-242.

Casaburi R, Wasserman K, Patessio A, Ioli F, *et al*. A new perspective in pulmonary rehabilitation: anaerobic threshold as a discriminant in training. *Eur Respir J* 1989, **(suppl 7):**618s-623s.

Guyatt GH, Berman LB, Townsend M, Pugsley SO, Chambers LW. A measure of quality of life for clinical trials in chronic lung disease. *Thorax* 1987, **42:**773-778.

Howell JBL. Breathlessness. In: Brewis, RAL, Gibson GJ, Geddes DM, eds. *Respiratory medicine*. London: Ballière Tindall; 1990:221-228.

GENERAL READING

Hudson LD, Tyler ML, Petty TL. Hospitalisation needs during out patient rehabilitation programme for severe COA. *Chest* 1976, **70:**606-610.

Jones NL, Jones G, Edwards RHT. Exercise tolerance in chronic airways obstruction. *Am Rev Resp Dis* 1971, **103:**477-490.

Kaplan RM, Feeny D, Revicki DA. Methods for assessing relative importance in preference based outcome measures. *Quality of Life Res* 1993, **2:**467-475.

Mahler DA, Weinberg DH, Wells CK, Feinstein AR. The measurement of dyspnea: contents, interobserver agreement and physiological correlates of two new clinical indexes. *Chest* 1984, **85:**751-758.

Medical Research Council. *Committee on research into chronic bronchitis: instructions for use on the questionnaire on respiratory symptoms.* Devon: W J Holman; 1966.

Office of Population Censuses and Surveys mortality statistics: England and Wales 1992 series DH no19. London:HMSO; 1993.

Patessio A, Casaburi R, Carone M, Appendini, L *et al.* Comparison of gas exchange, lactate, and lactic acidosis thresholds in patients with chronic obstructive pulmonary disease. *Am Rev Resp Dis* 1993, **148:**622-626.

Rochester DF. Effects of COPD on the respiratory muscles. In: Cherniack NS, ed. *Chronic obstructive pulmonary disease.* Philadelphia: WB Saunders; 1991:134-157.

Whipp BJ, Pardy RL. Breathing during exercise. In: Fishman AP, ed. *Handbook of physiology, Section 3. The respiratory system.* Baltimore: Williams and Wilkins Company 1986, **3:**605-629.

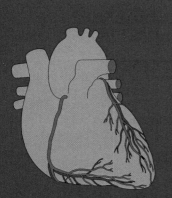
THE TRANSPLANTATION UNIT

CHAPTER OUTLINE

- Heart transplantation
- Lung transplantation
- Heart-lung transplantation
- Physiotherapy and transplant surgery

- Pre-operative phase
- Post-operative phase
- Rejection
- Effects and benefits of exercise

INTRODUCTION

Within 30 years, heart and lung transplantation has been transformed from an almost impossible dream to an every-day reality that is now practised in transplant centres throughout the world.

The human body has an innate ability to eject and destroy foreign protein, which therefore permanently threatens the transplanted organs with rejection, hence the need for all transplant recipients to receive lifelong immunosuppressive drugs. While ensuring the survival of the graft, immunosuppression has undesirable side effects that render the recipient liable to infection and malignancy. The perfect immunosuppressive agent prevents the body from rejecting the transplanted organs, maintains the normal responsiveness of the immune system to infection and malignancy, and has minimal or no side effects. Such a drug has yet to be discovered. Until that day, transplantation must be veiwed as a palliative treatment despite the remarkably long periods of survival achieved by some recipients. Five-year survival figures for heart transplants are in excess of 60%, while 40% of heart transplant patients survive 10 years. The leading causes of death after intrathoracic organ transplantation are rejection, infection and side effects from antirejection therapy.

HEART TRANSPLANTATION

HISTORY

The first human heart transplant was performed by Professor Christian Barnard in Cape Town, South Africa on the 7th December, 1967, using techniques developed in the laboratories of Norman Shumway at Stanford University, USA. The first recipient died of overwhelming infection 18 days after the transplant. In 1968, 102 transplant procedures were carried out world-wide. The average survival of these cases was 29 days.

The enthusiasm for transplantation rapidly waned because of the poor early results. Transplant activity continued in a few transplant centres scattered around the world, most notably at Stanford. However, early survival figures remained disappointingly low with less than half the transplanted patients alive at 1 year due to infection and graft rejection. By the late 1970s, survival figures of 65% at 1 year were achieved. Further significant improvements in survival figures followed the discovery of cyclosporin with its selective immunosuppressive properties, and the introduction of endomyocardial biopsy enabling early detection of rejection.

By 1996, 300 heart transplants were carried out annually in the UK, and approximately 3000 transplants were performed annually world-wide.

INDICATIONS FOR HEART TRANSPLANTATION

Transplantation of the heart is offered to patients with end stage cardiac disease with extensive myocardial damage that has proved refractory to aggressive medical therapy, where the life expectancy of the patient is less than 12 months.

Heart muscle damage is most commonly caused by extensive myocardial infarction and viral infections as well as excessive alcohol intake. Chronic severe aortic valve regurgitation can severely damage the heart muscle so as to negate the benefit of valve replacement. Pregnancy is very rarely complicated by postpartum cardiomyopathy, which proves fatal in a high proportion of cases. Other causes of heart muscle damage include chemotherapeutic agents, infiltration of the heart muscle by iron and amyloid deposits, and granulomata of sarcoid.

Recipient Selection

Strict criteria are applied to the selection of candidates for transplantation due to the scarcity of donor organs, the cost of the transplant operation (estimated at £25 000 in the UK) and the side effects of immunosuppressive therapy. Patients on transplant waiting lists should be ill enough to need a transplant and well enough to stand the rigors of the postoperative period, and expect a good functional result.

A typical heart transplant candidate is a patient with severe heart failure, causing an unacceptable quality of life from disabling symptoms in spite of appropriate tailored medical therapy.

The patient must be without any other systemic disease that would in itself shorten life expectancy or increase the risks of side effects from the immunosuppressive drugs. The recipient must be negative for HIV and hepatitis and have no malignant disease. Heart transplantation is not normally offered to patients over the age of 60; there is no lower age limit. Transplant in the paediatric age group is covered in Chapter 19. The presence of active infection and ulcer disease is a relative contraindication, and severe peripheral or cerebrovascular disease, even if asymptomatic, disqualifies the patient. Diabetes with end organ damage, i.e. neuropathy or severe peripheral vascular disease, is a contraindication to transplantation. However, diabetics controlled by oral hyperglycaemic drugs or insulin, in the absence of complications of diabetes, are considered for transplantation. Patients with severe pulmonary hypertension who do not respond to vasodilator therapy are not suitable candidates for orthotopic heart transplantation but may be suitable for heterotopic 'piggy back' (i.e. the patient's heart is not removed) or heart–lung replacements. Persistent drug or alcohol misuse disqualifies candidates from consideration for heart transplantation. A history of serious non-reactive psychiatric disturbance which may result in life-threatening non-compliance is a contraindication to transplantation.

Donor Selection

The success of any transplant operation is highly dependent on the function of the donor organ and appropriate matching to the recipient. The discrepancy between the demand for and the supply of donors is illustrated by the fact that in the USA it is estimated that as many as 35 000 patients could benefit from transplantation. However, the number of heart transplants performed annually in the USA does not exceed 2500. Not all potential organ donors are suitable intrathoracic organ donors; 60% have unsuitable hearts and 85% unsuitable lungs. Currently, donors up to the age of 55 are considered for heart transplantation. Potential donors must have two sets of brainstem death tests performed within the space of 12 hours by two consultants who are not members of the transplant team. These tests must not be done in the presence of hypothermia, shock, drug overdose, and electrolyte, acid–base or glucose abnormalities. The donor must be negative for HIV and hepatitis and have no malignant disease; however, primary brain tumours do not preclude intrathoracic organ donation. Only then is an offer of donation made to the transplant team for careful assessment and management.

The heart donors have to be assessed carefully to exclude the presence of coronary artery disease or severe left ventricular hypertrophy. The process of brain death is accompanied by profound haemodynamic and metabolic changes which can severely damage the heart and eventually result in cessation of all cardiac activity despite supportive measures including ventilation. The vast majority of patients satisfying brainstem death criteria develop cardiac and circulatory arrest within 72 hours despite conventional support.

All cardiac donors must have a normal electrocardiogram (ECG) and preferably a normal echocardiogram. They must not be on inotropic support exceeding 5–10 µg/kg/min of dopamine or equivalent doses of other inotropes, to sustain a satisfactory blood pressure with normovolaemia. The donor recipient weight mismatch must not exceed 20–30%, provided the pulmonary vascular resistance is within normal limits; in cases where there is elevation of the pulmonary vascular resistance an oversized donor organ will be required. The donor and recipient must be blood group compatible.

HARVESTING AND PRESERVATION OF THE DONOR HEART

Harvesting of the heart is most frequently carried out as part of a multiorgan retrieval. The donor, who is usually intubated and ventilated, is taken to the operating room. Ideally, the cardiac harvesting team should be at the donor hospital before the removal of the donor to the operating room, having assessed the patient in the Intensive Care Unit (ICU) and carried out any additional haemodynamic measurements, and instituted fluid or drug treatment so as to optimise the function of the donor heart. The abdomen and chest are prepared. An incision extending from the suprasternal notch to the pubis is made. The sternum is divided. Following opening of the pericardium the heart is inspected and a search is made for areas of contusion of the heart or atheroma of the coronary arteries as well as disease or damage to the valves or the septum. A note is made of the vigour of cardiac contraction and distension of the ventricles and atria. Tapes are placed around the superior and inferior venae cavae. The findings of the harvesting team are communicated to the recipient hospital. The abdominal organ harvesting team begins dissection of the abdominal organs in preparation for their removal. Once all preparations are completed the cardiac team proceeds to excise the donor heart. Clamps or ties are placed on the superior and inferior vena cavae. The superior vena cava is tied at a distance above its junction with the atrium and divided. The inferior vena cava is divided, blood is aspirated from the pericardial cavity, the aorta is cross-clamped and 1 litre of St Thomas' cardioplegic solution at 4°C is run into the aortic root with a large bore needle. Concurrent with this is the application of topical cold saline into the pericardium. Once this has been completed the heart is elevated out of the pericardium, and the pulmonary veins divided individually followed by division of the pulmonary artery at its bifurcation. The aorta is divided below the cross-clamp. The heart is then placed in a bowl of cold saline, and rapidly inspected for the presence of any patent foramen ovale. The valves are examined. The heart is then placed in a polythene bag containing cold saline in an icebox for transport to the recipient hospital by the harvesting team with the minimum delay so as to reduce the graft ischaemic time. As the operative mortality of cardiac transplantation progressively rises with increasing graft ischaemic time, every effort is made to reduce the time gap between harvesting and implantation.

THE RECIPIENT OPERATION

At the recipient hospital, the patient is taken to the operating room on receipt of information from the harvesting team indicating satisfactory function of the donor organ. Anaesthesia is induced. A median sternotomy is performed and preparation is made for the institution of cardiopulmonary bypass by cannulating the superior and inferior venae cavae as well as the aorta. Upon arrival of the heart and after the preparation of the donor organ, cardiopulmonary bypass is established. The aorta is cross-clamped. The recipient heart is then removed, leaving about 1 cm of the main pulmonary artery before its division and 2–3 cm of the aorta distal to the clamp, as well as leaving the posterior part of both atria which the venae cavae and the pulmonary veins drain. The donor heart is then brought out of the icebox and implanted by suturing the trimmed donor left and right atria to the recipient residual left and right atria and anastomosing the pulmonary artery and aorta to those of the recipient. The aortic cross-clamp is removed and air is evacuated from the cardiac chambers. The heart is resuscitated for a period on bypass. Bypass is then discontinued with the help of inotropic drugs to reduce pulmonary vascular resistance and increase the rate of the heart and its contractility. Early right ventricular dysfunction is not uncommon following implantation. This in its mildest form responds to augmentation of inotropic support but may require the institution of more vigorous therapeutic measures, such as pulmonary vasodilators and,

occasionally, the use of mechanical right ventricular assist. Failure of the left ventricle is a less common occurrence and is most frequently caused by inadequate preservation of the heart. Treatment is along the usual lines with the use of inotropes and occasionally an intra-aortic balloon pump. In very rare cases hyperacute rejection leads to severe irreversible graft failure.

IMMUNOSUPPRESSION

Immunosuppression is for life following heart transplantation. Soon after heart transplantation, immunosuppression is at its highest since the incidence and dangers of rejection are at their peak. Cytolytic agents such as rabbit antithymocyte globulin and OKT3 are used in addition to cyclosporin, azathioprine and prednisolone. Cytolytic drugs are very rarely used outside the immediate post-operative phase and for resistant rejection. Most centres employ cyclosporin, azathioprine and prednisolone to maintain immunosuppression.

Cyclosporin is a plant-derived selective immunosuppressive drug with a substantial number of side effects such as renal impairment, hypertension, hirsutism, tremors and gingival hyperplasia (growth of the gums). Cyclosporin can be administered orally or parenterally. Dosage levels are adjusted according to measurement of the cyclosporin level in the serum. Cyslosporin levels can be significantly affected by concurrent administration of certain drugs.

Azathioprine interferes with DNA synthesis by the lymphocytes, which constitutes the main agent for rejection. Bone marrow depression is a side effect of the drug. The drug dosage needs to be reduced if the white cell count is below 5000.

Steroids are non-selective immunosuppressives; prednisolone is most often used. Steroids have a long list of side effects such as the development of hypertension, the exacerbation of diabetes, weight gain, truncal obesity, osteoporosis, acne and hirsutism. They are used as the first line in the treatment of an acute rejection episode.

EARLY POST-OPERATIVE MANAGEMENT

This differs little from that received routinely by cardiac surgery patients, except for the use of immunosuppressive drugs and reverse barrier nursing techniques.

In the majority of cases the grafted organ functions well with resultant improvement in the patient's circulation. Patients can usually be taken off the ventilator the following day. The majority of heart transplant patients can be extubated within 24 hours.

The impact of the well-functioning transplanted heart on the patient's haemodynamics is remarkable. A sense of well-being is restored and convalescence is, by and large, unremarkable. However, the more ill the patient is pre-operatively the more protracted is the recovery. Occasionally the transplanted heart does not function adequately. The right ventricle of the transplanted heart is unaccustomed to coping with high pulmonary arterial pressures. These pressures are often elevated in transplant patients. The pulmonary artery pressure is further elevated by cardiopulmonary bypass, hypoxia and hypercapnia. This may lead to failure of the right ventricle with subsequent inadequate filling of the left side of the heart, and low blood pressure. Right heart failure can be successfully treated in the majority of cases with inotropic drugs and, on occasion, with the use of pulmonary vasodilators. Occasionally mechanical assistance of the failing right ventricle is necessary, but it is rarely successful.

Rejection

Immunosuppressive drugs need to be administered on a lifelong basis to control and treat rejection. Since the introduction of cyclosporin, the detection of rejection following transplantation has been dependent on a regular and periodic histological assessment of samples obtained from the heart using ultrafine biopsy forceps introduced through the internal jugular vein. Sampling is carried out under fluoroscopic control. Severity of the rejection can be gauged by examination under the microscope. Resolution of rejection under treatment can be monitored by repeat biopsy. The biopsy schedule is as follows: weekly for 6 weeks, fortnightly for the next 3 months, monthly up to the next 6 months, and at 3-monthly intervals thereafter. Biopsies are also performed whenever rejection is suspected.

Infections

The management of transplant patients is similar to walking a tightrope. Too much immunosuppression results in demolishing the immune system and exposing the patient to infection. Inadequate immunosuppression results in rejection and damage to the transplanted organ.

Infections in transplant patients are most frequently bacterial, with viral infections the second commonest. The most serious and frequent of these infections is cytomegalovirus (CMV) infection which, in a normal individual, causes subclinical infection. However, in immunosuppressed patients this can cause substantial morbidity and, until recently, has caused significant mortality. Fungal infections, which are rare in normal individuals, constitute 17% of infections in the transplant patient. Organisms such as *Toxoplasma* and *Pneumocystis* cause subclinical infection in the non-immunosuppressed population. However, in transplant patients they can cause severe and occasionally fatal illness. Early detection and aggressive management of the infection are of paramount importance in transplant patients.

LONG-TERM COMPLICATIONS

Graft Atherosclerosis

Graft artherosclerosis is the main cause of death in long-term survivors after heart transplantation. The disease process occurs with increasing frequency with the passage of time after transplantation. The distribution of coronary artery disease is significantly different from that normally seen in the general population. Heart transplant patients can sustain myocardial infarcts without experiencing pain, although in some, due to re-innervation, vague chest pain can be experienced. Graft atherosclerosis is not suitable for treatment by either bypass surgery or angioplasty in the vast majority of cases and ultimately leads to the death of the patient from extensive damage to the myocardium. The only effective treatment is re-transplantation.

Malignancies

The incidence of malignancies is up to 100-fold higher in transplant patients than in the normal population. The more intense the degree of immunosuppression, the higher the frequency. Heart transplant patients have a significantly higher incidence of malignancy than renal transplant patients who are less immunosuppressed. Skin malignancies are common after transplant, and should be biopsied and treated early. Lymphoproliferative malignancies are the second most common tumour developing after organ transplants. Their development is thought to be linked to a viral infection. Some of these tumours respond to a reduction in the level of immunosuppression while others require chemotherapy. Organs such as the lung, colon, kidney and liver are possible sites for tumour development.

CURRENT STATUS OF HEART TRANSPLANTATION

Just over 35 000 patients have so far undergone heart transplantation. In 1982, 190 transplantations were performed world-wide. In 1994, over 3500 heart transplants were performed in 271 centres throughout the world. Coronary artery disease and cardiomyopathy are the two main indications for transplantation. Actuarial survival at 1, 5 and 10 years following transplantation is 80%, 60% and 40%, respectively. Survival beyond 20 years is not known.

FUTURE OF HEART TRANSPLANTATION

The scarcity of organs limits the availability to only a highly selected fraction of the potential recipients. The use of artificial and animal hearts is an obvious solution. However, the use of either has severe limitations and drawbacks.

Artificial Hearts

Artificial hearts have been used successfully in a few hundred patients as a bridge to transplantation. However, their use as totally implantable, permanent devices has been tried in only a few patients.

Artificial hearts used as a bridge to transplantation is a practical reality. Their use as a permanent replacement of the heart must still be considered as experimental. Artificial hearts are still extremely costly. Systemic embolism and infection are not uncommon with these devices. The problem of a suitable and convenient power supply to these devices has yet to be satisfactorily solved although major steps have been taken in that direction.

Xenotransplantation

A primate heart was used by James Hardy in 1964 in the first heart transplant ever performed. The heart functioned for an hour before hyperacute rejection caused it to fail. Since then a few xenotransplants have been attempted but none survived more than a few days. There are major immunological barriers and ethical considerations to be solved before xenotransplants can become a reality. Although primates are an obvious source of donor organs, such animals are scarce and their use as a source of donor organs is open to strong moral objection; let alone the obvious discrepancy in size between an adult and a small primate, and the real possibility of transmission of infections from primates to humans. Pigs are an obvious source. They can be bred in a germ-free environment. Using genetic engineering techniques it is possible to breed pigs that possess inhibitors of human complement on the lining of their blood vessels, thus reducing the incidence and severity of hyperacute rejection which has so far been the main barrier to successful animal to human transplantation. The indications are that organs from genetically engineered pigs will be used in clinical transplantation in the near future. It remains to be seen whether such xenotransplants will be successful in clinical practice. Clearly, success in this endeavour would revolutionise the practice of transplantation. However, one must not underestimate the immunological barriers that still have to be crossed before that most elusive of goals becomes a reality.

LUNG TRANSPLANTATION

HISTORY

Lung transplantation has become an established modality for the management of end stage lung disease. In 1963, Hardy performed the first human lung transplantation without success. Between 1963 and 1983, 60 single lung transplants were performed with no long-term survivors. In 1983, the first long-term success with human single lung transplant was achieved by Cooper in Toronto. On 9th March, 1981, Bruce Reitz successfully transplanted a heart–lung block into a 45-year-old woman who became the first long-term survivor after a heart–lung transplant. Heart–lung transplantation was initially used exclusively in patients with pulmonary vascular disease usually secondary to congenital heart disease. It is only in the past few years that this procedure has been extended to patients with intrinsic lung disease. Double-lung transplantation and sequential bilateral lung transplantation were introduced by the Toronto group in early 1986.

PHYSIOLOGICAL CHANGES OF THE TRANSPLANTED LUNG

The lung is the only solid organ that is continuously exposed to atmospheric contaminants after transplantation. The risk of nosocomial infection therefore is high. In addition, other sources of infection are contained within the recipient that magnify the risk, e.g. the sinuses of patients with cystic fibrosis. Vagal fibres innervating the lung are divided during the transplant operation. This occurs at the level of the trachea for heart–lung transplantation, or at the level of the main stem bronchus for single-lung or bilateral single-lung transplantation. Because of the division of the vagal fibres, the cough reflex is absent. The lymphatic drainage of the lung is also divided. This may contribute to prolonged pleural drainage or the early accumulation of pleural effusions after chest tube removal, and secondary lung collapse.

VENTILATION AND PERFUSION

Blood flows preferentially to transplanted lung with its lower pulmonary vascular resistance. Perfusion scans show that over 95% of the blood flows into the transplanted lung in patients with pulmonary hypertension who undergo single-lung transplantation. The pulmonary artery pressure drops from systemic levels to near normal early after the transplantation. This decrease in right ventricular afterload leads to improvement in right heart contractility, decreased right ventricular dilation and a decrease in tricuspid regurgitation. However, ventilation is split between the transplanted and the native lung. This ventilation–perfusion mismatch becomes an acute clinical problem should the patient retain secretions and so impair ventilation in the transplanted lung, which receives nearly all the flow. Single-lung transplantation performed for emphysema may be complicated by hyperinflation of the native more compliant lung, with compression of the transplanted lung and cardiac embarrassment.

IMMEDIATE FUNCTION OF THE TRANSPLANTED LUNG

Ischaemic injury due to suboptimal preservation of the transplanted lung is largely responsible for early graft dysfunction. This is clinically manifest by hypoxaemia and pulmonary oedema, and radiologically by pulmonary infiltrates, perihilar flaring and pleural effusions. In addition, patients who undergo single-lung transplantation for pulmonary hypertension may show reperfusion oedema due to the increased blood flow through the transplanted lung.

INDICATIONS FOR LUNG TRANSPLANT
Recipient Selection

These procedures are offered only to those patients with end stage lung disease who have the best opportunity for long-term survival with capacity for full rehabilitation. With the availability of these procedures, careful tailoring of the transplant procedure for a specific disease entity and specific individuals has also developed as an important consideration.

All patients must have end stage pulmonary or cardiopulmonary disease leading to severe impairment of quality of life with a life expectancy of less than 2 years. Patients, although terminally ill, should be otherwise fit and free of other disease. Stability and a firm commitment to the idea of transplantation and a willingness to comply with the rigorous and often invasive medical management are prerequisites for placement on a transplant waiting list.

All patients undergo a thorough assessment of cardiopulmonary status including pulmonary function studies, quantitative ventilation and perfusion scans, and determination of lung compliance, exercise tolerance and supplemental oxygen requirements. ECGs are performed with Doppler-assisted calculation of pulmonary artery pressure.

11

Coronary angiography and right and left ventriculography are performed when clinically indicated for male patients above the age of 40 and female patients above the age of 45 years. All patients undergo a thorough psychological and sociological assessment before acceptance.

Absolute contraindications to heart–lung and lung transplantation include significant systemic or multisystem disease, active or systemic infection (excluding the lungs), significant hepatic and renal disease not attributable to cardiac output or hepatic congestion, morbid obesity or malnutrition, current tobacco or drug misuse, psychiatric illness, surgical or chemical pleurodesis (may not contraindicate single-lung transplantation), age above 50 for heart–lung and sequential double-lung transplantation and above 60 for single-lung transplantation, positivity for HIV and hepatitis B, and patients harbouring multiresistant organisms in the lung.

Donor Assessment

Only 10–15% of cardiac donors meet the strict criteria for acceptable heart–lung or lung donors. Most lung donors are also acceptable heart donors. Donors should ideally be under the age of 45 although donors up to 55 can be considered if otherwise suitable. There should be no history of cardiac or pulmonary trauma. Donors should have minimal or negative smoking history with a normal ECG and echocardiogram. Low dose inotropic support is acceptable. A clear chest film is a prerequisite. Bronchial aspirates should be clear with no fungi, yeasts or Gram-negative organisms. Satisfactory gas exchange as manifested with a partial pressure of arterial oxygen (PaO_2) greater than 13.3 kPa on 40% FiO_2 or a PaO_2 greater than 53.3 kPa on 100% inspired oxygen is mandatory, as is a peak inspiratory pressure of less than 4 kPa at 15 ml/kg tidal volume (V_T). A close size match between the recipient and the donor is essential for heart–lung and double-lung transplantation, as oversizing will result in atelectasis and hypoxaemia. For single-lung transplantation, especially on the left side, oversizing is allowed, the oversized lung having adequate room for expansion by depressing the diaphragm and the underlying stomach. Matching the donor and the recipient is based on measurements of chest X-rays or on the basis of predicted vital capacity. Organs from individuals positive for HIV or hepatitis B and C are not acceptable, neither are lungs from donors with extracranial malignancy.

HARVESTING HEART-LUNG BLOCK

The heart–lung block is removed from a multiorgan donor after taping and occluding the superior vena cava and the aorta. Cooling of the heart and lungs is achieved by simultaneously running 1 litre of cold cardioplegia into the aortic root and 4 litres of EuroCollins solution into the pulmonary artery of a 70 kg donor. The left atrial appendage is amputated to decompress the left side of the heart and prevent pulmonary oedema. The lung is ventilated while the fluid is running in. The superior and inferior venae cavae as well as the aorta are transected. The trachea is stapled and divided. The heart–lung block is dissected from the posterior mediastinum and the oesophagus. The heart–lung block can be used as such or it can be split into its three components ensuring adequate length of vascular cuffs and bronchi. The organs are then placed in plastic bags containing cold preservation solution and transported to the recipient hospital in an icebox.

SINGLE-LUNG TRANSPLANTATION

Single-lung transplantation is the procedure of choice for patients with pulmonary fibrosis, older patients with emphysema, patients with sarcoidosis or asbestosis with end stage pulmonary disease, and for selected patients with primary and secondary pulmonary hypertension with good left ventricular function and easily correctable congenital defects.

Single-lung transplantation is infrequently used in retransplant operations on patients who have undergone heart–lung transplantation previously and developed bronchiolitis.

Single-lung transplantation is specifically contraindicated in patients with bilateral septic lung conditions and those with irreversible right ventricular dysfunction.

Anaesthetic Considerations

Any discussion of surgical technique would be incomplete without addressing the challenging problems that these patients present to the anaesthetist. Preparation for operation includes positioning of a pulmonary artery flotation catheter in the non-transplanted lung. Additional monitoring includes pulse oximetry, arterial line, and continuous carbon dioxide monitoring of expired gases. Partial veno-arterial extracorporeal bypass (see Chapter 20) using a microporous membrane oxygenator is available for patients who cannot be adequately ventilated, become hypoxaemic, or develop haemodynamic instability during one-lung anaesthesia. Such partial bypass, using femoral cannulation, is required occasionally during single-lung transplantations for pulmonary fibrosis, and is rarely required in patients with emphysema.

Surgical Technique

A standard posterolateral thoracotomy is performed through the 5th intercostal space. The main pulmonary artery is encircled and temporarily clamped early in the procedure. If haemodynamic stability and gas exchange are maintained, the procedure is continued without cardiopulmonary bypass. The recipient lung is removed, leaving an adequate length of pulmonary artery and veins. The bronchus is divided just above the origin of the upper lobe orifice with minimal dissection to avoid disruption of the arterial supply to the bronchial anastomosis. The donor bronchus is trimmed two rings proximal to the origin of the upper lobe, and an end-to-end anastomosis created using continuous suture for the membranous portion and interrupted suture for the cartilaginous portion. Vascular clamps are placed on the recipient left atrium and pulmonary artery while performing the vascular anastomosis. Fibreoptic bronchoscopy is performed to evaluate the airway and document a satisfactory anastomotic lumen.

DOUBLE-LUNG TRANSPLANTATION

In bilateral sequential lung transplantation, the patient is placed in the supine position and the chest is opened through a clamp-shell incision extending from one mid-axillary line to the other. Bypass is frequently used for bilateral sequential lung transplantation. The presence of adhesions complicates the operative procedure. Patients with primary pulmonary hypertension rarely have any significant adhesions as do patients with Eisenmenger's syndrome (see page 302). The presence of extensive adhesions increases the length of operation and the amount of blood loss. The use of the bilateral thoracotomy incision greatly facilitates access to the inaccessible areas of adhesions and potential bleeding. The recipient lungs are removed and the donor lungs sequentially implanted using a technique identical to single-lung transplantation.

Following completion of the operation, bypass is discontinued, the lungs ventilated and the chest closed. The bilateral thoracotomy incision is a particularly uncomfortable incision. An epidural catheter is placed once the clotting abnormalities subsequent to cardiopulmonary bypass have returned to normal.

POST-OPERATIVE CARE FOR LUNG TRANSPLANT RECIPIENTS

Following lung operations, all patients are ventilated with positive end expiratory pressure (PEEP) and the lowest possible inspired oxygen compatible with adequate oxygenation. Diuresis is encouraged to reduce the tendency towards the development of pulmonary oedema. Throughout the early post-operative phase, volume loading with clear fluids is avoided. Blood volume is maintained with colloid infusion. Patients are extubated on the basis of clear chest X-ray and satisfactory gas exchange.

HEART–LUNG TRANSPLANTATION

INDICATIONS

Heart–lung transplantation is the treatment of choice for patients with:

- Pulmonary hypertension and severe right ventricular dysfunction due to uncorrectable congenital heart disease (Eisenmenger's syndrome).
- Primary pulmonary hypertension with ventricular dysfunction.
- Cases with severe concurrent cardiac and pulmonary disease.

SURGICAL TECHNIQUE

After median sternotomy and institution of total cardiopulmonary bypass, the heart is removed in the same fashion as for orthotopic heart transplantation. Each lung is then removed separately preserving the phrenic, the vagi and the recurrent laryngeal nerves. The trachea is divided immediately above the carina. Meticulous haemostasis in the posterior mediastinum must be achieved. The combined heart–lung graft is then positioned in the chest. The tracheal anastomosis is performed first. The donor right atrium is then opened to match the recipient atrial cuff. After completion of the right atrial anastomosis, the donor and recipient aorta are trimmed and anastomosed end-to-end.

COMPLICATIONS OF LUNG TRANSPLANTATION

Early Post-operative Complications

Haemorrhage and graft dysfunction are the leading causes of early morbidity and mortality following heart–lung transplantation. Patients undergoing heart–lung transplantation with adhesions due to infection or previous surgery are prone to haemorrhage. Airway complications due to tracheal anastomosi breakdown are unusual due to the retention of coronary to bronchial collateral flow through the intact posterior pericardium in the heart–lung block.

Immunosuppression

Immunosuppression in heart–lung and lung transplantation is broadly similar to that used for cardiac transplantation. Centre to centre variations exist in the usage of cytolytic therapy and steroid dosages. Cyclosporin therapy is commenced as soon as renal function is satisfactory. Patients with cystic fibrosis need much larger and more frequent doses of oral cyclosporin given to achieve satisfactory blood level.

Rejection

Rejection in the early post-operative phase after heart–lung and lung transplantation is frequent and often symptomatic in contrast to its incidence and asymptomatic nature early on after heart transplantation. Furthermore, acute lung rejection can be very rapidly progressive and lead to a marked deterioration in the patient's clinical condition within the space of a few hours. Symptoms of rejection include fever, lethargy and shortness of breath. Auscultation of the chest often reveals bilateral basal crackles. Pulse oximetry shows desaturation often despite oxygen therapy. There are infiltrates, septal lines and effusions on chest X-ray. Infections of the lung after transplantation are a major cause of morbidity and mortality. Signs and symptoms of infection can often mimic rejection although the presence of a productive cough and purulent sputum is more in favour of infection. In rejection, cough is usually non-productive. Differentiation between rejection and infection which may co-exist requires broncho-alveolar lavage (BAL) and transbronchial biopsy. Multiple biopsies from multiple segments of the transplanted lungs are obtained for histological examination. Rejection is considered to be present if there are no organisms in the BAL and if histological changes of acute rejection are present on the biopsy specimen. Treatment of acute rejection consists of a 3-day course of prednisolone 15 mg/kg/day. This treatment usually results in prompt improvement of symptoms, both clinical and radiological, within the space of 24 hours. Repeated episodes of rejection or failure of resolution, despite steroid therapy, require more aggressive therapy with cytolytic agents

In heart–lung recipients, pulmonary rejection is far more frequent than cardiac rejection. Transbronchial biopsies are carried out at increasing intervals following heart–lung and lung transplantation and whenever it is clinically indicated on the basis of a 20% decrease in the daily measured forced expiratory volume in 1 second (FEV_1) or with the development of symptoms and signs suggestive of rejection. Transbronchial biopsy is a relatively safe procedure. However, occasionally it can result in the production of a pneumothorax which may require a chest tube insertion for its treatment. Haemorrhage from a transbronchial biopsy is uncommon but can be troublesome. The incidence of this complication can be reduced by attending to any clotting disorder before proceeding with the biopsy.

Late Complications

Infection of the lung after transplantation is a major source of morbidity and mortality. The lung is exposed to contamination through its free communication with the atmosphere, as well as being liable to infection from other sources such as the nasal sinuses of patients with cystic fibrosis. The infections are most frequently caused by bacteria, followed by viruses, particularly CMV, and less commonly fungi and protozoa. Unless diagnosed and treated early, infections in immunosuppressed patients can have catastrophic consequences. Hence early detection and aggressive treatment are of paramount importance. Close and regular clinical, radiological and microbiological surveillance of the patient with early resort to transbronchial biopsy and BAL will lead to early diagnosis and appropriate treatment for bacteriological, fungal or viral infection.

Airway Problems

Tracheal anastomosis in heart–lung transplantation has historically been relatively free from the problems that plague anastomosis in single-lung transplantation, due to better blood supply of the anastomosis contained in the heart–lung block that comes from the circumflex coronary artery. The commonest anastomotic problem encountered these days is narrowing at the site of the bronchial anastomosis in single or bilateral sequential lung transplantation. However, this complication is unusual and is treated by the insertion of a stent across the bronchial stricture. The problem presents with dyspnoea, and is reflected by significant deterioration in the FEV_1.

A major complication of heart–lung and lung transplantation is the development of irreversible widespread and severe obliteration of the small air passages in the lung. This is a rapidly progressive inflammatory disorder of unknown aetiology. Progressive, often irreversible, deterioration in lung function affects a substantial proportion of heart–lung and lung transplant patients. The incidence varies from 10 to 54%. The disease mostly presents towards the end of the first year although it can occur at any time after the first month. The chest X-ray appearances are not helpful. Transbronchial biopsy is not invariably diagnostic. The diagnosis rests on progressive deterioration of lung function. Occasionally the progress of the disease may be halted by augmentation of immunosuppression. However, in the majority of cases the disease progresses inexorably and leads to recurrence of the symptoms which initially prompted transplantation. The only available and effective treatment for patients with a progressive form of this disease is re-transplantation.

RESULTS IN HEART-LUNG AND LUNG TRANSPLANTATION

Currently, heart–lung transplant recipients can expect 70% survival at 1 year and 60% at 3 years. The results are not significantly different for cystic fibrosis patients treated with heart–lung transplantation. It is interesting to note that cystic fibrosis does not recur in the transplanted lungs. With single-lung transplantation, survival rates of 67% at 1 year, 58% at 2 years and 50% at 3 years have been noted in nearly 2500 patients. Bilateral lung transplantation has a similar survival record at 2 years. The vast majority of patients undergoing double-lung transplantations are younger patients with emphysema and cystic fibrosis in whom the operation is rapidly replacing heart–lung transplantation as the procedure of choice.

FUTURE DEVELOPMENTS IN LUNG TRANSPLANTATION

The scarcity of donors and the significant mortality of recipients on waiting lists, as well as the desire of close relatives of small transplant patients to donate parts of their lungs, led to the development of lobar transplantation with the adult transplanted lobe functioning as a single-lung transplant. This procedure has been carried out in a small number of patients successfully. The procedure has merits in that it alleviates the donor shortage problem and provides the transplant recipient with a somewhat better matched organ. Long-term results are awaited. If favourable, the use of the procedure is likely to increase despite the ethical problems involved in using live donors.

PHYSIOTHERAPY AND TRANSPLANT SURGERY

Cardiopulmonary transplantation is accepted as a proven therapy for end stage heart and lung disease. In recent years particularly, some relaxation of criteria combined with improved selection and management of both donor and recipient has increased the number of transplants that it is possible to carry out with the available donor offers. Improvements in organ preservation, immunosuppressive regimens, and the prophylaxis, diagnosis and treatment of infective complications have increased the numbers and longevity of the transplant population. The physiotherapist has therefore an opportunity to work and carry out research within a dedicated multidisciplinary team in an expanding and challenging setting with patients who have sometimes complex management problems.

PRE-OPERATIVE PHASE

TREATMENT

Potential transplant recipients are admitted for 3–5 days for assessment before any offer of surgery. This period may be extended if necessary to optimise the patient's condition before investigations or to observe the effects of change in medication. These patients will be seen by most members of the multidisciplinary team, i.e. physician, surgeon, transplant nurse specialist, transplant co-ordinator, dietitian, medical social worker and physiotherapist. Necessary medical investigations will be carried out. The patient and his or her spouse/partner will receive information regarding the operative, post-operative and early out-patient follow-up, and be able to view the hospital transplant facilities. During discussion, anxieties about transplantation which have no real basis in fact can be relieved.

PHYSIOTHERAPY

Aims

The aims of pre-operative physiotherapy are to:
- Reduce anxiety about the post-operative phase through discussing post-operative goals.
- Maintain muscle strength and exercise tolerance.
- Regain joint range and muscle extensibility, and improve posture.
- Offer support with advice about activities of daily living, social activities and relaxation techniques.
- Build a rapport with the patient and his or her partner.
- Provide documentation for future reference.

The written assessment will consist of the patient's present condition, relevant medical history, social history, physical capabilities, mobility, need for walking aids, lung function and attitude to transplantation, and is kept on record if the patient is accepted on to the transplant programme. Active cycle of breathing techniques, forced expiratory technique, positioning and supported cough are taught. Respiratory assessment will be followed by chest clearance as necessary. Even at this late stage, patients using inhalers should have their technique checked. The position of incisions, intravenous catheters and 'drips', drains and endotracheal tubes, and types of analgesia will be explained. It is explained that in lung transplantation, the lungs will be denervated below the level of the anastomosis with the result that there may be decreased awareness of the presence of secretions.

All patients for transplant will be New York Heart Association (NYHA) scale grade 4, i.e. symptoms at rest. They may be emotionally depressed as many have long-term disease and increasing exercise limitation. Most worrying are those patients who have no future goals and view transplant as a delay in their inevitable demise. These patients will be less motivated to comply with rehabilitation and may make a less than optimal recovery. Exercise may be anathema to some patients and every opportunity should be taken to educate the patient regarding the importance of exercise on health and fitness, not only in the immediate post-operative period but also in the long-term. The patient can then make an informed choice about changing his or her post-transplant lifestyle to include regular exercise. It is important to include the partner in these discussions as his or her anxiety and disapproval of the rehabilitation programme will hinder even the most determined of patients.

Advanced heart (or lung) failure may result in multi-organ insufficiency from hypoxia, muscle and adipose tissue loss, hypoalbuminaemia, malabsorption, nausea and vomiting and anorexia. Risk of mortality and post-operative complications increase with each of these problems. For the same ejection fraction of 15% in stable cardiac patients, exercise tolerance may vary. The reasons for the variance are not only due to haemodynamic dysfunction; non-cardiac factors such as muscle deconditioning also influence exercise capacity. Patients in advanced congestive cardiac failure have disordered muscle metabolism with rapid depletion of phosphocreatine and greater intracellular acidosis during exercise (Stratton et al., 1994). These changes may also cause decreased exercise performance. A simple pre-operative exercise regimen complements optimal medical therapy and improvement in nutritional status to prepare the patient for the physical stress of the post-operative period. The patient will also be taking a more active role in the maintenance of his or her health. As a result a few high compliers have improved muscle strength and therefore exercise tolerance when they are admitted for transplant. There is no potential for improvement in cardiac or lung function at this stage but there may be some peripheral adaptation with increase in capillary and mitochondrial densities and a drop in minimum vascular resistance in skeletal muscle (Astrand and Rodahl, 1986). Independence returns more quickly after surgery particularly if leg strength is maintained. Following a simple exercise regimen from the pre-operative period helps to reduce anxiety about exercising post-operatively.

HEART PATIENT ASSESSMENT

Potential heart and heart–lung recipients are taught a simple regimen of breathing exercises. Patients in controlled heart failure may still have some pulmonary congestion and be more vulnerable to chest infections. Chest clearance is also taught with techniques outlined above, which may be repeated at home if necessary. The patient is educated to recognise the onset of a chest infection and to seek treatment promptly so that the risk of being rendered unsuitable when called for transplant is minimised. A home exercise regimen will be prescribed according to individual needs, and may include a leg muscle strengthening, walking or exercise cycle. These exercises can be taught while oxygen saturation is monitored. If the patient has been prescribed oxygen, this should always be used during exercise. A few patients who have continued to enjoy an active hobby up to the onset of serious illness manage to maintain their exercise tolerance through engaging in this preferred activity.

HEART–LUNG AND LUNG PATIENT ASSESSMENT

A 6 minute walk test is a useful addition to the assessment, particularly of potential heart–lung and lung transplant patients. This gives an accurate and reproducible assessment of the patient's exercise tolerance so that repeat tests during the waiting period can determine deterioration.

Ideally, potential lung or double-lung transplant recipients are assessed for transplant earlier in the disease process than are possible heart transplant recipients. This may allow for a more intensive exercise programme, although it is not unknown for a patient with long-term disease to have flexion contractures of the hips and knees because of sitting for most of the day. Inactivity will compound osteoporosis through steroid therapy. All patients will be instructed in breathing control, thoracic mobility exercises, light loading weight work, and quads, upper limb and trunk exercises. A regimen incorporating these exercises can be graded according to difficulty starting with exercises in supported long sitting, progressing to unsupported sitting and standing. Exercises are timed and carried out using a pulse oximeter so that the pace and number of repetitions within the timed interval is controlled by the rate at which the patient oxygen-desaturates during the exercise. Rest between each exercise is indicated by how long it takes for oxygen saturation to return to resting levels. Exercise can then be carried out at home at the same pace with the same timed rests between. Patients are advised always to exercise using oxygen if it has been prescribed. Symptoms of oxygen desaturation are discussed, i.e. not to continue with an exercise if excessive breathlessness, dizziness, palpitations or visual disturbance are experienced. Patients are instructed not to exercise if they are more than usually unwell or have an acute infection, and to exercise at the time of day when they feel at their best.

FOLLOW-UP

Exercise regimens are reviewed on an out-patient basis through contact with the patient's local hospital or community physiotherapist. Concomitant soft tissue and orthopaedic problems may be addressed at the same time. Exercise follow-up can also be accomplished by correspondence, with the patient filling in exercise charts. Contact can be maintained through the establishment of regular pre-operative support group meetings. Further detailed information regarding treatment and lifestyle post-operatively can be discussed as well as encouraging the patient to maintain social contacts. Advice regarding activities of daily living can be given. Relaxation techniques can also be taught at this forum, to the patient and his or her partner, taking the form of relaxation tapes or the teaching of massage techniques with or without the use of essential oils.

POST-OPERATIVE PHASE

TREATMENT

Aims of Post-operative Treatment

The aims of post-operative treatment are to:

- Remove and clear secretions from the airways.
- Assist weaning from the ventilator.
- Establish a good breathing pattern.
- Increase exercise tolerance and muscle strength, and continue to correct posture.
- Encourage independence.
- Begin the patient education programme.

Initial treatment progress is summarised in Table 11.1. These stages of treatment are typical of a routine heart or lung transplant patient post-operatively; heart–lung and double-lung transplant patients will lag behind by a few days. Treatment progress is entirely dependent on the patient's medical condition.

All transplant patients should have daily sputum samples sent for culture and sensitivity while they have a productive cough. Previous chest surgery may give rise to adhesions involving the recurrent laryngeal, vagus or phrenic nerves, that may cause these nerves to be damaged during further surgery. Chest physiotherapy techniques may have to be modified to accommodate these problems. Patients who have been unable to lie flat for years may take some time and reassurance to become confident enough to tolerate some chest drainage positions (Table 11.2).

Lung transplant patients are more vulnerable to pneumothorax and this should be borne in mind where positive pressure techniques are employed. Epidural or epipleural analgesia is employed for the first 3–4 days in addition to a morphine infusion. The physiotherapist may be able to provide a transcutaneous nerve stimulator where necessary to supplement pain relief. Occasionally, use of nasal intermittent positive pressure ventilation (NIPPV) may be made to aid the weaning process, preventing reintubation and reliance on long-term formal ventilation. Once patients with previously septic conditions such as cystic fibrosis or bronchiectasis have been extubated, nasopharyngeal suction should be avoided. Oropharyngeal suction should be applied if necessary. These patients have the same pathogenic organisms in their sinuses as once colonised their explanted lungs. Inevitably these organisms may migrate to the new lung, and nasopharyngeal suction could make this a certainty. As the patient is heavily immunosuppressed early in the post-operative period, these organisms may prove difficult to eradicate.

DIFFERENTIAL LUNG VENTILATION

Differential lung ventilation may be indicated after single-lung transplantation for emphysema if intermittent positive pressure ventilation (IPPV) is needed for more than a few hours. Gas delivered through the endotracheal tube under pressure will follow the path of least resistance into the remaining emphysematous lung because of the lack of elastic recoil of the lung tissue. This leads to hyperinflation, mediastinal shift, arrhythmias, and crushing of the new lung.

Differential lung ventilation (DLV) can be achieved by using a double lumen endobronchial tube which is divided lengthways by a central septum. A tracheal cuff is inflated above the carina, allowing the opening to ventilate one lung. The distal end of the tube is curved and cuffed, the tip passing into the right or left main bronchus. Once the bronchial cuff is inflated the lung is isolated from the other in terms of ventilation. Appropriate modes of ventilation can be applied to each lung; for example, the native lung may have a lower respiratory rate and V_T, and no PEEP delivered compared with the transplanted lung.

The ventilatory observations must be charted separately for each lung.

Daily treatment progress		
Post-operative day 1	On Intensive Care Unit	Respiratory assessment and chest physiotherapy as necessary Passively or actively assisted, or active movements as appropriate Document on patient's exercise chart
Post-operative days 2–3		Respiratory assessment, etc. as above Institute postural drainage where appropriate Chart increase in active movements Active transfer to chair Static pedals
Post-operative days 3–4	On ward	Chest treatment as above Independent transfers taught Add exercises in standing Short walk p.m.
Post-operative days 4–7		Chest treatment as appropriate Static cycle, increase walk distance and active exercise Stairs Patient documents exercise on chart

Table 11.1 **Daily treatment progress.**

Some observations on post-operative chest treatment	
Heart transplant	Median sternotomy Treatment as for open heart surgery, may be posturally drained if necessary
Heart–lung	Median sternotomy Check the level of the anastomosis with the anaesthetist/surgeon May be afforded some protection by position of endotracheal tube Postural drainage where necessary
Double lung	Trans-sternal incision More haemodynamically stable immediately postoperatively than heart–lung if the heart remains innervated Cardiac denervation can occur Postural drainage where necessary
Single lung	Thoracotomy incision Careful monitoring of fluid balance is needed as ease of circulation through the new lung may allow fluid overload to occur Differential lung ventilation may be required Postural drainage as required

Table 11.2 **Some observations on post-operative chest treatment.**

During physiotherapy, the native lung will be temporarily hyperinflated if bag squeezing is employed. This may quickly result in changes in heart rate and rhythm and a drop in blood pressure, indicating compression of the heart owing to mediastinal shift. This should resolve once DLV is recommended. If it does not, bag squeezing to the native lung may be contraindicated for subsequent treatments. Before and after treatment, observations of V_T, oxygen saturation and airways pressure may indicate that the problems are due to the tube being dislodged. If this is suspected it should be reported to the duty anaesthetist without delay.

Long suction catheters are needed to traverse the bronchial arm of the endobronchial tube. Owing to the small diameter on each side of the tube's central septum, size 10–12 catheters are used. This may lead to difficulties where excessive or tenacious secretions are present. If bronchoscopy becomes necessary to remove secretions, the patient must be extubated and re-intubated after the procedure.

Samples of sputum obtained during physiotherapy should be labelled as to whether they are from the right or left lung.

It is not possible to support the endobronchial tube satisfactorily if the patient is left in side lying and therefore positioning is restricted to supine lying leading to difficulties in mobilising and clearing secretions.

During this immediate post-operative period, the patient may be assessed many times during the day by various members of the transplant team. It is vital that all observations and changes in the patient's condition noted by the physiotherapist are conveyed to the rest of the team. As the patients are immunosuppressed they will be vulnerable to infection, particularly during the first 3 months, and the physiotherapist should be vigilant in looking out for signs and symptoms of the onset of infection. As well as bacterial infection, this group of patients are subject to infection with mycobacterial, viral, fungal and protozoal organisms.

Aims of Rehabilitation

The aims of rehabilitation are to:
- Continue to increase exercise tolerance and muscle strength.
- Continue with joint mobilisation and posture correction where necessary.
- Educate the patient to recognise and report significant symptoms.
- Give written advice with explanation regarding resumption of activities of daily living.
- Increase the patient's confidence to increase his or her own exercise programme.
- Facilitate independent activity and return to previous hobbies/occupation.

Heart patients will exercise in the physiotherapy gymnasium from 5 to 7 days after transplant, following the first endomyocardial biopsy to detect any rejection. Transbronchial biopsies via bronchoscopy are not carried out on the heart–lung and lung transplant patients until 3 weeks

post-operatively unless there is an indication of rejection. Therefore these patients come to the gymnasium as soon as they are independent of oxygen or are able to carry out a programme of exercises on oxygen without a deleterious drop in their oxygen saturation. At this stage patients are encouraged to dress each day in clothing appropriate for exercise. As soon as possible, they will walk independently to each department for the day's investigations, and will become self-medicating on the ward. Walking in the hospital grounds is encouraged. All patients, except those who live nearby, spend a week or more in bungalows in the hospital grounds before being discharged home. They may also leave the hospital vicinity to shop or socialise as their individual case dictates. These practices encourage patients to think of themselves as individuals working towards good health and independence rather than as patients dependent on hospital staff. The patient's partner is always invited to accompany the patient to each department in order to increase his or her knowledge and confidence about transplant, and to encourage the patient in his or her endeavours.

New transplant patients need constant reassessment as most progress quite rapidly at this stage. Patient education begins with the effects of denervation of the heart and the importance of warm up and cool down activities for all groups of patients. Exercise will be aimed at strengthening specific muscle groups, gradually increasing resistance using proprioceptive neuromuscular facilitation (PNF) techniques, light weights and then a multigym. More dynamic aerobic exercise is added with use of the treadmill, step ups and cycling with resistance. Weight resistance and repetitions/time taken for an exercise are recorded on the patient's exercise chart, and an extra exercise or a few extra repetitions can usually be added each day so that the patient can see his or her progress in writing. Arm exercises are included as pain and wound stability allow. If the patient is unable to progress his or her exercises or has to cut back, he or she may be rejecting and enquiries should be made regarding other relevant symptoms. Once rejection is confirmed, the significance of the symptoms is discussed with the patient. In this way the patient will learn to recognise what is significant. This is one of the hardest and most worrying aspects of transplantation for new patients.

REJECTION

During a severe acute rejection episode when the myocardium is oedematous and is subject to cellular infiltration and myofibre injury, exercise is restricted to limit permanent myocardial damage. There are no typical chest X-ray appearances of lung rejection, although there may be a visible increase in infiltrates and the hilar regions (hilar flare) in established rejection. There will also be decreased gas exchange, worsening lung function tests and increased shortness of breath, and temperature in the absence of infection. On confirmation by transbronchial biopsy, augmenting immunosuppression gives rapid improvement. Once these patients are largely pain free, a pocket spirometer is issued so that the patient begins to monitor and report changes in the peak expiratory flow rate (PEFR), FEV and forced vital capacity (FVC). In conjunction, they are taught to use an effective huff to detect the presence of secretions in the denervated lung below the level of the anastomosis. A productive huff should be followed up with appropriate drainage techniques and the quality and quantity of secretions reported immediately. (Heart transplant patients referred for rehabilitation who are a few years post-operative will need to be carefully screened and exercise tested before any programme of vigorous exercise, as diffuse widespread coronary disease may have developed as part of a chronic rejection process. As the heart is denervated, this will not be heralded by warning anginal pain.) Recording of ECG, heart rate, oxygen saturation and blood pressure is taken before exercise.

Signs of Rejection

Signs of rejection include:

- A rise in temperature above 37°C, which is sustained.
- Ankle swelling, general fluid retention and decreased urine output.
- A sudden weight gain of 2 kg or more over 2 consecutive days.
- Shortness of breath on exertion.
- Generally feeling unwell.
- Mood swings.
- Fatigue at a level of exercise which does not usually cause a problem.
- Lack of appetite.
- Bronchospasm or coughs.
- Heart–lung and lung transplant patients may notice a 10% or more decrease in spirometry values.

As the heart rate and blood pressure response to exercise is attenuated where there is cardiac denervation, these values cannot be used to determine end points for exercise. For all patients the Borg Scale of rate of perceived exertion (RPE) is used instead. As this is introduced to the patient in the pre-operative phase, the patient will have become used to using it for self-monitoring purposes. It will become useful to gauge the level of activity at home and in the work situation, and to help to pitch activity at the right level when resuming an exercise programme following an episode of rejection. Following warm up exercises with stretches, exercise intensity is gradually increased, working at levels 9–11 (very light to light), and increasing in the middle of the programme to level 13 (somewhat hard) (see page 141). Before discharge home, a comprehensive written discharge summary, with appropriate contact telephone numbers, covering all aspects of medical follow-up, self-care, work and social activities is discussed with the patient. Guidelines of activities (Table 11.3) which allow time for the chest to heal are taken from this.

Patients should gain permission from the transplant officer before resuming contact sports such as karate and rugby. Patients are also advised to avoid public swimming baths, Turkish baths and saunas for the first 3–6 months after surgery because of the risk of infection. Some single-lung transplant patients (those treated for emphysema) have found that the imbalance between their new and remaining lung causes their non-operated side to roll uppermost in the water so that it is more difficult to maintain their chosen stroke or position in the water.

On Discharge

Before discharge, ongoing rehabilitation needs and realistic goals are discussed. Some emphasis is placed on the American College of Sports Medicine guidelines (1990) regarding the need for aerobic exercise to be undertaken at least three times a week for 20–30 minutes in order for benefit to be derived. Some patients will need further supervision and will be referred to their local hospital, others feel confident and sufficiently motivated to continue on their own or use their local leisure facilities, in which case a letter is supplied to enable them to approach the resident instructor. This transplant centre has an established transplant games team that participates in all of the annual transplant games and tournaments. Patients often become drawn into these activities because of the camaraderie only to find that they have become committed to the weekly practice sessions.

EFFECTS AND BENEFITS OF EXERCISE

Thoracic organ transplant patients have impaired physical fitness for a number of reasons. In addition to those discussed earlier, drug therapy with corticosteroids and diuretics decreases bone mineral content, accelerating osteoporotic changes which may have begun after the menopause, through ageing and inactivity. Corticosteroids also exacerbate lean tissue loss. Some antibiotics are known to cause tendinitis, which may lead to spontaneous tendon rupture. Cardiac denervation gives rise to resting tachycardia and decreased left ventricular ejection fraction, and contributes to subnormal exercise tolerance. There is a possibility that there is residual left ventricular dysfunction related to the process of brain death in the donor, organ preservation at the time of transplantation and subsequent episodes of cardiac rejection (Banner et al., 1989). Resting hypertension may be present as a result of renal tubular dysfunction caused by cyclosporin therapy or as a result of persisting chronic elevation of noradrenaline levels which occurred in pre-operative congestive cardiac failure.

In the normal individual at the outset of dynamic exercise, cardiac output will increase through the immediate rise in heart rate by sympathetic stimulation and a simultaneous increase in stroke volume. In the denervated heart, there is no immediate rise in heart rate through sympathetic stimulation during the first stage of exercise. The resting tachycardia implies a low stroke volume, therefore there is potential for some increase in cardiac output through increased stroke volume of up to 20%. This is brought about by muscle pump action of the working limbs and respiratory muscle pump action of increased ventilation increasing pre-load (Frank–Starling mechanism) (Pflugfelder et al., 1987).

Ten minutes into dynamic exercise, circulating plasma catecholamine levels have risen but their chronotrophic action is insufficient to increase myocardial contractility to the same degree as sympathetic stimulation. Heart rate and blood pressure responses to exercise are therefore attenuated and are not used to determine end limits during exercise therapy.

On ceasing exercise, there is no vagus nerve to moderate the heart rate. Endogenous catecholamines remain in the circulation for 10–15 minutes before being broken down (Yusef *et al.*, 1989). Decreased venous return coupled with a persisting tachycardia during this period can cause a drop in cardiac output below baseline levels. It is therefore important for the patient to perform cool down exercises following activity which has raised the heart rate.

Despite differences in cardiac dynamics, exercise training has potential for improving the quality of life of transplant patients. Benefits are similar to those seen in normal subjects. Heart rate, blood pressure, minute ventilation and RPE are decreased at submaximal workloads. Heart rate and blood pressure are reduced at rest. At exhaustion, peak heart rate, peak power output, peak rate of oxygen consumption (VO_{2max}) are increased but less so than in normal controls (Pflugfelder *et al.*, 1987; Kavanagh *et al.*, 1988; Keteyian *et al.*, 1989). Some

reversal of bone loss and myopathic changes will also take place. The patients also enjoy an enhanced sense of wellbeing as rehabilitation progresses.

Studies of untrained cardiac recipients and matched normal controls undergoing exercise with increasing workloads showed that the transplant recipients terminate exercise at a lower heart rate, with lower blood lactate levels and respiratory exchange ratio. These findings are indicative of limitations of non-oxygen-dependent peripheral skeletal muscle during exercise performance. Consequently, strengthening of peripheral muscle seems to be the major contributor to the effects observed after training. Peripheral adaptation accounts for improved power output and, because of later onset of anaerobiosis, reduced RPE and minute ventilation during submaximal exercise (Kavanagh *et al.*, 1988). Rehabilitation programmes should therefore aim to increase muscle strength as well as cardio-respiratory endurance.

In a study of 36 orthotopic heart transplant patients, Kavanagh (1988) noted that eight highly compliant subjects had a decreased heart rate at rest following training. Vagal inhibitory tone cannot be responsible for this decrease as there is no evidence that reinnervation of the heart occurs.

Guidelines for activity	
Up to 6 weeks post-operatively	Do not lift anything weighing more than 11–22 kg. Avoid carrying shopping and picking up babies and toddlers. Avoid the weight of heavy shop and freezer doors. Begin light activities in the house including light washing by hand, ironing small items, bed making, washing dishes and gentle sweeping. Keep RPE during activity at 9–12
At 6 weeks post-operatively	Driving may be resumed (gain permission from the transplant officer). Start lifting slightly heavier weights; increase gradually. Still avoid the handling of heavy items of wet washing, i.e. pulling them out of a washing machine, and changing bedclothes. RPE up to 12 when exercising
At 8 weeks post-operatively	You may resume hanging out the washing, folding sheets and changing bed linen and light work in the garden, e.g. planting and weeding using a trowel—avoid excess weed pulling, and wash hands thoroughly afterwards. RPE up to 13
At 12 weeks post-operatively	You may travel on public transport. Gardening can now include digging, hoeing and raking. Resume sports, e.g. cycling, swimming, bowling and putting and practise golf swing, fishing and dancing. Allow RPE up to 13
At 16 weeks post-operatively	Resume walking a dog on a lead. Gardening may include mowing the lawn and hedge cutting. Sports may include golf, badminton, tennis and jogging. It is not recommended that you take up jogging as a new pastime. RPE 13 (somewhat hard) to 15 (hard)
RPE, rate of perceived exertion using the Borg Scale	

Table 11.3 Guidelines for activity.

It may be that with training there is a significant reduction in effort-induced levels of serum noradrenaline or that there is a down-regulation in sensitivity of myocardial β-receptors.

The physiological consequences of lung denervation have been discussed earlier in this chapter. Recipients of heart–lung transplants have an exercise capacity and cardiac dynamics similar to those of matched cardiac transplant recipients (Banner et al., 1989). Because these two groups show similar performance, the overall exercise limitation is likely to be related to circulatory and cardiac causes rather than the lungs. No ventilatory limitation to exercise has been found in heart–lung or lung transplant patients (Miyoshi et al., 1990; Grassi et al., 1993; Levy et al., 1993). Ventilation and oxygen uptake increase immediately on exercise to normal or even exaggerated levels (Banner et al., 1989) in the absence of normal circulatory response to exercise. This goes against the concept that ventilation is causally linked to right ventricular output and work. Levy and co-workers (1993) found indications that double-lung recipients following vigorous rehabilitation showed superior peak exercise capacity compared with heart–lung and single-lung recipients, but the study group was too small to demonstrate statistical significance.

CONCLUSIONS

In the initial period following a straightforward recovery from transplant, the patient may feel miraculously better. Euphoria combined with an overnight increase in exercise tolerance and ability to cope with activities of daily living leads especially the least debilitated patients to think that they are 'cured' and that the treatment phase is over. Without a rehabilitation programme patients may be discharged without realising how unfit they are and that they could improve much further. On discharge, because of low peak oxygen uptake, attempts at exercise above the level already experienced are terminated quickly by fatigue. Discouraged, the patient would become weaker with further lean tissue loss and ever decreasing exercise tolerance, anxiety and depression. It is essential that the physiotherapist's role as an educator and rehabilitation facilitator is carried through from the pre-operative period to beyond the immediate post-operative phase to maximise the cost effectiveness of the transplant programme and the quality of the outcome for the patient.

REFERENCES

Astrand PO, Rodahl K. *Textbook of work physiology*, 3rd ed. New York: McGraw-Hill; 1986.

Banner NR, Lloyd MH, Hamilton RD, Innes JA, Guz A, Yacoub MH. Cardiopulmonary response to dynamic excercise after heart and combined heart-lung transplantation. *Br Heart J* 1989, **61(3):**215-223.

Grassi B, Ferretti G, Xi L, *et al*. Ventilatory response to excercise after heart and lung denervation in humans. *Respir Physiol* 1993, **92(3):**289-304.

Kavanagh T, Yacoub MH, Mertens DJ, *et al*. Cardiorespiratory responses to exercise training after orthotopic cardiac transplantation. *Circulation* 1988, **77(1):**162-171.

Keteyian S, Purves PD, McKensie FN, Kstuck WJ. Exercise following cardiac transplantation: recommendations for rehabilitation. *Sports Med* 1989, **8(5):**251-259.

Levy RD, Ernst P, Levine SM, *et al*. Exercise performance after lung transplantation. *J Heart Lung Transplant* 1993, **12:**(1 pt 1):27-33.

Miyoshi S, Truloch EP, Schaefers HJ, Hsieh CM, Patterson GA, Cooper JD. Cardiopulmonary exercise testing after single and double lung transplantation. *Chest* 1990, **97(5):**1130-1136.

Pflugfelder PW, Purves PD, McKensie FN, Kostuk WJ. Cardiac dynamics during supine exercise in cyclosporine-treated orthotopic heart transplant recipients: assessment by radionuclide angiography. *J Am Coll Cardiol* 1987, **10(2):**336-341.

Stratton JR, Dunn JF, Adamopoulos S, Kemp GJ, Coats AJ, Rajagopalan B. Training partially reverses skeletal muscle abnormalities during exercise in heart failure. *J Appl Physiol* 1994, **76:**1575-1582.

Yusef S, Theodoropoulos S, Dhalla N, *et al*. Influence of beta blockade on exercise capacity and heart rate response after human orthotopic and heterotopic cardiac transplantation. *Am J Cardiol* 1989, **64:**646-641.

GENERAL READING

Baue A, Cooper JA, eds. Lung transplantation. In: *Glenn's thoracic and cardiovascular surgery*, 5th ed. Connecticut: Appleton Lange; 1991:441-457.

Brown ME, Oyer PE. Donor heart-lung retrieval. In: Phillips MG, ed. *Organ procurement, preservation, and distribution in transplantation*. Richmond: William Byrd Press; 1991:90-95.

Emery RW, Pritzker MR, eds. *Cardiothoracic transplantation. Cardiac surgery: state of the art reviews*. Philadelphia: Hanley and Belfus; 1988:**2(4)**.

Emery RW, Pritzker MR, Eales F, eds. *Cardiothoracic transplantation II. Cardiac surgery: state of of the art reviews*. Philadelphia: Hanley and Belfus; 1989:**2(3)**.

Kaiser LR, Cooper JD. The current status of lung transplantation. *Adv Surg* 1992, **25:**259-307.

Kempeneers G, Noakes TD, van Zyl-Smit R, *et al*. Skeletal muscle limits the exercise tolerance of renal transplant recipients: effects of a graded exercise training program. *Am J Kidney Dis* 1990, **16(1):**57-65.

Reichart B, Jamieson SW. *Heart and heart-lung transplantation. Orthotopic and heterotopic techniques*. Munich: Verlag-Schulz; 1990.

Renlund DG, Bristow MR, Lee HR, O'Connell JB. Medical aspects of cardiac transplantation. *J Cardiothorac Anesth* 1988, **2:**500-512.

Report of the Medical Consultants on the Diagnoses of Death to the President's Commission for the Study of Ethical Problems in Medicine. *JAMA* 1981, **246:**2184-2186.

Smith JA, McCarthy PM, Sarris GE, Stimson EB, Reitz BA, eds. In: *The Stanford manual of cardiopulmonary transplantation*. London: Futura; 1996.

Starnes VA, Baldwin JC, Harjula A. Combined heart and lung transplantation: the Stanford experience. *J Appl Cardiol* 1987, **2:**71-89.

Thompson ME, ed. *Cardiac transplantation*. Philadelphia: FA Davies; 1990.

Young JB, Leon CA, Lawrence EC, Whisennand HH, Noon GP, DeBakey ME. Heart replacement for terminal cardiac disease: cardiac transplantation and mechanical sustenance of the cardiovascular system—Part I. *Baylor Cardiol Ser* 1989, **12(2):**4-27.

Young JB, Leon CA, Lawrence EC, Whisennand HH, Noon GP, DeBakey ME. Heart replacement for terminal cardiac disease: cardiac transplantation and mechanical sustenance of the cardiovascular system—Part II. *Baylor Cardiol Ser* 1989, **12(3):**4-27.

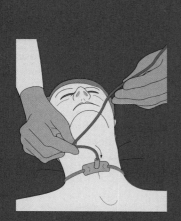

12
M Danton, J A McGuigan
& M Smith

THORACIC TRAUMA

CHAPTER OUTLINE

- Basic mechanisms of traumatic injury
- The chest wall
- The pleural space
- The diaphragm
- The heart
- The lungs
- The trachea and major bronchi
- The cervical trachea
- Thoracic aortic rupture
- The oesophagus
- The thoracic duct
- Management techniques
- Physiotherapy and the chest trauma patient
- Physiotherapy management

BASIC MECHANISMS OF TRAUMATIC INJURY

In the assessment of thoracic trauma, an appreciation of the mechanism of injury is important as the pattern of injury is dependent on the type of insult sustained. Injury to the thorax can result from blunt or penetrating trauma.

Blunt trauma to the chest causes injury by compression/crushing or deceleration. Compressional force results in physical deformity of the tissue, and when this exceeds the limits of elasticity and viscosity, injury ensues. This mechanism of injury typically causes fractures to the skeletal frame comprising the ribs, sternum and vertebrae. With increasing force, contusion of the underlying lungs and heart occurs. Extreme compressional force can injure the descending thoracic aorta. Deceleration injury, typical of vehicular trauma, causes injury by inducing a state of relative motion within a structure. The classic example of this mechanism is tearing of the aortic isthmus, the junction between the arch and the descending thoracic aorta. The descending thoracic aorta is fixed to the left paravertebral gutter by parietal pleura in contrast to the aortic arch which is untethered and relatively free to move. On abrupt deceleration, the reduction in velocity of forward motion of the thorax and descending aorta is less than that relative to the arch, inducing shearing forces maximally applied to the isthmus.

The type of injury induced by penetrating trauma is dependent on the velocity, mass and area of impact of the penetrating object. Low velocity injuries, stab wounds and handguns, cause direct laceration to the tissue and when a vital organ, such as the heart, lungs or great thoracic vessels, is penetrated this can prove fatal. With high velocity penetrating injuries the kinetic energy is dissipated as the missile decelerates, causing cavitation in the surrounding structures. This cavitational injury tends to have a greater effect when the missile penetrates dense tissue such as the liver.

INITIAL ASSESSMENT AND MANAGEMENT

The priority of resuscitation is to establish a patent airway and achieve adequate lung ventilation and sufficient cardiac output for vital organ perfusion. Airway patency can be compromised by trauma to the face and neck. In patients in whom there is upper airways obstruction, stridor and hoarseness may be evident. Patients in whom ventilation is compromised present with respiratory distress. The patient will frequently be confused, restless and often difficult to manage due to a combination of pain and hypoxia. The rate of breathing is significantly increased and intercostal muscle retraction and use of accessory muscles of respiration are initiated as the work of breathing increases.

Establishment of an airway may be achieved by various methods appropriate to the clinical situation. A simple oro- or nasopharyngeal airway can be readily inserted, and is of particular benefit in patients with a depressed level of consciousness due to a co-existing head injury. In this situation the tongue tends to flop back occluding the larynx, and a correctly positioned airway prevents such movement. In patients where there is a likelihood of aspiration of material, e.g. blood, mucus, vomitus, or in whom the possibility of mechanical/assisted ventilation is required, orotracheal intubation with a cuffed endotracheal tube is employed. The correct positioning of such a tube requires the clinician to extend the neck in order to visualise the larynx, and in patients with a suspected cervical spinal injury this can be hazardous. In such a situation nasotracheal intubation may be preferred as neck extension is not required for its placement. With severe facial or laryngeal trauma, oral or nasal intubation may not be possible and surgical access to the trachea is required. The procedure of choice is the tracheostomy, in which a lower midline transverse neck incision is made, the trachea identified and an opening made between the second and fourth tracheal rings. The trachea is then directly intubated with a cuffed tracheostomy tube (see page 97 for examples of airways).

Following establishment of a secure airway, attention should be turned to impaired ventilation. The chest is carefully inspected for reduced and paradoxical movements, as occur with flail segments (see below). Penetrating wounds and surgical emphysema should be noted. Auscultation of the chest may detect decreased air entry into one hemithorax. Provided the patient's condition is not *in extremis*, an erect anteroposterior film chest X-ray should be quickly performed in the emergency room. Pneumothorax or haemothorax should be treated by a correctly placed intrapleural drain; this will allow the lung to re-expand. Pain, caused by chest wall trauma, rib fractures, etc., is another common cause of impaired ventilation, and should be adequately controlled. However, excessive systemic narcotic analgesia may lead to central nervous depression and consequently reduced breathing so a careful balance must be achieved, particularly in the elderly patient who is sensitive to such medication. If following these measures ventilation is not adequate for the patient, mechanical ventilation may be required.

An inadequate cardiac output is determined by the presence of a weak and thready pulse, tachycardia and hypotension with cool peripheries. Following thoracic trauma this is the result of either inadequate venous return to the heart, or direct injury to the heart causing myocardial contusion and cardiac failure. Inadequate venous return is commonly a consequence of blood loss and hypovolaemia exacerbated by excessive fluid restriction. It can also occur with mediastinal displacement following tension pneumothorax

when the venous return to the heart is obstructed. Cardiac tamponade, in which blood escapes from a penetrated/injured heart into the pericardial cavity, will cause impaired venous return by compressing the atria, impeding their filling. Clinical examination of the jugular venous pressure (JVP) will give reliable information as to the cause of inadequate venous return because in hypovolaemia the JVP will be low, whereas in tension pneumothorax, pericardial tamponade or cardiac failure it will tend to be elevated.

Good venous access should be established and the administration of fluid adequate to replace the lost circulating volume and improve cardiac output. Advanced trauma life support (ATLS; American College of Surgeons) protocols advise 2 litres of clear fluids (crystalloid and colloid) as the initial fluid followed by blood transfusion if further circulatory expansion is required. Certain reservations have been expressed in this practice, particularly in the setting of major thoracic trauma. In a patient who has sustained a stab wound to the heart, or aortic rupture, such rapid transfusion may provoke a secondary haemorrhage with devastating results. A relatively stable hypotensive young patient may re-bleed and exsanguinate as a consequence. Furthermore, such clear fluids have no oxygen-carrying capacity and have little effect on correcting tissue hypoxia. Finally, transfusion of large volumes of clear fluids may contribute to the development of adult respiratory distress syndrome (ARDS), a common sequel in the multiply injured patient. It is therefore advocated that the judicious transfusion of intravenous fluids is employed in thoracic trauma. Blood, because of its oxygen-carrying capacity, should be used early in the resuscitation. Blood transfusion is not without its own inherent risks. Future developments in alternative oxygen-carrying fluids may provide safe alternatives.

THE CHEST WALL

The chest wall comprises skin and subcutaneous tissue, a skeletal frame consisting of the ribs, sternum, vertebral column and musculature. The chest wall has two principal functions: firstly, protection of the underlying thoracic organs, and, secondly, a mechanical role in ventilation. Whenever significant trauma to the chest wall take place, injury to the underlying thoracic organs can occur which is of greater importance. Injury to the chest wall can result from both blunt and penetrating trauma.

RIB FRACTURES

Rib fractures result commonly from blunt trauma. The amount of force required to break ribs is dependent on the age of the patient and the particular rib(s) involved. Children's ribs are elastic and require considerable force before fracture will occur, whereas in the elderly patient, often with osteoporotic bone, only minimal force is needed. Fractures involving the first two ribs indicate major force as they are short, strong bones protected by the scapula, clavicle and chest wall musculature.

A diagnosis of rib fracture is suggested by a history of blunt thoracic trauma, chest wall pain aggravated by deep inspiration or coughing, and localised tenderness or crepitus. Postero-anterior chest X-ray will define the number of ribs involved, particularly when the fractures are posteriorly located and, most importantly, may indicate any injury to the thoracic organs. The pleural space can fill with blood from intercostal vessel injury or air escaping from a lung injury. Lung and cardiac contusion can result. Low rib fractures can be associated with liver and splenic injury, particularly in children. With fractures of the first and second ribs, aortic arch and great vessel injury should always be considered. When significant injury to the intrathoracic organs has been eliminated, management is addressed to the rib fracture injury. Pain induced by fractured ribs causes splinting of the involved chest wall area due to reflex muscle spasm. If extensive, this will impair lung ventilation, eventually resulting in atelectasis. The cough reflex is also inhibited, allowing secretions to build up and superimposed pneumonia to develop. These complications will develop more readily in elderly patients, particularly those with underlying chronic lung disease. Principles of treatment are control of pain by local and/or systemic analgesia, and physiotherapy to re-expand the atelectactic lung segments and to clear pulmonary secretions. Physiotherapy is discussed later.

FLAIL SEGMENTS

When trauma is severe, each rib can fracture at two sites, producing a flail segment in which that part of the chest wall becomes functionally isolated from the rest. The flail segment moves paradoxically during respiratory movements, being sucked in during inspiration and pushed out in expiration, resulting in hypoventilation of the underlying lung segments. The underlying lung is usually contused by the original injury, further aggravating the respiratory embarrassment. The principles of treatment are similar to those for simple rib fractures but the ventilation status of the patient is carefully monitored. The early institution of epidural anaesthesia may prevent respiratory deterioration. However, if ventilation becomes inadequate with deterioration in the blood gases, mechanical ventilation will be necessary. Surgical internal fixation of the flail segment may reduce the required period of ventilation.

STERNAL FRACTURE

Sternal fracture is relatively uncommon but is seen with increasing frequency in car accidents. This tends to occur with seatbelt injuries or compression by the steering wheel. As the required force to cause sternal fracture is large, intrathoracic injury should be considered, particularly myocardial contusion. Sternal fracture can be caused by sudden thoracic flexion without impact. The forces required are large if the sternum is fractured in this way, and there is frequently a wedge fracture of a thoracic vertebra.

THE PLEURAL SPACE

In the normal state the visceral and parietal pleurae lie in contact, separated only by a thin film of fluid. Their principal function is to keep the chest wall and the lung in apposition while allowing relative movement between them during the ventilatory cycle. If air (pneumothorax) or blood (haemothorax) enters this pleural cavity the lung separates from the chest wall, collapsing under its own inherent elasticity.

PNEUMOTHORAX

Pneumothorax is the presence of air within the pleural cavity and commonly follows both blunt and penetrating trauma. Three types of pneumothorax are recognised, namely, simple, tension and open.

Simple Pneumothorax

Simple pneumothorax typically results from air escaping into the pleural cavity after underlying lung injury as a consequence of laceration by fractured ribs or a penetrating object. The amount of air entering the pleural cavity will determine the degree of lung collapse and resultant respiratory compromise. Small, superficial lacerations in an otherwise healthy lung will result in a small air leak which tends to seal quickly. In this situation the degree of lung collapse will be small and respiratory compromise minimal. Conversely, major lung injury following an extended or deep laceration will cause a large and continuing air leak leading to complete lung collapse and respiratory difficulties. Peripheral lung trauma also causes prolonged leaks in emphysematous lungs.

The clinical manifestations of simple pneumothorax depend upon the degree of lung collapse and the pre-morbid status of the patient. Patients suffering from chronic lung disease will become distressed with a minor pneumothorax, whereas fit patients can often tolerate complete lung collapse without respiratory distress at rest. The clinical presentation is of acute pain and dyspnoea. Pain will result from injury sustained to the chest wall and parietal pleura, which is richly supplied with pain fibres. The pain will be localised to an area of the chest wall and typically aggravated by deep inspiratory movements or coughing. Examination may reveal visible signs of chest wall trauma, bruising and skin laceration. Chest wall movements on the injured side will be reduced compared with the normal side as the underlying lung will fail to expand. Surgical emphysema may be detected as a crepitus sensation on palpating the chest wall. This sign is produced by air in the subcutaneous tissue escaping from the pleural cavity via the torn parietal pleura. Percussion of the chest will reveal the affected side to be resonant or hyperresonant in comparison with the other normal side. Finally, on auscultation of the chest, breath sounds on the affected side will be reduced as a consequence of reduced air entry into the collapsed lung. The diagnosis of pneumothorax is confirmed by plain chest X-ray which demonstrates separation of the visceral from the parietal pleura of the chest wall.

Pneumothorax sustained as a result of trauma is usually treated by insertion of a chest drain into the pleural cavity. This is because a traumatic lung injury is often associated with a delayed or continuing air leak, and an initial minimal lung collapse may later prove fatal. Furthermore, if the patient requires positive pressure ventilation, this will exacerbate the air leak and result in a life-threatening tension pneumothorax.

Tension Pneumothorax

Tension pneumothorax is a medical emergency. It usually develops as a result of a flap in the visceral pleura acting as a one-way valve allowing air to enter the pleural cavity on inspiration without being able to escape during expiration. As the volume of air within the pleural cavity increases, the lung collapses. A continuing build-up of air will displace the mediastinum to the opposite side, compressing the contralateral lung, causing severe respiratory embarrassment. Furthermore, as the mediastinum becomes displaced the inferior vena cava kinks as it crosses the diaphragm. Venous drainage to the heart is impaired and an acute reduction in cardiac output follows.

Tension pneumothorax presents as haemodynamic instability and impaired ventilation. The patient is agitated and uncontrollable, with cyanosis and increasing respiratory distress. The reduction in cardiac output is manifested by hypotension, tachycardia and cool peripheries. Examination reveals signs of pneumothorax on the injured side and deviation of the trachea to the contralateral side. Once recognised, treatment is instituted without delay as cardiovascular collapse can be imminent. Time is not wasted by obtaining radiological confirmation of the diagnosis. The tension can be quickly relieved by insertion of a large bore needle into the affected chest cavity, through the second intercostal space in the midclavicular line. Upon entering the pleural cavity, air escapes quickly under tension and the patient's condition is seen to improve rapidly. When stable, a chest drain can then be inserted under controlled conditions.

Open Pneumothorax

Open pneumothorax occurs following penetrating chest injury in which the wound edges do not approximate and air moves into and out of the pleural space with each inspiration and expiration. The amount of air moving is dependent on the size of the chest wall defect. If the defect is larger than the cross-section of the trachea then the air will move more easily through the defect, causing marked impairment of ventilation. Clinically the condition is recognised by a characteristic sucking sound produced on inspiration. When the diagnosis is made, the wound should be immediately covered with a sterile dressing. This has the effect of converting an open pneumothorax into a safer and easier controlled closed pneumothorax. A chest drain is then placed in the affected pleural cavity.

HAEMOTHORAX

Haemothorax, blood within the pleural cavity, is a frequent consequence of both blunt and penetrating trauma.

Commonly it is the result of chest wall injury where bleeding arises from rib fractures or traumatised intercostal vessels. Superficial lung parenchymal lacerations can also result in significant bleeding. Injury to major vessels such as the aorta, pulmonary arteries and vein will result in massive blood loss with the patient *in extremis*.

The clinical consequences of haemothorax result from blood loss, impairment of lung mechanics and chronic effects such as retained clot and fibrothorax. With significant or ongoing blood loss from the circulation into the pleural cavity, the patient will develop circulatory shock manifested by an unstable blood pressure, tachycardia, sweating, pallor and cold extremities. As blood collects within one or both pleural cavities, lung expansion becomes restricted, resulting in hypoventilation with hypoxaemia and hypercapnia. Chronically, if the blood is not removed from the pleural cavity it will clot and then become organised into a fibrin peel on the lung surface causing lung trapping. The blood clot can also become infected and give rise to an empyema.

Clinical examination may reveal signs of haemodynamic instability with significant blood loss. On examination of the chest, the trachea may be deviated away from the affected side with blood in the pleural cavity, causing contralateral mediastinal displacement. The injured haemothorax will be dull to percussion and reveal reduced air entry. The chest X-ray appearance of haemothorax is that of any fluid collection within the chest cavity, and is dependent on the volume of blood within the pleural cavity and the position of the patient when the X-ray is taken. Approximately 200 ml of blood is required before the haemothorax becomes radiologically evident. When the X-ray is taken in the erect position, the blood will be seen as an area of dense opacity with a meniscus. In the supine position, often taken when the patient is haemodynamically unstable, a generalised haze on the affected size is observed as blood spreads along the paravertebral gutter. With massive haemothorax the affected side will appear as a 'white out' completely obscuring the lung, irrespective of the patient's position.

Management consists of fluid resuscitation of the patient as required. The haemothorax is treated by draining the pleural cavity with an intrapleural chest drain. This will drain blood from the pleural cavity, allowing the lung to expand and thus improve ventilatory mechanics. Furthermore, it will allow assessment of the rate of continued blood loss which will dictate further management. Ideally, the chest drain is placed in the 6th intercostal space, in the midaxillary line, and directed posterobasally which is the dependent aspect of the pleural cavity. When correctly placed, blood will drain, often 1 or 2 litres, which represents that already 'lost' from the circulation, and thus no haemodynamic deterioration will occur. With a massive haemothorax or significant ongoing blood loss, blood can pour from the drain, causing circulatory collapse. In such situations the drain should be temporarily clamped until haemodynamic control is achieved.

In the majority of cases, bleeding into the pleural cavity settles spontaneously due to the muscular nature of the chest wall arteries which tend to constrict, preventing further blood loss. Similarly, lung lacerations, if superficial, will become haemostatic, particularly when the lung is re-inflated following successful chest drain insertion. However, in 10% of patients with haemothorax, surgical exploration is required to control ongoing blood loss. These patients will have continued drainage in excess of 200 ml/h and often haemodynamic instability.

If the haemothorax is not drained, the blood will eventually clot after a period of 24 hours, and chest drain insertion will be ineffective. Retained clot, which is an excellent bacterial culture medium, can become infected, leading to an empyema. This life-threatening complication becomes increasingly likely if repeated attempts are made to aspirate blood, as additional opportunities to cause infection arise. Clot can also organise into a fibrin peel which coats the lung surface, thus trapping the lung, tethering it and preventing full expansion. This can lead to permanent reduction in pulmonary function and exercise capacity. In such a situation whereby drainage of the acute haemothorax has been neglected, surgical exploration of the pleural cavity to remove blood clot may be required to avoid such long-term complications.

THE DIAPHRAGM

Most frequently, traumatic injury to the diaphragm is the result of blunt trauma.

BLUNT INJURY

The usual mechanism of injury is a sudden increase in intra-abdominal pressure relative to the intrathoracic pressure. The left hemidiaphragm is the most vulnerable, accounting for 68% of all significant diaphragmatic injuries. The right hemidiaphragm is protected by the liver and accounts for 25% of diagnosed injuries. Rupture of the pericardial diaphragm can occur on rare occasions.

Following major diaphragmatic rupture, the abdominal contents, small bowel, spleen and liver can become displaced into the thoracic cavity. This can result in mediastinal displacement with subsequent impairment of venous return to the heart and a falling cardiac output. The lung becomes compressed on the affected side, reducing ventilation. If the pericardial diaphragm is injured, abdominal contents can enter the pericardial cavity, compress the heart and induce tamponade.

Clinically, such patients present with abdominal pain, haemodynamic instability and respiratory distress. The diagnosis is frequently confirmed by plain chest X-ray, which will reveal displaced abdominal contents in the thoracic cavity. Such major injuries to the diaphragm are often associated with concurrent intra-abdominal organ injury and splenic or liver trauma.

With lesser degrees of trauma the diaphragmatic rupture is small, not permitting abdominal contents to enter the thoracic cavity.

In the acute situation, the diaphragm heals without obvious clinical significance, and such small ruptures often go undetected. However, the diaphragm is weakened at this site and later rupture may occur months or years after the acute event. As with the acute rupture, bowel contents become displaced and in so doing may become twisted, resulting in bowel obstruction and ischaemia. Classically, the patient will describe upper abdominal pain, nausea and vomiting, and a history of abdominal trauma.

Confirming the diagnosis of diaphragm injury may prove difficult. Chest X-ray may reveal elevation of the affected hemidiaphragm, with an irregular contour. Displaced bowel may be seen in the hemithorax or indicated by nasogastric tube displacement. A barium swallow will confirm the presence of bowel within the thorax. The diaphragm can be directly visualised by a thoracoscope.

With large diaphragmatic rupture and significant displacement of bowel, the haemodynamic and respiratory distress can be relieved in part by passage of a nasogastric tube. This will decompress the displaced bowel, thereby reducing its volume and pressure effect on the lungs and mediastinum. In addition, decompressing the bowel will reduce the risk of bowel wall ischaemia, infarction and perforation.

Surgical repair of the diaphragm is performed via either the abdominal or thoracic approach. In the acute situation the abdominal approach is favoured because of the possibility of co-existing abdominal organ injury. Chronic, i.e. longer than 7 days, and right-sided diaphragmatic injuries are usually approached through a thoracotomy. The principle of treatment is to reduce the abdominal contents and to close the diaphragm defect.

PENETRATING INJURY

This can occur when the site of injury is below the fourth rib anteriorly or the upper quadrant of the abdomen. Commonly, there will be associated injury to intrathoracic or abdominal organs, which will account for the clinical presentation. As the diaphragm defect is small with penetrating as opposed to blunt trauma, intrathoracic displacement of bowel is less extensive.

THE HEART

Cardiac injury occurs commonly after blunt trauma and accounts for a preponderance of deaths in the immediate post-injury period. The spectrum of blunt cardiac injury is wide, ranging from minor subclinical wall motion abnormalities to devastating heart rupture producing immediate death.

BLUNT INJURY

Blunt injury of the heart is most commonly the result of compression by the sternum as a result of a direct blow to the anterior chest wall as in a 'steering wheel injury'. As the left ventricle lies anteriorly, it is the most common area of the heart to be involved in such injury. Compression-induced cardiac injury can also follow sudden elevation in intra-abdominal pressures by transmission through the diaphragm, especially following lap-belt injuries. Anatomically, the heart is part fixed to the thorax (the inferior vena cava traverses the diaphragm, and the left atrium is held by the pulmonary veins) and is part suspended, relatively free to move within the pericardial cavity. With such an anatomical arrangement, sudden deceleration can result in cardiac injury by shearing forces across points of fixation or by impaction of the heart against adjacent structures.

Myocardial contusion is the commonest result of blunt cardiac injury. Pathologically, this is characterised by areas of myocardial cell necrosis, haematoma formation and acute inflammatory cell infiltrate. The epicardial surface is typically most affected but the injury can extend to full wall thickness with increasing force. If the patient survives the acute insult, the area of injury heals by scar formation, leaving a permanent regional wall movement deficit.

Minor contusional injuries result in regional wall abnormalities due to loss of contractile function. With increasing severity, the pumping function of the cardiac chamber becomes compromised and cardiac failure will ensue. The anteriorly placed left ventricle is frequently the site of such injury. Cardiac arrhythmias are a common sequel and range from mild conduction abnormalities to ventricular fibrillation and electromechanical dissociation. The diagnosis of contusion is often difficult to confirm. Standard assessment involves a 12 lead electrocardiogram (ECG) and cardiac monitoring, measurement of specific enzymes (creatinine kinase myocardial band and troponin), and echocardiography. Cardiac rupture resulting from severe blunt trauma is often fatal. Death can result from pericardial tamponade, air embolism and, when the pericardium is torn, exsanguination. The right ventricle is the most frequent chamber involved, followed by the left ventricle, right atrium and left atrium. The diagnosis is suspected in a patient who has sustained blunt thoracic injury and presents with the clinical signs of tamponade, hypotension, distended neck veins and muffled or distant heart sounds. If the pericardium is open, hypovolaemic shock with massive haemothorax will develop. Coronary arteries may be injured by blunt trauma, leading to intimal injury with acute thrombosis, laceration, arteriovenous fistulae and pseudoaneurysm formation. The most frequently involved vessel is the left anterior descending artery.

PENETRATING INJURY

Penetrating trauma is commonly the result of gunshot or stab wound injuries. The incidence of this injury is increasing with the continual rise in inner city violence.

When the heart is penetrated, the acute manifestation is bleeding. The heart is enclosed in a tough fibrous sac, the pericardium, and the clinical presentation of cardiac bleeding depends on the integrity of the pericardium. If the pericardium has been widely torn, bleeding from the heart will escape from the pericardial cavity into the pleural space. The patient will show signs of hypovolaemic shock, tachycardia, hypotension and low JVP. Chest X-ray may reveal a large haemothorax. Such patients require rapid fluid and blood replacement and urgent surgical exploration to control bleeding.

Patients in whom the pericardium is intact present with cardiac tamponade. In this condition blood escapes from the injured heart and collects within the pericardial cavity. The continuing accumulation of blood compresses the cardiac chambers, particularly the right and left atrium, impeding their filling. Venous return to the heart is reduced and cardiac output falls. The classic signs of pericardial tamponade, Beck's triad, consist of hypotension, muffled heart sounds and elevation of the jugular venous pulse. As little as 150 ml blood loss can induce significant tamponade. In a stable patient, the diagnosis can be confirmed by non-invasive measures, particularly echocardiography.

The condition is a life-threatening emergency requiring immediate relief. In the emergency room this can be performed by the technique of pericardiocentesis. This consists of percutaneous aspiration of blood, which is carried out using a needle guided from the subxiphoid area into the pericardial cavity. Further injury to the heart is a potential risk. Another approach consists of creating a window, where the pericardium is exposed through a subxiphoid skin incision.

When the tamponade has been relieved, repair of the cardiac injury must be performed. The heart is approached through a median sternotomy or anterior thoracotomy. Injuries include perforation of cardiac chambers, particularly the right ventricle and atrium. Coronary artery injury, resulting in myocardial ischaemia and infarction, requires cardiopulmonary bypass, which will also be required for perforation of the intraventricular septum and other complex cardiac injuries.

THE LUNGS

PULMONARY CONTUSION

Pulmonary contusion results from blunt trauma to the thorax. When the lung is traumatised there is disruption of the air passages and vasculature. Haemorrhage occurs, permeability is increased and this results in extravasation of fluid from the intra- to the extravascular space. This process is a natural response to any acute injury as it allows the transport of inflammatory cells to the site of damage which combat infection and commence the repair process of damaged tissue. However, within the lung this fluid collects in the interstitial and alveolar spaces, causing arteriovenous shunting and hypoxaemia. The diagnosis of pulmonary contusion is usually based on radiological and blood gas findings. On chest X-ray, pulmonary contusion appears as patchy areas of pulmonary infiltrate and is usually well localised to areas of lung that underlie the chest wall injury. Blood gas analyses in the presence of established contusion are characterised by hypoxaemia. Because loss of pulmonary capillary permeability is part of the pathogenesis of pulmonary contusion, the oedema and physiological derangement evolves over time and, typically, the radiographic appearances and hypoxaemia increase over the first 24–48 hours.

Patients with significant contusion and increasing hypoxia require mechanical ventilatory support. The use of prophylactic antibiotics in the management of lung contusion is controversial. There is no convincing evidence that antibiotics prevent pneumonia only in cases where aspiration pneumonia is likely to develop. Another contentious issue in the management of pulmonary contusion is fluid management. In order to discourage the extension of intravascular fluid, it appeared logical to administer colloid-type fluids and diuretics to 'dry out' the contused lung. Unfortunately, the damaged microvasculature cannot maintain a colloid osmotic gradient, and contusion is not effectively treated by this approach. In such patients, measurement of the pulmonary artery pressure, which indicates cardiac filling pressures, allows the clinician to administer enough fluid for adequate perfusion without causing pulmonary oedema due to fluid overload.

THE TRACHEA AND MAJOR BRONCHI

BLUNT INJURY

Blunt trauma resulting in tracheobronchial injury is rare, and usually follows car accidents. It may also result from direct chest crush injury or falls from a great height. Typically, the injury occurs in isolation without co-existing trauma to other organs, rib fractures occurring in only 50% of such patients. The mechanism of injury is not fully understood but sudden elevation in intra-abdominal pressure or torsional movements around the carina have been proposed as possible factors.

Within the trachea, the commonest injury is a linear laceration in the membranous wall or in the area of the carina. If such injuries are not surgically repaired, granulation tissue growth in the area can result in tracheal stricture. Complete bronchial disruption results in retraction of the bronchial ends and total obstruction of the airway. The lung segment supplied by the isolated bronchus becomes atelectatic but is sterile and therefore does not become infected. This is in contrast to a partial bronchial disruption which results in stricture, and the supplied lung segment often become chronically infected as a result.

Clinically, bronchial injuries can be divided into two groups: those in which the mediastinal pleura is disrupted and those in which the pleura remains intact. In the first group, such patients present with a large air leak arising from the injured airway. A pneumothorax develops and persists despite the insertion of a chest drain. Subcutaneous and mediastinal emphysema occur and generally the patient is in severe respiratory distress. The second group in which the pleura remains intact have surprisingly few symptoms or signs. If a pneumothorax develops it is often small and resolves quickly following drainage. Minor haemoptysis may occur from bronchial artery injuries. The segments of lung supplied by the bronchus become atelectactic but, provided the patient has normal pre-injury lung function, this may not cause significant problems. In the elderly or patients with diminished pulmonary reserve, the loss of lung segment function will result in increasing

dyspnoea. Patients with partial bronchial disruption that heals with stricture formation often develop a unilateral wheeze and cough, and are sometimes misdiagnosed as asthmatic. The stricture invariably causes repeated infection in lung segments supplied by the strictured airway, and this can eventually destroy the lung tissue.

In order to make the diagnosis of tracheobronchial injury, the clinician must keep a high index of suspicion. Chest X-ray may reveal pneumothorax, air in the mediastinum, dropped hilum or undetectable bronchial air shadow. In the asymptomatic patient, where the pleura remains intact, the acute chest X-ray is often normal. Where one suspects bronchial injury, the procedure of choice is bronchoscopy in order to visualise the defect directly in the bronchial mucosa. If the diagnosis has not been made, chest X-ray a week or so later will reveal collapse of the supplied lung segments. This appearance is often considered the result of retained secretions, but bronchoscopy at this stage will reveal obstruction of the bronchial lumen by granulation tissue and blood clot, and inability to advance the scope beyond this to visualise the distal lobar bronchus.

The management of acute tracheobronchial injuries consists of early surgical repair. This requires close collaboration between surgeon and anaesthetist because the patient's ventilation must be sustained in the uninjured lung while the bronchus is repaired. Post-operatively, effective clearing of airways secretions is essential for healing. If the diagnosis has been missed, late bronchial repair can sometimes be performed, but as the area is encased in fibrotic scar tissue the procedure is technically difficult.

PENETRATING INJURY

Penetrating trauma resulting in tracheobronchial injuries continues to increase. Except for the cervical region, tracheobronchial injuries are usually caused by gunshot wounds. The depth of the tracheobronchial tree renders these structures safe from stab wound trauma.

Clinical presentations vary but major airways trauma is suggested by rapidly progressing subcutaneous emphysema, pneumothorax with continuing air leak, massive haemoptysis and abnormal phonation. Penetrating trauma to the tracheobronchial tree is commonly associated with major vascular injury.

If haemorrhage is not a significant finding, bronchoscopy, contrast studies of the oesophagus and aortography should be performed. The unstable patient, however, requires immediate thoracotomy to control the bleeding.

THE CERVICAL TRACHEA

BLUNT INJURY

Blunt injury to the cervical trachea is caused by several mechanisms. Acute hyperextension of the neck can result in tracheal rupture. The injury can result, for example, from rope contact-pressure across the anterior cervical area; this usually disrupts the trachea between the cricoid and first tracheal ring. Injury may also be induced by direct crush force to the neck.

Clinical signs of tracheal injury include stridor indicating airways obstruction, hoarseness as a result of recurrent laryngeal nerve involvement and haemoptysis.

The management consists of airways establishment as the first priority. Endotracheal intubation may be possible, but if difficulties are encountered tracheostomy is performed. The trachea is then surgically repaired.

PENETRATING INJURY

In penetrating trauma to the cervical trachea, other neck structures which are closely related are often simultaneously involved, e.g. carotid artery, jugular vein and oesophagus. Patients present with stridor, cyanosis, dyspnoea and, with vessel injury, bleeding. Management consists of intubation to control airways thus preventing further aspiration of blood. Surgical exploration is performed to control bleeding and repair the tracheal defect.

THORACIC AORTIC RUPTURE

Injury to the thoracic aorta is typically caused by severe blunt trauma. It represents a major thoracic emergency with a high mortality rate. The condition has increased in frequency due to the rising incidence of high speed vehicular accidents.

The commonest aortic injury involves disruption of the aortic wall in the area of the isthmus. The isthmus is the anatomical junction between the relatively mobile aortic arch and the fixed descending aorta, fixed by intercostal vessels and pleura to the posterior chest wall. Following a severe decelerating force, such as occurs with a 'head-on' car accident, these two areas of the aorta decelerate at different rates. This motion induces a shearing force in the aortic wall maximally in the area of the isthmus. The intima and media of the aortic wall disrupt initially but the integrity of the aorta can be maintained by the strong outer adventitial layer. With greater degrees of force, the complete wall ruptures and massive haemorrhage ensues. Falls from great heights causing vertical deceleration and crush injuries can cause aortic rupture, particularly of the ascending portion of the aorta.

The majority of patients who have sustained an aortic wall injury die at the scene of the accident because of complete wall disruption and exsanguination. Those that survive have a wide variety of clinical presentations. Furthermore, such injuries to the aorta are commonly associated with trauma to the central nervous system, skeletal system and abdomen and, as a result, complicate the clinical presentation. Pain is caused by an expanding haematoma in the aortic wall. This haematoma has a mass-like effect and can obstruct the oesophagus, causing dysphagia, or distort the left main bronchus and left recurrent laryngeal nerve, causing hoarseness. Blood flow in the aortic lumen can become obstructed and result in ischaemia of the spine, left arm and lower body. Clinical examination may detect differences in amplitude between the right and left radial pulses. A systolic murmur results from turbulent flow over the injured aortic wall. Acute co-arctation syndrome, where upper limb hypertension occurs, results from compression of the aortic lumen. A rare but valuable sign is bruising in the neck, representing extravasation of blood from the injured aorta into the neck tissues.

Rupture of the ascending aorta is usually immediately fatal. In this injury the aortic valve configuration is distorted, leading to valvular incompetence. Blood escaping from the aorta can track retrogradely into the pericardial cavity causing tamponade. The expanding haematoma may impinge on the coronary arteries and induce myocardial ischaemia. However, often no clinical signs may be evident so the clinician must retain a high index of suspicion in order to identify this condition.

Chest X-ray may reveal several clues leading to suspicion of aortic injury, for example mediastinal widening greater than 8 cm (in the adult) at the aortic knuckle. The aortic knuckle itself may become blurred and indistinct due to expanding haematoma. The trachea and oesophagus are displaced to the right. Additional signs include left pleural effusion and fracture of the first and second ribs. Once suspected, definitive diagnosis of aortic wall injury may be obtained by angiography, computerised tomography (CT) scanning and transoesophageal echo.

These investigations can be performed only in a haemodynamically stable patient.

When the diagnosis of aortic rupture is suspected or established, initial management consists of control of blood pressure, as any sudden increase may precipitate full rupture and exsanguination. Intravenous fluids are administered judiciously. Pain control is optimised and the patient gently sedated, then transferred to theatre for surgical repair of the aortic injury. However, if at any time haemodynamic collapse occurs, immediate surgical intervention to control haemorrhage becomes necessary.

THE OESOPHAGUS

The oesophagus is that part of the alimentary tract between the oropharynx and the stomach. Anatomically it is divided into three areas, namely, cervical, thoracic and intra-abdominal. There are four mechanisms of injury to the oesophagus, namely, penetrating, blunt, barotrauma, and ingestion of corrosive materials.

BLUNT INJURY

Blunt, compressional type forces are recognised as a cause of serious oesophageal injury. This injury is commonest in the cervical oesophagus but has been documented in the thorax and peritoneal oesophagus. Direct blows to the neck encountered in boxing or steering wheel injuries have been implicated. As with penetrating trauma, injury to the great vessels and trachea/larynx is commonly associated with this type of injury. Major compressional force to the thorax is required to cause oesophageal injury and tends to be seen in younger individuals whose elastic vessels are more resilient to such forces.

Vigorous external cardiopulmonary resuscitation (CPR) and the Heimlich manoeuvre have resulted in iatrogenic blunt oesophageal injury.

PENETRATING INJURY

Direct injury is the result of a penetrating object such as a knife or bullet. The cervical oesophagus is the area most frequently injured by this mechanism as it is accessible from the body surface. Within the neck the oesophagus lies in close proximity to the trachea, larynx and great vessels, and these structures can also be injured by the penetrating object. In the thorax and abdomen the oesophagus is surrounded by vital structures and therefore more protected from such injury. Penetrating injuries to the thoracic oesophagus are often associated with lethal injury to the heart or great vessels.

Iatrogenic perforation of the oesophagus is caused by endoscopy and various therapeutic manipulations of the oesophagus. The oesophageal mucosa can be visualised by rigid and flexible endoscopes, perforation being more common with the latter. Injury is more likely to occur when the oesophagus is diseased by inflammation or tumour infiltrate, which renders the wall more friable. In patients presenting with dysphagia, a contrast study of the oesophagus before endoscopy is recommended as this will delineate the site of obstruction and reduce the risk of perforation.

Therapeutic manipulations of oesophageal strictures by bougie, pneumatic dilation or laser are associated with a risk of perforation.

Perforation can also occur as a result of the ingestion of a foreign body. A wide variety of ingested objects has been described as the result of accident, suicide attempts or psychiatric acts. The objects tend to lodge in areas of anatomical narrowing of the oesophagus, the cricopharyngeal area, the hiatus and where the oesophagus crosses the left main bronchus. Those objects particularly likely to cause perforation are sharp, e.g. broken dentures, safety pins and razor blades. Removal of the foreign body, usually by rigid endoscopy, is hazardous and can cause perforation in itself.

BAROTRAUMA

Barotrauma may injure the oesophagus by intrinsic or extrinsic forces.

Boerhaave's syndrome describes a postemetic oesophageal rupture. It arises as a consequence of intrinsic barotrauma induced by vomiting against a closed glottis. Typically, such patients will have a full stomach, having ingested a large meal often in the presence of alcohol. There then follows a sudden urge to vomit which is restrained completely or in part by voluntary contraction of oropharynx muscles. This leads to a rapid elevation in intraluminal oesophageal pressure, which results in rupture. The site of perforation is usually the lower third of the oesophagus on the left side, and the gastro-oesophageal contents spill into the left pleural cavity.

Blast injuries, typically seen in military or industrial situations, can cause extrinsic barotrauma to the oesophagus.

The blast injury transmits a pressure wave across the body, the energy of which is adsorbed by the tissues. Hollow organs are particularly vulnerable as energy adsorption is maximum where a gas/tissue interface exists.

Oesophageal penetrating and blast injuries are commonly associated with damage to the heart, great vessels or trachea. These injuries dictate the acute clinical presentation, and a co-existing oesophageal injury may go undetected. In isolated oesophageal perforation the classic symptom is pain and, for cervical injury, dysphagia and odynophagia (pain on swallowing). The pain is typically severe, unremitting and localised to the intracapsular region, being similar to that of acute aortic dissection or myocardial infarction, conditions with which the injury is often confused. Clinical examination is often unrewarding revealing tachycardia and sweating, and tachypnoea associated with painful stress. Subcutaneous emphysema in the cervical subcutaneous tissues is a highly specific and valuable sign of oesophageal perforation, and results from air escaping from the oesophagus and tracking along mediastinal tissue planes into the neck. If the condition is undiagnosed and allowed to progress, gastro-oesophageal contents accumulate in the mediastinal tissues and pleural cavities. Contamination results in mediastinitis. The patient may succumb to overwhelming sepsis after the initial insult.

The diagnosis is usually confirmed by radiological investigation. Chest X-rays reveal air within the mediastinal or cervical tissues. Pneumothorax or pleural effusion may be present. Confirmation is obtained by contrast studies of the oesophagus. Usually a water-soluble contrast medium is swallowed and the area of injury identified as the material leaks from the oesophageal lumen.

Oesophageal injury carries a high mortality rate, which increases with delay in establishing the diagnosis and institution of treatment. Therefore, the goal is to suspect the injury, confirm the diagnosis, and initiate treatment.

In the setting of major thoracic trauma, where injury to other organs has occurred, oesophageal rupture may be easily overlooked. As time elapses, mediastinal contamination increases and the patient develops systemic sepsis and ultimately multisystem organ failure if the perforation is not managed.

Attempts to close the oesophageal perforation surgically have met with varying success. Often such patients with sepsis and other thoracic injuries present a high operative risk for major thoracic surgery. In addition, the oesophageal wall around the perforation becomes friable and oedematous, making suture closure of the defect insecure and liable to break down. Surgical closure may be successfully achieved if the defect is closed within 24 hours of injury as the systemic sepsis will not be established and the oesophageal wall is still healthy. Such closures are reinforced by mobilising vascularised tissue, intercostal muscle, pleura or omentum, and covering the defect. After 24 hours from the time of injury, the principle of treatment consists of nil by mouth, good hydration, nutritional support by enteral or parenteral nutrition, and drainage of the area of oesophageal perforation. Three tubes are surgically placed to drain the stomach, lower oesophagus and relevant pleural cavity, respectively. This will remove the local contamination and allow the oesophageal perforation to heal.

THE THORACIC DUCT

Following blunt or penetrating injuries, the thoracic lymphatic duct may be damaged. Thoracic duct injuries are usually detected after the first few days of trauma. They require surgical repair if the volume is high and persistent.

MANAGEMENT TECHNIQUES

PAIN RELIEF

Adequate relief of pain is a fundamental priority in the patient who has sustained chest trauma, particularly in the spontaneously ventilating patient. Pain is often the result of chest wall injury, or rib and sternal fractures, and in order to control the pain, movement of the affected part of the chest wall is reflexly inhibited. This will cause hypoventilation of the underlying lung segments, and atelectasis and hypoxia as a consequence. Furthermore, the cough reflex is suppressed, allowing secretions to gather which may become infected, ultimately resulting in pneumonia. If it is extreme, untreated chest wall pain causes hypoxia, hypercapnia, carbon dioxide narcosis and even respiratory arrest.

There are a variety of approaches to controlling pain in the patient with chest wall trauma. In the young, fit patient with trivial injuries, non-steroidal anti-inflammatory agents may suffice. Narcotic analgesics administered parenterally are the agents of choice for more severe injuries or in the elderly infirm patient. Parenterally administered medication, besides relieving pain, also causes respiratory depression. Its use requires careful titration of enough medication to control pain without undue inhibition of respiratory drive. Patient-controlled analgesia (PCA) devices that allow the patient, within limits, to administer his or her own analgesia are valuable. When properly managed they allow adequate pain relief with minimal respiratory depression, and prevent intermittent periods of inadequate pain relief. Regional and local nerve blocks have a major role to play. Intercostal block can be of benefit in patients with one or two rib fractures as it provides pain relief without associated respiratory depression. The disadvantage of such an approach is that the duration of action is short and that therefore it must be repeated frequently. Furthermore, there is the risk of intravascular injection of an anaesthetic agent or the creation of a pneumothorax. Also, repeated injection in the presence of haematoma can lead to chest wall infection or empyema.

Epidural analgesia provides excellent control of pain. The catheter is introduced into the epidural space in the thorax or lumbar region and the anaesthetic agent delivered. Local anaesthesia such as Marcain can provide excellent pain control but may significantly impair blood pressure. Opiate agents seem to offer advantages of good analgesia with minimal haemodynamic upset. Furthermore, such agents, because of their short halflife, tend not to migrate from the site of injection and are less likely to cause depression of the respiratory centre. Epidural catheters are not without complication, e.g. infection and haematoma formation. Some patients may develop pruritus, ileus or urinary retention. Ideally, epidural analgesia requires the patient to be monitored in a high dependency unit (see Chapter 7 for more details on pain relief).

ANTIBIOTIC THERAPY

The use of antibiotics in the management of chest trauma is not clearly defined. While some would recommend the use of prophylactic antibiotics to prevent septic complications of chest trauma, the majority are against this. Prophylactic antibiotics have been demonstrated to be beneficial in the subgroup of patients who require chest tube thoracostomy as they appear to reduce infective complications, including empyema.

The use of prophylactic antibiotics does not reduce the incidence of infection and may allow the emergence of resistant strains. Where obvious infection exists, clinically indicated by pyrexia, rigors and elevation of the leucocyte count, antibiotic therapy should be commenced, dictated by the infective agent responsible. Repeated sampling of blood, sputum, urine, and other potential areas of infection is essential in order to isolate the infective agent. From this, an antibiotic sensitivity of the bacterium can be obtained and the appropriate antibiotic antimicrobial agent used.

If the organism is not identified, the clinician is guided by the knowledge of factors responsible for the infection, such as oesophageal perforation, as to which is the most likely causative agent. Furthermore, the time in which the clinical sepsis develops is important as an infection that develops after several days in hospital is likely to be nosocomial and thus have a different infective agent and antibiotic profile from a community acquired infection. In general, courses of antibiotics should be short, i.e. 4 to 5 days.

CHEST DRAINS

Chest drains are frequently employed in the management of thoracic trauma. A drain consists of a tube placed into the pleural cavity and connected to an underwater seal. This arrangement acts as a one-way valve, allowing air and fluid to drain out.

Chest drain insertion is indicated in the treatment of pneumothorax and haemothorax. By draining the affected pleural cavity the lung re-expands and ventilation is improved. In patients who require positive pressure ventilation, chest drain insertion should be considered early because of the risk of tension pneumothorax.

The technique of insertion is important as iatrogenic injuries following chest drain insertion are frequently reported. The skin incision is made in the midaxillary position above the nipple line, to avoid diaphragm injury. The subcutaneous fat and intercostal muscle layers are divided by blunt dissection. The parietal pleura is then breached and a finger introduced to examine the pleural cavity and any adhesions that may be present. For a pneumothorax, a 22–28 French gauge drain is placed into the pleural cavity and advanced towards the apex. For haemothorax, a 24–32 French gauge drain is inserted. Following insertion, the drain is secured and attached to the underwater seal. Air or blood can then be seen to drain freely. Confirmation of the position of the chest drain is carried out by chest X-ray.

In the patient who presents *in extremis* due to tension pneumothorax, time may not permit the insertion of a chest drain. The tension can be quickly relieved by placing a 14 French gauge intravenous needle into the pleural cavity in the midclavicular line in the 2nd intercostal space. Air will be heard hissing out as the tension is relieved. Formal chest drain insertion can then be performed. Care is required in draining a haemothorax as decompression of the pleural cavity may provoke a secondary haemorrhage. In such situations the drain may be relieved slowly or clamped until haemodynamic stability is achieved. Ongoing blood loss from the chest drain is an indication for surgical exploration of the thorax.

CHEST SECRETIONS

Following chest trauma, there is increased production of bronchial secretions. Removal of such secretions is essential to avoid atelectasis and infection. The patient should have good pain control in order to cough freely and co-operate well with physiotherapy. Bronchodilators and nebulised saline given at regular intervals help with expectoration of secretions. While gentle chest vibrations, postural drainage and incentive spirometry are the mainstay of preventive physiotherapy, it is necessary on occasions to resort to mechanical suction of the airways. In its simplest form, a nasopharyngeal airway is placed which allows a suction catheter to be passed into the upper airway (Figure 6.8, p97). This will stimulate a cough reflex and aspirate the upper airways. The nasotracheal airway should be used only as a short-term measure as it is uncomfortable for the patient and interferes with normal breathing and coughing.

The use of the mini-tracheostomy has been a significant advance in the treatment of retained secretions. This is covered later in the physiotherapy section.

Where lobar collapse has occurred because of retained secretions occluding a bronchus, fibreoptic bronchoscopy is employed to visualise the obstructing mucous plug directly and then to aspirate it. Bronchoscopy is typically used in the ventilated patient where the bronchoscope can be easily introduced into the airway via the orotracheal tube. Bronchoscopy is not without side effects of hypoxia, cardiac arrest and hypotension, and therefore should be carried out by a skilled operator.

EMERGENCY ROOM THORACOTOMY

Penetrating injuries to the heart and great vessels are now more common in inner city areas. Such injuries are rapidly fatal if not identified and treated urgently.

Patients frequently arrive in the accident and emergency department in a moribund condition; there is not time for transfer to the operating theatre and prompt surgical exploration may be life saving.

In this situation, the diagnosis of heart or great vessel injury is made clinically; time does not permit for investigations. The site of penetration is typically between the anterior axillary line and above the epigastrium; in about 65% of cases entry is to the left of the sternum. There may be signs of cardiac tamponade or haemorrhagic collapse.

In the stable patient, further tests may be performed. Patients who are haemodynamically unstable are transferred immediately to the operating theatre. On admission, some patients are tachycardiac and semiconscious. Where there is loss of blood pressure, or the patient has become lifeless during transit to hospital, surgical exploration in the accident and emergency department may be life saving.

The heart and great vessels are exposed through a median sternotomy or an anterolateral thoracotomy. The principle of treatment is to relieve cardiac tamponade, and control bleeding by simple measures such as digital compression. When the patient's condition has stabilised, he or she is transferred to the operating theatre for definitive repair of the injury.

Survival figures for emergency room thoracotomy range from 35 to 61% for stab injuries, and from 21 to 26% for gunshot wounds.

CONCLUSION

Injury to the chest continues to be a major cause of trauma-related morbidity and mortality. An appreciation of the basic mechanisms of blunt and penetrating injury is important in the evaluation of such patients. Initial management is concerned with control of the airways and establishment of adequate ventilation and cardiac output. When stabilised, a detailed assessment of the patient is required to detect injuries such as ruptured diaphragm and penetrated oesophagus as these are deceptive in their initial presentation. By contrast, tension pneumothorax and penetrating cardiac wounds are immediately serious and life threatening, demanding urgent surgical intervention for a successful outcome.

PHYSIOTHERAPY AND THE CHEST TRAUMA PATIENT

In an acute unit with a busy accident and emergency department, the likelihood of seeing patients with chest trauma is high. The injuries can be to the chest alone or with multiple fractures to the long bones and pelvis for example. If there are accompanying injuries, this may impede chest physiotherapy because of difficult access to the chest due to a severely injured humerus or a fractured spine.

Depending on the geographical area of the hospital, there may be a high incidence of mining injuries or multiple trauma from car accidents, gunshot wounds or stabbings. In industrial regions that use heavy mobile equipment there could be crush injuries to the chest.

On an average night in Cape Town, an accident and emergency department will receive many patients with stab injuries to the chest and patients with gunshot wounds, so the need to discharge straightforward cases quickly, e.g. patients with pneumothorax or haemothorax is important.

PHYSIOTHERAPY MANAGEMENT

The major input of physiotherapy is early mobilisation. This is facilitated by adequate analgesia.

Common forms of analgesia are morphine-based infusions or epidurals. The use of entonox and transcutaneous nerve stimulation is determined by the individual physiotherapist. Details of pain control are discussed in Chapter 7 and although they relate to post-operative cases, the same applies to chest trauma. The physiotherapy problems arising from chest trauma cases are atelectasis, sputum retention, chest infections and pulmonary embolism. Pulmonary embolism can occur through poor perfusion and contused lung tissue, atelectasis through sputum retention and immobility, and chest infections through inadequate ventilation and insufficient clearance of secretions.

The role of the physiotherapist is to encourage the patient to expand the lungs, and to assist in expectoration of sputum. Further assessment of the chest for early signs of atelectasis, consolidation, sputum retention and infection is essential. Wound support is important to aid coughing, and use of adequate humidification to loosen secretions and moisten upper airways is recommended. This is particularly the case in patients who require oxygen therapy, as oxygen dries the mucosa and makes the secretions tenacious and difficult to clear. Methods of humidification are discussed in Chapter 6

Physiotherapy techniques employed in patients with chest trauma are similar to those used in patients with respiratory problems, with the exclusion of percussion and rigorous vibrations. In Stoke on Trent, the use of a mechanical vibrator has been found to be beneficial, as the patients can tolerate the vibrations over the rib fractures or thoracotomy scar, or close to a chest drain. Typically, the vibrator is placed on top of a folded towel on the surface of the chest. Used in conjunction with postural drainage positions and incentive spirometry, the clearance of secretions is usually successful as is the management of atelectasis.

SPUTUM RETENTION

If a patient has difficulty in expectorating and develops sputum retention, there is a need to assess whether nasopharyngeal or oral suctioning is necessary. On auscultation, the patient has decreased breath sounds and inspiratory and expiratory wheeze or crackles. If excessively severe, there may be reduced movement of the chest on the side of the retention. Blood gas analysis demonstrates poor gaseous exchange, and so if the decision is to suction the secretions then the discomfort and distress caused to the patient are considered. The use of the mini-tracheostomy tube is popular in most units, and offers easy access for suctioning with a size 10 suction catheter. With the patient supine, the mini-tracheostomy is inserted via a small incision near the cricothyroid cartilage under a local anaesthetic. Once *in situ*, the patient is sat up and suctioning may take place (Figure 12.1). The technique will force the patient to cough and therefore there is attendant pain but the procedure causes less panic and less barotrauma compared with suctioning via an oral airway. Many units use the

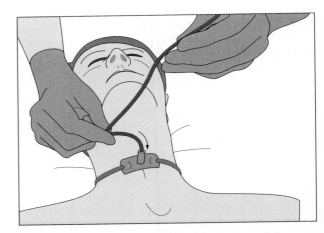

Figure 12.1 Patient being suctioned via a mini-tracheostomy.

nasopharyngeal airway, placed in the nostril and remaining *in situ* until resolution of the condition.

Most patients with chest problems, will not tolerate the head-down position but are happy with side-to-side or forward sitting. It is best if the patient is sat out of bed early, and then mobilised as soon as possible. We encourage patients to sit out of bed on the day of admission, with mobilisation a few hours later or at least by the next morning.

If the patient has intercostal drains *in situ*, assessment of the underwater seal drains is as important as the chest assessment. If bubbles pass through the fluid when the patient coughs or, worse still, while talking or exhaling, then this indicates a residual pneumothorax, and the position of the chest drain needs to be re-evaluated. Bubbling with minimal effort suggests a bronchopulmonary fistula and, in the patient with chest trauma, the need to exclude a ruptured bronchus, bulla or trachea is evident. If a patient has the chest drain attached to a wall suction unit to assist in the re-inflation of the lung, then mobilisation can be achieved by use of an exercise bike, step-ups on a single step, walking on the spot, sitting to standing, or walking within the confines of the suction tube extension. Typically, patients with poor lung compliance have more difficulty in re-expanding their lungs, for example, patients with chronic pulmonary airways disease, and they tend to require suction on their chest drains.

Assessment of a chest X-ray will determine the position of the drain in the thorax, whether the lung is inflated or, in the case of a haemothorax, whether the drain is low enough in the hemithorax to drain the blood. Now is a good time to employ postural drainage positions to aid the removal of unwanted air or blood if the patient is capable. Typically, if the pnemothorax persists, especially with a bronchopleural fistula, the potential of an operation is high, e.g. repair of the bronchus or a bullectomy. If the patient has a persistent pleural effusion that does not drain, and the fluid is a source of infection, an empyema may develop. In such cases, the need for surgery to evacuate the fluid is considered, e.g. decortication or pleurectomy. These procedures are discussed in Chapter 7.

SEVERE CHEST INJURIES

More severe injuries to the chest may involve multiple rib fractures with a flail segment, i.e. a mobile section of chest wall that presents paradoxical movement on inspiration and expiration. The patient should be closely monitored for signs of respiratory failure as the mechanics of respiration are affected by the incomplete chest wall. In such cases, the use of positive pressure support, with continuous positive airway pressure, biphasic positive airway pressure, or formal ventilation via an endotracheal tube, may be necessary. The use of pressure support via a face or nose mask has often obviated the need to ventilate patients and place them in an Intensive Care Unit (ICU), but care must be taken to exclude the possibility of an unresolved pneumothorax or a non-functioning chest drain before positive pressure is applied to the chest as this can cause increased pneumothorax or, worse, tension pneumothorax. If the patient becomes distressed or shows an increase in surgical emphysema while subjected to positive pressure ventilation, the status of his or her chest should be reviewed and, until the problem is solved, the positive pressure removed.

Patients requiring an ICU bed as a result of their injuries will be treated as described for the critically ill patient (see Chapter 6). More serious injuries such as a ruptured trachea, oesophagus or diaphragm (possibly as a result of a crush fracture of the pelvis), and lung laceration, would need the attention of the cardiothoracic surgeon to assess whether surgery to repair the injury were needed (see below).

FRACTURED STERNUM

An impact sufficient to fracture a sternum, a direct blow from a steering wheel in a car accident, for example, can also cause myocardial contusion. Such patients will be assessed for signs of cardiac trauma and monitored with an ECG for approximately 24 hours. They can then be mobilised when the doctor in charge permits. Following this, routine mobilisation using stairs and exercise on the ward will apply.

RUPTURED BRONCHUS, TRACHEA AND OESOPHAGUS

Early diagnosis of a ruptured oesophagus can be instigated by viewing the chest X-ray with common findings of mediastinal and/or neck tissues surgical emphysema. Confirmation is by oesophagoscopy and barium swallow, which will reveal the site of the tear. The presence of a pleural effusion may indicate leakage from the oesophagus into the pleural space. A ruptured trachea can present with the patient having stridor due to tracheal stenosis, and a ruptured bronchus with the patient having a persistent pneumothorax; confirmation is by bronchoscopy.

RUPTURED AORTA

A ruptured aorta is treated as an emergency as the patient often presents with severe hypovolaemia and shock. Confirmation is by aortography or CT scan.

Injury sufficient to cause mediastinal damage needs the expertise of the cardiothoracic surgeon, and repair is often by operation. If the patient undergoes a thoracotomy or sternotomy, then the physiotherapy requirements are similar to those discussed in Chapter 7, depending on the stability of the patient.

CONCLUSION

Early physiotherapy intervention is beneficial for patients with chest trauma, and this is greatly helped by adequate pain control. The physiotherapist is often the person assessing the pain control in conjunction with the nursing and medical staff, and also monitoring the respiratory status of the patient on a regular basis. Early mobilisation will help prevent respiratory complications. Patients who are immobilised because of their injuries tend to be at risk of chest complications, and therefore are a high priority for the physiotherapist.

GENERAL READING

Feghali NT, Prisant LM. Blunt myocardial injury. *Chest* 1995, **108:**1673-1677.

Guth AA, Pachter L, Kim U. Pitfalls in the diagnosis of blunt diaphragmatic injury. *Am J Surg* 1995, **170**.

Hood, Boyd, Culliford. *Thoracic trauma.* 1989.

Kshettry VR, Bolman RM. Chest trauma—assessment, diagnosis and management. *Clinics Chest Med* 1994, **15(1)**.

Parry GW, Morgan WE, Salama FD. Management of haemothorax. *Ann R Coll Surg Engl* 1996, **78:**325-326.

Roxburgh JC. Emergency room thoracotomy, is it ever justified? *Ann R Coll Surg Engl* 1996, **78:**327-330.

Saadia R, Levy RD, Degiannis E, Velmatios GC. Penetrating cardiac injuries—clinical classification and management strategy. *Br J Surg* 1994, **81:**1572-1575.

Sabiston FC. *Surgery of the chest*, 6th ed. 1995.

Westaby S. Resuscitation in thoracic trauma. *Br J Surg* 1994, **81:**929-931.

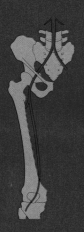

13 P Morgan & R Morgan

VASCULAR SURGERY

CHAPTER OUTLINE

- Peripheral arterial occlusive disease
- Clinical presentation of chronic ischaemia
- Medical management of PAOD
- Complications of vascular surgery
- Physiotherapy after vascular

- reconstructive surgery
- Lower limb amputations
- Abdominal aortic aneurysm
- Carotid artery disease
- Venous diseases of the lower limb
- Rehabilitation of the amputee

INTRODUCTION

Atheroma is among the commonest causes of death in the Western developed world. Its presentation is varied, ranging from cerebrovascular disease, lower leg arterial occlusions to coronary artery disease. The development of atheroma is discussed in Chapter 9. Peripheral arterial occlusive disease (PAOD) can present as:
- Occlusive disease.
- Aneurysmal disease.
- Embolic disease.

Each of these will be described along with its treatment.

PERIPHERAL ARTERIAL OCCLUSIVE DISEASE

Occlusive disease is the most common presentation of PAOD. Here, atheromatous lesions have led to stenoses or occlusions in the arteries, hence insufficient blood flows into the distal limbs. At times of exercise, the oxygen requirements and removal of waste products of metabolism from the limb distal to the lesion becomes increasingly difficult. This gives rise to muscle ischaemia distally, and usually results in pain on exercise. When this pain occurs at rest and is not corrected, irretrievable tissue loss with gangrene will occur. The ischaemic tissue is very

prone to infection and super-added infection is commonplace. This adds to the tissue loss and may ultimately cause loss of the limb. PAOD in the renal vessels may lead to renal hypertension and renal failure. Visceral vessel occlusion gives rise to reversible bowel ischaemia or mesenteric angina, and may progress to bowel infarction.

PATHOPHYSIOLOGY OF MUSCLE ISCHAEMIA

The arterial flow to the essential tissues, e.g. brain, kidneys, liver, adrenals and thyroid, is constantly high. Other tissues, e.g. skeletal muscle, require very little flow at rest, and massive flow under stress.

If stenosis limits flow, then the metabolism in the distal skeletal muscle becomes anaerobic much earlier than would otherwise be the case. Metabolites build up in the muscle inducing extreme vasodilation and subsequent muscle pain. Initially this occurs only under stressed conditions and disappears quickly on resting. This is often referred to as intermittent claudication, describing the discomfort or disability associated with exercise, and there is no permanent damage to skeletal muscle.

If the arterial disease is very severe and little or no blood can enter the muscles, then the pain becomes persistent even at rest. This symptom is an indicator of severe PAOD or critical ischaemia. Critical ischaemia is defined as either an ankle brachial pressure index (ABPI) of less than 0.2, an ankle pressure less than 50 mmHg, or a toe pressure less than 30 mmHg, as measured by Doppler ultrasonography (see below).

COLLATERAL CIRCULATION

Arterial occlusions in the aorto-iliac or femoro-popliteal segments are very common and may cause only minimal discomfort due to the development of a collateral supply. Numerous, small, muscular and cutaneous vessels develop to circumvent the occluded arterial segment over a period of years, and the limb is almost asymptomatic. Occlusions that occur suddenly do not give the limb time to compensate and such acute ischaemia often leads to limb loss.

Mild to moderate exercise encourages collateral development, and training programmes for these patients are commonplace. Excellent results have been obtained, the patients being able to walk increasing distances after a period of training. Although the skeletal muscle of the leg is not permanently harmed by exercise or training, the muscle ischaemia releases a blood-borne metabolite which may damage distant tissues such as the heart and lungs, but conclusive evidence is lacking.

ANEURYSMAL DISEASE

In aneurysmal disease, the arterial wall begins to give way and stretch. It is far more common in the larger arteries, i.e. the aorta, iliac, femoral and popliteal vessels, than it is elsewhere in the arterial tree. It is less common than occlusive disease but no less dangerous, as rupture of an aneurysm of a large vessel can result in massive haemorrhage and the patient's death.

The causes of aneurysm are:
- Atheroma.
- Connective tissue disorder.
- Mycosis.
- Syphilis.
- Trauma.
- Iatrogenic, e.g. catheter puncture sites or at arterial anastomoses following vascular surgery.

TRUE ANEURYSM

A true aneurysm results from a weakness in the arterial wall, and tends to be fusiform in shape. True aneurysms are commonly caused by atheromatous degeneration of the medial arterial layer with consequent passive dilation. The lining of the aneurysm consists of atheromatous material and platelet thrombus compressed into a more solid mass by the intraluminal pressure. On close examination of a cross-section of the aneurysm, all layers of the original artery can be identified.

FALSE ANEURYSM

A false aneurysm does not show any of the normal arterial layers on sectioning. It usually forms as a result of localised damage to the arterial side wall. The escaping blood forms a haematoma which then, as further flow is forced into it, organises into a fibrous stromal capsule.

The aetiology of false aneurysms is primarily iatrogenic, often caused by arteriography, angioplasty or cardiac catheterisation.

EMBOLIC DISEASE

Embolic disease results if an artery has an ulcerated or roughened surface onto which tiny fragments become dislodged and block the circulation distal to the lesion. In the internal carotid artery this gives rise to transient ischaemic attacks or strokes. This kind of lesion is less common in the distal circulation but a popliteal artery aneurysm can progressively occlude the calf vessels by repeated emboli.

RISK FACTORS IN THE DEVELOPMENT OF PAOD

Risk factors in the development of PAOD include:
- Smoking.
- High serum cholesterol/lipid concentrations.
- Hypertension.
- Elevated fibrinogen levels.
- Age, e.g. PAOD patients under 55 years of age have the worst prognosis.

CLINICAL PRESENTATION OF CHRONIC ISCHAEMIA

INTERMITTENT CLAUDICATION

Intermittent claudication is the commonest manifestation of PAOD, affecting more than 5% of men over the age of 50 years. Depending on the extent and level of the disease, the patient may present with buttock and thigh claudication and calf or foot claudication, either singly or in combination. The most common, calf claudication, is easily recognised as a cramping pain in the calf that can be consistently reproduced by the same degree of exercise, and completely relieved by a minute or so of rest. These cramp pains are not to be confused with those that occur at night in older patients; these have no known vascular basis.

Patients with more proximal disease distribution, i.e. aorto-iliac, usually suffer from buttock and thigh claudication. This sensation is more of an aching or weakness rather than pain, therefore spinal cord compression and nerve root irritation should be eliminated. Proximal aorto-iliac occlusions can also give rise to Leriche's syndrome, i.e. buttock claudication and loss of erectile function.

ISCHAEMIC REST PAIN

Ischaemic rest pain is one of the most severe that any patient can experience. It typically begins as a nocturnal pain of disturbing severity involving the foot and the toes. Even high dosage narcotic analgesia may not provide relief. Patients sleeping in the horizontal position are typically awakened by this pain, and attempt to find relief by walking. Some find dangling the leg out of the bed improves the perfusion pressure to the distal foot, temporarily relieving the pain. This method is not advisable as it precipitates ankle oedema and further arterial compromise.

If rest pain is allowed to go unchecked, pregangrenous changes in the toes and then overt gangrene will follow. The progression from rest pain to gangrene and tissue loss may take days, weeks, months or even years, dependent on the degree of collateral circulation.

CLINICAL PRESENTATION OF ACUTE LOWER LIMB ISCHAEMIA

There are three presentations of acute ischaemia:
- Fixed venous staining anaesthetic limb, with function loss and pain in the proximal musculature. This is an unsalvageable limb and primary amputation is required, as revascularisation of such bulky ischaemic muscle will often result in severe acidosis for the patient, and possible death.
- Marble white anaesthetic limb, with loss of function. This should result in a very urgent operation as permanent tissue loss is imminent. Immediate angiography is necessary, and a reconstructive procedure may be considered.
- Painful, blotchy, blue limb with some change in sensation, and maintaining a slight degree of movement. A limb in this state will require some hours of investigation and non-operative treatment, e.g. thrombolysis.

MEDICAL ASSESSMENT OF PAOD

Firstly, when making a medical assessment of PAOD, it is necessary to exclude causes such as musculoskeletal pain, spinal disc pain, diabetic peripheral neuropathy, spinal claudication or reflex sympathetic dystrophy.

The following stages need to be considered:
- Does the patient have significant PAOD?
- Which segments of the arterial tree are involved?
- How severe is the arterial disease, and is the limb threatened?
- Complex disease affecting more than one segment—which is the more significant and which should be treated first?
- To plan formally for further investigation and treatment as required.

Objective assessment of the disease will include one or more of the following tests:

DOPPLER ULTRASONOGRAPHY
Doppler ultrasound pressure measurement is the first investigation for assessing PAOD in both the upper and lower limbs. The handheld instrument is applied to the patient's skin over the target artery, providing an audible signal proportional to the velocity of the blood within the artery. Doppler ultrasound can detect pressures as low as 20 mmHg. The ABPI is calculated by comparing the ankle artery pressure with the brachial artery pressure measured in an asymptomatic limb. This gives a reproducible index of disease severity.

In a normal subject, the ABPI would be 1.1, with an ankle pressure of 130 mmHg and a brachial pressure of 120 mmHg.

A patient with moderate PAOD may have an ankle pressure reduced to 60 mmHg, whereas the brachial pressure would be maintained at 120 mmHg. This equals an index of 0.5.

In a patient with severe occlusive disease, the ankle pressure would be only 30 mmHg; this would give an index of 0.25. This equates with critical ischaemia and imminent limb loss if the situation is not corrected.

Doppler ultrasound does have its limitations, especially if the arteries are calcified or thick walled and incompressible. This circumstance occurs very commonly in patients with diabetes or vasculitis, when falsely high pressures will be observed resulting in an underestimation of the severity of the disease.

TREADMILL TESTING
Testing a patient on a treadmill is a highly reliable method of separating true vascular pain from others. This is achieved by testing the patient before and after a short period of exercise; if the Doppler ultrasound detects a decrease in pressure then vascular insufficiency is suspected, whereas the pressure remains unchanged if the vasculature is normal.

MAGNETIC RESONANCE IMAGING
Magnetic resonance imaging (MRI) is particularly useful for intracerebral, carotid and aortic studies.

HELICAL COMPUTERISED TOMOGRAPHY
The 3D images produced by helical computerised tomography (CT) can be rotated through any axis for viewing; it is also possible for helical CT to provide an image of the flow within a vessel.

ANGIOGRAPHY
In angiography, radiopaque contrast is introduced in to the artery proximal to the stenosed section. Angiography is less accurate than MRI because the views are uni- or biplanar. It has a recognised risk of haemorrhage, thrombosis and false aneurysm, and up to a 7% risk of stroke in carotid cannulation.

MEDICAL MANAGEMENT OF PAOD

ANTIPLATELET AGENTS
Aspirin

In doses of 75 mg or 150 mg, aspirin decreases the incidence of cardiac and cerebrovascular events and increases survival rates. The majority of patients would now be placed on aspirin either pre-operatively or certainly post-operatively for reconstructive surgery or angioplasty.

Dipyrimadole

Dipyrimadole stabilises platelets and decreases their adhesion, aggregation, and release of metabolite rich granules.

Antilipid Drug Therapy

Reduction of serum cholesterol and low density lipoprotein may have a long-term beneficial effect on the development of atherosclerosis, but long-term studies have not yet shown clear survival advantages. Antilipid drugs increase the risk of death from malignancy.

Prostacycline Analogues

Prostacycline analogues given as an intravenous infusion to patients with critical ischaemia improve the limb salvage rate in the short term, but further studies of longer duration will be necessary to decide their ultimate place.

SURGICAL MANAGEMENT OF PAOD

INDICATIONS

The most common relative indication of PAOD is incapacitating claudication. Before intervention for incapacitating claudication is considered, the patient's work must be affected and their mobility limited to approximately 100 yards of level walking.

Critical ischaemia, including rest pain, pregangrene or established gangrene with tissue loss, constitutes an absolute indication for intervention. This could take the form of revascularisation or amputation. Many more patients are now undergoing revascularisation procedures rather than primary amputation. A proportion of vascular reconstructions will fail and lead to either secondary reconstruction or secondary amputation. When considering which procedure to use, multiple factors have to be taken into account. These include:

- Mobility pre-operatively, e.g. independent, chair-bound, bed-bound etc.
- Medical history.
- Concurrent disease.
- Previous vascular surgery.
- Patient expectation.
- Social support.
- Patient age and motivation.
- Quality of life: amputation, although keeping the patient alive and pain free, does have significant detrimental effects on body image and social interactions. Patients who undergo successful revascularisation do not experience these problems.
- The minimal intervention necessary, to render the patient symptom free or improved.

SEGMENTAL APPROACH TO VASCULAR RECONSTRUCTIVE SURGERY FOR PAOD

When considering intervention by either angioplasty or reconstruction, the arterial system is divided into functional segments. These are:

- Aortic (supra/infrarenal).
- Aorto-iliac (common/external).
- Femoro-popliteal (above/below-knee).
- Trifurcation (crural).
- Distal (ankle/foot).
- Microvascular (digital/arteriolar).

The segments refer to sections of the arterial tree which lend themselves to surgical bypass. Patients who present with critical ischaemia will have occlusions in at least two functional segments. Those with claudication will usually have one occlusion. In patients with disease involving two levels, the proximal segment must be treated first or a distal segment reconstruction will fail.

INTERVENTIONAL RADIOLOGICAL TECHNIQUES

PERCUTANEOUS TRANSLUMINAL BALLOON ANGIOPLASTY

Percutaneous transluminal balloon angioplasty (PTA) is the procedure of first choice, and is used successfully in 40% of patients presenting to the vascular surgeon. The technique is more successful in stenoses than in occlusions, and in short lesions and large proximal vessels with high flow rates. Angioplasty of the proximal iliac arteries in patients with a single arterial lesion can give excellent symptomatic relief in 60–70% of patients over 5 years.

Patients who are at risk from surgery would be offered balloon angioplasty even if the lesion is high risk, as the morbidity and mortality from PTA are significantly less than for surgery.

PTA requires a team approach between vascular surgeons and radiologists. Performed under local anaesthesia, a guide wire is passed through the artery, and a deflated balloon between 2–10 mm in diameter positioned across the narrowing or occlusion, and expanded with a mixture of saline and radiographic dye. This is held in place for a minute and the balloon is then deflated.

Advantages of PTA

The advantages of PTA are that it is:
- Safe.
- Quick.
- Cost effective.
- Durable in selected patients.

Complications

The complications of PTA include:
- Haematoma.
- Arterial embolisation.
- Arterial thrombosis.
- Arterial rupture.
- Puncture site infection.

PERCUTANEOUS TRANSLUMINAL STENTING

In percutaneous transluminal stenting, the balloon is inflated and a cylindrical stent of metallic wire is placed into the vessel in a collapsed form. The stent then either expands itself to a predetermined diameter or is stretched from within with an angioplasty balloon to hold the walls of the artery apart. Percutaneous transluminal stenting is used for long occlusions, stenoses or recurrence after previous PTA.

PERCUTANEOUS TRANSLUMINAL STENT GRAFTING

In percutaneous transluminal stent grafting, a graft is anchored in position at both ends within the artery by stents. This new procedure has been used for repair of abdominal aortic aneurysm.

THROMBECTOMY

On occasion, large arterial occlusions occur suddenly as a result of thrombosis or embolus; occlusions resulting from emboli are easier to extract. The commonest sites of occlusions are the femoral or brachial arteries. These vessels are removed either through an arteriotomy or by using a balloon extraction catheter. The balloon can cause further intimal damage, therefore these patients require anticoagulation post-operatively. After removing thrombi from a damaged artery, the underlying stenosis remains, and bypass procedures may be required.

BYPASS PROCEDURES

Surgical bypass is considered under the same functional segmental approach as used for radiological intervention. Three factors affect the graft patency. These are:
• Run in.
• Run off.
• Graft.

If any of these three factors is compromised, the graft will fail.

RUN IN

The proximal segment of occlusive disease should always be treated first, ensuring that the run in, or flow, to any distal graft is maximised. Grafts to the proximal vessels which have higher flow rates and larger anastomoses allow more room for minor technical error without compromising the flow. Hence proximal grafts have higher long-term patency rates than distal grafts with lower flow rates.

RUN OFF

The run off refers to the arterial tree below the point of insertion of the graft. If the run off is good, i.e. into patent vessels, the highest possible flow rate is maintained in the graft itself. If the run off is poor, e.g. stenosis distal to the graft, then the long-term outlook for the graft will be poor.

GRAFT MATERIAL

In high flow situations, such as aortic or iliac reconstructions, the graft material is less important than in situations of low flow, such as distal grafts. The two most common materials used for grafting are dacron and autogenous vein (the long saphenous is the usual vein used).

For intra-abdominal work, dacron is used, the former being employed far more commonly. For femoro-femoral cross-over grafts and axillo-bifemoral grafts, dacron is the most commonly used material. For most infra-inguinal bypasses, autogenous vein has a higher patency rate in the long term than any synthetic graft material. Synthetics have to be used if the vein is unavailable or of very poor quality. Long bypasses from the femoral artery to ankle level must be constructed from vein or they will inevitably fail early. In shorter bypasses in the lower limb, PTFE and dacron are being used more frequently. Lower limb arteries are shown in Figure 13.1.

PSEUDO-INTIMAL HYPERPLASIA

In pseudo-intimal hyperplasia, the normal single layered vascular endothelium is disrupted (or non-existent in synthetic grafts) and is replaced by a multilayered fibrotic cell mass which has none of the normal biochemical properties of endothelium. As the lesion progresses, it protrudes into the graft lumen, and stenosis or occlusion occurs. Many grafts fail because of the development of this condition.

Oral aspirin limits the rate of progression of pseudo-intimal hyperplasia but unfortunately does not halt it completely.

AORTO-BIFEMORAL BYPASS

Aorto-bifemoral bypass is used when the aorta and common iliac vessels are simultaneously diseased or occluded causing bilateral and severe symptoms in both legs. This procedure has an excellent long-term patency rate of 75% at 5 years, with much improved exercise tolerance. The patient has wounds in both groins and is generally hospitalised for up to

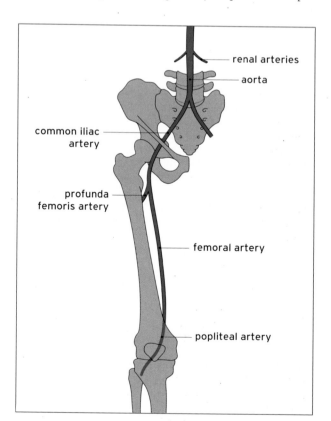

renal arteries
aorta
common iliac artery
profunda femoris artery
femoral artery
popliteal artery

Figure 13.1 Lower limb arteries.

10 days. The initial post-operative period requires close control of systolic blood pressure to prevent excessive tension at the anastomotic sites. Post-operative ileus is common. Mobilisation can begin on day 3 or 4 post-operatively.

FEMORO-FEMORAL EXTRA-ANATOMIC BYPASS

In a patient with unilateral iliac occlusion, the femoro-femoral bypass graft receives blood from one groin passing subcutaneously across the front of the abdomen to the other groin. This procedure requires dissections in both groins but no abdominal incision, and therefore can be performed under spinal or regional anaesthesia. This is a preferred procedure to aorto-bifemoral bypass after angioplasty of the most suitable iliac lesion, as the morbidity and mortality are substantially less.

AXILLO-FEMORAL (OR BIFEMORAL) EXTRA-ANATOMIC BYPASS

The axillo-femoral (or bifemoral) extra-anatomic bypass is used for limb salvage procedures only in very unwell patients with extensive aorto-iliac disease and failed angioplasty.

INFRA-INGUINAL BYPASS SURGERY

Bypasses from the common femoral artery in the groin to sites more distal in the lower limb are among the most common reconstructive procedures performed in vascular surgery. The segmental approach applies within the lower limb.

Femoro-popliteal (Above-knee)

The femoro-popliteal bypass is undertaken between the common femoral artery and the most proximal part of the popliteal artery using PTFE, dacron or the long saphenous vein reversed. Incisions are made in the groin and on the inner thigh above the knee. These procedures have a low mortality rate and a 70–80% patency rate at 5 years.

Femoro-popliteal (Below-knee)

On many occasions the superficial femoral and proximal popliteal artery are both occluded, and the latter becomes patent again below the level of the knee joint. A reversed long saphenous vein graft, or a long saphenous vein graft *in situ* (the venous valves have to be disrupted for this procedure), has a better long-term patency rate than when prosthetic material is used, but bypass grafts that cross the knee joint have a poor long-term survival compared with those which do not.

Femoro-crural Bypass

The popliteal trifurcation situated approximately 8–10 cm below the knee joint is a very common site for arterial occlusion, especially in diabetic patients. The long-term patency rate of this procedure in the order of 20–50% at 5 years.

Femoro-distal Bypass

The femoro-distal bypass was developed as an alternative to amputation to preserve the foot in patients with extensive disease in the lower limb. It is technically difficult, but is a successful distal bypass which saves the limb (sometimes amputation of the toes or transmetatarsals) and maintains mobility and quality of life to a far higher degree than a major amputation. Patency varies widely from 15 to 50% at 5 years.

COMPLICATIONS OF VASCULAR SURGERY

Complications of vascular surgery include:
- Haemorrhage.
- Haematoma.
- Thrombosis.
- Infection.
- Nerve injury.
- False aneurysm.
- Graft morphology, i.e. dilation, degeneration, stenosis, intimal hyperplasia, atherosclerosis, elongation and kinking.
- Remote ischaemia.

PHYSIOTHERAPY AFTER VASCULAR RECONSTRUCTIVE SURGERY

Physiotherapists have a role in reinforcing the lifestyle changes that may prevent disease progressing in patients that have undergone vascular reconstructive surgery. However, in common with many general surgery procedures, physiotherapy treatment is not normally required for patients undergoing elective vascular reconstructive surgery. These patients are mobilised by the nursing staff and are discharged home early. The patients likely to be referred for active physiotherapy management fall into two main categories: those with respiratory problems and those with mobility problems.

Acute respiratory problems are most common in patients having the more proximal bypass procedures and, in particular, when concurrent pulmonary pathology, e.g. chronic obstructive pulmonary disease (COPD), is present or when the patient is a current smoker. Treatment methods will depend on identification of the problem, but often attention to humidification and adequate analgesia is the primary action.

Patients whose mobility has been delayed by one of the complications listed above are the second group of patients that are likely to be referred to the physiotherapist. Pain, reduced muscle strength from immobility, and reduced joint range from swelling are the problems likely to be encountered. Before selecting a treatment method, the physiotherapist will need to take into account any limitations imposed by the surgeon to maintain integrity of the graft, and the degree of blood flow impairment to the affected limb.

LOWER LIMB AMPUTATIONS

Despite many advances in interventional radiology, surgical techniques and medical management of patients with PAOD, amputations still constitute a significant proportion of a vascular surgeon's workload. Too often patients present late when established gangrene has already affected one or more toes. Minor amputations of toes are common following successful reconstructive surgery.

Major amputation is performed as a primary procedure, or as a secondary procedure following revascularisation.

PRIMARY AMPUTATION

Primary amputation accounts for up to 30% of the major amputations performed because a patient has usually presented late to the surgeon when the affected limb is irretrievably damaged. Revascularisation of necrotic limbs can precipitate death, making amputation the only safe option. Lower limb arterial thrombosis is an indicator of poor general health, and survival rates from these amputations are poor; more than half of these patients die from co-morbidity within a year of their operation.

SECONDARY AMPUTATION

Secondary amputation is the major amputation after attempts at reconstruction or radiological intervention have failed.

Revascularisation of an ischaemic limb with a subsequent minor amputation provides the patient with a far better quality of life than a primary amputation.

MAJOR AMPUTATIONS OF THE LOWER LIMB

Hindquarter Amputation

Hindquarter amputation is a rare procedure that is required after extensive trauma to the pelvis and lower limb, with devascularisation and infection of the hip and thigh musculature. There is a significant mortality from blood loss and consequent infection associated with the procedure. The operation involves removing the hemipelvis, the hip joint and the lower limb.

Femoral Disarticulation

Femoral disarticulation is another rare procedure, used after infection in the thigh muscles, e.g. gas gangrene. The femur is removed from the acetabulum, and the entire length of the limb is lost. Mobilisation after such a procedure is difficult in the young patient and impossible in the elderly.

Above-knee Amputation

Amputations through the mid-femur are common in vascular surgical practice. The profunda femoris artery usually remains patent, even in the presence of a totally ischaemic distal limb, and provides the muscle in the upper thigh with collateral circulation; therefore healing is not problematic. Unfortunately, only 25% of patients will achieve full mobility following the procedure and rehabilitation.

Technique

Equal anterior and posterior myoplastic flaps are constructed at the site of amputation, and the femur is sectioned 5–20 cm above the knee joint. The flaps are approximated and the skin is closed primarily. The femoral artery and vein are ligated and the sciatic nerve sectioned high to prevent any mechanical damage to its cut surface resulting in stump pain, a significant problem post-operatively at the time of mobilisation.

The above-knee stump does not bear weight, which is borne through the pelvis directly, and an above-knee prosthesis usually requires a supporting strap around the waist and over the shoulder. Mobilisation on such a prosthesis is difficult as the proprioception from the knee joint is lost. A mechanical knee joint is required for sitting and other occasions where the knee needs to be bent. There are many designs of standard prosthesis for this amputation site.

Gritti-Stokes Amputation

In patients where a prosthetic limb is not an option and length of femur is important for balance, amputation may be performed at the knee joint. The patella is drawn backwards and sutured over the cut surface of the femur distally. This kind of amputation is not favoured by prosthetists as a weight-bearing prosthesis is very difficult to fit onto the rather broad end of the intercondylar part of the femur.

Below-knee Amputation

Below-knee amputation is the most common type of major amputation performed. Combined with revascularisation, a severely ischaemic limb may be salvaged at this level. A revascularisation procedure that converts a patient from an above-knee amputee to a below-knee amputee is considered a more promising procedure as the below-knee amputations offer a greater chance of independence.

Technique

The tibia and fibula are sectioned 10–12 cm below the knee joint with the formation of a long myoplastic flap of gastrocnemius. This flap is brought forwards over the end of the sectioned bones to be sutured into place. The fascia and muscles are sutured across the anterior surface of the tibia to cover the tibial and fibula bone ends. The skin is closed primarily. On mobilisation, the weight is borne through the tibial tuberosity.

In a well-motivated patient, a well-fitting prosthesis on a good below-knee stump, with knee joint proprioception, can give normal mobility even over rough ground. Independent mobility can be expected in a high proportion of these patients (>80%).

Symes Amputation

Amputation through the tarsal bones with preservation of the heel pad can follow attempts at revascularisation of a severely ischaemic limb with pre-existing necrosis of the forefoot. Symes amputation preserves proprioception at ankle level allowing the patient to guide the limb more accurately during walking. No prosthesis need be worn for short walks within the home, and a supporting prosthesis within a built-up boot is all that is necessary for use outside on normal terrain. Unfortunately, the healing rate in PAOD patients who have had a Symes amputation is poor.

Transmetatarsal Amputation

The transmetatarsal amputation has become much more common since the advent of distal bypasses. Loss of all the toes requires very little prosthesis either for indoor or outdoor use. Some support is occasionally necessary within the shoe of the patient for optimal mobility. Transmetatarsal amputations as primary amputations tend to have a very poor outcome in large vessel peripheral vascular disease but are more commonly performed in patients with diabetic peripheral microvascular occlusions where they heal very well.

Sympathectomy

Sympathectomy was the mainstay of surgical management before the introduction of direct arterial surgery. It is based on the premise that severing the sympathetic fibres to a limb will increase its blood supply, as the supply of blood to the skin is regulated in part by the sympathetic outflow. The arteriolar plexuses are constantly held in a state of mild vasoconstriction in a normal subject. Hence severing these fibres will result in vasodilation.

Lumbar sympathectomy

Lumbar sympathectomy is now performed percutaneously by fluoroscopically placed phenol injection, under local anaesthesia. It is effective in only a small proportion of patients with critical limb ischaemia, is very limited in diabetic autonomic neuropathy and does not improve patients with intermittent claudication. It therefore remains a very limited tool in the treatment of PAOD.

Cervical sympathectomy

In the upper limb, surgery to divide the cervical plexus entails a complex dissection in the root of the neck, which is potentially hazardous to the patient. Cervical sympathectomy is effective in improving the blood supply to the fingers but its effects are temporary, and Horner's syndrome (drooping eyelid, pupil contraction and loss of sweat function on the affected side) is a common complication. Thoracoscopic cervical sympathectomy is durable and safer, and results in an arm and hand which are much warmer and drier than pre-operatively.

ABDOMINAL AORTIC ANEURYSM

TREATMENT INDICATIONS

Repair of aneurysm should be undertaken when the operative risks are outweighed by the risks associated with conservative management. Rupture of the aneurysm is associated with a prohibitive death rate, 90–95% in the community, and 50% if patients are fortunate enough to reach hospital. The diameter of the aneurysm is directly proportional to the rupture rate. At 4 cm, the rupture rate is very small (1–2% per year) but at 8 cm there is a 50% chance of rupture within a year. Patients who have an abdominal aortic aneurysm greater than 5.5 cm are offered elective repair, if their general medical condition permits. The operative risk is considerable at 2% to 8% but mortalities of 15% or more are common in high risk patients with co-morbidity such as ischaemic heart disease, lung disease or renal disease.

SURGICAL REPAIR

The accepted method of treatment for abdominal aortic aneurysm is resection and replacement with a dacron graft. This usually necessitates a midline incision and transperitoneal approach to the aorta. The graft can be either a straight tube in the simpler procedures, or a bifurcated graft for the more complex aorto-bi-iliac or bifemoral bypasses required for extensive aorto-iliac aneurysms.

The aneurysm may extend proximally to involve the renal artery origins. The procedure includes reimplantation of the renal arteries into the new graft. This procedure is associated with a higher incidence of post-operative renal failure as both kidneys are rendered ischaemic during reimplantation.

PERCUTANEOUS TRANSLUMINAL STENT GRAFTING

Percutaneous repair of infrarenal abdominal aortic aneurysms by the use of a graft stent combination has been performed in selected patients who have a prohibitive risk from general anaesthesia and conventional repair. This type of correction is still undergoing evaluation. The procedure involves a large catheter, containing two stents attached to a very thin-walled graft, being pushed into position from a femoral artery into the aorta above the aneurysm. The proximal stent is then placed just below the renal arteries, the graft unfurled within the aneurysm, the distal end of the graft placed into the bifurcation, and the graft then anchored thereby expanding the second stent. The stents form blood-tight seals at either end, and blood therefore passes into the new graft not the aneurysm.

CAROTID ARTERY DISEASE

Strokes are responsible for 11% of all deaths in the UK, and 2.5% of the annual NHS expenditure. Of the 200 strokes per 100 000 population in the UK, 20–30% are related to carotid disease.

PRESENTATION OF CAROTID DISEASE

Carotid disease can give rise to symptoms from either emboli or flow restriction.

Emboli

Atheroma is particularly common at the bifurcation of the common carotid. Plaque that forms in the internal carotid artery is in direct line with the cerebral circulation. Any platelet thrombus on the plaque's surface may embolise distally into the brain via the middle cerebral artery, giving rise to transient ischaemic attacks. These can be typical transient hemiplegias on the contralateral side to the artery involved, speech problems or cognitive function loss. Alternatively, embolisation of the ophthalmic artery (amaurosis fugax) causes temporary blindness on the ipsilateral side. Typical amaurosis is described as a black curtain coming either down or up through the field of vision. This leaves the patient totally blind for a short period of time. Recovery is usually complete unless the emboli occur frequently, in which case permanent blindness may result.

Cerebral Flow Restriction

Isolated unilateral internal carotid occlusion may have no symptoms whatsoever. Where one internal carotid is occluded and the other is significantly stenosed, patients will present with cerebral ischaemia, characterised by ill-defined neurological symptoms, e.g. memory loss, loss of cognitive function, lack of concentration, etc. These symptoms will occur despite an adequate Circle of Willis, as the vertebral arteries alone are insufficient to maintain cerebral flow. Correction of the stenosed carotid vessel often improves these patients by restoring an adequate arterial blood pressure to the Circle of Willis.

'Asymptomatic' Carotid Disease

Carotid disease may be detected in the pre-operative assessment for another major surgical procedure such as coronary artery bypass grafting or aneurysm surgery. If the major surgery could compromise cerebral circulation, these patients may benefit from prior endarterectomy or even a combined surgical procedure.

Carotid Endarterectomy

Patients presenting with a transient ischaemic attack (TIA) or non-disabling stroke with stenosis greater than 70% of the internal carotid artery are offered endarterectomy, which will reduce the subsequent stroke rate by 75% over 3 years.

The technique requires a pre-sternomastoid incision. The internal, external and common carotid vessels are controlled with vascular clamps. As the cerebral circulation is interrupted during the time of endarterectomy, a temporary shunt is used to maintain cerebral blood flow. The diseased arterial wall is removed leaving as smooth a surface as possible. If the vessel is small, a patch angioplasty is then performed using either saphenous vein or dacron. The shunt is then removed before re-establishing cerebral blood flow. Post-operatively, the systolic blood pressure is closely controlled to protect both the arterial suture line and the cerebral tissue from extremes of perfusion.

VENOUS DISEASES OF THE LOWER LIMB

SIMPLE VARICOSE VEINS

These are the most commonly seen venous problem. Long saphenous varicosities tend to occur on the medial aspect of the leg from the thigh to the ankle, and short saphenous varicosities begin below the knee from the sapheno-popliteal junction in the popliteal fossa, running along the track of the sural nerve, and tending to appear more laterally on the calf. The aetiology of varicose veins is unknown but abnormalities in the collagen of either the vein wall itself or the valve leaflets have been suggested.

Treatment

If the sapheno-femoral (or sapheno-popliteal) junction is competent, then local sclerotherapy is likely to be effective. Otherwise, vein stripping from knee to thigh would be the treatment of choice. These procedures are performed as a day case, and early mobilisation is essential.

If the deep venous system is patent, then removal of the superficial veins will decrease the venous pressure in the lower leg; however, surgery is not recommended when there is occlusion of the deep venous system.

ACUTE DEEP VEIN THROMBOSIS

Acute deep vein thrombosis (DVT) occurs commonly after surgery despite the use of anti-embolic stockings and the administration of subcutaneous heparin. Certain procedures, e.g. hip replacement, carry a very high incidence of DVT, in the order of 60%. The incidence is also higher in patients with malignancy, or undergoing pelvic procedures.

Thrombosis is thought to occur during surgery or in the very early post-operative period. Mobility is limited and venous stasis allows thrombosis to form behind the deep venous valve leaflets, which then extends into the lumen of the vein. This occlusion gives rise to peripheral oedema, local tenderness and redness—the typical clinical presentation of a DVT. If unchecked, the process progresses to give more ankle oedema and increasing pain on walking. The clot organises over the next week or so, and the vein wall then produces substances which lyse the clot to give varying degrees of resolution. If lysis acts primarily on the periphery of the clot, the latter is freed to move within the vein and possibly give rise to a pulmonary embolus (see Chapter 10). This typically occurs 10 days after the onset of thrombosis but the majority of cases resolve without embolus.

There are three possible outcomes of DVT:

- Resolved acute thrombosis: this is the most common outcome where, within 3–4 weeks, the limb becomes asymptomatic.
- Venous valvular incompetence: as the clot lyses, some or all of the deep venous valves may become incompetent. The resulting venous hypertension leads to ongoing damage to the vein resulting in further thrombosis and valvular damage.
- Long-term venous occlusion: the resolution process results in occlusion of the deep vein. During exercise, the venous pressure in the calf and lower leg increases and the patient complains of a bursting claudication-type pain in the calf. (This venous claudication must be distinguished from pain secondary to PAOD.) Subsequently, the perforating veins fail, increasing the pressure on the skin of the lower calf and giving rise to ulceration.

Treatment of the Post-phlebitic Limb

A post-phlebitic limb is one presenting with venous hypertension, valvular incompetence or occlusion in the deep vein and/or perforator disease. It is assessed with Doppler ultrasound, giving accurate localisation of reflux in the superficial or deep veins.

13

The mainstay of treatment for peripheral venous hypertension is the application of well-fitting support stockings which will relieve much of the discomfort and oedema which trouble these patients.

Deep Vein Surgery

Surgery on the deep veins is limited to bypass procedures which decompress the venous system. The long saphenous vein from the contralateral limb is swung across subcutaneously in front of the pubis and its distal end anastomosed into the deep venous system of the symptomatic limb. The long saphenous vein of the donor leg has within it a competent set of valves which will allow flow of blood out of the symptomatic limb, decreasing venous pressure.

Direct surgery on the deep venous valves has been attempted but abandoned owing to poor results.

PERFORATOR DISEASE

Perforator veins connect the deep and superficial venous systems. They pass through the deep fascia of the limb, which acts as a valve to direct blood from the superficial into the deep system.

This valvular function may be lost if the vein becomes dilated or is subject to vastly increased venous pressure. Pressurised blood passes through to the superficial system, and increases pressure in the skin vessels. This venous hypertension will restrict the removal of harmful metabolites from the skin and its subcutaneous tissue, compromising its nutrition and resulting in atrophy of the skin and damage to the subcutaneous tissues (lipodermatosclerosis).

Surgical Treatment

An endoscope is passed beneath the deep fascia of the calf, and the perforating veins are isolated and clipped. The scar is small and sited well away from the diseased skin of the lower calf.

VENOUS LEG ULCERATION

Venous leg ulceration is the final stage of venous disease, where deep vein and/or perforator disease exists. Increased venous pressure in the lower limb damages the skin and its subcutaneous tissues. Lipodermatosclerosis will occur and the typical 'inverted champagne bottle' appearance of the lower leg will develop.

Small amounts of blood will escape from damaged skin capillaries, causing the brown 'venous staining' commonly seen in these patients' limbs, and the development of 'venous eczema'. The staining is irreversible but the eczematous changes respond to external compression treatment.

Treatment

The application of compression to the ulcer is essential to its healing, but not by support hosiery as exudation is common. A four layered dressing has been developed to provide a substantial amount of absorbency in conjunction with a high level of compression. The bandaging is left undisturbed for up to 10 days in order to allow the fragile epithelialisation process beneath to progress undisturbed. The vast majority of purely venous ulcers heal rapidly with this approach.

REHABILITATION OF THE AMPUTEE

Once it has been decided that amputation is the most appropriate course of treatment, the surgeon will discuss this option with the patient. The therapists need to be informed to enable them to commence their pre-operative assessment and treatment. They can also offer support and information about the routine to be followed before, during and after the operation.

PRE-AMPUTATION ASSESSMENTS
Physical Assessment

Patients who undergo amputation due to vascular disease are generally over 65 years of age and usually have numerous medical conditions or multiple physical problems. It is therefore very important to assess the patient's physical status as a whole.

Points to consider are:
- How active have they been over the past years, months or weeks?
- What sort of lifestyle do they have at present, or wish to achieve?
- What amount of assistance is required for them to walk or to be transferred? Do they use walking aids?
- What is their normal walking pattern, and is mobility and independence limited by other medical factors, or pain?
- Have they needed to use a wheelchair for short/long distances?
- What is the condition of their other leg?
- What medication are they on?

A physical assessment can establish muscle strength, joint range of movement, skin tone, skin temperature and sensation. However, in accordance with the patient's emotional and physical condition it is important to find out what he or she finds acceptable. Most patients who are awaiting an amputation are pleased to discuss their general health and undergo a physical examination, so long as they are made aware of the importance of giving accurate information to the therapist. The assessment is an opportunity for patients to ask questions, as this can help them to gain further understanding of the many factors that are involved in their recovery and mobility following the operation.

During the assessment, it is important a relationship of trust and respect is built up between patient and therapist.

Information can be gained by observation and in discussion with relatives and carers. This may require a series of visits rather than one long detailed assessment. It must be remembered that this is often a very frightening experience and there are many emotional as well as physical factors to be considered.

Emotional Assessment

Everybody reacts differently to the knowledge that an amputation is going to be necessary. Although most patients are confused and upset by the realisation that they will need to lose all or part of their limb, not everyone will react in this way. Some patients who have been experiencing excruciating pain from a useless limb may actually be relieved that the amputation is going to take place. They may look upon the amputation as a positive treatment to an unresolvable problem. This should be encouraged because indeed they may be able to have a much more active and pain free life following amputation.

For most people a range of emotions are expressed, from anger and resentment to a feeling of loss and uselessness. The therapists as members of the team have a large part to play in helping patients to acknowledge and express their emotions, and to help them to understand what to expect once the amputation has taken place. Much of the fear is fear of the unknown.

Patients need to feel in control of the situation. By understanding what to expect before, during and after the operation, uncertainty can be reduced. However, be guided by the patients. Estimate how much information they want pre-operatively. It may be sufficient for them that a therapist is available if they have any questions, rather than to be given extensive information that they may not be ready to take in.

Social Assessment

Each patient will have his or her own set of priorities. One of the factors which will have a large influence on these priorities will be home circumstances.

Points to consider are:

- Where is the home situated, both geographically and in relation to relatives and carers?
- What is the design of the home, e.g. flat, bungalow, three-storey house? Will the patient be able to return there after the amputation operation?
- What support networks are available, e.g. neighbours, friends?
- Where is the patient's work and/or social life situated?
- What local authority or voluntary organisations are in the area to offer support, e.g. home help, meals on wheels, support groups, day centres?
- What is the patient's financial position, and should he or she be seeking advice on allowances and benefits?

Pre-operatively it may not be appropriate to go into a detailed assessment of the patient's home surroundings and social circumstances. However, assessment is a process rather than a single treatment. Relatives, carers and ward staff should all be included in this process. They can contribute to your understanding of the situation, and will be working with you and the patient both pre- and post-operatively.

PRE-OPERATIVE TREATMENT

An active programme of pre-operative treatment may not be possible due to the patient's medical condition. In this circumstance, one or more alternatives may be appropriate. These include:

- Strengthening the muscles.
- Preserving joint mobility and decreasing the likelihood of oedema. Active exercise is the ideal method of treatment, although passive stretching may be used.
- Teaching transfers. A standard pivot transfer using the unaffected leg is often used.
- Teaching independent movement in bed.
- Maintaining ability to walk wherever possible.
- Ordering the wheelchair.
- Teaching wheelchair mobility. This will be the most effective and safest means of mobility immediately following the amputation.
- Explaining to the patient that phantom limb sensation may be experienced, i.e. the sensation that part or all of the amputated limb is still present.
- Showing the patient an artificial limb if it is appropriate.
- Finding out if the patient would like to meet someone who has already had an amputation so as to gain further understanding and insight.

Through the therapist's assessment and treatment, valuable information on which to base the level of amputation can be obtained.

POST-OPERATIVE TREATMENT

It is recommended that the older amputee is mobilised on the first or second day post-operatively, if his or her general medical condition allows. Wheelchair mobility is recommended as it is safer than hopping, lessening the risk of falls and overuse of the remaining leg. Below-knee amputees will require a stump board for their wheelchair. Correct pressure-relieving cushions and mattresses may need to be considered, and education regarding positioning, weight transference and skin care reinforced.

Other treatment may include:

- An exercise routine appropriate to the patient's abilities.
- Practice with transfers and wheelchair mobility.
- Prevention of contractures and oedema. For a person with a below-knee amputation, the knee should rest in full extension. After above-knee amputation both passive and active hip extension should be encouraged.

Dressing practice can be commenced by the occupational therapist as soon as the patient feels able. Patients should be encouraged to perform as many activities of daily living as possible. The independence achieved will give the patient a physical and psychological boost. He or she should be encouraged to look at, handle and move the residual limb. Some people find it easier than others to do this. You should be guided by the patient, and developments should proceed at his or her own pace.

After removal of the wound drain, the programme of exercise can be increased. This can take place either on the ward or in the physiotherapy department, individually or in group sessions. Treating patients in groups allows them to learn from each other's experiences.

Pneumatic Post-amputation Mobility (PPAM) AID

The penumatic post-amputation mobility (PPAM) aid is the most commonly used early walking aid. It comprises a basic metal frame, inflatable air bags which come in two sizes—for below-knee and above-knee amputees—a small inner cushion bag and a foot pump.

The PPAM aid can be used while the sutures are still in the wound provided that the wound is healing satisfactorily.

This aid helps the physiotherapist to assess a patient's potential for wearing an artificial limb. It can reduce stump oedema, allow the patient to experience walking, and provide a psychological boost.

The PPAM aid is not as effective for above-knee amputees. The Femurett may be a better option both for assessment and as a walking aid. It is not, however, used to reduce stump oedema.

Home Visit

As patients become physically stronger, they may either return to their own home or be transferred to a rehabilitation unit. If a patient is to return home, a home visit from an occupational therapist will usually be required. The occupational therapist organises this with the patient and the relatives and carers. It can be of great value for the physiotherapist and/or any relevant community based staff also to take part in this visit.

The occupational therapist will be assessing how the patient functions within the home environment and support network. Through discussion and experimentation, the patient and the other people present on the visit will be able to decide what needs to be achieved before a successful discharge can take place. Points to consider include:

- The position of the property and access.
- Suitability for wheelchair access.
- Carer network.
- Transfers to and from chair, bed, toilet, commode and bath as applicable.
- Adaptations and equipment required.
- Method of heating.
- Community services needed.

The visit will help to form treatment plans for the future, realise strengths/limitations—both personal and geographical—and assist in the formation of realistic goals. This assessment is part of a continuing process and assesses only the patient's adaptation to the situation at that time.

Referral to a Prosthetic Centre

Referral to a prosthetic centre will depend upon the patient's physical and emotional health. Some patients do not wish, or are unable, to wear a limb, and have a full and varied lifestyle as wheelchair users. Points to consider are:

- The patient's wishes.
- Will he or she be physically and intellectually capable of using a prosthesis?
- Is the patient ready for prosthetic rehabilitation?
- Does he or she fully understand the effort involved in learning to use a prosthesis?
- Is he or she appropriately motivated?

Prosthetic centre working with local hospital services

There are many ways of providing rehabilitation services for amputee patients. They may:

- Attend out-patient physiotherapy and occupational therapy at the local district general hospital, and attend the prosthetic centre to see the rehabilitation consultant, prosthetist, nurse, psychologist or counsellor.
- Attend out-patient physiotherapy and occupational therapy, and see the staff from the prosthetic centre at satellite clinics or at the local district general hospital.
- Attend the prosthetic centre for all the out-patient therapy and prosthetic care.
- Have a bed in a rehabilitation unit attached to the prosthetic centre, and receive an intensive rehabilitation and prosthetic programme.

The availability of services locally and the patient's preferences will be important in deciding which rehabilitation programme is followed.

Provision of a prosthesis

Each prosthetic centre has its own procedures. There are, however, three main stages in the provision of the patient's first prosthesis. These include:

- Measuring and casting the residual limb.
- The fitting—alterations can be made to the limb to ensure comfort and correct alignment.
- Delivery of the finished prosthesis.

This process should take a maximum of 10 days but may be longer if several adjustments are required at the fitting stage. Patients will need to bring the same pair of comfortable shoes on each visit.

Stump socks and shrinkers

A stump sock is worn to provide protection and cushioning, which makes the prosthesis more comfortable. It allows some air to circulate around the skin, while absorbing perspiration. Stump socks are made of several different materials: wool, wool mix, cotton (both flat weave and terry towelling) and nylon. A combination of stump socks may be required to allow for stump shrinkage. Up to three woollen socks are thought to be acceptable before socket adjustment is required. If the stump increases in size due to swelling or weight gain, it is advisable to reduce the number or thickness of the stump socks.

A stump shrinker is a shaped stump support to provide even pressure over the stump, decrease oedema and encourage optimal shaping of the soft tissue. A range of sizes is available.

The silosheath is also used. This is a prosthetic sheath impregnated with gel and formulated with a medical grade mineral oil. It dissipates shock and vibration and helps to eliminate abrasions on the residual limb.

GAIT RE-EDUCATION

Gait re-education is a detailed process. Initially it involves the use of parallel bars, progressing (dependent on the patient's capabilities) to fully independent walking and running. There are many different levels of ability and mobility grades (Table 13.1). For some patients, very limited mobility within the home may be the aim, or indeed they may use the limb only to assist them in transfers.

If the patient can master walking with or without walking aids, he or she may be able to be instructed in how to do some/all of the following activities:

- Walking up and down stairs.
- Negotiating slopes, curbs, pavements and uneven surfaces.
- Manoeuvring in and out of a car.
- Using a supermarket trolley.
- Carrying objects either for work or for pleasure.
- Pursuing a hobby or sport, e.g. cycling, running, fishing, bowls.
- Returning to or re-training for a job which entails physical activity.
- Climbing, e.g. ladders.

Further home assessments may be required by the occupational therapist, as the patient regains his or her independence. Different assistive equipment may be required such as stair, grab and external rails.

EMOTIONAL ADJUSTMENT

Some health regions provide counselling or psychology services at their prosthetic centres and these can be of benefit to those patients having difficulty adjusting emotionally following their amputation.

REGAINING INDEPENDENCE

Rehabilitation aims to return the patient to an acceptable lifestyle with maximum independence and dignity. For each individual the level will be different, but areas which deserve consideration are:

- Activities of daily living.
- Mobility—both wheelchair and prosthetic.
- Driving.
- Finances—benefits and allowances.
- Employment.
- Hobbies.
- Holidays.
- Relationships.
- Emotional adjustment.

CARE OF THE UNAFFECTED LEG

Smoking

Current smokers need help and encouragement to stop.

Diet

Care needs to be taken to ensure a balanced nutritious diet, to maintain a constant weight. Excessive weight gain or loss can adversely affect the comfort and fit of the prosthesis. Prostheses have upper weight limits and cannot be used by obese individuals.

Skin Care

A proper skin care routine should be emphasised. This includes:

- The foot being washed daily, with particular care taken with drying.
- A doctor being contacted if there are any red areas or broken skin on the leg or foot. If the skin is dry, a little cream may be applied if prescribed.
- Wearing comfortable footwear that is not too restricting. Insoles should be securely attached. Sandals with straps are best avoided because they do not give the required support and protection.
- Avoiding creased or tight socks and stockings—socks or stockings with elastic tops are not recommended. Natural fibres are best because they allow ventilation. They should be washed regularly
- Having the toenails cut straight across and not too short. This is best done after a bath or soak when the nails have softened. Patients with diabetes and or PAOD should

Table 13.1 Harold Wood/Stanmore mobility grades.

Harold Wood/Stanmore mobility grades	
I	Limb wearing abandoned or use of cosmetic limb only
II	Wears prosthesis only for transfers or to assist nursing. Walks only with therapist or carer
III	Indoor walker using only walking aids, e.g. sticks, crutches, walking frame
IV	Indoor and outdoor walking, though with regular use of walking aids
V	Independent indoor and outdoor walking with no walking aids, except for confidence or to cover difficult terrain or weather conditions
VI	Normal unrestricted walking

have their toenails cut by a chiropodist. Corns or hard skin should also be treated by a chiropodist.

- Checking the temperature of the bath, avoiding extremes of temperature. Excessive heat should be avoided, such as an unwrapped hot water bottle or sitting directly in front of a fire.
- Keeping the leg raised on a stool when sitting to assist venous return and reduce the likelihood of oedema. While dependent, care must be taken to avoid striking any sharp objects.
- Keeping the legs uncrossed when in the lying position. Excessive or continuous pressure on the healing area should be avoided, along with pressure from bedclothes on the toes if this makes them sore.

CARE OF THE RESIDUAL LIMB

Care of the residual limb includes:
- Washing and thoroughly drying the limb daily.
- Using a clean stump sock daily.
- Avoiding creams or talcum powder unless advised or prescribed by a doctor as they can irritate the skin.
- Daily examination for any skin changes.

FOLLOW-UP

Follow-up is routinely carried out during the first 12 months after the amputation. This occurs at the:
- Vascular surgeon's out-patient clinic.
- Prosthetic centre if a prosthesis is provided.
- Physiotherapist and occupational therapist departments.

Although community services are often organised before discharge, it is important to ensure that equipment and services arrive according to plan. If they prove to be insufficient or inappropriate then a new plan of action can be devised quickly, thus reducing the risk of an avoidable re-admission.

CONCLUSION

In conclusion, the aim is for an efficient and needs-based service that is of sufficient adaptability and comprehensiveness that the patient's quality of life can be maintained or even improved.

GENERAL READING

Cheshire NJW, Wolfe JHN, Barradas MA, Chambler AW, Mikhailidis DP. Smoking and plasma fibrinogen lipoprotein and serotonin are markers for post-operative infra-inguinal graft stenosis. *Eur J Vasc Surg* 1996, **11**:479-486.

European working group on critical leg ischaemia. Chronic critical leg ischaemia. *Circulation* 1991, **84(suppl 4)**:1-26.

Fowkes FGR. Epidemiology of atherosclerotic arterial disease in the lower limbs. *Eur J Vasc Surg* 1988, **2**:283-291.

Fowkes FGR, Lowe GDO, Housley E, *et al.* Cross-linked fibrin degradation products. Progression of peripheral arterial disease and risk of coronary heart disease. *Lancet* 1993, **342**:82-86.

Housley E. Treating claudication in 5 words. *BMJ* 1988, **296**:1483-1484.

Ross R. The pathogenesis of atherosclerosis—an update. *New Engl J Med* 1986, **314**:488-500.

Smith I, Franks PJ, Greenhalgh RM, Poulter NR, Powell JT. The influence of smoking cessation and hypertriclyceridaemia on the progression of peripheral arterial disease and the onset of critical ischaemia. *Euro J Vasc Endovasc Surg* 1996, **11**:402-408.

Wiseman S, Kenchington G, Dane R, *et al.* Influence of smoking and plasma factors on patency of popliteal vein grafts. *BMJ* 1989, **299**:643-646.

SECTION 3

ON-CALL

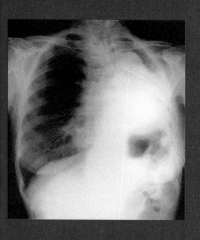

14 M Smith

ON-CALL PHYSIOTHERAPY

CHAPTER OUTLINE

- **Responding to a call**
- **Problem solving**
- **Chest auscultation**
- **The neurological patient**

- **The intensive care patient**
- **Physiotherapy treatment methods**
- **Auditing on-call episodes**

INTRODUCTION

In most hospital centres, there is an on-call physiotherapy service available in the evenings and at weekends to cater for emergency chest conditions. As a rule, the medical officer responsible for the patient will initiate the request to contact the physiotherapist on-call for the night or weekend. However, depending on the physiotherapy department's protocol for the on-call service, a sister or staff nurse in charge for the shift can also call out the physiotherapist, especially if he or she is an experienced clinician. The service also caters for patients who are particularly chesty and who have needed intensive chest physiotherapy during the day, and who therefore may need treatment during the night.

Each physiotherapy department should have a documented policy for its call-out procedure which will give guidance to both the physiotherapist on duty and the multi-disciplinary team making the call.

The aim of this chapter is to provide guidelines for the newly qualified physiotherapist on his or her first call out, and to give examples of typical reasons for using the service. Inappropriate referrals and the method of dealing with such situations will be addressed.

The most common fear of inexperienced physiotherapists is the feeling of inadequacy in an emergency situation. As a rule, the junior physiotherapist will have some respiratory knowledge, and his or her department will offer an in-service training programme to enhance their skills and continually bring them up to date with their respiratory

knowledge. No doubt the senior respiratory clinicians will offer their services and advice if asked or a pre-arrangement can be made so that the junior member of staff has the reassurance that the senior physiotherapist will be available to help, or at least be at the end of the telephone.

Although the member of staff calling for your help may have given a clinical presentation of the patient's condition, there will be the need to assess the problem yourself. This chapter offers advice on how to assess conditions quickly and to eliminate problems that do not require the assistance of a physiotherapist.

RESPONDING TO A CALL

The procedure for responding to a call should be as follows:
- Be polite.
- Get a brief but accurate history from the caller—even on the telephone a clinical picture will take shape, and advice can be offered as to whether you need to visit the patient immediately or at all. For example, if the caller states that the patient is wheezy and this is the only symptom, then bronchodilator therapy can be suggested and the caller asked to telephone later if the patient has not responded to the treatment. If the decision is to see the patient, then the physiotherapist may suggest use of a saline nebuliser while they are en route to the hospital if, by the description of the caller, the problem seems to be sputum retention. Request that the post-operative patient has analgesia before your arrival.

- Ensure the availability of the patient's notes, chest X-rays, blood gas reports (if possible) and suction catheters with suction equipment. Some wards may not have the need for this equipment on a daily basis, e.g. rheumotology, and this impedes the speed of the physiotherapy treatment.
- On meeting the patient, what is the first impression? Is it necessary to treat the patient immediately? If possible, time should be spent reading the notes and observation charts, and assessing the patient's cardiovascular, renal, neurological and respiratory systems. An objective assessment is necessary to establish the severity of the situation—commonly, increasing tiredness, pain, distress, cyanosis and, worse still, lapses of consciousness. Signs of respiratory distress and failure are covered in Chapters 2 and 6.
- Having assessed the patient, will the condition respond to physiotherapy? Examples of when physiotherapy is beneficial or of no use are given below.
- Again, having assessed the patient, is the problem one that will benefit from chest physiotherapy, e.g. post-operative atelectasis and sputum retention in a compliant, stable patient, aspiration of vomit in a patient with head injuries? Following treatment, re-assess the patient and offer advice to the nursing staff on, for example, positioning the patient, adequate humidification and further signs of deterioration where your input would benefit.
- It is difficult to refuse a call out unless it is clear that physiotherapy is of no benefit, for example, if the diagnosis is a definite pulmonary embolus or a pneumothorax. In the latter case, it is fair to suggest that once the chest drain is *in situ* the doctor may telephone you if there is still a problem that will benefit from physiotherapy. If the call out is inappropriate, allow the physiotherapist in charge of that area to deal with the problem the next day, and possibly remind the staff of the protocols for use of the facility.

The next part of the chapter will cover common scenarios for call out and problem solving. As an inexperienced clinician, the prospect of dealing with the unknown is daunting, but if the physiotherapist adheres to an organised format of assessment, and establishes a treatment plan, successul problem solving follows. Calling upon the experience of a senior colleague is not a weakness but an acknowledgement of your limitations; for example, if the patient is tiring and intermittent positive pressure ventilation is indicated but you do not have experience in using the equipment, then ask for the patient to be referred to the anaesthetic team. If an oesophagectomy patient, in whom airway suction is contraindicated, has sputum retention, ask for a mini-tracheostomy to be inserted and then treat the patient. But if the patient's condition is beyond physiotherapy intervention, then refer to the doctor in charge.

EXAMPLES OF APPROPRIATE CALL OUT
Case 1
Mr Smith is a 67-year-old known smoker who underwent emergency surgery for a perforated bowel 2 days ago. He now presents with a pyrexia, irritating cough with obvious sputum, evidence of left lower lobe atelectasis on chest X-ray and dropping oxygen saturation.

Case 2
Mrs Morris is a longstanding chronic bronchitic who has been admitted through casualty with infective exacerbation of her condition. She is on Ventolin nebulisers and is well humidified but still has difficulty in expectorating. Her blood gas analysis is reasonable with a pH of 7.38, partial pressure of carbon dioxide (PCO_2) of 6.2 and partial pressure of oxygen (PO_2) of 9.0 on 28% inspired oxygen. She is awake and co-operative but she is tiring.

Case 3
Miss Davis is a 20-year-old with head injuries who is unconscious and has vomited past her nasogastric tube. The nursing staff have resited her tube but she now has an increased respiratory rate with dropping oxygen saturation, and clinically there are signs of infection in her middle and right lower lobe confirmed by chest X-ray.

EXAMPLES OF INAPPROPRIATE CALL OUT
Case 1
Mr Symmonds is 70 years old and has been admitted to hospital with increasing shortness of breath and left-sided chest pain. His clinical picture is of a left lower lobe pneumonia with air bronchogram on chest X-ray suggesting severe consolidation of the lobe and air trapping. He has a persistent dry cough and is not expectorating.

Here, chest physiotherapy is of no benefit until the pneumonia starts to resolve, and despite the patient's obvious respiratory problem, the advice can be given over the telephone to increase the patient's analgesia and to improve the patient's oxygen concentration if possible.

Case 2
Mrs Morris (see above) has deteriorated and now has a blood gas analysis of pH 7.28, PCO_2 of 8.5 and PO_2 of 6.3 on 35% inspired oxygen. She is very distressed and has lapses in consciousness.

Although your assessment establishes that she has sputum retention with bilateral lower lobe atelectasis, any major chest physiotherapy may cause her to have a respiratory arrest, and therefore no intervention is advisable. This type of situation is a difficult one as the problem is for the physiotherapist to solve. Therefore, your assessment is of value as your intervention could be dangerous.

Case 3
Mr Henry underwent elective surgery for repair of an abdominal aortic aneurysm. Post-operatively, he has become short of breath, is cold and clammy and has a 'bubbly' chest. On examination, he has a urine output of 500 ml for the day and has received 3 litres of saline intravenously. His central venous pressure is 17 cmH$_2$O, and on auscultation there are fine crackles posteriorly and he is expectorating frothy sputum; hence the call out.

Here the obvious problem is fluid overload, and the medical team need to reassess his diuresis. The problem is not a physiotherapy one.

Further examples of appropriate and inappropriate referrals are given in Table 14.1, but even if the problem is not amenable to physiotherapy some advice may be offered to the referrer on positioning the patient to maximise ventilation/perfusion ratio (V/Q) matching.

PROBLEM SOLVING

The method of approach for problem solving is to think of the obvious. Your objective assessment is as important as the subjective assessment, as the seriousness of the situation is established early on in the intervention. As mentioned above, the state of consciousness is a good indication of the patient's condition, excluding electively sedated or neurological patients. If the patient is awake, oriented and co-operative, there is time to assess the situation formally. If the patient is clearly distressed or tired or lapsing into a semi-conscious state, then the problem is more serious and a quick assessment is necessary. A thorough clinical presentation of the patient's condition by the doctor in charge will give you the relevant information and therefore your respiratory assessment can follow.

As mentioned in Chapter 6, an overall analysis is as important as the chest assessment. Bearing this in mind, assess the patient's temperature, fluid balance, blood gas analysis where available, chest X-ray and medication. Take into account the oxygen requirement and the presence of drips and drains.

CHEST AUSCULTATION

It is fair to say, the more experienced the clinician, the more accurate his or her auscultation skills. The medical picture will already give you an idea of the problem and whether physiotherapy is of use, and chest auscultation should confirm the diagnosis. Often, chest sounds can indicate a variety of conditions, and the skill is to establish the correct diagnosis; for example, interstitial crackles may be a result of pulmonary oedema. But is the problem cardiogenic or non-cardiogenic as in the adult respiratory distress syndrome (ARDS) or lung tissue infection? Again, if there is an accurate history and an analysis of the data is available, the cause should already be known.

The following is a brief resumé of types of breath sounds to aid the diagnosis (see also pages 35–37).

INTERSTITIAL CRACKLES: PULMONARY

- Infection, localised, e.g. lobar.
- Fibrosis, widespread—diagnosis evident from history.
- ARDS, widespread—diagnosis evident from history.

INTERSTITIAL CRACKLES: CARDIAC

- Gravitational, e.g. if the patient is upright, the crackles are in the lower lobes; if the patient is supine, the crackles are posterior.

WHEEZE: PULMONARY

- Expiratory: bronchospasm, e.g. asthma or irritative, as in aspiration of vomit or inhalation of smoke.
- Inspiratory and expiratory: obstruction of the major airways, e.g. inhalation of foreign body or tenacious secretions or tracheal stenosis causing stridor. The noises occurring due to secretions will disappear after the patient expectorates.

WHEEZE: CARDIAC

- Expiratory: severe pulmonary oedema obstructing the airways, often with interstitial crackles.

N.B. The treatment of the above conditions varies wildly; the pulmonary condition calls for bronchodilator therapy whereas the cardiac problem may require diuretics and inotropic support. Also, with ARDS, the mode of treatment may be anti-inflammatories and antibiotics.

Table 14.1 Examples of appropriate and inappropriate call outs.

Examples of appropriate and inappropriate call outs	
Physiotherapy problem	Not a physiotherapy problem
Post-operative atelectasis	Fluid overload
Acute lobar atelectasis	Pleural effusion
Chronic obstructive pulmonary disease with exacerbation	Undrained pneumothorax
	Lung tissue disease, e.g. fibrosis
Aspiration	Frank haemoptysis
Resolving consolidation	Pulmonary embolus

LOSS OF BREATH SOUNDS OR DIMINISHED BREATH SOUNDS

- Pneumothorax: if the patient is clearly distressed, tachycardiac, tachypnoeic and cyanosed, it is important to exclude a pneumothorax. If there is time, then a chest X-ray will confirm the diagnosis; however, if the picture is a tension pneumothorax then the situation is critical and must be acted upon immediately.
- Pleural effusion: confirm the diagnosis with a chest X-ray, preferably with the patient sitting or standing up.
- Atelectasis: often the patient has evidence of secretions, and there is improvement after physiotherapy. Atelectasis is also confirmed on chest X-ray.

INCREASED OR BRONCHIAL BREATH SOUNDS

- Consolidated lung tissue, e.g. pneumonia, fibrosis (may have interstitial crackles): confirm on chest X-ray.
- Collapse and consolidation, e.g. untreated post-operative atelectasis: usually improves with physiotherapy, with better breath sounds after treatment.

THE NEUROLOGICAL PATIENT

All the above applies if the patient is self-ventilating, despite the patient being unconscious. In patients with cerebral oedema, e.g. head injuries, hyperventilation is one sign of cerebral irritation, so it is important to distinguish this symptom from respiratory distress caused by other problems. If the patient cannot communicate, the history should be obtained from relatives or ward staff. If the patient has a neurological condition whereby the gag reflex is absent, then exclude aspiration. The same applies with the intubated patient where there may be a cuff leak.

THE INTENSIVE CARE PATIENT

The intensive care patient has been discussed earlier in Chapter 6, but there are a few additional tips to consider regarding the ventilated patient. If the patient is paralysed and sedated, then check the ventilator's airway pressure to ensure that there is no pneumothorax. With the pressure-cycled ventilators, lung compliance is registered and the patient's tidal volume varies, so the risk of pneumothorax is reduced. With volume-cycled ventilators, high airway pressures may indicate pneumothorax, bronchospasm, tube obstruction, coughing, intubation of a main bronchus (commonly the right), significant lobar collapse and the patient breathing against the pre-set respiratory cycle of the ventilator. Secretions alone rarely increase the airway pressure unless they are tenacious and copious.

The physiotherapy assessment is no different than for an unventilated patient; however, access to the chest may be impeded by drips, drains and the inability to move the patient because of the instability of the condition. All efforts must be made to assess, in particular, the posterior aspect of the chest, as many supine ventilated patients develop lower lobe problems.

PHYSIOTHERAPY TREATMENT METHODS

Physiotherapy techniques are discussed in Chapter 6, and listed in Table 14.2.

Table 14.2 Chest physiotherapy methods and adjuncts.

Chest physiotherapy methods and adjuncts	
Conscious patient	**Unconscious/sedated/ventilated patient**
Positioning	Positioning
Active cycle of breathing	Suction
Incentive spirometry	Manual hyperinflation
Postural drainage	Postural drainage (modified if ventilated)
Percussion	Percussion
Shaking/vibrations	Shaking/vibrations
Suction	
Non-invasive positive pressure ventilation	

AUDITING ON-CALL EPISODES

In Stoke on Trent, the use of an on-call form facilitates the physiotherapist's approach to the patient, and is also used as an audit tool to analyse typical reasons for call out and to measure the number of inappropriate referrals (Figure 14.1). As a result of the audit, the number of inappropriate call outs has reduced as medical and nursing staff are now aware of the correct use of the service and what conditions are best dealt with by chest physiotherapy.

Patient's name:	Ward:
Unit No:	Consultant:
Age/DOB:	Date:
Time of call out:	Time left home:
Time of arrival to patient:	New patient ☐ Yes ☐ No Date of admission:
Treatment time:	Time back home:
Who called you out:	Mileage:
Their job title:	Known potential call out:
☐ Emergency ☐ Useful non-emergency ☐ Inappropriate	
Physiotherapist:	Signature:

HPC

Diagnosis   **Prognosis** Good/Fair/Poor

Relevant PMH

Medication

☐ Inotropes   ☐ Diuretics   ☐ Analgesia   ☐ Bronchodilators

☐ Respiratory stimulants   ☐ Antiarrhythmics   ☐ Other ....

Oxygen therapy

% O_2 .... Delivery (eg mask) ....

Humidification

☐ Yes   ☐ No   Type ....

Fluid balance

☐ Positive   ☐ Negative

Blood gases

FiO$_2$ .... PH .... PCO$_2$ .... PO$_2$ ....

BX .... SBC .... SATS ....

Date ....

Time ....

Figure 14.1 Example of an on-call form facilitating the physiotherapist's approach to the patient (page 1).

Ventilation

☐ Spontaneous ☐ CPAP .... cm H$_2$0 ☐ Nasal (mask) ventilation ☐ Tracheostomy

☐ Other ....

ITU/HDU Patients

☐ Intubated ☐ Paralysed ☐ Sedated

Ventilator type .... Mode .... Rate ....

☐ PEEP .... cm H$_2$0 ☐ Pressure support .... cm H$_2$0

Monitoring - ECG (high/low) .... CVP (high/low) .... BP ....

Pulmonary artery pressure (high/low) .... SaO$_2$ .... ICP ....

Other ....

CXR

Date .... Findings:

Patient Assessment

☐ Distressed ☐ Audible secretions ☐ Wheezy ☐ In pain

☐ SOB ☐ Cyanosed ☐ Conscious level ....

Auscultation

Treatment

Reassessment

Auscultation

Instructions for continuing care

Figure 14.1 Example of an on-call form facilitating the physiotherapist's approach to the patient (page 2).

GENERAL READING

Anderson A. *ABGS-Six easy steps to interpreting blood gases. Am J Nurs* 1990
90(8):42-45.

Hough A. *Physiotherapy in respiratory care, a problem solving approach.* 2nd
ed. Stanley Thornes; 1997.

Webber BA, Pryor JA. *Physiotherapy for respiratory and cardiac problems.*
Edinburgh: Churchill Livingstone; 1996.

SECTION 4

PAEDIATRIC MANAGEMENT

15 D Glover

PAEDIATRIC RESPIRATORY ANATOMY/ PHYSIOLOGY

CHAPTER OUTLINE

- Pre-natal development
- Post-natal development

- Differences in respiratory anatomy
- Differences in respiratory physiology

INTRODUCTION

Infants and children are anatomically and physiologically different from adults, and therefore physiotherapists working in the field of paediatric respiratory care require both specialist knowledge and specialist skills. This chapter describes the development of the respiratory system, and the infant–child–adult differences in relation to anatomy and physiology, to enable the reader to understand the principles of the physiotherapy management of children.

DEVELOPMENT OF THE RESPIRATORY SYSTEM

The respiratory system of babies born after 37 weeks' gestation is usually sufficiently advanced in its development to enable independent respiration. However, growth and development of the lungs continue throughout childhood.

PRE-NATAL DEVELOPMENT

This progresses through four stages (Inselman and Mellins, 1981).

Embryonic Stage (3–5 Weeks' Gestation)
At 3 weeks' gestation, the trachea develops as a bud from the anterior part of the oesophagus. First division branching of this bud occurs to form the two major bronchi, which in turn divide to produce the major lung branches. This stage is complete by 5 weeks' gestation.

Pseudoglandular Stage (6–16 Weeks' Gestation)
During this period all the conducting airways as far as terminal bronchioles are formed. After 10 weeks there is also development of cartilage, lymphatic vessels, cilia and the pulmonary circulation (Avery and Fletcher, 1974; Yu, 1986). The pulmonary artery communicates with the aorta via the ductus arteriosus. At birth this duct should close.

Canalicular Stage (17–24 Weeks' Gestation)
From 17 weeks' gestation the respiratory bronchioles and alveolar ducts begin to develop and mature, until at 24 weeks the two main types of cells which will line the alveoli appear (Campiche *et al.*, 1963). The lung starts to fill with fluid—not amniotic fluid but fluid produced by the lung itself—which is necessary to give shape and volume to the distal lung units. Without this fluid the lungs would fail to develop fully (Avery *et al.*, 1981). There is also rapid maturation of the lung capillaries during this stage.

Terminal Sac Stage (24 Weeks' Gestation to Term)
During this final stage of fetal lung development, the alveolar sacs are formed, creating the potential for independent respiration should the baby be born prematurely. The two different types of cells lining the alveoli are called type I and type II pneumocytes, and have very different roles to play. Type I pneumocytes cover about 96% of the alveolar surface and are responsible for the production of surfactant. Surfactant is a phospholipid which reduces surface tension within the alveolus, thus preventing its collapse on expiration. It is therefore

essential for the mechanics of independent respiration. Small amounts of surfactant have been identified in cells as early as 23 weeks' gestation, but surfactant is not delivered on to the alveolar surface until 30 weeks (Gluck and Kulovich, 1973). The process of birth and initiation of breathing also helps to stimulate the production of surfactant (Gluck *et al.*, 1967).

POST-NATAL DEVELOPMENT

Chest Shape

The ribs of the newborn infant are horizontally placed in relation to the sternum and vertebral column, and the transverse diameter of the thoracic cage equals the antero-posterior diameter. As the infant grows, and begins to develop an upright posture, the ribs develop a more oblique angle and the transverse diameter of the rib cage increases. The adult chest shape is achieved by 3 years of age (Oppenshaw *et al.*, 1984).

Airways

At birth there is no further increase in the number of airways formed but there is growth and development in their size.

In the first few years of life there is a significant increase in the diameter of the larger, more proximal airways (Hislop and Reid, 1974). The smaller, more distal airways do not increase in diameter until nearer 5 years of age.

Alveoli

Both the number and size of alveoli continue to increase post-natally. At term there are approximately 150 million alveoli (Hislop *et al.*, 1986). Much of the growth in number of alveoli occurs during the first 12 months. By 4 years of age, the adult number of 300–400 million may exist, although growth can continue until 7 years of age. After 3 years of age, when most of the alveoli have been formed, the alveoli continue to increase in size until the chest wall stops growing (Pang and Mellins, 1975).

Collateral Ventilation

Collateral ventilation is the means by which a distal lung unit can be ventilated despite blockage of its main airway.

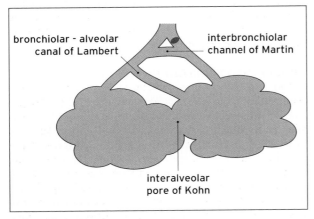

Figure 15.1 Collateral ventilatory pathways.

bronchiolar - alveolar canal of Lambert

interbronchiolar channel of Martin

interalveolar pore of Kohn

This is achieved by a network of interconnecting pathways linking different structures (Figure 15.1).

Respiratory bronchioles are linked by channels of Martin. Canals of Lambert connect respiratory and terminal bronchioles with alveoli and their ducts; and adjacent alveoli are joined by openings in the alveolar wall, called pores of Kohn (Menkes and Traystman, 1977). However, none of these pathways exists at birth. The pores of Kohn develop between years 1 and 2, and the canals of Lambert do not appear until about 6 years of age.

DIFFERENCES IN RESPIRATORY ANATOMY AND PHYSIOLOGY OF INFANTS AND CHILDREN

ANATOMY

Larynx

In the newborn infant, the larynx is positioned high up, so most breathing takes place via the nasal passages. The larynx descends with age but for the first few months of life its high position enables the infant to feed and breathe simultaneously. Obstruction of the nasal passages of infants therefore compromises breathing considerably and increases the already high resistance to inspiration that the nasal passages offer. However, it is no longer believed that infants are purely nose breathers (Rodenstein, 1987).

Lymphatic Tissue

Enlarged tonsils and adenoids in the infant may be the cause of, or exacerbate, upper airways obstruction. The relatively large tongue may also be a contributing factor.

Airways

The diameter of an infant's trachea is only about one-third that of an adult. This makes the resistance to inspiration higher and therefore the work of breathing greater. Further narrowing of the airway may occur if there is localised swelling. This may be a result of trauma caused by invasive procedures such as endotracheal intubation or suction. The effect of such swelling on the airway size will be much greater in the infant.

Throughout the infant's lung the smaller calibre of the airways means higher resistance to air flow, but especially in more distal regions where airway diameter does not increase until about 5 years of age. Up until this time the peripheral airways resistance can be four times greater than that of an adult. This higher peripheral airways resistance is further exacerbated by respiratory infections which cause inflammation of the airways, e.g. bronchiolitis.

Bronchial Walls

The bronchial walls are supported by cartilage, which begins to develop from 12 weeks' gestation and continues throughout childhood. The cartilaginous support of an infant's airways is therefore much less than that of an adult, and predisposes the airways to collapse.

The bronchial walls contain proportionally more cartilage, connective tissue and mucous glands than do those of adults, but less smooth muscle; this makes the lung tissue less compliant.

The high proportion of mucous glands in the major bronchi of infants make the airways more susceptible to mucous obstruction.

The lack of bronchial smooth muscle, particularly in the smaller bronchioles, may be one reason for the lack of response to bronchodilators under the age of 12 months. The β-receptors in infants are also immature, which further reduces any response to β-adrenergic bronchodilator therapy.

Cilia
At birth the cilia are poorly developed, which increases the risk of secretion retention, especially in the premature infant. The airway obstruction caused by secretions in a neonate is much greater than in an adult whose airways are relatively large.

Alveoli
The smaller alveolar size of an infant makes the infant more susceptible to alveolar collapse, and the smaller number of alveoli reduces the area available for gaseous exchange.

Internal Organs
The heart and other organs are relatively large in infants, leaving less space for lung expansion.

Rib Cage
The ribs of an infant are horizontally placed compared with the more oblique angle of adults. This altered rib cage configuration is coupled with the fact that the intercostal muscles are poorly developed in infancy. Therefore 'bucket handle' rib movement seen in older children and adults is not possible. This, in turn, reduces the infant's ability to increase either the anteroposterior or transverse diameter of the chest. This limitation to chest expansion consequently limits the infant's ability to increase lung volume, which can then be achieved only by increasing the respiratory rate.

Diaphragm
The angle of insertion of the infant diaphragm is more horizontal than in the adult, and therefore works at a mechanical disadvantage. However, the diaphragm is the main muscle of inspiration in the infant, since the intercostals are poorly developed at this stage. Ventilation in the infant is therefore more affected by impaired diaphragmatic function, e.g. abdominal distension, than in the adult.

PHYSIOLOGY
Compliance
Compliance is the force required to inflate the lungs (see Chapter 1).

Lung compliance
The lung compliance of a child is comparable to that of an adult, being directly proportional to the child's size.

However, compliance is reduced in the infant because of the high proportion of cartilage in the airways. The premature infant who lacks surfactant demonstrates a further significant decrease in compliance.

Chest wall compliance
The chest wall of an infant is cartilaginous and therefore very soft and compliant in comparison with the more calcified and rigid adult structure. The intercostals are also less well equipped to stabilise the rib cage during diaphragmatic contraction. As a result, when the demands on the diaphragm increase, e.g. in respiratory distress, the increased force of the diaphragmatic contraction is less easily counteracted by the intercostals, and the chest wall is drawn in, reducing the overall efficiency of respiration.

Closing Volume
The closing volume is the lung volume at which closure of the small airways occurs. This volume plus the residual volume, i.e. the volume of gas left in the lungs following maximum expiration, is known as the closing capacity (CC). In the adult, CC is less than functional residual capacity (FRC), i.e. the volume of gas left in the lungs following tidal expiration, whereas in the infant it is greater than FRC.

The higher closing volumes apparent in infants are due to greater chest wall compliance and reduced elastic recoil of the lungs than in the adult. Therefore, airway closure may occur before the end of expiration, e.g. during expiratory chest vibrations, putting the infant at a much greater risk of developing widespread atelectasis, especially in the presence of lung disease, where lung volume is further reduced.

In the event of respiratory distress, the infant grunts on expiration, adducting the vocal cords in an attempt to reduce the amount of gas expired, thus maintaining a higher FRC and minimising alveolar collapse (Pang and Mellins, 1975). Re-inflation of alveoli, once collapsed, is more difficult in the infant, who has to work considerably harder to overcome the effects of the compliant chest wall.

Collateral Ventilation
Another predisposing factor to the development of atelectasis in the infant is the poorly developed interconnecting pathways which, in the adult, enable collateral ventilation to take place (see Figure 15.1).

Ventilation and Perfusion
In the adult, both ventilation and perfusion are preferentially distributed to the dependent lung. The best gas exchange and ventilation–perfusion match (see Chapter 1) will therefore be in the dependent region of the lung (Zack et al., 1974). In the infant, however, ventilation is preferentially distributed to the uppermost lung (Davies et al., 1985), whereas the perfusion remains best in the dependent regions. This leads to greater gas exchange in the uppermost lung (Heaf et al., 1983) but an imbalance between ventilation and perfusion (Bhuyan et al., 1989). This becomes more clinically significant if, in unilateral

lung disease, the affected lung is positioned uppermost for postural drainage of retained secretions, thereby impairing ventilation in all lung areas.

The difference in ventilation distribution between infants and adults is most likely due to the more compliant rib cage of the infant which compresses the dependent areas of lung. In addition, while in the adult the weight of the abdominal contents provides a preferential load on the dependent diaphragm and therefore improves its contractility, in the infant this does not happen. The effect on both hemidiaphragms is similar due to the abdomen being so much smaller and narrower (Davies *et al.*, 1985). It has been shown in adults that, when the diaphragm is inactivated, e.g. when ventilated under anaesthetic, the ventilation distribution changes to that of an infant (Rehder *et al.*, 1972). It is not yet known exactly when the ventilation distribution in the infant changes to that of an adult, but it may be as late as 10 years of age.

Oxygen Consumption

Infants have a higher resting metabolic rate than adults and consequently have a higher oxygen requirement. This also means that infants will develop hypoxia more quickly.

Response to Hypoxia

An infant responds to hypoxia with bradycardia and pulmonary vasoconstriction whereas the adult becomes tachycardic and there is systemic vasodilation. The bradycardic response in infants is probably due to myocardial hypoxia and acidosis.

Muscle Fatigue

The respiratory muscles of infants tire more quickly than those of adults due to a much smaller proportion of fatigue resistant muscle fibre (Keens and Ianuzzo, 1979). There are two main muscle fibre types, type I and type II. Type I muscle fibres are slow twitch, high oxidative and slow to fatigue. Type II fibres are fast twitch, slow oxidative and tire quickly. Of the muscle fibres in the adult diaphragm, 55% are type I compared with only 30% in the infant. Premature infants tire even more easily as, at 24 weeks' gestation, only 10% of their muscle fibres are fatigue resistant (Muller and Bryan, 1979). Excessive muscle fatigue results in apnoea. By 12 months of age the number of type I fibres equals that of an adult.

Rapid Eye Movement (REM) Sleep

During rapid eye movement (REM) sleep there is tonic inhibition of the infant's intercostal muscles such that the rib cage is even less well equipped to counteract the contraction of the diaphragm during inspiration (Muller and Bryan, 1979). This reduces the efficiency of respiration, increases the work of breathing and predisposes the infant to apnoeic episodes. The premature infant is most at risk, spending up to 20 hours a day asleep, 80% of which may be REM sleep compared with 20% in adult sleep.

Breathing Pattern

Irregular breathing patterns are common in newborn infants, especially if premature, and may result in apnoea. Short spells of apnoea can be considered normal in these circumstances, but need careful monitoring.

CONCLUSION

The respiratory anatomy and physiology of infants and children is very different from that of adults. An infant with pulmonary pathology cannot have the principles of adult management directly transposed to the paediatric setting. Therefore, the management of acutely ill children has become a highly specialised area of respiratory physiotherapy, where the inexperienced therapist will require the support and supervision of an experienced paediatric physiotherapist.

Normal paediatric vital signs					
Age	Pre-term	Birth (full term)	1-3 years	3-10 years	Adult
Heart rate (beats/min)	120-200	100-200	100-180	70-150	60-80
Blood pressure (mmHg)	70/40	80/40	100/65	115/60	120/80
Respiratory rate (breaths/min)	40-60	30-40	25-30	15-20	12-16
PaO_2 (kPa)	7-10	8-11	9-12	12-14	12-14

Table 15.1 **Comparison of normal paediatric vital signs with adult values.**

REFERENCES

Avery ME, Fletcher BD. Lung development. In: Fletcher BD, ed. *The lung and its disorders in the newborn infant*. Philadelphia: WB Saunders; 1974:1-21.

Avery ME, Fletcher BD, Williams RG. *The lung and its disorders in the newborn infant*, 4th ed. Philadelphia: WB Saunders; 1981.

Bhuyan U, Peters AM, Gordon I, Helms P. Effect of posture on the distribution of pulmonary ventilation and perfusion in children and adults. *Thorax* 1989, **44**:480-484.

Campiche MA, Gautier A, Hemandeg EI, Raymond A. An electron microscope study of the foetal development of the human lung. *Pediatrics* 1963, **32**:967-994.

Davies H, Kitchman R, Gordon I, Helms P. Regional ventilation in infancy. *New Engl J Med* 1985, **313**:1626-1628.

Gluck L, Kulovich MV. L/S ratios in amniotic fluid and abnormal pregnancies. *Am J Obstet Gyn* 1973, **115**:539-552.

Gluck L, Motoyama EK, Smits HL, Kulovich MV. The biochemical development of the surface activity in the mammalian lung. *Pediatr Res* 1967, **1**:237-246.

Heaf DP, Helms P, Gordon I, Turner HM. Postural effects on gas exchange in infants. *New Engl J Med* 1983, **303**:1505-1508.

Hislop A, Reid L. Development of the acinus in the human lung. *Thorax* 1974, **29**:90-94.

Hislop A, Wigglesworth JS, Desai R. Alveolar development in the human foetus and infant. *Early Hum Develop* 1986, **13**:1-11.

Inselman LS, Mellins RB. Growth and development of the lung. *J Pediatr* 1981, **98**:1-15.

Keens TG, Ianuzzo CD. Development of fatigue resistant muscle fibres in human ventilatory muscles. *Am Rev Respir Dis* 1979, **suppl. 119**:139-141.

Menkes HA, Traystman RJ. Collateral ventilation. *Am Rev Respir Dis* 1977, **116**:287-309.

Muller NL, Bryan AC. Chest wall mechanics and respiratory muscles in infants. *Ped Clin North Am* 1979, **26(3)**:503-516.

Oppenshaw P, Edwards S, Helms P. Changes in rib cage geometry during childhood. *Thorax* 1984, **39**:624-627.

Pang LM, Mellins RB. Neonatal cardiorespiratory physiology. *Anaesthesiology* 1975, **43(2)**:171-196.

Rehder K, Hatch DJ, Sessler AD, Fowler WS. The function of each lung of anesthetised and paralysed man during mechanical ventilation. *Anesthesiology* 1972, **37(1)**:16-26.

Rodenstein DO, Kahn A, Blum, *et al*. Nasal occlusion during sleep in normal and near miss for sudden death syndrome in infants. *Bull Eur Physiopathol Respir* 1987, **23**:223-226.

Yu VYH, ed. Development of the lung. In: *Respiratory disorders of the newborn*. Edinburgh: Churchill Livingstone; 1986:1-7.

Zack MB, Pontoppidan H, Kazemi H. The effect of lateral positions on gas exchange in pulmonary disease. *Am Rev Respir Dis* 1974, **110**:49-55.

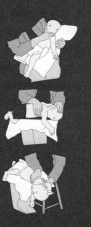

16 SA Prasad

PAEDIATRIC RESPIRATORY DISEASE

CHAPTER OUTLINE

- Assessment of respiratory status
- Physiotherapy techniques
- Respiratory tract infection
- Acute epiglottitis
- Pertussis

- Bronchiolitis
- Pneumonia
- Bronchiectasis
- Inhaled foreign body
- Asthma

INTRODUCTION

Respiratory disease in children differs significantly from that in adults, both in terms of the conditions seen and the medical, nursing and physiotherapy management. Optimal care of respiratory disease in infancy and childhood depends on a multidisciplinary approach. A close working relationship between all members of the care team, support services, the child and the family is essential.

One of the most challenging aspects in the treatment of children compared with adults is the need and ability to communicate effectively with both the child and their family. The hospital environment, which may appear unfamiliar and frightening to the child, often has to be faced at times of considerable anxiety when a family is already burdened by the stress of having a sick child. Physiotherapy itself may also seem to cause distress, and it is essential that the child and family are handled with care and respect, and given careful explanations of the indications for intervention and the treatment techniques being used.

The first section of this chapter will outline a paediatric respiratory assessment; this can be adapted to any situation where the physiotherapist encounters an infant or child, either in hospital or in the community, and whatever concurrent pathology is present. Additional information concerning the assessment of a child on the paediatric Intensive Care Unit (ICU) or infant on the neonatal unit can be found in Chapters 18 and 20, respectively. Physiotherapy treatment techniques are described in the second section of this chapter. The third section describes the common pulmonary pathologies found in the paediatric age group, together with specific points for the physiotherapist. The management of cystic fibrosis for which physiotherapy plays such a major part is considered in Chapter 17.

ASSESSMENT OF RESPIRATORY STATUS

HISTORY
Medical Notes
The details relating to the present condition, as well as relevant birth history and medical history, and family and social history, should be elicited from the patient's medical records.

Relevant Investigations
Relevent investigations in infants and children include chest X-ray and arterial blood gas analysis. In the latter there is a lower partial pressure of oxygen in arterial blood (PaO_2) compared with adults, rising from about 8 kPa at birth to adult levels around 8 years of age.

Full blood counts, bacteriological results and pulmonary function tests should be referred to as appropriate.

Subjective Examination

A history should be taken from the parents and child where appropriate to determine the child's presenting status. The following issues should be considered:

- Onset and type of symptoms.
- Details of symptoms, e.g. cough, sputum, wheeze, dyspnoea.
- Exercise tolerance.
- Pain.
- Relevant environmental factors, e.g. passive smoking and household pets.

It is also important to make a brief assessment of the neurological and motor development of the child, recording the achievement of relevant milestones. This may, particularly in chronic disorders, reveal previously unrecognised mild neurological impairment or developmental disorders. If these are present, then referral to the paediatrician, the neurological physiotherapy team or other specialists is appropriate.

Discussion with other Team Members

Medical and nursing staff should be consulted to gain accurate information regarding the current status of the child, or any recent changes in condition or management strategies. This should also include ascertainment of the stability of the child in response to handling, feeding regimens (whether oral, enteral or intravenous) and timing of feeds. Knowledge of these factors will determine optimal timing of physiotherapy intervention.

PHYSICAL EXAMINATION

Before the commencement of any physical examination, the type and degree of any respiratory support required (such as oxygen therapy), baseline values of vital signs (normal values are listed in Chapter 15) and necessity for pain relief should be noted. Physical examination should include inspection, palpation and auscultation (Table 16.1).

Inspection

Respiratory rate and pattern should be noted, bearing in mind that this is variable according to sleep state and wakefulness. Tachypnoea is seen in states of decreased respiratory compliance, and also in the presence of metabolic acidosis. Signs of respiratory distress should be looked for carefully (Table 16.2). These include retraction of the chest wall (subcostal, intercostal or sternal), inspiratory or expiratory stridor (indicating significant narrowing or obstruction of the larynx or trachea), grunting (an expiratory sound caused by partial closure of the glottis in order to slow expiration, increase functional residual capacity (FRC) and maintain alveolar patency) and the presence of nasal flaring (enlargement of the anterior nasal passages in order to reduce airways resistance). The colour of the peripheries and mucous membranes should be observed for evidence of cyanosis. Pallor is commonly seen in infants with respiratory distress, and may be a sign of hypoxia. The presence of asymmetrical chest movement, structural abnormalities and any digital clubbing should also be noted.

Abdominal distension in an infant or small child may significantly impair respiratory function, as the diaphragm

Physical examination of a child with respiratory disease		
Inspection	**Palpation**	**Auscultation**
Activity/conscious level	Pain/tenderness/swelling	Breath sounds
Breathing rate/pattern	Expansion	Stridor
Respiratory effort	Crepitus	Wheeze
Recession: subcostal	Subcutaneous emphysema	Crackles
intercostal	Tracheal position	Pleural sounds
sternal		
Nasal flaring		
Stridor		
Grunting		
Clubbing		
Cyanosis		
Structural abnormalities		

Table 16.1 **Physical examination of a child with respiratory disease. (Modified from Prasad and Hussey, 1995a.)**

(the main respiratory muscle in this age group) becomes mechanically disadvantaged. Observation of the behaviour of a child can also indicate respiratory status. Irritability and distress may be early signs of hypoxia, and the child in severe respiratory distress may be listless, withdrawn and inactive. However, a child who is upright, happy and playing is rarely distressed.

Palpation

This allows any observed abnormalities to be confirmed or further investigated. Additionally, areas of pain and tenderness can be detected. The position of the trachea (normally midline or slightly to the right) should be checked and any 'tugging' noted. Placing the hands on the chest also allows the examiner to assess expansion and symmetry of chest movement. Crepitations over the lung fields may also be noted. Percussion of the chest wall may be performed in order to assess resonance.

Auscultation

Auscultation of the chest is used to determine the presence and character of breath sounds, adventitious sounds and sometimes vocal resonance (see Chapter 2). In the infant and young child, auscultation may be difficult due to the easy transmission of sounds and the relatively high respiratory rate. Upper airway secretions in older infants and children may cause transmitted or referred crackles on auscultation over the lung fields. Wheezing, though commonly caused by bronchoconstriction, may also be due to retained secretions which partially occlude and therefore cause narrowing of small airways.

PHYSIOTHERAPY TECHNIQUES

Safe and effective physiotherapy management of infants and children with respiratory disorders requires an understanding of the treatment aims, thorough assessment and the judicious use of appropriate techniques (Prasad and Hussey, 1995a). The same chest physiotherapy techniques employed in adults can be used in children and generally the same contraindications apply. Treatment should not be routine, and should be performed only when indicated. However, in patients with chronic sputum production, e.g. cystic fibrosis, bronchiectasis and primary cilial dyskinesia, daily regimens are usually necessary. It is important that timing of treatment is carefully planned and treatment should be given before feeds or not before at least 1 hour following a feed.

POSITIONING

Careful positioning of infants and children can be used both to optimise lung function (ventilation and perfusion) and to enhance bronchial clearance. The supine position can compromise lung function (Dean, 1985). Even in the very sick infant or child, it is usually possible to obtain a good side-lying position. This releases the diaphragm from the pressure of the abdominal viscera allowing for more effective basal expansion, and facilitates drainage of secretions from the uppermost part of the lung. In infants, ventilation has been shown to be preferentially distributed to the uppermost lung regions (Davies et al., 1985), therefore a child with unilateral lung disease may not tolerate the side-lying position with the affected lung uppermost. Treatment positions may have to be modified to account for this, or it may be necessary in the acutely ill child to increase the level of inspired oxygen during treatment in order to maintain adequate oxygenation yet apply effective therapy.

The prone position is advocated in infants and children as it has been shown to improve gas exchange, reduce gastro-oesophageal reflux and reduce energy expenditure, particularly in the neonatal age group. In the sitting position, lung volume and FRC are increased; however, to ensure optimal benefit from this position it is important that the child is well supported and does not slump forward. This position also allows the child to observe his or her environment from a normal perspective and encourages activities of play, both of which are essential to gain normal cognitive and motor development. This is especially important in the child who has significant recurrent or chronic respiratory problems.

POSTURAL DRAINAGE

The use of gravity to assist drainage of pulmonary secretions from the more peripheral to central airways is widely used in paediatric practice (Figure 16.1). However, it should be noted that newborn infants are better oxygenated in a slightly head up position (Thoresen et al., 1988). Children with abdominal distension do not tolerate the head down position, as their respiration relies heavily on the diaphragm, which cannot work effectively if put at a further mechanical disadvantage. In the infant and small child with chronic respiratory disease, it is particularly important to facilitate drainage of the apical segments of the upper lobes, as youngsters of this age

Signs of respiratory distress
Tachypnoea (infant >70 breaths/min) (older child >40 breaths/min)
Rib cage distortion: subcostal recession intercostal recession sternal retraction
Expiratory grunting
Nasal flaring
Tracheal tug
Cyanosis
Pallor
Tachycardia
Restlessness/irritability
Reduced activity—inability to feed or cry

Table 16.2 Signs of respiratory distress.

group tend to spend most of their time in lying positions rather than upright.

PERCUSSION AND VIBRATIONS

Manual techniques such as chest percussion and vibrations aim to enhance both large and small airway clearance. Chest percussion is generally very well tolerated, particularly in infants and small children. Application of chest percussion using a small sized anaesthetic mask is sometimes preferred for infants. Single handed percussion is usually more practical in the paediatric age group but the rate at which it is performed depends very much on the therapist's personal bias. Vibrations can also be very

effective in facilitating bronchial clearance in small children where the chest wall is very compliant, provided that the respiratory rate allows them to be applied effectively. In those who are tachypnoeic, the expiratory phase is often too short to allow effective application of this technique.

Similar contraindications apply when using these techniques in children as in adults. It is important to ensure that patients do not have a low platelet count or coagulopathy as petechiae or localised bruising may arise. Patients with any mineral deficiency may be susceptible to rib fracture. Percussion may exacerbate bronchoconstriction in children who are wheezy or susceptible to bronchospasm (Prasad and Hussey, 1995b).

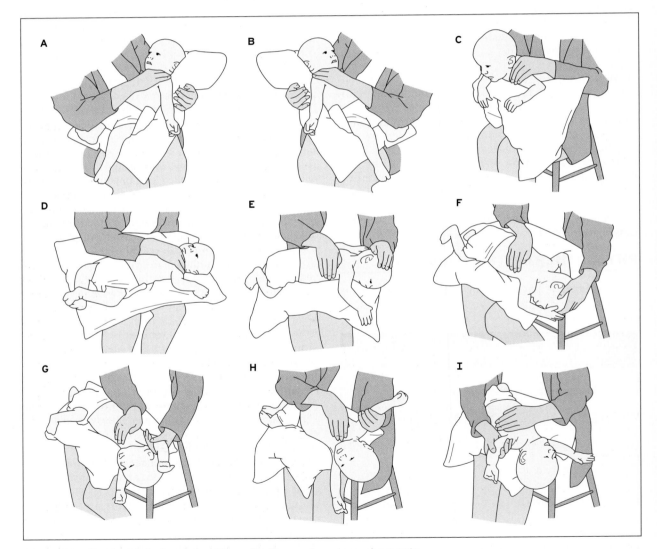

Figure 16.1 Postural drainage positions for the various lung segments.
(A) Apical segment left upper lobe, (B) apical segment right upper lobe, (C) posterior segments of the upper lobes (slight head up tilt and a quarter turn to either side to differentiate left and right), (D) anterior segments upper lobes, (E) apical segments lower lobes, (F) posterior basal segments lower lobes, (G) lateral basal segment right lower lobe (with the position reversed to right side lying the right medial basal and left lateral basal segments of the lower lobes would be drained), (H) right middle lobe, (I) lingular.

BREATHING EXERCISES AND COUGHING

It is usually possible to encourage some form of breathing exercises in children from about 2 years of age. Usually this would take the form of play, using bubbles, paper windmills or perhaps incentive spirometry. As the child grows, more formal techniques using thoracic expansion exercises and huffing can be introduced. By 4 years of age most children can be effectively taught the active cycle of breathing techniques (ACBT) (Partridge *et al.*, 1989).

It is rarely possible to ask a child below the age of 18 months to 2 years to cough effectively on command, and children less than 4–5 years of age are usually unable to expectorate secretions. In the infant and small child, if positioning or manual techniques have not induced a cough then it is possible to stimulate coughing by gentle application of sideways pressure with a finger to the trachea. Apposition of the pliable tracheal walls stimulates the cough reflex. However, this technique should be applied only in experienced hands and with extreme care as it can induce bradycardia. If effective clearance cannot be achieved by any of the above methods, airway suction may be necessary.

AIRWAY SUCTION

Nasopharyngeal suction is frequently necessary in infants and small children with retained secretions (see page 285).

CONCLUSION

The treatment modalities described in this section are not an exhaustive list. The older child able to take an active role in treatment may be taught to use a positive expiratory pressure mask, an active cycle of breathing or a graded exercise programme. Accurate assessment will determine which treatment modality is required for the presenting pulmonary pathology. The following section will describe the commonly seen pulmonary pathologies to allow the physiotherapist to treat them effectively and to understand when physiotherapy is not appropriate.

PAEDIATRIC PULMONARY PATHOLOGY

CONGENITAL MALFORMATIONS OF THE LUNG

Congenital abnormalities of the lung in children are rare but include lung cysts and lobar emphysema. Although some cases may be detected antenatally at ultrasound scanning, more commonly they present in the postnatal period with the development of recurrent respiratory signs and symptoms. If managed conservatively these conditions do not require physiotherapy intervention except where there is superimposed infection. If treated surgically, however, physiotherapy may be indicated postoperatively if there are problems with sputum retention.

RESPIRATORY TRACT INFECTION

Respiratory tract infections are the commonest cause of illness in children. Worldwide, they are reported to result in 4–15 million deaths per year in children under the age of 5 years. Epidemiological factors such as age (infancy and preschool years) and low socio-economic status, malnutrition, air pollution and passive smoking are known to predispose to frequent and severe infection. In the UK, respiratory diseases comprise about half of all illnesses in children under the age of 5 years. Most of these are mild; however, approximately 5% are more serious and the highest morbidity and mortality from lower respiratory tract disease occurs in the first year of life.

The nature and management of respiratory infection can be categorised into upper respiratory tract infection (involving the ears, nose, throat, pharynx and sinuses) and lower respiratory tract infection (involving the larynx, trachea, bronchi, bronchioles, alveoli and pleura) (Dinwiddie, 1996a).

UPPER RESPIRATORY TRACT INFECTIONS

Upper respiratory tract infections are very common in children, the most frequently affected areas being the nose and throat. The majority of infections are viral. They present with pyrexia, associated with poor feeding and signs such as sneezing, coughing and rhinorrhoea. Antibiotics are not indicated due to the viral nature of the illness, and management involves controlling the pyrexia with, for example, paracetamol and encouragement of fluid intake. Occasionally, these infections are bacterial and if symptoms are persistent antibiotics may be helpful.

Another very common illness, particularly in the preschool child, is ear infection such as otitis media. The child often presents with an acute febrile illness and constantly rubs his or her ears or, if older, complains of severe pain. In severe cases, spontaneous perforation of the tympanic membrane may occur. Treatment involves controlling the pyrexia and pain with, for example, paracetamol and antibiotic therapy. Inflammation and infection of the adenoids and sinuses are also seen in infants and children. In the case of adenoids, if infection is recurrent and adenoidal hypertrophy causes upper airway obstruction, adenotonsillectomy is indicated. There is no indication for chest physiotherapy in the management of upper respiratory tract infection.

LOWER RESPIRATORY TRACT INFECTIONS

Laryngotracheobronchitis (Croup)

Laryngotracheobronchitis is a common cause of acute laryngeal obstruction in childhood. It is frequently seen between the ages of 6 months and 4 years and is due to viral infection of the larynx, trachea and bronchi. Inflammation of the mucosa and submucosa leads to narrowing of the subglottic area and, due to the relatively small diameter of the airways, may significantly impair ventilation (Phelan *et al.*, 1994a). In its severest form laryngotracheobronchitis may cause respiratory failure and necessitate admission to a Paediatric Intensive Care Unit (PICU).

Clinically, the child usually presents with slow onset of a harsh sounding cough during 1 or 2 days of coryzal symptoms and pyrexia. An inspiratory stridor develops, and, as the inflammation increases so narrowing the subglottic area, the stridor worsens and is accompanied by signs of respiratory distress. These include subcostal and sternal recession, tachypnoea and restlessness. If airway obstruction becomes very severe and hypoxia develops, the child becomes irritable and cyanotic. In the majority of cases, signs of airway obstruction subside after 1 or 2 days though the dry barking cough may persist for up to 2 weeks.

Milder cases of croup can be managed at home. It has been advocated that extra humidity is helpful, for example sitting with the child in a steamy bathroom or boiling a kettle; however, there is no objective evidence for the benefits of this. In the more severely affected child, admission to hospital is required and humidified oxygen is administered if there is evidence of hypoxia. A policy of minimal handling should be adopted, pyrexia should be controlled and adequate fluid administration ensured. There is evidence that systemic or inhaled steroids are beneficial in the management of this illness. Only a small percentage of children with croup go on to require intubation or ventilation. A few children, however, do suffer from recurrent episodes of croup (Dinwiddie, 1996a).

Physiotherapy management

There is no indication for physiotherapy in this group of patients unless they require intubation and/or ventilation, when treatment may be required if suction alone fails to clear secretions or if there is superimposed infection.

Acute Epiglottitis

The incidence of acute epiglottitis has been decreasing dramatically since the introduction of vaccination in infancy. However, it remains an extremely dangerous condition, usually caused by *Haemophilus influenzae*, and most commonly occurs between the ages of 6 months and 6 years. It has an acute onset, with pyrexia, sore throat and toxicity. This progresses rapidly to respiratory obstruction, with inspiratory stridor and signs of severe respiratory distress. The child often holds the neck in the extended posture to facilitate air flow through the obstructed airway. Acute and fatal airway obstruction can occur at any time (Dinwiddie, 1996a). The child requires urgent transfer to the operating theatre where there are experienced personnel available to directly visualise the epiglottis and intubate to relieve obstruction. Rarely, when intubation fails, it is necessary to perform emergency tracheostomy. Treatment is then supportive until the oedema has reduced.

Physiotherapy management

There is no indication for physiotherapy unless secretion retention develops following intubation.

Pertussis

Pertussis, more commonly known as whooping cough, is caused by the organism *Bordetella pertussis*. Its incidence has fallen over the past few decades due to the introduction of immunisation. However, due to adverse publicity regarding side effects, the uptake of immunisation fell in the 1970s and 1980s but has since recovered with the knowledge that cerebral damage is an extremely rare complication occurring in approximately 1 in 10 000 cases. Pertussis occurs in epidemics at intervals of 3–4 years. The mucosal lining from the trachea down to the bronchioles becomes congested and oedematous. The organism attaches to the ciliated epithelial cells and there is a marked decrease in cilial activity; eventually necrosis and sloughing of the cells occurs, producing a thick sticky mucus.

Clinical presentation usually includes a 7–10 day coryzal illness followed by onset of a classic 'whooping' cough. The cough is paroxysmal and may be triggered by crying, feeding or any other disturbance. Short bursts of coughing occur without an inspiratory pause between each burst; during these bouts there is acute facial congestion and, if the spasms are severe, cyanosis follows. At the end of the coughing spasm there is an indrawing of air characterised by the typical whoop. In infants and small children these coughing bouts can lead to an apnoeic spell or may result in vomiting. This spasmodic phase usually lasts for 6–8 weeks but can be longer, and the condition is sometimes described as the '100 day cough'. It is not uncommon to develop a secondary bacterial infection and pneumonia. The chest X-ray in more severe cases shows patchy overinflation together with other areas of collapse or consolidation.

The majority of cases of pertussis can be managed at home. Attention should be paid to fluid intake and nutrition. Antibiotics do not actually affect the course of the disease but may be valuable in reducing infectivity. In the more severe cases, as well as general supportive measures, careful nursing is of prime importance. Minimal handling and a quiet environment reduce disturbances which may precipitate coughing. A small number of infants will require intubation and ventilation due to severe apnoeic spells and respiratory failure.

Physiotherapy management

During the acute phase of the illness, physiotherapy alone will serve no purpose other than to precipitate paroxysmal coughing (Parker, 1993). If the condition is severe enough to warrant intubation and ventilation, however, physiotherapy plays an important role in aiding removal of the tenacious secretions blocking the small airways. It should be noted, however, that the patient may require additional sedative and or paralysing agents to prevent bouts of coughing during treatment.

Following the acute stage of the illness there may be persistent lobar collapse. This can be readily treated with postural drainage, manual techniques of percussion and vibration with breathing exercises as appropriate. In the older child, the active cycle of breathing techniques (described later) should be used. It is important to teach the parents/guardians treatment techniques if the child is discharged before any radiographic changes have cleared.

Bronchiolitis

Acute viral bronchiolitis is the commonest serious acute lower respiratory tract infection in infants. It affects children in the first year of life, most frequently in the first 6 months. Seasonal epidemics occur between October and March. In 70% of cases the condition is caused by the respiratory syncytial virus (RSV). This produces an acute inflammatory response in the bronchioles. The submucosa becomes congested and inflamed and there is disruption of the airway architecture with small airways obstruction (Dinwiddie, 1996a). The lack of collateral ventilation in the lungs of infants contributes to the development of atelectasis and hyperinflation. Ventilation–perfusion mismatch leads to hypoxia and hypercapnia.

Presentation includes difficulty in feeding, a fever, coryza and a dry sounding cough. Tachypnoea develops as the disease progresses, and the infant becomes wheezy and shows signs of respiratory distress. Auscultation reveals widespread fine inspiratory crackles and expiratory wheeze. Typical radiographic changes include hyper-inflation with patchy collapse or pneumonic consolidation.

Management is mainly supportive—the infant should be nursed in a head up position or even upright to assist respiration, and humidified oxygen should be administered via a head box as required. Oxygen saturation should be measured closely, and infants with severe disease will require nasal continuous positive airway pressure (CPAP) or even intubation and respiratory support. Attention should be paid to fluid intake, and enteral feeding (via naso- or orogastric tubes) may be required where the infant is unable to feed normally. In severe circumstances, fluid intake should be maintained intravenously. Antibiotics are unhelpful as the aetiology is viral, but are required in the presence of secondary bacterial infection. An inhaled antiviral agent, ribavirin, may be effective in reducing the duration and severity of disease but is an expensive form of treatment with a complicated mode of delivery. Its clinical use is therefore limited to children with impending severe respiratory failure or other underlying cardiopulmonary or immunodeficiency disorders. The vast majority of infants with bronchiolitis appear to make a full clinical recovery. However, at follow-up, an increased incidence of recurrent wheeziness is reported.

Physiotherapy management

In the acute stages of the disease, infants respond very poorly to handling, and there is no indication for chest physiotherapy. Webb and co-workers (1985) reported no positive benefit from chest physiotherapy on the course of bronchiolitis. If the condition is severe enough to necessitate ventilation, physiotherapy may be given, following thorough assessment if there are problems with secretion retention, or relevant radiographic changes.

Pneumonia

Pneumonia is most commonly caused by RSV in the infant and, similarly, other pathogens in the younger child tend to be viral. However, in older children in addition to viral pneumonias, bacterial infections become increasingly common. The child usually presents with a fever, dry cough and tachypnoea, and can be very sick. Chest X-ray shows consolidation.

Management is supportive with attention to fluid intake, and humidified oxygen is administered if necessary. As differentiation between viral and bacterial agents relies on microbiological cultures, wide spectrum antibiotics are usually prescribed at presentation.

Physiotherapy management

Where there is consolidation on chest X-ray there is often no sputum production and physiotherapy is therefore of no benefit. However, sputum retention can be a problem both in the early stages of the disease and also during resolution. Postural drainage and percussion are appropriate techniques to use, and in the younger child suction may also be necessary. In the older child, the active cycle of breathing techniques can be used.

Bronchiectasis

Bronchiectasis is a condition where there is chronic infection associated with persistent cough and sputum production. Factors which contribute to the development of bronchiectasis are listed in Table 16.3.

Management includes vigorous treatment with physiotherapy, physical exercise and antibiotics during bronchopulmonary exacerbations. Occasionally, if the area of disease is very localised, persistently collapsed and infected, but the rest of the lung fields appear healthy, lobectomy may be indicated.

Table 16.3 Factors predisposing to bronchiectasis.

Factors predisposing to bronchiectasis
Recurrent lower respiratory tract infection associated with:
poor nutrition
immunodeficiency
chronic aspiration (feeding/swallowing problems)
Previous inhalation of foreign body

Physiotherapy management

Daily chest physiotherapy with particular attention to the affected area is advised. The active cycle of breathing techniques with gravity-assisted positioning or other independently performed treatment modalities, e.g. positive expiratory pressure, is extremely useful. These will be discussed in Chapter 17.

Inhaled Foreign Body

Foreign material may be aspirated into the bronchial tree resulting in either acute or chronic symptomatology, depending on the material aspirated and the length of time it has been present in the respiratory tract (Dinwiddie, 1996b).

Inhalation of a foreign body into a child's airways is a common problem, and occurs most frequently between the ages of 1 and 3 years. Foodstuffs are most common, especially peanuts and pieces of fruit or vegetable, but small plastic or metal objects may also be aspirated. Commonly, the foreign body will pass through the larynx and lodge in one or other main stem bronchus (most commonly the right), though smaller objects may penetrate as far as the right middle lobe bronchus or occasionally the left lower lobe bronchus. Parents may report a sudden onset of coughing and gagging and, if left unattended, this may progress to persistent coughing and wheezing caused by the offending object partially occluding the airway. Foodstuffs such as peanuts are particularly irritating and secondary pneumonic changes occur distal to the obstruction. Auscultation often reveals a reduced breath sound over the affected are, and wheezing may be heard. If acute inhalation is suspected, inspiratory and expiratory chest X-rays should be performed, and classically the expiratory film shows overinflation of the other lung with decreased lung markings on the affected side. If the event goes unwitnessed the pneumonic changes developing distal to the obstruction will be demonstrated as consolidation on the chest X-ray along with loss of lung volume, indicating collapse.

Treatment consists of urgent bronchoscopy and removal of the offending article. Antibiotics are used for the associated bacterial contamination of the airway and the inflammatory pneumonic process which occurs (Dinwiddie, 1996b). It has been shown that there can be persistent residual damage to the lungs of children who have inhaled a foreign body (despite complete resolution of chest X-ray appearances), and this is related to the length of time the object has been present in the airway.

Physiotherapy management

Attempting to remove a foreign body from the airway by using chest physiotherapy is contraindicated. It is neither effective nor safe and may result in complete obstruction of the trachea (Parker, 1993; Phelan *et al.*, 1994b; Prasad and Hussey, 1995a).

Following bronchoscopic removal of the foreign body, physiotherapy may be important in clearing excessive secretions, particularly if the object has been in the airway for some time and secondary bacterial infection has occurred. Postural drainage, percussion and vibrations can be used safely and effectively once the object has been removed from the respiratory tract.

Asthma

Asthma is common in children (affecting between 10% and 20%) and has been defined as 'episodic wheeze and/or cough in a clinical setting where asthma is likely and other rarer conditions have been excluded' (Warner *et al.*, 1992). The disease follows a naturally remitting and relapsing course and is very variable in severity. Wheezing occurs as a result of bronchial hyperactivity where the bronchial smooth muscle over-reacts to a wide variety of stimuli. The muscle in the bronchial wall then hypertrophies. In addition, there is an inflammatory response in the mucosa and submucosa. Wheezing may be triggered by a wide variety of factors including respiratory tract infection, exercise, smoke, atmospheric pollutants, inhaled or ingested allergens and emotional factors. Hereditary factors also play an important role in the development of asthma. A child is more likely to develop asthma if other members of the close family are asthmatic or atopic. Many children with asthma also have other atopic features such as eczema.

Treatment varies according to the individual and the severity of the disease. Mild infrequent asthma is treated by intermittent bronchodilator therapy. Those children who are more severely affected with more frequent attacks require prophylactic treatment with sodium cromoglycate and inhaled steroids as well as broncho-dilators. Babies may be given oral bronchodilator preparations but generally all drugs should be administered by inhalation. In infants, bronchodilators are often delivered via a nebuliser in addition to oral preparations, though a metered dose inhaler (MDI) with a spacer device can be used. Children over the age of 2 can use a conventional MDI and spacer device. From about 5 years of age, children are able to use a rotahaler, diskhaler or turbohaler to deliver powdered preparations of drugs. Nebulised drugs will still be required for more severe attacks when inhalation may be difficult. Children with a severe attack of asthma may require admission to hospital for more intensive therapy. A minority of children who do not respond to the usual drug regimens will go on to require intubation and ventilation.

Physiotherapy management

During an acute attack, physiotherapy has little place in the management of asthma. Treatment is not indicated and if applied is likely to exacerbate bronchoconstriction. Even in the ventilated patient treatment cannot be performed until bronchospasm has been controlled. Though excess secretions are common in this condition, patients rarely need chest physiotherapy intervention to manage them. However, those who develop persistent areas of lung collapse following an asthma attack can be treated with postural drainage and percussion, or preferably, when old enough, should use the active cycle of breathing techniques. If this is a recurring problem then parents should be instructed in chest physiotherapy techniques.

Physiotherapists in some centres may be involved in educating the parents and child about the condition and its treatment, particularly in relation to administration of inhaled drugs, although this is frequently done by a clinical nurse specialist.

Physical exercise is important to maintain general fitness in children with asthma, who may have a tendency to be physically inactive. It is important that in those with exercise-induced asthma, physical exercise is preceded by bronchodilator therapy. Some physiotherapists are involved in organising and conducting exercise classes for children with asthma; these include not only physical activities, e.g. swimming and progressive exercise programmes, but also postural awareness, breathing control

and education on drug therapy. These classes are particularly helpful for children with severe asthma from both a physical and psychological perspective as these children often lack confidence and are afraid to exercise.

CONCLUSION

Respiratory disease in children is different from that in adults. The assessment and treatment of infants and children requires:

- The development of trust with the child and his or her family.
- Understanding of the disease process.
- Knowledge of the child's stage of development.
- A close working relationship with the multidisciplinary team and support services.

REFERENCES

Davies H, Kitchman R, Gordon I, Helms P. Regional ventilation in infancy. *New Engl J Med* 1985, **313:**1626-1628.

Dean E. Effects of body position on pulmonary function. *Physical therapy* 1985, **65:**613-618.

Dinwiddie R. Respiratory tract infection. In: Dinwiddie R, ed. *The diagnosis and management of paediatric respiratory disease*, 2nd ed. London: Churchill Livingstone; 1996a:103-134.

Dinwiddie R. Aspiration syndromes. In: Dinwiddie R, ed. *The diagnosis and management of paediatric respiratory disease*, 2nd ed. London: Churchill Livingstone; 1996b:247-260.

Parker AE. Paediatrics. In: Webber BA, Pryor JA, eds. *Physiotherapy for respiratory and cardiac problems*. London: Churchill Livingstone; 1993:281-318.

Partridge C, Pryor JA, Webber BA. Characteristics of the forced expiration technique. *Physiotherapy* 1989, **75:**193-194.

Phelan PD, Olinsky A, Robertson CF. Clinical patterns of acute respiratory infections. In: Phelan PD, Olinsky A, Robertson CF, eds. *Respiratory illness in children*. London: Blackwell Scientific; 1994a:58-64.

Phelan PD, Olinsky A, Robertson CF. Pulmonary complications of inhalation. In: Phelan PD, Olinsky A, Robertson CF, eds. *Respiratory illness in children*. London: Blackwell Scientific; 1994b:252-267.

Prasad SA, Hussey J. Assessment of the child with respiratory disease. In: Prasad SA, Hussey J, eds. *Paediatric Respiratory care–a guide for physiotherapists and health professionals*. London: Chapman & Hall; 1995a:56-66.

Prasad SA, Hussey J. Chest physiotherapy techniques. In: Prasad SA, Hussey J, eds. *Paediatric respiratory care–a guide for physiotherapists and health professionals*. London: Chapman & Hall; 1995b:67-104.

Thoresen M, Cavan F, Whitelaw A. Effect of tilting on oxygenation in newborn infants. *Arch Dis Child* 1988, **63:**315-317.

Warner JO, Gotz M, Landau LI, *et al.* Asthma: a follow up statement from an international paediatric asthma consensus group. *Arch Dis Child* 1992, **67:**240-248.

Webb M, Martin JA, Cartlidge PHT, *et al.* Chest physiotherapy in acute bronchiolitis. *Arch Dis Child* 1985, **60:**1078-1079.

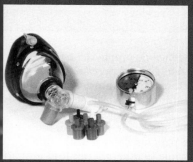

17 SA Prasad
CYSTIC FIBROSIS

CHAPTER OUTLINE

- Basic defect
- Presentation of cystic fibrosis
- Physiotherapy
- Active cycle of breathing techniques

- Positive expiratory pressure
- Physical exercise
- Terminal care
- Heart-lung transplantation

INTRODUCTION

Cystic fibrosis (CF) is the most common serious inherited chest disorder in the white population. In the UK in 1993, there were 6000 cases of CF (40% being adults). It is estimated that in the UK approximately 300 infants per year are born with CF, which is equivalent to 1 in 2500 births. This is an autosomal recessive genetic disorder which means that there is a 1 in 4 chance of CF occurring in each pregnancy where both parents are carriers of the genetic defect (the carrier rate being approximately 1:20). The genetic abnormalities were discovered in 1989, and the defect lies on the long arm of chromosome 7. The commonest defect is known as the δF508 mutation, which accounts for approximately 68% of CF genes. A number of other mutations have since been discovered, some of which are more commonly seen in certain ethnic groups. Generally, the correlation of genotype and disease severity has not proved to be very helpful in terms of clinical management (Dinwiddie, 1996).

BASIC DEFECT

The abnormal genes code for a protein known as the cystic fibrosis transmembrane conductance regulator (CFTCR), and the defect results in abnormal ion transport across the cell membrane. Principally, this is a defect of chloride transport but sodium and water transportation are also defective. These abnormalities result in the elevation of sodium and chloride, and give the classic salty taste typical of these infants when kissed. The excessive saltiness of sweat forms the basis of the standard diagnostic tool, the sweat test, which is still widely used. However, since the genetic defect has been isolated, diagnosis is also by genetic analysis of a blood sample. Diagnosis can also be reliably made prenatally. Couples can, if there is a known history of CF in the family, be screened before pregnancy to assess carrier status. If both are carriers of a known mutation, chorionic villus sampling at 11–12 weeks' gestation, or amniocentesis at a later gestation, can be used for diagnosis.

The disease principally affects the respiratory tract and the digestive system. Other systems, however, can also be involved and lead to problems such as diabetes and hepatic cirrhosis. With increasing longevity these disorders are becoming more common. Affected males are usually infertile, while female patients have slightly impaired fertility. The disease is lifelong and results in early death. When the condition was originally described in the mid 1930s, life expectancy was less than 2 years. Currently, the median survival is 29 years in the best centres; however, the predicted survival of a CF child born in the 1990s is likely to be greater than 40 years (Frederikson et al., 1996).

PRESENTATION OF CYSTIC FIBROSIS

CF can present in many different ways because of its effects on various systems. Meconium ileus is the commonest clinical presentation at birth (accounting for about

10–15% of cases). The infant fails to pass meconium after birth due to bowel obstruction by inspissated intestinal secretions. This is sometimes successfully managed conservatively, but surgical intervention may be required to relieve obstruction. Other modes of presentation in infancy include failure to thrive despite a good appetite, a history of loose offensive stools and recurrent respiratory tract infections.

DIGESTIVE SYSTEM

The majority of patients with CF have some degree of pancreatic insufficiency, which results in malabsorption. Reduced bile salts in the duodenum further impair fat absorption. The resulting poor nutritional status can then affect growth and lower resistance to infection. These patients are also known to have a higher total energy expenditure than normal individuals and they therefore have increased nutritional requirements (120–150% of the recommended daily allowance). Children with CF should have a normal diet which is high in energy (with a normal or increased fat content). High calorie drinks can be very helpful in supplementing intake. In addition, patients need to take pancreatic enzymes (in powder form for infants and later as capsules) with every meal and snack to improve fat digestion. Vitamin A, B, C, D and E supplementation is given routinely, and, for those with significant liver disease, vitamin K may also be necessary. In the more advanced stages of lung disease it may not be possible to maintain weight using the above measures. In this situation children may benefit from enteral feeding via nasogastric tube in the short term or, if longer-term enteral feeding is necessary, via gastrostomy.

RESPIRATORY SYSTEM
Pathophysiology
The lungs, though normal at birth, rapidly become inflamed and colonised with pathogenic organisms. This leads to production of thick sticky secretions, which impair mucociliary clearance and increase the risk of chest infection. By the age of 3 months, approximately 50% of patients with CF are symptomatic in some way, and by the age of 8 months 50% will have developed respiratory symptoms (Dinwiddie, 1996). Recurrent infection leads to obstruction of small airways by mucous plugging. The airways become progressively damaged and distorted, and collapse leads to air trapping, persistent infection and eventually chronic bronchiectasis. In the late stages of the disease, pulmonary hypertension develops and the right side of the heart fails. Figure 17.1 shows the progression of lung disease in CF. Currently, there is considerable interest in the underlying pathophysiology of the lung disease and particularly in the inflammatory response which occurs from a very early stage in the disease process.

Pseudomonas is a pathogen often seen in patients with CF. Once established in the lungs it is almost impossible to eradicate. On initial culture it requires aggressive treatment with oral and nebulised antibiotics. If it is regularly cultured from sputum, treatment should be tailored to the individual's needs. This may include prophylactic nebulised antibiotic therapy, with additional preparations as required, or a rigorous structured programme of regular intravenous treatment. Recently, a more virulent species, *Burkholderia cepacia*, has emerged as a major pathogen in patients with CF. The clinical course after culture of this organism is variable; some patients carry it with little change in their condition, while in others it can lead to rapid decline.

Management
The aim of treatment is to minimise the effects of intercurrent infection, to clear the lungs of obstructive and damaging secretions, and to delay the onset of bronchiectasis. The strategies used in pulmonary management include chest physiotherapy and physical exercise, mucolytic agents to reduce the viscosity of sputum, bronchodilator therapy to control any concomitant bronchial hyper-reactivity, and antibiotics. Antibiotics may be administered either on a long-term prophylactic basis or episodically to treat infection. Milder infections can be treated with oral antibiotic therapy but more severe infections will require intravenous therapy.

PHYSIOTHERAPY

Chest physiotherapy is an integral part of the management of CF. In the short term, clearing obstructive bronchial secretions improves ventilation and in the long term it is hoped that removal of these purulent secretions delays the progression of damage to the airways. An outline of various aspects of the physiotherapy management of CF can be seen in Table 17.1

INFANTS AND YOUNG CHILDREN
Once the diagnosis has been ascertained, daily chest physiotherapy should be implemented. This should include a general regimen of postural drainage and chest

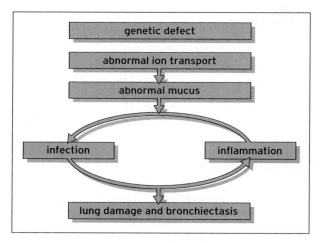

Figure 17.1 Progression of lung disease in cystic fibrosis.

percussion. Positions of drainage should include alternate side lying and prone with a head down tip, and supine flat. The sitting position is also important in the infant to drain the apical segments of the upper lobes. If there are particular radiological changes, more specific postural drainage positions will be necessary. As the child grows and is upright for a significant portion of the day, drainage of the apical segments can be omitted from the regimen. In the presence of infection or broncho-pulmonary exacerbation, it is important that the frequency of treatment is increased; this may be necessary up to four times per day (Dinwiddie and Prasad, 1995). Initially, treatment can be performed on the parent's lap, but as the child grows use of a foam wedge or a postural drainage frame is more appropriate.

Both parents should be taught the techniques. This will require a careful and sensitive approach at a time when they are not only trying to come to terms with the diagnosis, but are being given a huge amount of information regarding the disease and its management. It is also important (particularly if diagnosis is made at a specialist centre) that the local hospital and community teams are fully informed so that they can provide appropriate follow-up and support.

As the child grows, breathing exercises can be instituted, initially as play and later more formally as part of the treatment programme. By the age of 4 most children can perform forced expiratory manoeuvres (huffing), and breathing exercises/control and are therefore able to play an active part in their own treatment.

OLDER CHILDREN

As life expectancy has increased considerably in patients with CF, the majority now live well into adulthood. It is important that older children and adults are able to experience full and independent lifestyles. Daily chest physiotherapy places a tremendous burden on the patient and family, and it is important that treatment is efficient and effective yet causes the least possible disruption to the patient's lifestyle. Partial or non-adherence to treatment is well recognised in chronic illness of any type. In CF, it is widely reported that physiotherapy is the least practised treatment despite the fact that, in addition to medication and attention to diet, it is essential to help maintain the patient's wellbeing. The teenage years can be a difficult time for normal children and an even greater burden for children with chronic diseases such as CF. It is often at this age, when patients are being encouraged to take more responsibility for their own treatment, that problems with compliance lead to significant stress within the family. Continuing education with regard to the condition and its treatment, along with the formation of an 'alliance' between the therapist and patient/family, is important in influencing compliance during difficult stages.

Older children and adults should for the most part be able to manage their disease independently, and to achieve this aim several chest physiotherapy techniques have been developed (Table 17.2) which allow patients to be completely independent in their treatment (Prasad, 1993).

ACTIVE CYCLE OF BREATHING TECHNIQUES

The active cycle of breathing techniques (ACBT) is a cycle of breathing control, thoracic expansion exercises and the forced expiration technique (FET) (Webber and Pryor, 1995). Breathing control is used between the more active components of the cycle and is normal tidal volume breathing at the patient's own comfortable rate, with the chest and shoulders relaxed. Thoracic expansion exercises are deep breaths which emphasise inspiration. The increase in lung volume facilitates collateral ventilation and allows air to flow behind secretions and assist in mobilising them. The forced expiration technique comprises one or two forced

Role of the physiotherapist in the management of cystic fibrosis at three stages of the disease		
Newly diagnosed patient	**Acute exacerbation**	**Out-patient review**
Assessment	Intensive chest physiotherapy	Lung function testing
Parental patient education	Inhalation therapy	Review/revision of technique
Instruction of treatment techniques	Exercise as appropriate	Instruction of new technique (if appropriate)
Advice regarding exercise	Physiotherapy adjuncts: periodic facial CPAP/IPPB if appropriate	Advice on exercise
Advice/provision of domiciliary equipment	Psychological support	Review/advice on domiciliary equipment
Psychological support		Psychological support

Table 17.1 **Role of the physiotherapist in the management of cystic fibrosis at three stages of the disease.**

expirations (huffs) from mid to low lung volume to loosen and clear peripheral secretions. Huffing is combined with breathing control to avoid any potential in air flow obstruction that can be caused by forced expiratory manoeuvres.

ACBT is usually performed in appropriate gravity-assisted positions, and the cycle is adapted to the individual patient. Thoracic expansion exercises may be accompanied by chest percussion, though it has been shown that this is not a necessary part of treatment provided the other techniques are performed properly. Many patients do, however, report considerable subjective benefit from percussion. An example of a cycle of treatment is shown in Figure 17.2.

POSITIVE EXPIRATORY PRESSURE

Positive expiratory pressure (PEP) is a treatment technique in which positive pressure is applied to the airways during expiration, usually via a face mask (Figure 17.3). The positive pressure keeps central and peripheral airways open, and collateral ventilation is improved; hence there is said to be a positive effect on lung clearance and gas exchange (Falk and Anderson, 1991). The PEP mask consists of a mask, one-way valve and resistors of various sizes which are placed into the expiratory port of the one-way valve to achieve PEP. The level of PEP achieved is monitored by a pressure gauge placed between the valve and resistor. The patient should be assessed by an experienced therapist for the resistor of appropriate size, which is one that achieves a PEP of 10–20 cmH$_2$O during expiration. Treatment is performed in a sitting position, and the patient breathes through the mask for 10–12 tidal volume breaths. Expiration will be slightly active but must not be forced. The mask is then removed from the face and huffing, breathing control and coughing are performed. The cycle is then repeated until maximal clearance is achieved.

OTHER MODALITIES

Other independently performed chest physiotherapy modalities include a modification of the PEP technique, known as high pressure PEP. In this technique after careful assessment (requiring full lung function testing equipment) and training, the patient performs a full forced expiration through the PEP mask after 7–8 of the normal tidal volume breaths described earlier. This maintains patency of the small airways, and allows evacuation of trapped gas from previously closed airways, thereby enhancing sputum clearance and reducing hyperinflation.

Table 17.2 Independently performed chest physiotherapy techniques.

Independently performed chest physiotherapy techniques
Active Cycle of Breathing Techniques (ACBT)
Positive Expiratory Pressure (PEP)
High Pressure PEP
Autogenic Drainage (AD)
Flutter
Exercise

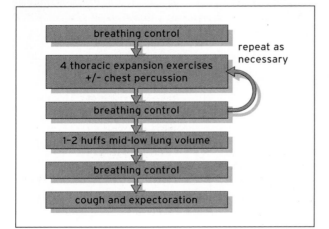

Figure 17.2 An example of a treatment cycle of the active cycle of breathing techniques (ACBT).

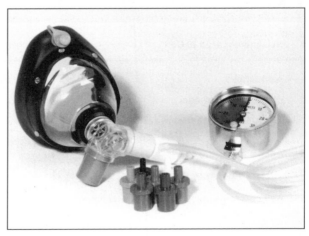

Figure 17.3 The positive expiratory pressure mask.

Autogenic drainage in its original form is a three phase breathing regimen where controlled breathing at different lung volumes (low, mid and high) is used to achieve the highest possible expiratory air flows without causing airway collapse. Forced expiration and coughing are avoided and secretions are mobilised from the periphery of the lung during the period of low lung volume breathing.

The flutter valve is a relatively recently introduced technique, consisting of a pipe-shaped device inside which a steel ball rests within a cone. On expiration through the device, air flow is initially impeded by the ball, but as the pressure rises within the system the ball is lifted out of the cone. The pressure is then released and the ball falls back into the cone. This results in application of a variable PEP within the airway, and production of endobronchial pulses, the vibratory effect of which enhances mucus clearance.

These techniques, though widely used throughout Europe and America, are less frequently used in the UK (Samuels *et al.*, 1995) and are therefore not described in detail here. However, it is essential that physiotherapists who are regularly involved in the care of patients with CF should be aware of these techniques in order to tailor treatment to an individual's needs. There is no one best method of chest physiotherapy, and the modality selected should take into account the patient's age, respiratory status and social and psychological circumstances, and be one that provides maximum therapeutic value for that individual.

PHYSICAL EXERCISE

Exercise is a very important part of the management of CF. The beneficial effects of regular exercise include improved cardiorespiratory fitness, muscle power and joint mobility and an improvement in one's sense of wellbeing and self-image. However, in order to maintain these benefits exercise must be continued on a regular long-term basis. Patients with severe disease should not be discouraged from exercise within their own capabilities. It may be necessary to administer supplementary oxygen therapy for those with a forced expiratory volume in 1 second of less than 50% predicted, as oxygen desaturation may be significant during exercise in these patients.

Exercise has also been reported as having a beneficial effect on sputum clearance. Most recent studies have shown it to be complementary to, rather than a replacement for, chest physiotherapy (Bilton *et al.*, 1992). There are, however, a few patients in whom sputum production is minimal and exercise alone may be sufficient to maintain respiratory status. Children should be actively encouraged to take part in all sporting activities both in and out of school, and it is rarely necessary to institute formal exercise programmes.

TERMINAL CARE

Physiotherapy intervention during the later stages of the disease will, to a large extent, be supportive rather than active. However, advice can be given regarding positioning, particularly with regard to breathlessness. In certain circumstances it may also be appropriate to use adjuncts to physiotherapy such as facial continuous positive airway pressure (CPAP) to assist secretion clearance, and in adults intermittent positive pressure breathing (IPPB) can also be helpful. The child can often be made significantly more comfortable by clearing even relatively little in the way of secretions.

HEART-LUNG TRANSPLANTATION

Heart–lung transplantation or lung transplantation may be an option for those patients with severe advanced lung disease who have a life expectancy of less than 12 months. However, the number of donor organs is relatively small and therefore careful patient selection is vital in order to achieve the best results. Criteria for referral for assessment, the assessment process, and management of children undergoing transplantation are described in detail in Chapters 11 and 20.

CONCLUSION

Physiotherapy plays an important role in the management of respiratory disease in CF. From birth through childhood, adolescence and adulthood each stage brings its own problems. After a lifetime of intervention, terminal care can be very difficult for the physiotherapy team to deal with emotionally, but the aim remains unchanged: to ensure the best quality of life for the patient.

REFERENCES

Bilton D, Dodd ME, Abbott JV, *et al*. The benefits of exercise combined with physiotherapy in the treatment of adults with cystic fibrosis. *Respir Med* 1992, **86:**505-511.

Dinwiddie R. Cystic fibrosis. In: Dinwiddie R, ed. *The diagnosis and management of paediatric respiratory disease*, 2nd ed. London: Churchill Livingstone; 1996:197-245.

Dinwiddie R, Prasad SA. Cystic fibrosis. In: Prasad SA, Hussey J, eds. *Paediatric respiratory care-a guide for physiotherapists and health professionals*. London: Chapman & Hall; 1995:159-174.

Falk M, Anderson JB. Positive expiratory pressure (PEP) mask. In: Pryor JA, ed. *Respiratory care*. London: Churchill Livingstone: 1991;51-63.

Frederikson B, Lanng S, Koch C *et al*. Improved survival in the Danish centre treated cystic fibrosis patients. *Pediatr Pulmonol* 1996, **21:**153-158.

Prasad SA. Current concepts in physiotherapy. *J R Soc Med* 1993, **86(suppl. 20):**23-29.

Samuels S, Samuels M, Dinwiddie R, Prasad S. A survey of physiotherapy techniques used in specialist clinics for cystic fibrosis in the UK. *Physiotherapy* 1995, **81:**279-283.

Webber BA, Pryor JA. Physiotherapy. In: Hodson ME, ed. *Cystic fibrosis*. London: Chapman & Hall; 1995:347-357.

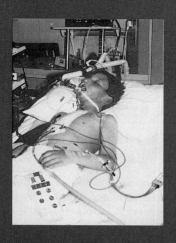

18 S Davey & A Magnay

THE PAEDIATRIC INTENSIVE CARE UNIT

CHAPTER OUTLINE

- The PICU environment
- Admission to the PICU
- Monitoring and life support equipment in the PICU
- Clinical problems

- Physiotherapy in the PICU
- Assessment of the paediatric intensive care patient
- Indications for physiotherapy
- Physiotherapy techniques

INTRODUCTION

Paediatric intensive care is a multidisciplinary field addressing the needs of children who have sustained, or are at risk of sustaining, life-threatening single or multiple organ system failure due to disease or injury. The Paediatric Intensive Care Unit (PICU) concentrates facilities for the maximum surveillance and support of vital systems in children with acute, but potentially reversible, impairment of major organ function. Quality of survival is of prime consideration.

The PICU is characterised by:
- Continuous specialised nursing.
- Continuous specialised medical supervision.
- Specialised monitoring and therapy.
- Immediate access to specialised equipment and laboratory and radiological services 24 hours a day.

The overall objective is to decrease mortality and morbidity of critically ill and injured children, and simultaneously provide a sensitive and effective support for their families.

THE PICU ENVIRONMENT

WORKING WITH CHILDREN AND THEIR PARENTS

Children become ill rapidly, and often recover quickly. However, illness in a child is usually very distressing to the family and often to hospital staff, as well as to the child. Ill children may exhibit fearful or terrified behaviour, may cry and be difficult to console, and may be unable to express their fears or needs. They may be unco-operative, and are usually frightened of strangers. These factors compound the difficulties of assessing and managing the ill paediatric patient.

An honest, gentle, calm, reassuring approach is crucial to win the co-operation of the child and parents, and the full support of the child's nurse. Management of pain, anxiety and restlessness requires non-pharmacological as well as pharmacological measures. A child-friendly environment includes appropriate decor, children's toys and familiar sights and sounds, including the parents. The greater part of the patient's care can be carried out with the parents present, which usually reassures the child. Full reasonable explanations to parents and the child often help the patient understand what to expect (including discomfort), especially if it is realised that any treatment should speed a recovery.

WORKING AS PART OF THE MULTIDISCIPLINARY TEAM

Good communication skills are important between professionals working in the stressful environment of the PICU. However, inappropriate conversations and laughter between professionals near an ill child are usually not well received by self-aware children or their parents.

Careful documentation of current treatment plans, with a problem-oriented approach, is important for team communication. This will assist all members of the team to have a clear grasp of the roles played by the different members of the multidisciplinary team. Important conversations with parents should always take place with the bedside nurse present, as the final common path of the multidisciplinary team. Controversial or difficult discussions, especially breaking bad news, should first be discussed with the medical and nursing members of the team, who may be in a better position to advise about preparation and timing for such discussions with the parents and child.

The unique environment of the PICU has ideally a child-friendly environment where the medical and psychological needs of the ill child and stressed family are addressed by a multidisciplinary team familiar with the patterns of illness and behaviour they may encounter.

KNOWLEDGE BASE OF STAFF

- Respiratory physiology of the preterm and term infant and older children, in particular the unique aspects of the anatomy and physiology, and the major differences between children and adults.
- Normal and abnormal cardiovascular anatomy and physiology in the newborn infant and older child, and how this information relates to the critically ill child.
- Problems of cardiorespiratory instability during care of critically ill children, and the factors which may lead to worsening or improvement of stability.
- Current views on the importance of maintaining adequate cerebral perfusion pressure (CPP), and controlling intracranial pressure (ICP) in the injured brain, e.g. after trauma, or infective or metabolic insults.
- Familiarity with the PICU environment, equipment and monitoring. This includes problems that may arise with interpreting monitors, or the safe use of the PICU equipment.

- Education and training of medical, nursing and allied professional staff in the care of critically ill children is a major objective within the PICU.

ADMISSION TO THE PICU

The clinical workload within the PICU depends on admission rate and the clinical case mix unique to each unit. For instance, the presence or absence of a cardiothoracic surgery programme will have a profound effect on the ratio of elective admissions to acute unplanned admissions (Table 18.1), the average duration of intensive care, and the range of problems seen by the physiotherapist. A tertiary PICU ideally will see a minimum of 250 admissions per year, up to 2000 per year in the largest of the North American PICUs. Depending on the stability of the patient and the intensity of the medical interventions required for the support of the patient, there may be a nurse to patient ratio of 1:2, increasing to more than 2:1 for the most demanding patients.

Patients may be admitted electively, following planned surgery, for example, or as emergency admissions. The development of paediatric intensive care transport teams has resulted in improved communication between non-tertiary intensive care units and tertiary PICUs, which enables optimal stabilisation and safe timely transfer of critically ill children to tertiary centres. The thrust of paediatric emergency medicine is to recognise the potentially ill child early, and to prevent progression of illness to organ failure.

The mortality rate for children admitted to the PICU depends on case mix and criteria for admission, but is recognised to be low (approximately 15%) compared with the adult ICU (AICU; approximately 55%) and neonatal ICU (NICU; approximately 60% for infants <1000 g).

The duration of PICU stay also depends on case mix and criteria for admission and discharge, but is recognised to be short (averaging 4.5 days in the UK) compared with

Table 18.1 Comparison of the case mix between two complementary tertiary paediatric Intensive Care Units (PICUs).

Comparison of the case mix between two complementary tertiary paediatric Intensive Care Units (PICUs)		
	% of admissions in one year	
Category of admission	PICU 1	PICU 2
Acute medical	64	8
Cardiac surgery	0	65
Paediatric surgery	12	17
Neurosurgery and trauma	12	4
Neurology	12	2
Oncology	0	9
Hepatology	0	4

the AICU and NICU. The survivors from the PICU live longer than survivors from the AICU, and have a lower handicap rate than the survivors from the NICU. Taking into consideration the shorter intensive care stay, lower morbidity and mortality, and longer useful survival following discharge, the cost effectiveness of intensive care is therefore greatest for PICUs (Shann, 1995).

MONITORING AND LIFE SUPPORT EQUIPMENT IN THE PICU

As in AICUs, all PICU beds will be equipped with multi-channel monitoring facilities for electrocardiography, respiration, non-invasive and invasive blood pressure monitoring, central venous pressure (CVP) monitoring and non-invasive transcutaneous oxygen monitoring and/or oxygen saturation (PO_2) monitoring. Transcutaneous carbon dioxide monitoring, end tidal carbon dioxide monitoring and continuous invasive oxygen saturation monitoring are present in some, but not all, PICUs.

Haemodynamic monitoring by pulmonary artery balloon flotation catheters (Swan–Ganz) is less often employed in PICUs because of technical problems of scale and patient size, but the majority of PICUs will use such techniques from time to time, when appropriate.

Invasive ICP monitoring via intraparenchymal or intraventricular fibreoptic pressure sensor is commonly employed for unconscious trauma patients or those at risk of secondary brain injury from either raised ICP or falling CPP.

Cerebral function monitoring, using 2- or 3-channel electroencephalogram continuous recording, is sometimes helpful in identifying seizure activity in selected patients if they are pharmacologically paralysed and therefore cannot be clinically assessed for control of seizures. Such monitors are continually evolving and pose significant problems of interpretation and unproved clinical benefit.

RESUSCITATION EQUIPMENT

Any professional participating in the care of critically ill patients should be familiar with the layout of the PICU and the location and use of emergency resuscitation equipment. Many PICUs will maintain a resuscitation trolley with a selection of paediatric-sized airway, breathing and circulation equipment, a defibrillator/electrocardiograph (ECG) monitor with paddles for small patients, and a selection of resuscitation drugs.

Airway and Breathing

Oral and nasopharyngeal airways should be available. Correct sizing before use is important. An oral airway should match the distance from the centre of the patient's mouth to the angle of the jaw. A nasopharyngeal airway (and also an endotracheal tube) should have an internal diameter calculated from (age in years/4) + 4 mm. Alternatively, a tube the diameter of the patient's fifth finger is likely to be approximately correct.

Masks for bag-valve mask ventilation may be circular (universal fit) for neonates up to about 15 kg, or shaped for larger children. A correctly fitting mask must allow free air entry into both the nose and mouth while retaining a seal.

Bags for manual ventilation are of two types:

Self-inflating bag-valve devices
Self-inflating bag-valve devices, e.g. Laerdel and Penlon, may have a pressure-limiting safety valve set to limit at 35 cmH$_2$O. However, in spite of the safety valve, with forceful squeezing it is possible to generate peak inflating pressures as high as 70 cmH$_2$O, which is excessive and may cause catastrophic pulmonary air leak. Manual inflation pressures should be sufficient to generate visible chest movement.

The advantages of self-inflating bags include:
- Relative ease of use.
- General safety.
- The ability to inflate the lungs even if there is no piped gas flow.

The main disadvantage in the PICU is the inability to generate positive end expiratory pressure (PEEP) or sustained breaths. For this reason, the self-inflating bags are usually confined to the resuscitation trolley, and are not routinely employed by the bedside for advanced airway management.

Open circuit T-piece bags
Open circuit T-piece bags come in various sizes, i.e. 250 ml, 500 ml, 1 litre and 1.5 litres. They have an open tail, and are deflated unless there is a gas flow and a seal (such as a properly fitted mask or an endotracheal tube). Dependent on the patient's size, fresh gas flow is set at 8–15 litres/min, with flow from the inspiratory limb of the T-circuit into the patient limb of the T-circuit. The bag controls the rate of flow out of the exhaust limb of the T-circuit. Manual control of PEEP requires gentle pinching of the open tail to maintain the desired pressure. Inflation requires squeezing the bag, with pressure maintained to sustain the breath for the required duration. The technique requires considerable practice, and is most safely managed by incorporating a pressure manometer into the circuit for accuracy and training.

The advantage of T-piece circuits is that the breath characteristics are precisely controlled by the operator, including generating PEEP, sustained breaths, and assessment of the degree of limitation of expiratory flow. Therefore they are the choice for bedside deployment for advanced airway management in the PICU.

The disadvantages of the open circuit T-piece bag include:
- Its relative difficulty of use.
- The potential for inexperienced users inadvertently to generate sustained high pressures.
- The need for piped gas flow.
- The need for a good mask seal to inflate the bag.

Intubation equipment may be required as an emergency, and comprises:

- Suction, i.e. catheters and hard plastic sucker.
- Oxygen, bag and mask.
- Airway, i.e. endotracheal tube with an introducer, laryngoscope and Magill's forceps.
- A resuscitation trolley with a drugs tray.
- Monitoring equipment, e.g. ECG, PO_2 monitoring, blood pressure monitoring.

Airway and Vascular Access: 'Tube Security'

Children are prone to attempt removal of vital airway equipment, vascular access and monitoring equipment, and urinary catheters. It is essential that attention is regularly paid to fixation of endotracheal tubes and invasive monitoring lines. Interventions such as physiotherapy or repositioning the patient are typically when accidents may happen, and all staff should be vigilant on these occasions. Poor fixation should be addressed before commencing such manoeuvres. Premedication with short-acting drugs such as fentanyl, midazolam, ketamine or propofol will often be necessary to improve analgesia and sedation cover for interventions which may be painful or increase arousal to the detriment of the patient. It is not usually appropriate to restrain patients with ties to prevent accidents. Calm reassurance and other non-pharmacological measures are also important, along with appropriate basal levels of pharmacological sedation and anxiolysis.

MECHANICAL VENTILATORS

It is beyond the scope of this chapter to give an account of all the products now available in PICUs for ventilatory support of patients ranging from infants to adults. A few centres have specialised in alternative approaches to ventilation, i.e. extracorporeal membrane oxygenation (ECMO) or negative pressure ventilation; these techniques are described in Chapter 20. The basic principles of conventional invasive positive pressure ventilation (PPV) are summarised here.

Lungs can be inflated with a set inflation pressure (pressure limited), or they can be filled with a set volume (volume cycled). The two approaches achieve similar end results, but employ different ventilator designs and have different problems which may need to be considered in the context of the patient's actual needs.

Endotracheal Tube Leak

In children under 12 years of age, the narrowest part of the airway is the cricoid ring. To avoid damage to this area, uncuffed endotracheal tubes are usually used in such children. A small leak around the tube is expected on inspiration. Historically, this led to difficulties with deploying volume-cycled ventilation in small patients, in whom an unknown and varying proportion of the breath could leak around the tube rather than inflate the lung. In addition, the volume 'lost' into the distensible ventilator circuit could not easily be quantified. For these reasons, neonatal and infant ventilation traditionally employed pressure-limited ventilation, e.g. Bourns, Dräger, Sechrist, Infant Star and SLE2000. Larger infants and children would usually have received volume-cycled ventilation. Modern ventilator strategies, including permissive hypercapnia, have led to a greater proportion of older patients receiving pressure-limited ventilation via multipurpose ventilators, with correspondingly less obsession with control of minute ventilation in the majority of patients.

Typical volume-cycled ventilators deployed in the PICU include the Servo 900 series, Servo 300 series, and Adult Star (paediatric module). All have the capacity for selecting from a number of ventilation modes, including volume-cycled or pressure-limited modes, and some have specialised weaning modes such as continuous positive airway pressure (CPAP) plus pressure support, or volume support. The choice of ventilator modes is large, reflecting the need to customise the ventilation and weaning strategy to the needs of the individual child. The ventilator tubing's dead space is highly significant to the weaning modes, e.g. a 5 ml dead space in the circuit can increase an infant's dead space by 100%. Care must be taken to ensure that tidal volumes are sufficient to allow the air/oxygen mix to reach the alveoli for gas exchange to take place.

Volume-cycled Ventilation

In volume-cycled ventilation:

- A PEEP is prescribed.
- A set tidal volume is prescribed, e.g. maximum 10 ml/kg (usually 5–7 ml/kg) per breath.
- The inspiratory time is prescribed by manipulating the inspiratory flow rate, and possibly other breath characteristics including the flow curve.
- A rate is prescribed to generate a minute ventilation of 100–200 ml/kg/min.
- The inspiratory phase is initiated either by time triggering, i.e. controlled mandatory ventilation (CMV), or by patient triggering, i.e. synchronised intermittent mandatory ventilation (SIMV). The expiratory phase is initiated either by reaching the end of the set volume (CMV, SIMV), or by patient triggering (in the case of sensed breaths over and above the mandatory breath rate). The peak airway pressures generated by the breath depend on the airway resistance and the inspiratory flow, the size of the endotracheal tube leak, and the airway compliance and how close to the limits of distensibility the lung volumes are being inflated.

Pressure-limited Ventilation

In pressure-limited ventilation:

- A PEEP is prescribed.
- An inspiratory pressure is prescribed, i.e. for normal lungs 10–12 cmH$_2$O above the PEEP, and for stiff lungs as high as 30 cmH$_2$O above the PEEP.
- A rate is prescribed.
- Inspiratory time is set.
- The inspiratory phase is initiated either by time triggering (CMV), or by patient triggering (SIMV). The expiratory phase is initiated either by time cycling (CMV, SIMV), or by patient triggering (in the case of sensed breaths over and above the mandatory breath rate).
- Each breath delivered has a set peak pressure. The tidal volume delivered with each breath depends on whether

there is limitation of inspiratory or expiratory flow caused by too short an inspiratory or expiratory time in the presence of a long time constant, the airway compliance and on how close to the limits of distensibility the lungs are being inflated.

High Frequency PPV

It is now recognised that volume distension, rather than pressure, is the main cause of ventilator-induced lung injury (Dreyfuss et al., 1988). It is also recognised that ventilation at low lung volumes can augment lung injury because of mucosal injury resulting from the shear force of repeated opening of small airways, which then close at the end of the respiratory cycle (Muscedere et al., 1994). The ideal form of ventilation would therefore appear to be low V_T, and high frequency ventilation around an optimally recruited lung volume. This can be achieved by employing high frequency jet ventilation or oscillation ventilation, at breath rates well above physiological respiratory rates. The ventilators used produce time-cycled, pressure-limited breaths at frequencies typically between 4 and 18 Hz. The expiratory time constant of the lung will be longer than the expiratory phase of each breath, resulting in limitation of expiratory flow and low V_T. This is partially overcome by ventilator design, employing an active expiratory phase effectively assisting the expiratory component of the breath, plus allowing an expiratory phase longer than the inspiratory phase (I:E ratio 1:2 or more). The importance of airway resistance in limiting V_T at high frequencies is crucial to understanding the limitations of this ventilation strategy. High frequency ventilation cannot be used in asthma, bronchiolitis or other conditions with high airway resistance. Airway secretions can also severely impair gas exchange, so adequate humidification and judicious (infrequent) physiotherapy are of paramount importance.

Clinical trials of high frequency strategies have shown benefit compared with conventional ventilation for premature neonates with the severest lung problems, especially those with developing pulmonary barotrauma such as pulmonary interstitial emphysema or pneumothorax (Keszler et al., 1991). Older children (Arnold et al., 1994) and adults undoubtedly respond to this form of ventilation in adult respiratory distress syndrome (ARDS), but study data are limited in adults. Controlled trials have shown benefit only if there is attention to maintaining adequate lung volumes, typically by adjusting mean airway pressure to keep the diaphragm at the level of the ninth rib posteriorly on chest X-ray. A protocol for re-inflating the lungs and recruiting alveoli by manual sustained inflation is also useful to prevent hypoxaemia and instability following suction.

Monitoring Respiratory Mechanics

Many ventilators now incorporate software, of varying usefulness, for monitoring the flow and volume characteristics of each breath. Stand-alone modules also exist. Improved monitoring of flow and volume allows estimates of airway resistance and compliance, and the ability to assess changes in lung mechanics following adjustments

in PEEP. The graphic displays also indicate if there is limitation of inspiratory or expiratory flow, which may indicate the need for lengthening the expiratory time.

MONITORING OF ARTERIAL GASES
Oximetry

Continuous transcutaneous pulse oximetry is an established technique in the PICU. It is based on the physical principle that oxygenated and deoxygenated haemoglobin have different light absorption spectra at red and infrared frequencies. The proportion of oxygenated haemoglobin in the pulsatile component of the light path is reported as oxygen saturation. Correct interpretation requires adequate pulsation (pulse pressure >20 mmHg), a correctly positioned probe with no external light interference, and exclusion of movement artifact (Poets et al., 1996). High saturations (98–100%) may be associated with dangerously high oxygen tension (>12.5 kPa) in preterm infants, in whom the risk of retinopathy of prematurity may be increased by high arterial oxygen levels. Saturations below 92% leave little reserve for further deterioration, which may be associated with increased risk of secondary brain injury following head trauma.

Transcutaneous Oxygen Monitoring

Transcutaneous oxygen ($Ptc.O_2$) electrodes measure the partial pressure of arterial oxygen (PaO_2) through the skin. The electrode is heated to 44°C, which alters the crystalline structure of the stratum corneum of the skin. This permits transcutaneous oxygen diffusion to the electrode. In preterm neonates, the electrode may need repositioning every 2–4 hours to prevent skin burns. Readings become reliable 15 minutes or so after repositioning, provided the skin site is suitable and the correct amount of contact gel is used. The instruments available will predict the PaO_2 to within 1.3–2.0 kPa 95% of the time in stable preterm neonates under optimal conditions. However, some reports have suggested that 15% of hypoxaemic episodes (<6.7 kPa) are missed by $Ptc.O_2$ monitoring (Poets et al., 1996). The 90% response time for identifying sudden falls in saturation may be as long as 1 minute, although it will fall faster if there is a co-existing fall in skin perfusion (Poets et al., 1991). If there is concern about the accuracy of the $Ptc.O_2$ reading, it should be checked against an arterial blood gas.

Transcutaneous Carbon Dioxide Monitoring

Transcutaneous carbon dioxide ($Ptc.CO_2$) electrodes measure the partial pressure of carbon dioxide ($PaCO_2$) through the skin. Typically, the sensor is heated to 42°C. The electrodes yield reproducible predictions of arterial carbon dioxide saturation, though they do tend to over-read. The correction factor provided by the manufacturer should improve the accuracy of the prediction of $PaCO_2$ although some PICUs feel it necessary to check the sensor accuracy in each individual patient against arterial blood gas values. Most reports indicate that the available instruments predict the $PaCO_2$ to within 0.8–1.2 kPa 95% of the time. The 90% response time is approximately 30–50 seconds (Merritt et al., 1981).

End tidal Carbon Dioxide Monitoring (Capnography)

End tidal carbon dioxide ($ETCO_2$) monitoring provides breath-by-breath analysis of exhaled carbon dioxide based on a sampling technique (mass spectrometry) or on infrared light absorption. The sampler or sensor is placed at the end of the endotracheal tube, adding slightly to the dead space (significant in infants) and adding extra weight to be borne by the tube fixation technique. This slightly increases the risk of accidental extubation or circuit leak.

Advantages include the immediate recognition of failed intubation or accidental extubation, and the warning of adverse trends in $PaCO_2$ in vulnerable patients, such as those receiving cerebral protection measures, especially during transportation or while receiving manual ventilation.

Disadvantages include the problems of interpretation of capnography in patients with pulmonary disease who may have non-uniform ventilation/perfusion (V/Q) matching throughout the lung. If the end tidal gas includes gas from poorly perfused alveoli, where little carbon dioxide has diffused into the air space, or the end tidal gas is contaminated by significant dead space gas, for example, in asthma, where limitation of expiratory flow leads to reduced escape of alveolar gas by the end of expiration, then the $ETCO_2$ value will be significantly and unpredictably lower than the $PaCO_2$. In practice, the technique reliably predicts only the $PaCO_2$ in 'normal' lungs, with uniform V/Q matching and uniform airway resistance.

OTHER EQUIPMENT FOR ORGAN SUPPORT OR MONITORING

Surface Cooling and Core Temperature Monitoring

Cerebral protection measures include the maintenance of a normal body temperature of 36–37°C. This may easily be carried out by servo-controlled water-filled cooling and warming blankets, attached to a free standing warmer/cooler and monitoring device. Core temperatures must be monitored by rectal or oesophageal probes. Axillary, tympanic and oral temperatures are not core temperatures and are poor predictors in the ill child, especially if the patient is receiving surface cooling.

CLINICAL PROBLEMS

RESPIRATORY SYSTEM

In many PICUs, respiratory support is the most frequent challenge. Infections with epidemic viruses such as respiratory syncytial virus (RSV) and parainfluenza, and other common community acquired viruses, account for many admissions during the winter months, causing bronchiolitis, laryngotracheobronchitis (croup) and viral pneumonia.

Bronchiolitis causes airway obstruction at the level of small bronchioles, resulting in areas of over-distended lung and areas of atelectasis. Affected children are usually infants, and may present with progressive respiratory failure, or exhaustion due to increased work of breathing. Mild hypoxaemia is surprisingly common and easily passes

unrecognised in this age group unless continuous transcutaneous monitoring is employed. Airway reactivity and pulmonary vascular reactivity are increased in bronchiolitis and are exacerbated by airway hypoxia, arterial hypoxaemia and unnecessary handling of the ill child. Feeding may be a major problem in the presence of significant tachypnoea and increased respiratory effort. Coughing and spluttering with feeds is an important sign of increased risk of aspiration and marginal respiratory reserve. In addition, ex-preterm infants, especially those who required treatment for apnoea of prematurity, may present with apnoeas later in infancy during intercurrent viral infections, especially RSV.

Bacterial pneumonia and respiratory failure due to severe systemic infection also occur more commonly in infants than in older children, due to the relative immaturity of their immunity. The increasing prevalence of congenital or acquired HIV in the paediatric age group has been associated with an increase in pneumonitis caused by *Pneumocystis carinii* seen in high dependency units and ICUs.

The acute lung injury syndrome, ARDS, occurs in the PICU following similar precipitating causes in children as in adults, although less commonly.

Management of Respiratory Illness

It is important to ensure adequate oxygenation to provide adequate oxygen delivery to vital organs and to minimise problems associated with labile pulmonary vascular resistance and airway resistance, especially in infants. However, in the sickest lungs requiring ventilatory support, it may be better to accept lower arterial oxygen saturation (PaO_2; 85–92%) under controlled conditions than to strive for 'normal' blood gases at the cost of ventilator-induced lung damage. The concept of permissive hypercapnia, and acceptance of mild hypoxaemia, is fundamental to the successful management of severe ARDS in all age groups (Hickling *et al.*, 1994).

Respiratory support can be non-invasive, employing positive pressure by mask or nasal prong, or negative pressure by perspex tank or cuirass, or invasive, employing an endotracheal tube via oral, nasal or tracheostomy routes.

The goals for respiratory support may differ for each patient, for example, to:
- Reduce the work of breathing.
- Improve alveolar recruitment and ventilation/perfusion matching, hence oxygenation.
- Control tidal ventilation for control of arterial pH and partial pressure of carbon dioxide ($PaCO_2$).
- Support left ventricular function by use of PPV.
- Protect the airway and allow airway toilet via a secure endotracheal tube.

Asthma and Conditions with Increased Airway Resistance

PPV may be transmitted to the pleural space and may impede venous return into the thorax, especially in normally compliant lungs. In the clinical settings of high airway resistance but relatively normal compliance, there will be a prolonged expiratory time constant. This occurs typically in asthma and bronchiolitis. Unless the expiratory time is sufficient to allow full expiration, this limitation of expiratory flow may lead to a high inadvertent intrathoracic PEEP, which will impede venous return to the heart and lead to a fall in cardiac output, which may be catastrophic. This can be overcome by lengthening the expiratory time and slowing the ventilation rate, and also by ensuring that the patient is adequately volume filled to keep central venous filling pressures high enough to overcome any inadvertent PEEP.

Slow ventilation rates are especially important during manual ventilation of patients who have a prolonged expiratory phase, when breath-stacking and inadvertent PEEP may occur unrecognised.

Asthma is also characterised by increased viscid secretions, which may cause airway obstruction. Airway toilet to remove large plugs may be a life-saving manoeuvre. However, airway reactivity in any acute respiratory illness may be exacerbated by handling and physiotherapy techniques. It is generally preferred to reserve chest physiotherapy to treat excessive mucus production, or specific areas with plugging and atelectasis.

Bronchodilator therapy may be nebulised into some paediatric ventilator circuits. Other circuits may require the incorporation of an additional customised section of tubing with a port for aerosol puffer administration. Manual ventilation through a nebuliser into the patient is also possible.

Stiff (Low Compliance) Lungs
In abnormal low compliance lungs, positive intrathoracic pressure may not be transmitted to the pleura or mediastinal structures, and so high levels of (intentional) PEEP or mean airway pressure may be haemodynamically well tolerated. In acute lung injury, e.g. ARDS, and in surfactant deficiency, the critical opening pressure of small airways and alveoli is elevated. Even after maximal lung volume recruitment, the airways are more prone to closure because of elevated critical closing (CC) volumes, i.e. the residual lung volume at which CC occurs. For these reasons, it is essential to maintain a PEEP above the CC volume in order to maintain alveolar recruitment, optimise ventilation/perfusion matching and minimise intrapulmonary shunting.

Alveolar recruitment manoeuvres include:
- Administration of adequate PEEP by mask, nasal prong or endotracheal tube.
- Sustained inflation manoeuvre.
- Natural surfactant replacement therapy.

Each may have a place in a child's respiratory plan in the PICU.

Chest Trauma
Chest trauma accounts for only 10% of major trauma in children. However, injuries to the lungs and mediastinal structures can rapidly compromise the airway, breathing and circulation, and therefore have a high associated morbidity and mortality. Management is directed first at identifying and treating acutely life-threatening conditions as a first priority, and then at identifying and dealing with potentially life-threatening problems. Airway obstruction and tension pneumothorax are the commonest life-threatening problems. Clinical recognition of pneumothorax, haemothorax and flail chest, and pulmonary contusion, cardiac tamponade and cardiac arrhythmia, are important skills for anyone caring for trauma patients in the PICU.

CARDIOVASCULAR SYSTEM
Heart failure in children is usually associated with congential heart disease (see Chapter 19) or multisystem failure, which is discussed below.

Congenital heart disease occurs in 0.8% of live births. The diagnosis is established by 1 week of age in approximately 40–50% of these, of whom some are diagnosed antenatally. Congenital structural anomalies are described in Chapter 19.

Improved cardiac surgery techniques and increasingly accurate pre-operative work-up have resulted in vastly improved outcomes for many congenital defects. Surgery is now more likely to be fully corrective rather than palliative, and is carried out at an earlier age. The majority of PICU admissions for cardiac surgery are less than 3 years of age. The median duration of intensive care stay is now approaching 1 day in the best centres, but depends on the precise surgical diagnosis.

Pre-operative problems including severe wasting, growth failure and pulmonary hypertension are now infrequent owing to improved pre-operative assessment and management. Post-operative complications of surgery and cardiopulmonary bypass are also infrequent but include cardiac arrhythmia or embolic stroke, and spinal infarction, acute renal failure or necrotising enterocolitis in infants, in addition to wound and mediastinal sepsis, and injury to the thoracic duct causing chylothorax. Pulmonary complications include lung contusion from handling thoracic structures, pulmonary oedema from left ventricular dysfunction, pulmonary embolism following insertion of prosthetic, allograft or xenograft material, and complications of mechanical ventilation including subglottic stenosis, and bronchopulmonary dysplasia following prolonged ventilation. Deep vein thrombosis is exceedingly rare in the paediatric population, and is most likely to be related to central venous line complication.

ECMO is now carried out in some units as a technique of bypassing the lungs and heart while supporting the circulation during cardiac surgery (see Chapter 20).

NEUROLOGICAL SYSTEM
The developing central nervous system (CNS) in the child is vulnerable to trauma, infection, neoplasia, epilepsy, metabolic disorders and congenital anomalies. Some children with non-traumatic neurological problems may have progressive disease with no chance of recovery with current knowledge, for example children with severe neurodegenerative metabolic disease such as Tay–Sachs disease, and may therefore not benefit from admission to the PICU. Others who are critically ill with a potential for recovery may be admitted to the PICU for intensive care

directed at protecting the injured or vulnerable CNS from secondary injury.

Head injury kills approximately 5.3 per 100 000 children per year. The head represents a relatively greater proportion of the body surface area in children (18%) compared with adults (9%). The head, face and neck are therefore more likely to be injured in paediatric trauma victims compared with adults.

Protecting the Injured or Vulnerable Brain

The therapeutic goals of protecting the injured or vulnerable brain comprise:

Preservation of brain function
Preservation of brain function implies:
- Attention to the ABCs, i.e. Airway, Breathing and pH control, and Circulation ensuring adequate circulating haemoglobin.
- Identification and treatment of life-threatening neurological crises, e.g. brain herniation, status epilepticus.

Relief of primary pathology
Relief of primary pathology includes:
- Glucose for hypoglycaemia.
- Anticonvulsants for status epilepticus.
- Antimicrobials for CNS infection.
- Neurosurgical intervention for space-occupying lesion, traumatic brain injury, vascular anomalies or hydrocephalus.
- Correction of metabolic disorders if possible.

Prevention of secondary brain injury
Prevention of secondary brain injury includes:
- Prevention of hypoxaemia.
- Prevention of thermal stress.
- Reduction of cerebral oxygen consumption, e.g. analgesia, anxiolysis and hypnosis.
- Maintenance of adequate CPP and cerebral blood flow.
- Prevention of elevated ICP, avoiding brain herniation.
- Avoiding hypo-osmolar stress by appropriate electrolyte and osmotherapy.
- Reducing the risk of seizures by appropriate anticonvulsant therapy.

Patients with a high risk of raised ICP and loss of autoregulation of cerebral blood flow may be managed with invasive ICP and CPP monitoring. Without invasive monitoring, clinical assessment of neurological status and conscious level is vital for identification of developing intracranial problems such as expanding haematoma, worsening cerebral oedema and falling cerebral perfusion. However, analgesia and deep sedation, with possible neuromuscular paralysis, reduces cerebral oxygen consumption and minimises the risk of noxious stimuli causing potentially catastrophic rises in ICP or falls in CPP. Furthermore, pyrexia is potentially damaging to the injured brain, and is almost inevitable following major trauma. Thermoregulation to maintain body temperature strictly within the normal range of 36–37°C is non-controversial, and is most simply and reliably carried out by surface cooling using a servo-controlled cooling/warming blanket in conjunction with regular antipyretic drugs. Shivering, with increased oxygen consumption, may occur unless neuromuscular paralysis is used. For these reasons, invasive intracranial monitoring is often employed to replace clinical assessment of conscious level in patients requiring cerebral protection measures during the acute phase of their illness.

Current opinion stresses the importance of maintaining ICP <20 mmHg to avoid brain herniation, and CPP (mean arterial pressure minus ICP) >60 mmHg in children and >70 mmHg in adults to ensure adequate cerebral blood flow. Prophylactic hyperventilation is now believed to be of no benefit, and may be harmful, to potentially recoverable areas of the injured or vulnerable brain. It is now recommended that $PaCO_2$ is strictly maintained within normal limits (4.5–6.0 kPa), reserving hyperventilation for acute treatment of raised ICP unresponsive to other measures, e.g. relief of painful stimuli or arousal, thermoregulation, osmotherapy and haemodynamic management.

Effective neurointensive care in heavily sedated or pharmacologically paralysed patients requires continuous monitoring of heart rate, arterial blood pressure, ICP, CPP, oxygen saturation, non-invasive $PaCO_2$ (transcutaneous or end tidal), core temperature and urine output, with frequent arterial gas and electrolyte measurements and minimal handling of the patient. Any interventions, especially airway toilet, may result in surges of ICP, which should recover within 5–10 minutes of the event. However, elevation of great magnitude, or longer than 10 minutes, should be prevented if possible, to reduce the risk of brain herniation. Pre-medication with a small intravenous dose of short-acting opiate, such as fentanyl (1–2 µg/kg), or intravenous lignocaine (1 mg/kg) may depress the ICP rise. Care should be taken to avoid turning the head as this may obstruct jugular venous flow, and to maintain a head up position of 30 degrees to reduce cerebral venous volume.

Protecting the Potentially Injured Spine

Only 1–2% of children with major trauma will have a spinal cord injury. The evaluation of children with major trauma initially includes a lateral radiograph of the cervical spine, along with an anteroposterior chest X-ray and anteroposterior pelvis X-ray, followed by a complete spinal X-ray series if indicated. However, approximately two-thirds of spinal injuries in children occur without radiological abnormalities (American College of Surgeons, 1993), due to differences in bony and ligamentous support of the spine in children compared with adults. Children require both radiological and clinical assessment to exclude spinal cord injury following major trauma. Cervical spine control requires midline stabilisation in the neutral position, maintained by both a semi-rigid collar and sandbags, with tapes across the forehead, to immobilise the neck properly. Thoracic and lumbar spine stabilisation implies a rigid board (with appropriate padding) and log-rolling technique to protect the spine during patient care or examination.

MULTISYSTEM FAILURE

In multisystem failure, each individual system is addressed according to the patient's need. For example, a child in septic shock with meningococcal disease with secondary acute renal failure may be acidotic, with poor left ventricular function, and may have massive capillary leakage of fluid into alveoli leading to respiratory failure due to hypoxaemia.

Respiratory support will employ PPV, PEEP set to maintain optimal lung volumes and alveolar recruitment above CC volumes, and tidal ventilation settings to avoid high peak distending pressures. Control of pH and $PaCO_2$ may be desirable to minimise cerebral oedema, but peak pressures may be limited to 30 cmH_2O to avoid barotrauma.

Left ventricular function will be supported with inotropic drugs and PPV, while appropriate filling of the circulation will be maintained by volume boluses. In this example, breaking into the ventilator circuit would be undesirable, could lead to abrupt pulmonary oedema and circulatory instability, and should be avoided except to clear mucus plugs. Following any break into the circuit for airway management, it might be necessary to perform a sustained inflation manoeuvre to re-recruit alveoli, using careful control with an open-circuit T-piece bag and pressure manometer to sustain an inflation pressure of 30 cmH_2O for 5–15 seconds before re-connection with the ventilator without loss of lung volume. Such airway manoeuvres should be performed only by properly trained and skilled operators.

Renal support can be provided by peritoneal dialysis, veno-venous haemofiltration and haemodialysis, which are all used in the PICU. Specialised peritoneal catheters or vascular access catheters are employed for these techniques. Heparinisation is usually required for vascular routes of renal support, which may have increased risks of unwanted oozing or bleeding.

PHYSIOTHERAPY IN THE PICU

Chest physiotherapy plays an important part in the management of critically ill infants and children on intensive care. It requires thorough initial and continuous assessment of each individual patient, clear identification of treatment aims, and an ability to modify treatment techniques appropriately. A multidisciplinary approach to patient care is essential and requires close co-operation and communication between all professionals, the child and family. Careful explanations of why physiotherapy is necessary and what it involves should always be given to parents before treatment of their child. Parents are encouraged to stay during treatment and are often a great help in reassuring and gaining the co-operation of a child that is awake or frightened.

Children with neurological problems or those who have a long stay in intensive care often require additional skills from the physiotherapist. Advice on how to maintain joint mobility and soft tissue length, positioning, and ways to encourage normal development in such an alien environment are often helpful to both nursing staff and parents.

In this chapter we discuss the respiratory assessment, indications for treatment, and treatment techniques, and the role physiotherapy plays in the management of conditions that result in the child being admitted to intensive care.

ASSESSMENT OF THE PAEDIATRIC INTENSIVE CARE PATIENT

The assessment of the child has been described in Chapter 16. The patient on PICU will require the following to be considered:

HISTORY

This will include the presenting history, birth history and any relevant medical history. It is also allows you to gather important information on social circumstances.

VENTILATION

Firstly, is the child ventilated or not? If ventilated then:
- What is the mode, ventilation rate, airway pressures (both PIP and PEEP) and level of inspired oxygen?
- What size is the endotracheal tube, to ensure the correct size of suction catheter is used?
  If the child is not ventilated, then:
- What is their respiratory rate and how much oxygen are they receiving? Is it via a mask or headbox?

DRUGS

Regarding medication:
- What drugs is the patient receiving and why?
- Is the patient paralysed or sedated? Is medication going to be adequate for treatment?
- Is the patient on any inotropic support? The dosage will indicate the unstable cardiovascular patient who may not tolerate treatment.
- Is the patient on bronchodilators and can these be given before physiotherapy?

VITAL SIGNS

Vital signs vary with age (Table 15.1, p256). Assessment of these includes:
- Temperature: a raised temperature or pyrexia can indicate infection, while a difference in core and peripheral temperatures of greater than 1°C may indicate poor peripheral perfusion thus poor cardiac output, and hence a patient that may not tolerate treatment.
- Heart rate and rhythm: as a general rule, a tachycardia is >180 beats/min and bradycardia <100 beats/min.
- Blood pressure and oxygen saturation, both from the chart (looking at the general trend of values) and from the monitor: hypotension indicates an unstable patient with poor cardiac output while hypertension may be due to inadequate sedation, or indicative of pain.
- Urine output: a reduced urine output may indicate poor renal perfusion, give further evidence of poor cardiac output, and may indicate impending renal failure.

CHEST X-RAY

Always examine chest X-rays closely before treatment. Note any areas of collapse, consolidation, hyperinflation or pneumothorax, pleural effusions, pulmonary oedema, or rib fractures. Infants are more prone to upper lobe collapse (particularly of the right upper lobe) than adults. A left lung collapse and/or right upper lobe collapse may be due to too long an endotracheal tube—the right main bronchus becomes intubated and consequently the left lung and right upper lobe receive no ventilation and collapse. It is therefore important to check the position of the endotracheal tube. In this case, treatment involves the tube being retracted, not physiotherapy.

ARTERIAL BLOOD GASES

Analyse these carefully to ascertain the acid–base status of the blood and to give an idea of gaseous exchange.

INVESTIGATIONS

What are the results of any investigations? Computerised tomography (CT) and magnetic resonance imaging (MRI) scans or EEG results may indicate problems with intracranial pressure (ICP). If the white cell count (WCC) is raised this may indicate infection—this may or may not be respiratory in origin. If the values for platelets, clotting or haemoglobin are low then treatment techniques may need to be modified.

INFORMATION FROM THE NURSE

A wealth of information will be obtained from talking to the nurse caring for the child. Is the child improving or deteriorating? Have there been any episodes of desaturation, bradycardia or apnoea? If so what provoked them? Is the child adequately sedated or paralysed? Is the pain adequately controlled? Has the patient had too much sedation and is therefore too drowsy to cough effectively? What are the secretions like, e.g. amount, colour, thickness, and ease of clearance? How does the child tolerate handling and suction? Was the patient stable following the last physiotherapy treatment, and does it seem to have helped or not?

OBSERVATION

Take care to look at the position of any incisions and all lines before handling the child. These may include wound and chest drains, peripheral arterial and venous lines, central venous lines, ECG leads, temperature sensor, probes for monitoring oxygen and carbon dioxide levels, a urinary catheter and ICP monitor.

The child may seem settled and asleep (either naturally or drug induced) or may be agitated due to pain, inadequate sedation or respiratory distress; this should be noted. What colour is the patient? Pale, grey or mottled may indicate hypoxaemia or poor cardiac output. In both the ventilated and non-ventilated child, assess respiratory rate and pattern by looking for any signs of respiratory distress. Look at the shape and movement of the chest. Is there asymmetry, hyperinflation, flattening or deformity? Note any noisy breathing such as stridor, snoring or grunting.

PALPATION

Examine the child's chest for equal chest expansion and for the presence of tactile fremitus, surgical emphysema or any tracheal deviation. Tactile fremitus may indicate the presence of secretions in the large airways while surgical emphysema may indicate small airway rupture or a pneumothorax. Tracheal deviation can really be assessed only in the self-ventilating child, and may indicate upper lobe pathology or pneumothorax.

AUSCULTATION

Breath sounds should be assessed for equality. Note any added sounds such as bronchial breathing, wheezes and crackles. Water in the ventilator tubing and air leaks around the endotracheal tube can produce deceptive noises. Transmitted airways sounds are often heard when secretions are present in the upper airways or endotracheal tube.

INDICATIONS FOR PHYSIOTHERAPY

Assessment will indicate the need for respiratory therapy. It may be that only advice to the nursing staff on positioning is required. Before considering active respiratory intervention there should be clear indications for treatment. These are:

- Retained secretions unable to be cleared with suction alone.
- Acute lobar or lung collapse from mucous plugging.

PHYSIOTHERAPY TECHNIQUES

SUCTION

Children who are intubated, have a tracheostomy or unable to cough effectively will require suction. Never regard suction as a routine, minor or non-invasive procedure as it can cause tracheobronchial trauma, hypoxia, atelectasis, bronchospasm, pneumothorax, bradycardia, hypotension, cardiac arrhythmias, apnoea and raised ICP (Young, 1984a) and induce vomiting. These complications can be minimised by good technique, careful consideration of pre-oxygenation, selection of catheter, and appropriate application of negative pressure. Observe heart rate, blood pressure and oxygen saturation before, during and after suction. Suction after a feed should be avoided (see treatment timing below).

Pre-oxygenation is useful as it can minimise the hypoxia and cardiovascular disturbances provoked by suction (Kerem et al., 1990). Increase the level of inspired oxygen via the ventilator for a couple of minutes before suction, or give manual hyperinflation with a bagging circuit. In the non-intubated child give extra oxygen via a headbox, face mask or bag, and anaesthetic mask.

Select a catheter that is made of an atraumatic material, and has more than one side hole, and a built-in control valve. Choosing the correct size is crucial. In infants and children, a guideline is that the outer area of the catheter should not occlude more than half the internal area of the endotracheal tube, but catheters smaller than size 5 French gauge are usually ineffective in removing tenacious sections. Generally, catheters between size 5 and 8 are used. For example, in an endotracheal tube (ETT) with an internal diameter of 3.0 mm:

area of ETT = πr^2

= $3.14 \times 1.5^2 = 7.065$ mm^2

The correct size of catheter to use is size 6 French gauge as this has an external diameter of 2.0 mm:

area of catheter = πr^2

= $3.14 \times 1.0^2 = 3.14$ mm^2

i.e. area of catheter is less than half the area of the ETT (see Table 18.2).

Negative pressure should be appropriate for each patient and checked before treatment. Recommended values are 60–90 mmHg for infants, 90–110 mmHg for small children and 110–150 mmHg for older children.

Keep suctioning time to a minimum to reduce the risk of hypoxia and possible bradycardia. A maximum suction time of 30 seconds in children and 15 seconds in neonates is mandatory (Young, 1984b). Bradycardias may occur due to hypoxia or as a vaso-vagal response. After extubation, children are prone to laryngeal spasm (usually just for a few hours), therefore take great care with suction. If they have post-extubation stridor then suction should probably be avoided. Avoid nasopharyngeal suction in children with cerebrospinal fluid (CSF) leakage or following nasal surgery. Following repair of tracheo-oesophageal fistula or oesophageal atresia, nasopharyngeal suction should be limited to a distance determined by the surgeon (usually 5 cm).

More recently, closed tracheal suction catheters have been used. They are useful in reducing hypoxia, especially in children who are difficult to ventilate and require high PIP and PEEP, as they do not require disconnection from the ventilator.

Suction via a Tracheostomy

Tracheostomy may be required in acute or chronic upper airway obstruction, or in children who require long-term ventilation. A few additional rules apply when caring for a child with a tracheostomy. Suction should be limited to no further than 0.5 cm beyond the length of the tube, and should never be performed through a speaking valve.

Secretions are often more copious and thicker than those aspirated from an endotracheal tube, and therefore instillation of saline before suction is advisable.

Nasopharyngeal Suction

Infants breath through their noses, therefore the nasal passages of non-intubated babies need to be kept clear of secretions. The catheter will stimulate the cough reflex and enable secretions to be cleared. Position all non-intubated infants in the side lying position before suction, to prevent them from aspirating vomit if they are sick. They should have their arms securely wrapped in a blanket during the procedure. Follow the same guidelines for catheter size and suction pressure as when endotracheal suction is being performed.

MANUAL HYPERINFLATION

Never use manual hyperinflation routinely. Children have delicate lung tissue that can easily be damaged. Use it only when there is an acute lung collapse from mucous plugging that has not responded to other chest physiotherapy techniques, or in situations where the child is too unstable to tolerate treatment on the ventilator. Use a paediatric re-breathing circuit. This consists of an open-ended bag of the appropriate size (500 ml for infants and small children and 1 litre for older children) and a pressure manometer with which peak inspiratory pressures are measured. Vary the flow of gas into the bag depending on the size of the child (4–6 litres per minute for an infant, up to 10 litres per minute in an older child).

Do not perform manual hyperinflation in someone with an undrained pneumothorax or low cardiac output. Only after discussion with the medical staff, can it be performed, with great care, in patients with surgical emphysema, raised ICP, severe bronchospasm, emphysematous bullae or cysts, following abdominal or thoracic surgery, and in patients who are difficult to ventilate, i.e. on high ventilator rates, high airway pressures and high concentrations of inspired oxygen. Too much hyperinflation can drop cardiac output. To avoid this, alternate one hyperinflation with two or three V_T breaths.

Table 18.2 Choosing the correct size of suction catheter for varying sizes of endotracheal tube.

Choosing the correct size of suction catheter for varying sizes of endotracheal tube		
Internal diameter of endotracheal tube (mm)	Recommended size of suction catheter (French gauge)	External diameter of catheter (mm)
2.5	5	1.7
3.0	6	2.0
3.5	7	2.2
4.0	8	2.7
4.5	8	2.7
5.0	10	3.3

If the child is on CPAP or a low ventilator rate, then it is often helpful to let him or her breathe spontaneously in between hyper-inflation to prevent 'blowing off' the respiratory drive. After finishing treatment and re-connecting the child to the ventilator it is imperative that you check the ventilator is working properly. Have the airway pressures risen? This can indicate that secretions still remain, the tubing is kinked or, more importantly, the child may have developed a pneumothorax. If there are no secretions on further suction and the tubing looks fine, then medical help should be sought immediately.

SALINE INSTILLATION

The instillation of normal saline (0.9%) into an endotracheal tube before suction or during physiotherapy is common clinical practice. It is thought to loosen thick secretions, elicit a cough in unparalysed patients and reduce tube blockage. However, there is little research to support this. The routine use of saline should therefore be avoided, but it can be useful in situations where secretions are thick and difficult to remove.

BRONCHOALVEOLAR LAVAGE

Bronchoalveolar lavage (BAL) is useful in acute lobar or lung collapse due to mucous plugging (Prasad and Hussey, 1995). It should be carried out only by experienced physiotherapists, usually with an anaesthetist present, as some patients tolerate the procedure poorly. It is usually necessary to pre-oxygenate the child before the procedure (often to 100%). Position the child in the reverse postural drainage position, i.e. left side uppermost and head down position, in order to treat a right upper lobe collapse, and turn the head the opposite way (to the left in this instance). This should allow selective intubation of the right main bronchus (Placzek and Silverman, 1983). A syringe of saline is attached to a catheter. Introduce the catheter into the endotracheal tube and inject the saline (2–5 ml in an infant, 5–10 ml in an older child). Quickly remove the catheter and re-connect the child to the ventilator or bagging circuit. After a few breaths (which allows the saline to reach the dependent part of the lung) turn the child into the correct postural drainage position (right side uppermost, head up in this instance). You can then carry out physiotherapy on the affected part of the lung. This will usually mean manual hyperinflation and vibrations followed by suction. If the procedure is well tolerated then repeat it again until the mucus plug is removed and the lobar or lung collapse is resolved.

BREATHING EXERCISES

In older children, these can be useful during weaning off ventilation, post-extubation and post-operatively. In young childen, blowing bubbles and using tissues, paper footballs and windmills is invaluable, while the older child can usually use paediatric incentive spirometers.

POSTIONING AND POSTURAL DRAINAGE

Positioning plays an important part in both the nursing and physiotherapy care of the acutely ill child. It can help clear secretions from the respiratory tract and improve ventilation/perfusion matching and arterial oxygen levels. It is also essential in relieving pressure areas and may help to avoid abnormal reflexes in a child with spasticity. If a child is nursed in the supine position for a long period of time (this may be out of necessity due to an acutely unstable condition), then mucous pooling and atelectasis tend to occur in the posterior lung bases. When possible, turn patients regularly to ensure that no particular lung region remains dependent for long.

It is well documented in infants and young children that ventilation is preferentially distributed to the uppermost lung (Davies *et al.*, 1985; Bhuyan *et al.*, 1989). It is crucial to consider this when positioning a child with unilateral lung disease. If you can position the patient with the good lung uppermost you improve gaseous exchange. However, during chest physiotherapy, you may need to place the 'bad' lung uppermost in order to drain secretions and re-expand areas of atelectasis. This can cause a drop in oxygen saturation. You may be able to avoid this by increasing oxygen. Sometimes, however, the child may be so unstable that toleration of any turning is poor, and you may have to make do with treating the child in alternative positions (quarter turn, supine or even with the normal lung uppermost).

Changing an infant from the prone to supine position should normally increase V_T, minute ventilation and arterial oxygen tension (Ciesla, 1989). This is thought to occur because of the chest wall being stabilised, and an improved co-ordination between the movement of the rib cage, diaphragm and abdomen. The prone position can therefore be useful in the management of the child having difficulty maintaining adequate oxygenation or proving difficult to ventilate. The head down position is rarely used in the treatment of infants and small children as they normally have lung pathology affecting the upper or middle lobes. It can occasionally be useful for treating older children with lower lobe problems. Remember, however, the normal contraindications such as raised ICP, cardiac instability, phrenic nerve palsy, gastro-oesophageal reflux and abdominal distension after neurosurgery or abdominal surgery and during peritoneal dialysis. When weaning from ventilation and when the child is no longer sedated, use the sitting position to aid removal of secretions, improve lung volumes and encourage normal development and play. Infants and small children can be sat in chairs such as the tumbleform chair, while older children should be encouraged either to sit up in bed or to get out into a comfortable chair.

Postual drainage is contraindicated if raised ICP or abdominal distension is present or if there is a risk of periventricular haemorrhage.

PERCUSSION AND VIBRATIONS

These techniques are described in Chapter 16.

It is important to note that percussion should be avoided in patients with a platelet count below 50 and vibrations below a count of 20, e.g. in leukaemia. Care is also required in patients with raised ICP, pleural effusions, bronchospasm, pulmonary haemorrhage, osteoporosis, burns or large areas of skin abrasions.

With high respiratory rates it is often easier to apply vibrations on every second or third exhalation. When an infant is ventilated it may be easier to watch the airway pressure dial on the ventilator to time the vibrations.

PRONGED CPAP

CPAP via a nasal prong is useful in infants with borderline respiratory failure, and also following extubation. The prong is effectively a short nasotracheal tube (cut to a length of 3–5 cm) attached to the normal ventilator circuit. Instillation of saline and manual hyperinflation are ineffective, and should not be attempted as the tube reaches only the pharynx. It can sometimes be difficult to perform suction and you should take care to avoid excessive trauma.

TREATMENT TIMING

Good communication with medical and nursing staff will avoid unnecessary handling of children in intensive care. Ideally, treatment should coincide with turning and nursing procedures. In unstable children it is often better to give short but frequent treatments as they tolerate this better. Treatment may be required just before extubation of a child and therefore close liaison with the anaesthetist is important.

Ideally treatment is best given about 30 minutes before a feed; a sick infant may need this rest before attempting to feed. Following a feed, treatment should be delayed for at least 45 minutes, and much longer in a child with gastro-oesophageal reflux or prone to vomiting.

PHYSIOTHERAPY MANAGEMENT OF RESPIRATORY CONDITIONS ON A PICU
Pneumonia

Children with pneumonia are occasionally admitted to intensive care for ventilation. This is most common in those with underlying cardiopulmonary disease, immunodeficiency, anaemia or chronic lung disease due to prematurity. As a general rule, if the pneumonia is consolidated then physiotherapy is of little value. Children that become productive may benefit from physiotherapy.

Aspiration Pneumonia

Repeated aspiration of saliva and food into the lungs can lead to recurrent lower respiratory tract infections and apnoeic episodes. Sometimes these require ventilatory support. Children with congenital upper airway or oesophageal abnormalities, swallowing inco-ordination or neurological deficit are at greatest risk. These children should be nursed and treated in the head up position as they often have gastro-oesophageal reflux.

Many children may also vomit and aspirate when unconscious or during resuscitation. This may account for the high incidence of respiratory complications following trauma.

Bronchiolitis

This acute viral infection, from which most infants will start to recover within 2–3 days, may result in severe respiratory failure requiring ventilation. Patients are often very unstable, can be difficult to ventilate and are often prone to pneumothoraces. It is important to understand what the virus does to the lungs. Initially, the epithelial cells lining the bronchioles become inflamed, swell and narrow the airways. Dead epithelial cells are shed and, together with the extra mucus produced, further block the already constricted airway. Meanwhile the cilia are being destroyed, mucociliary clearance becomes impaired, and the airways become more blocked. The airway obstruction leads to air trapping. Areas of hyperinflation and atelectasis develop causing reduced gaseous exchange.

In the acute phase, physiotherapy is usually contra-indicated. The main problem in this condition is the oedema of the bronchioles for which physiotherapy is useless. However, if there are excessive secretions which cannot be cleared effectively with suction, or new areas of lung collapse after intubation, then chest physiotherapy may be indicated. These patients often desaturate dramatically with handling and suction. It is therefore not surprising that they often tolerate physiotherapy poorly. Pre-oxygenation, bronchodilators before treatment and initially treating patients *in situ* may help. Try to avoid manual hyperinflation as patients are at high risk of developing pneumothoraces. However, they may be necessary if there are thick, tenacious secretions and cell debris adding to the lobar collapse.

Laryngotracheobronchitis (Croup)

This is a common condition of young children, most frequently seen between the ages of 6 months and 4 years (see Chapter 16). It causes acute swelling and oedema of the airway. Only the most severe cases develop significant laryngeal obstruction and respiratory failure requiring intubation and ventilation. Physiotherapy is indicated in the ventilated child only when there is difficulty clearing secretions or lobar collapse. It should not be required after extubation, and can be dangerous due to residual airway swelling.

Acute Epiglottitis

This is an extremely dangerous condition, most frequently seen between the ages of 2 and 4 years. Acute airway obstruction develops rapidly, with 60–70% of hospital admissions requiring intubation. Like laryngotracheobronchitis, physiotherapy is indicated only following intubation and in the presence of retained secretions or lobar collapse. Post-extubation physiotherapy should not be attempted. Occasionally, a child can suffer severe hypoxia due to prolonged airway obstruction or following a difficult intubation. This can result in brain damage. In the acute stages, chest physiotherapy may need to be adapted to prevent a further rise in ICP. Positioning, passive stretches, splinting and rehabilitation may also need consideration.

Pertussis (Whooping Cough)

This is an acute lower respiratory tract infection caused by *Bordetella pertussis*. It can be very severe in infants, often causing bronchopneumonia and respiratory failure requiring ventilation. Chest physiotherapy is contraindicated until the child is intubated, as any handling can initiate coughing spasms and apnoeic spells. Once intubated and ventilated, chest physiotherapy is useful in removing the very thick, tenacious secretions that often occur. However, unless the child is fully sedated and paralysed, it can still be difficult, causing paroxysmal coughing and desaturation. If manual hyperinflation is indicated chest physiotherapy needs to be performed with extreme care as it can exacerbate air trapping, bronchospasm and coughing. Following extubation, physiotherapy is often required for persistent lobar collapse.

Asthma

During an acute episode, ventilation may be required in children who, despite medication, develop significant respiratory failure. Physiotherapy, if indicated, should be carried out only following intubation, and when bronchospasm has been relieved. Percussion, saline instillation and suction are helpful in removing mucus plugs that often cause areas of lung collapse. Manual hyperinflation is often contraindicated as it can worsen areas of hyperinflation, increasing the risk of pneumothorax. It can also aggravate bronchospasm. Bronchodilators given before treatment may help reduce bronchospasm, together with warming saline before instillation. Always stop treatment if bronchospasm becomes significantly worse.

Smoke Inhalation

Children suffering from smoke inhalation will be admitted to intensive care for airway management. There is often both thermal and chemical damage to the epithelial lining of the tracheobronchial tree. This can result in severe upper airway obstruction, inflammation and necrosis of the smaller airways, and destruction of surfactant leading to atelectasis. Both can cause marked hypoxia. In addition, toxins such as carbon monoxide, which reduces the ability of the blood to carry oxygen, and hydrocyanic acid, which prevents the uptake of oxygen by the tissues, add to the general hypoxia. The physiotherapy management of these patients is complicated. Chest physiotherapy is vital in removing soot, necrosed cells, excessive secretions and often gastric contents secondary to aspiration. However, raised ICP, severe bronchospasm, burns to the chest, pulmonary oedema, ARDS and cardiovascular instability can complicate the management. You should remember that pulse oximeters are inaccurate in the presence of carbon monoxide poisoning.

Near Drowning

Drowning may be classified into three types: dry, fresh water or salt water.

Dry drowning occurs when the child's breath is held and no water is aspirated into the lungs. Although no respiratory complications are suffered, the child will often suffer profound hypoxia and secondary cerebral damage.

Aspiration of fresh water causes washout of surfactant, subsequent lung collapse and fluid overload as the hypotonic solution is drawn into the blood and tissues.

Salt water aspiration results in a chemical pneumonitis due to alveolar tissue injury together with pulmonary oedema as the hypertonic solution draws water out of the blood and tissues.

Aspiration of gastric contents is common, either during the acute episode or during resuscitation. As the apirate is likely to contain bacteria and vegetable matter from the water, this can further exacerbate the respiratory problems. Physiotherapy is beneficial in treating areas of collapse and in removing the debris from the lungs of these patients. It does, however, depend on the amount of cerebral oedema present, and may have to be modified or withheld to maintain an adequate CPP.

PHYSIOTHERAPY MANAGEMENT OF NEUROLOGICAL CONDITIONS ON A PICU

Head Injury

Children with severe head injuries may require ventilation to prevent secondary brain injury from raised ICP, hypoxia and hypercarbia.

It is important to maintain adequate perfusion to the brain at all times to prevent ischaemia. The adequacy of brain perfusion is measured by the CPP. CPP can be calculated by subtracting the ICP from the mean arterial blood pressure (MABP):

CPP = MABP – ICP (normal values, ICP = <15 mmHg)

CPP = 50–70 mmHg (Tasker & Prasad, 1995).

CPP is therefore a crucial parameter, and all attempts must be made to prevent either hypotension or elevating the ICP. Physiotherapy is not given routinely in these patients, but they do require regular assessment. Focal chest X-ray signs, deteriorating arterial blood gases or difficulty clearing secretions may indicate the need for treatment. Hypoxia will cause a rise in ICP. It is therefore important to pre-oxygenate, observe oxygen saturation throughout treatment, perform quick effective suction and to keep treatment sessions short. Bolus doses of sedating and or anaesthetic agents, e.g. thiopentone, may need to be given before treatment.

The head down position impairs venous return and raises ICP. It is therefore contraindicated except in very exceptional circumstances, i.e. lower lobe collapse leading to severe hypoxia. A 30 degree head up tilt, with the head midline, is recommended to aid cerebral drainage (Feldman et al., 1992). This is also the safest position for treatment. When the patient is stable, log-rolling may be allowed.

Slow percussion does not normally cause elevations in ICP and may actually lower it (Garradd & Bullock, 1986). Manual hyperinflation can be dangerous. Each inflation will cause a rise in the intrathoracic pressure. This in turn compromises cerebral venous return (increasing the ICP) and reduces systemic venous return (lowering cardiac output and hence blood pressure); these both decrease cerebral perfusion. However, it may be necessary when secretions are difficult to clear, to use manual hyperinflation to prevent hypoxia, or to keep treatment time to a minimum.

Non-accidental Injury

Occasionally, children are admitted to intensive care as a result of deliberate injury. Damage to the brain, often caused by being forcibly shaken, may be present along with other major injuries, fractures and bruises. Any health professional who deals with injured children must always be aware of the possibility of non-accidental injury and know what action to take if this is suspected. In some countries, including the UK, you will be under a legal obligation to comply with this. In many of these cases the shaking causes cerebral oedema, and physiotherapy treatment follows the guidelines given for a head injury.

Other Neurological Conditions

Children with a whole host of neurological conditions may require admission to intensive care for long- or short-term ventilation. This may be following spinal cord lesions, head injury, or Guillain–Barré syndrome, or for degenerative conditions such as spinal muscular atrophy and muscular dystrophy. These patients need regular assessment, and require close liaison with family and community staff. Chest physiotherapy should be given as necessary and stretches, either passive or active assisted, performed regularly.

OTHER CONDITIONS

Ingestion of Toxic Substances

A few children who accidentally ingest substances such as solvents can suffer such severe airway oedema that they require intubation. Often the child will vomit and aspirate the gastric contents, together with the toxic substance, into the lungs. Chest physiotherapy is useful if there are focal signs of collapse on chest X-ray. BAL may be helpful if there is difficulty clearing the lungs. Post-extubation, physiotherapy should not be needed.

Meningococcal Septicaemia

Meningococcal meningitis is a very severe disease. Many children develop septicaemia and multisystem failure as a result and are admitted to PICU in a very poor state. They may be suffering from circulatory and respiratory failure, renal failure, pulmonary haemorrhage, pulmonary oedema and ARDS, and develop areas of ischaemia on their skin. They often have raised ICP resulting in poor cerebral perfusion, and this may result in long-term brain damage. Chest physiotherapy is often inappropriate in the acute stages but may be necessary once the child's condition stabilises. Severe chest infections may develop, complicated by lung pathology as mentioned above. If raised ICP is an issue then treatment may need to be modified (as for a

head-injured patient). If areas of skin ischaemia are present, then positioning, gentle passive stretching and possibly splinting may be necessary following discussion with the plastic surgeon. As the child recovers, a programme of intense neuro-rehabilitation may be necessary with long-term follow-up in the community often required.

Post-operative

Following major operative procedures, children may be admitted to intensive care routinely or as a result of complications. This can take place following spinal, neuro-, cardiac, thoracic or abdominal surgery. The effects of anaesthetic gases, high levels of inspired oxygen, prolonged immobility, and splinting due to pain will affect adult and paediatric patients undergoing major surgery.

The patient undergoing elective surgery, and the family, will have been prepared for admission to the PICU, but in the event of emergency surgery this will not have been possible. Time needs to be taken to explain the procedures to gain the patient's and the family's confidence during this very stressful period.

Treatment will be based on the assessment findings. The techniques used may have to be modified in the event of an unstable haemodynamic status. Careful attention to pain management is required to gain the confidence of the patient.

CONCLUSION

This chapter illustrates the unique features of the PICU, and outlines the clinical setting familiar to professionals working within this stressful environment. An attempt has been made to review the clinical problems often encountered in the PICU, with an overview of the strategies used in the monitoring and support of critically ill children. The increased use of non-invasive monitoring where possible requires an understanding of the techniques employed, together with their limitations. Some insight is provided into the problems that may be encountered when interpreting monitored data.

In the final analysis, the most important information usually comes from attending to the child. Good clinical and communication skills are the essential toolkit for anyone working in the PICU.

Respiratory physiotherapy for infants and children on intensive care is always given in response to an assessed need, and is never routine. The acutely ill child can deteriorate very quickly and the physiotherapist must respond appropriately. Close co-operation between the multidisciplinary team can reduce the amount of potentially detrimental handling an acutely ill infant experiences. It is always neccesary to remember that a conscious child is likely to be very frightened in the enviroment of the PICU. Full explanations should be given to the child and the parents; perhaps the aid of a favourite toy or game can also help to win the child's co-operation.

REFERENCES

American College of Surgeons. *Advanced trauma life support provider manual*. 1993:275-276.

Arnold JH, Hanson JH, Toro-Figuero LO, Gutierrez J, Berens RJ, Anglin DL. Prospective randomized comparison of high frequency oscillatory ventilation and conventional mechanical ventilation in paediatric respiratory failure. *Crit Care Med* 1994, **22:**1530-1539.

Bhuyan U, Peters AM, Gordan I, Davies H, Helms P. Effects of posture on the distribution of pulmonary ventilation and perfusion in children and adults. *Thorax* 1989, **44:**480-484.

Ciesla N. Chest physiotherapy for special patients. In: Mackenzie CF, Imle CP, Ciesla N, eds. *Chest physiotherapy in the intensive care unit*, 2nd ed. Baltimore: Williams and Wilkins; 1989:254.

Davies H, Kitchman R, Gordan I, Helms P. Regional ventilation in infancy-reversal of adult pattern. *New Engl J Med* 1985, **313(26):**1626-1628.

Dreyfuss D, Soler P, Basset G, Saumon G. High inflation pressure pulmonary oedema. Respective effects of high airway pressure, high tidal volume and positive end-expiratory pressure. *Am Rev Respir Dis* 1988, **137:**1159-1164.

Feldman F, Kanter MJ, Robertson CS, *et al*. The effect of head elevation on intracranial pressure and cerebral blood flow in head injured patients. *J Neurosurg* 1992, **76:**207-211.

Garradd J, Bullock M. The effect of respiratory therapy on intracranial pressure in ventilated neurosurgical patients. *Aust J Physiother* 1986, **32(2):**107-111.

Hicking KG, Walsh J, Henderson S, Jackson R. Low mortality rate in ARDS using low-volume pressure-limited ventilation with permissive hypercapnia: a prospective study. *Crit Care Med* 1994, **22:**1568-1578.

Kerem E, Yatsiv I, Goitein J. Effect of endotracheal suctioning on arterial blood gases in children. *Intensive Care Med* 1990, **16:**95-99.

Keszler M, Donn SM, Bucciarelli RL, *et al*. Multicentre controlled trial comparing high frequency jet ventilation and conventional mechanical ventilation in newborn infants with pulmonary interstitial emphysema. *J Pediatr* 1991, **119:**85-93.

Merritt TA, Liyamasawad S, Boettrich C, Brooks JG. Skin surface CO_2 measurements in sick preterm and term infants *J Pediatr* 1981, **99:**782-786.

Muscedere JG, Mullen JBM, Gan K, Slutsky AS. Tidal ventilation at low airway pressures can augment lung injury. *Am J Respir Crit Care Med* 1994, **149:**1327-1334.

Placzek M, Silverman M. Selective placement of bronchial suction catheters in intubated neonates. *Arch Dis Child* 1983, **58(10):**829-831.

Poets CF, Martin RJ. Noninvasive determination of blood gases. In: Tocks J, Sly PD, Tepper RS, Morgan WJ, eds. *Infant respiratory function testing*, Chapter 16. New York: Wiley-Liss; 1996:411-443.

Poets CF, Samuels MP, Noyes JP, Jones KA, Southall DP. Home monitoring of transcutaneous oxygen tension in the early detection of hypoxaemia in infants and young children. *Arch Dis Child* 1991, **66:**676-682.

Prasad SA, Hussey J. Chest physiotherapy techniques and adjuncts to chest physiotherapy. In: *Paediatric respiratory care—a guide for physiotherapists and health professionals*. London: Chapman &Hall; 1995: 88-89.

Shann F. *Which way forward for the care of critically ill children?* CRD Report 1. The University of York NHS centre for reviews and dissemination, 1995.

Tasker RC, Prasad SA. Neurological intensive care. In: *Paediatric respiratory care—a guide for physiotherapists and health professionals*. London: Chapman &Hall; 1995:143.

Young CS. A review of the adverse effects of airway suction. *Physiotherapy* 1984a, **70(3):**104-106.

Young CS. Recommended guide lines for suction. *Physiotherapy* 1984b, **70(3):**106-108.

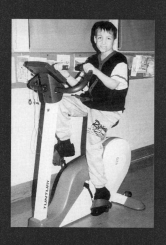

19 E Main

PAEDIATRIC CARDIOTHORACIC SURGERY

CHAPTER OUTLINE

INTRODUCTION

This chapter will cover the most significant congenital surgical conditions encountered by the paediatric physiotherapist. Only conditions that relate to chest and heart will be discussed. These are broadly: congenital lobar emphysema, diaphragmatic hernia, oesophageal atresia and tracheo-oesophageal fistula, exomphalos (gastroschisis and omphalocele), and congenital cardiac anomalies.

The physiotherapy treatment of the conditions described is never routine and will be dictated by the findings on assessment. There is generally little to offer pre-operatively, unless there is a specific problem which will be noted at the end of the relevant subsection. Post-operative care will be dictated by assessment indicating the presence of pulmonary secretions, loss of volume or increased work of breathing; again, particular points of note will be included. The differences in paediatric respiratory systems (See Chapter 15) should be noted as critical to the safe and effective treatment of paediatric patients.

CONGENITAL THORACIC DEFECTS

CONGENITAL LOBAR EMPHYSEMA

An abnormality of a lobar bronchus creates a one-way valve effect causing air trapping and overinflation of the affected lobe, most commonly the left and right upper and right middle lobes. The gross overinflation irreversibly damages the affected lobe, and normal surrounding lung is compressed with mediastinal shift to the contralateral side.

Surgical excision of the affected lobe is indicated if the infant is in respiratory distress. If this is found in the older child, conservative management may be more appropriate.

DIAPHRAGMATIC HERNIA

Diaphragmatic herniation refers to the abnormal fetal development of diaphragm resulting in abdominal contents being displaced into the thoracic cavity. Significant diaphragmatic hernias cause neonatal respiratory distress. They are often associated with other congenital abnormalities, such as persistent fetal circulation and abnormalities of the pulmonary vasculature. Hernias are usually large, on the left side and situated posteriorly. The abdominal contents may be seen in the thorax on chest X-ray. Ventilation techniques should avoid distending the gut with air as this would compromise respiratory effort even further. Sometimes these patients are managed with extracorporeal membrane oxygenation (ECMO) to stabilise them before surgery.

Treatment usually involves surgical closure of the diaphragm and restoration of the bowel into the abdomen, but this procedure is often associated with initial further deterioration in lung function. One or both lungs may be hypoplastic, which will severely reduce chances of survival since normal lung growth will not follow surgical replacement of bowel contents into the abdomen. Of those that present acutely in the neonatal period, only about half will survive, and those that do will generally have persisting problems with lung function and ventilation–perfusion abnormalities.

Physiotherapy
Physiotherapy has little to offer these often critically unstable babies pre-operatively. After surgery, head down postural drainage should be avoided.

OESOPHAGEAL ASTRESIA AND TRACHEO-OESOPHAGEAL FISTULA
Oesophageal atresia occurs in about 1 in 3000 births; 10% of affected infants have oesophageal atresia with a tracheal fistula and 80% a blind proximal oesophageal pouch and fistula between the trachea and distal oesophagus. The infant presents post-natally with dribbling from the mouth, episodes of choking, cyanosis and cough due to overflow of secretions into the larynx or trachea. It may be difficult to pass a nasogastric tube.

The treatment consists of surgical division of the fistula, and anastomosis of the ends of the oesophagus.

Physiotherapy
In the presence of recurrent or continuous aspiration before corrective surgery, physiotherapy treatment may be essential in clearing excessive secretions from the lungs and preventing pulmonary morbidity. Post-operatively, treatment will be dictated by the findings on assessment, but head down postural drainage should be avoided. Nasopharyngeal suction should never, in general, exceed the external distance between the nasal cavity and the ear. This catheter length is effective in producing cough, and the risk of traumatising the surgical repair is avoided.

GASTROSCHISIS AND OMPHALOCELE
These are relatively rare anterior abdominal wall defects so should not strictly be included in this chapter, but they have significant respiratory consequences so a brief word will be said about them.

Gastroschisis refers to the abdominal wall defect through which the midgut has prolapsed. The omphalocele usually contains liver as well as bowel, and affected infants frequently have other major anomalies.

In most cases, primary repair is preferred, with reduction of the bowel into the abdominal cavity. The increased abdominal pressure following surgery can lead to respiratory compromise in the infant in the immediate post-operative period. Some infants have impaired antenatal lung growth, and a proportion continue to have abnormal lung function during infancy.

Physiotherapy
Physiotherapy management pre-operatively will aim at reducing the risk of pulmonary complications, as these infants are nursed supine with very limited positional change due to the suspension of abdominal contents above the abdomen. Surgical reduction of bowel into the abdominal cavity will compromise lung function, but not in a fashion that will respond to physiotherapy treatment. Nursing in a slightly head up position may relieve the thorax of some of the weight of the abdominal contents, and reduce the work of breathing.

CONGENITAL CARDIAC DEFECTS

The physiotherapist working in a paediatric cardiac Intensive Care Unit (ICU) should have an excellent understanding of the nature of the cardiac defect and the type of repair that the child has had. This is essential in alerting the therapist to specific complications that may arise as a result of treatment, e.g. pulmonary hypertensive crisis, or facilitating decisions about whether a low oxygen saturation is as a result of blood shunting between the systemic and pulmonary circulations or whether it is due to a respiratory complication that will respond to physiotherapy treatment.

Cardiac defects are found in approximately 8 in 1000 live births, although only a third of these will require surgical intervention, the rest either resolving spontaneously or being not significant enough to require surgery. Operations are usually termed corrective or palliative depending on whether the surgery will offer a definitive treatment or simply temporary or extended relief of symptoms. The majority of operations are performed in the first year of life, with the result that the therapist most frequently encounters very small infants in the ICU; he or she should be confident and experienced in their management.

ACYANOTIC HEART DEFECTS ('PINK BABIES')

Defects in which left-to-right shunting is continuous or predominant will produce high pulmonary blood flow, and affected patients will eventually develop pulmonary vascular obstructive disease and pulmonary hypertension. Respiratory tract infections are common and respiratory failure may result from poor pulmonary compliance. With the exception of patent ductus arteriosus and simple atrial septal defects, the post-operative course of these patients may be prolonged, and pulmonary hypertensive events may complicate recovery (see page 298).

PATENT DUCTUS ARTERIOSUS

The ductus arteriosus is the fetal vascular connection between the main pulmonary trunk and the aorta, which should close shortly after birth. If it remains open, excessive blood shunts from the aorta to the lungs causing pulmonary oedema and, in the long term, pulmonary vascular disease. Symptoms may be mild or severe depending on the magnitude of the left-to-right shunt. Patent ductus arteriosus (PDA) occurs frequently in the premature infant and can be associated with difficulty weaning from ventilation and with congestive cardiac failure (see Chapter 20 for principles of neonatal care). Conservative treatment includes fluid restrictions or the use of indomethacin to promote duct closure. Surgical treatment involves ligation of the ductus arteriosus. If the child is not symptomatic, surgery can be delayed until the age of 4–5 years.

ATRIAL SEPTAL DEFECT

Atrial septal defect (ASD) is characterised by a hole in the septum that separates the left and right atria. It is one of the most common congenital cardiac defects. Types of ASD include:

- 'Ostium primum', now known as partial atrio-ventricular septal defect (AVSD; see below).
- 'Ostium secundum' of the foramen ovale, and commonly a superior vena caval defect, where one or more of the superior pulmonary veins drains into the superior vena cava.

Children with ASD are generally asymptomatic and diagnosis is usually made after murmur is discovered on routine examination. If left undiscovered, slow development of symptoms may occur with rising pulmonary artery pressure (PAP) and pulmonary vascular disease. Severe irreversible pulmonary hypertension is associated with clinical deterioration which cannot be relieved by corrective surgery. Heart–lung transplantation is then the only palliative option. Because of the severe late consequences of pulmonary hypertension, children usually have ASD repair before the age of 5 years via a midline sternotomy or right anterior thoracotomy. The defect is repaired on cardiopulmonary bypass with a pericardial or Gore-Tex patch or stitch, but umbrella or balloon devices may be used to close small round defects.

VENTRICULAR SEPTAL DEFECTS

Ventricular septal defects (VSDs) are the most common congenital cardiac lesion, defined by a hole in the septum that separates the left and right ventricles. VSDs can be found in conjunction with other cardiac defects, and the clinical presentation will depend on the size of the defect and on the presence or absence of other cardiac anomalies. More than half of all ventricular septal defects close spontaneously and do not require surgery. Undiagnosed VSDs will ultimately result in the development of severe pulmonary vascular disease whereafter corrective surgery will offer no relief. Infants may present with congestive cardiac failure, a history of repeated chest infections and failure to thrive. The older the child at presentation, the

more likely it is that pulmonary hypertension will have developed.

Surgical repair of VSDs is done through a midline sternotomy on cardiopulmonary bypass, and the hole may be closed through the right atrium (most commonly) or right ventricle, left ventricle or one of the great arteries. Although operative mortality approaches zero in most centres, multiple VSDs carry a higher risk, and conduction disturbances are common following repair.

ATRIO-VENTRICULAR SEPTAL DEFECT

This defect involves incomplete development of the inferior atrial septum, the superior ventricular septum and the atrio-ventricular valves. Symptoms vary in severity according to the magnitude and direction of the shunt and the extent of the ASD, VSD, valve incompetence or a combination of these. AVSDs may co-exist with other defects, major cardiac defects and Down syndrome.

Some patients may be asymptomatic despite high pulmonary vascular resistance (PVR) but a high left-to-right shunt will cause symptoms such as dyspnoea, recurrent chest infections and congestive heart failure.

Partial AVSD

Partial AVSD refers to an 'ostium primum' type of atrial septal defect above the mitral and tricuspid valves, which are displaced into the ventricles and may be incompetent. The development of pulmonary vascular disease is uncommon.

Complete AVSD

In the complete form of the defect there is one common atrio-ventricular valve between the right and left atrio-ventricular chambers. This valve has six leaflets and is continuous with the ASD above and VSD below. More than half the children with this defect will die within the first year of life because of pulmonary vascular disease if left untreated and almost all will have succumbed within 5 years.

Surgical repair on cardiopulmonary bypass is done through a median sternotomy. If pulmonary vascular disease is well established the defect is considered inoperable, and heart–lung transplantation may be offered.

Hospital mortality is 5%–6% in patients with straightforward AVSD but more than 10% in patients with major associated anomalies.

Conduction problems and valve incompetence may occur post-operatively.

TRUNCUS ARTERIOSUS

Truncus arteriosus is a defect characterised by a single arterial trunk arising from both ventricles from which the aorta and pulmonary arteries originate via a single semi-lunar valve. A VSD permits flow of mixed blood from both ventricles up the common trunk. Congestive cardiac failure and irreversible pulmonary vascular disease secondary to excessive pulmonary blood flow usually develops in early infancy. Untreated infants rarely survive beyond 1 year. Operative mortality is generally more than 10% at most centres. Surgery involves separation of the pulmonary arteries from the truncal artery and connection via a conduit to the right atrium, and the VSD is closed to divert the left ventricular flow up the aorta.

TOTAL OR PARTIAL ANOMALOUS PULMONARY VENOUS CONNECTION

This is a rare cardiac anomaly involving two or more pulmonary veins connecting anomalously to either the vena cava or the right atrium. The reduced left atrial pressure results in the foramen ovale remaining open post-natally, therefore mixed arterial and venous blood being transported systemically.

Most patients present in the first days of life with congestive cardiac failure and cyanosis. This defect is often accompanied by other congenital heart defects.

Early primary repair via median sternotomy on cardiopulmonary bypass is the treatment of choice. The operative mortality is over 10%, mostly because of pulmonary hypertensive events.

Many children go to theatre with pulmonary oedema and thus return with pulmonary oedema. Sternal closure may be delayed by the surgeon post-operatively.

PHYSIOTHERAPY

Physiotherapy treatment will depend on the findings at assessment. If the patient is a premature baby the principles of neonatal management, i.e. minimal handling and cautious treatment, are appropriate (see Chapter 20). Physiotherapy is rarely indicated following ASD repair or for older children having PDA ligation, as they are often mobile the following day.

The post-operative recovery after VSD, AVSD, truncus arteriosus and anomalous pulmonary venous connections operations may be prolonged and complicated by pulmonary hypertensive crises. Details of its management can be found on page 298. The introduction of nitric oxide therapy may help improve the outcome for these patients. High inspired-oxygen levels and heavy sedation initially are also helpful.

CYANOTIC HEART DEFECTS ('BLUE BABIES')

Right ventricular outflow tract obstruction with right-to-left shunting will produce low pulmonary blood flow. Cyanosis is always present and polycythaemia may be severe.

TETRALOGY OF FALLOT

The four components of Fallot's tetralogy (Figure 19.1) were classically described as:

- A large VSD.
- Right ventricular outflow (infundibular) obstruction.
- Right ventricular hypertrophy.
- Over-riding aorta.

Blood flow to the lungs is reduced and the child may present with cyanosis. Severity of symptoms will depend on the degree of obstructed pulmonary blood flow. The majority of infants are pink at birth and gradually become cyanosed as they grow. 'Spelling' episodes refer to the symptoms produced by periodic spasm of the infundibulum preventing any blood flow to the lungs. Infants become irritable and cry with increasing cyanosis and eventual breathlessness and loss of consciouness. At this point the spasm relaxes and the child gradually recovers. These may be dangerous events and the child may die during an episode, or suffer cerebral anoxia.

Older undiagnosed children may squat after periods of exercise; this appears to be an automatic physiological response in older children to reduce their oxygen debt, and, in the presence of cyanosis, it should alert the clinician to the possible diagnosis.

Some controversy exists about whether it is better to effect a primary repair or provide palliation in the form of a modified Blalock–Taussig (see below) shunt until the child is older. Corrective surgery requires closure of the VSD, resection of the hypertrophied infundibulum and reconstruction of the pulmonary arteries.

PULMONARY ATRESIA OR STENOSIS AND MAJOR AORTOPULMONARY COLLATERAL ARTERIES

The infant with pulmonary atresia may be cyanosed at birth and this may become rapidly worse as the ductus arteriosus closes. Palliation in the form of modified Blalock–Taussig shunt is the immediate treatment of choice with the primary goal of ensuring adequate blood flow to the lungs. Prostaglandins are used to keep the ductus arteriosus open until surgery. This condition may be accompanied by a hypoplastic or a hypertrophied right ventricle, or desaturated blood being supplied to the coronary arteries from the right ventricle.

Connections develop between the aorta and the pulmonary vessels, known as major aortopulmonary collateral arteries (MAPCAs), usually arising from the anterior surface of the aorta but occasionally originating from the carotids. They are high flow, high pressure vessels in which pulmonary vascular obstructive disease can develop.

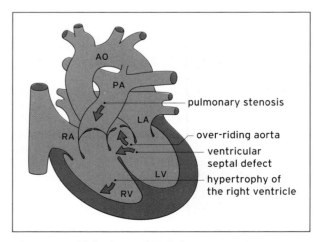

Figure 19.1 Tetralogy of Fallot.

Corrective surgery depends on the size of the right ventricle. A reasonable size can indicate removal of the obstruction and linkage of the right ventricle to the pulmonary arteries with ligation of the MAPCAs. A poorly developed right ventricle requires a bidirectional Glenn shunt or total cavopulmonary connection to relieve the left ventricle of having to cope with both systemic and pulmonary circulations.

In the absence of right ventricular hypoplasia and coronary anomalies, the mortality is very low.

TRANSPOSITION OF THE GREAT ARTERIES

Transposition of the great arteries is characterised by the aorta originating from the right ventricle, and the pulmonary artery from the left ventricle. Oxygenated pulmonary blood recirculates through the lungs without reaching the body and deoxygenated blood recirculates through the body without reaching the lungs. The two closed circulations would quickly lead to death, but there is usually a degree of mixing through the PDA and the sometimes associated anomalies, i.e. VSD and ASD. The infant usually becomes progressively cyanosed within the first day of life, and after diagnosis the ductus arteriosus is kept patent using prostaglandin E until surgery. If this does not provide adequate mixing of venous and arterial blood, an ASD is created during cardiac catheterisation.

The arterial switch operation has been performed with good results since 1985. It is usually undertaken in the first 2–3 weeks of life, and involves the repair of the great arteries by switching them back to their correct anatomical positions.

LEFT VENTRICULAR OUTFLOW TRACT OBSTRUCTIONS

COARCTATION OF THE AORTA

This defect is a narrowing of the aorta most commonly distal to the left subclavian artery and proximal to the junction of the ductus arteriosus (Figure 19.2). In a severe case, the infant will present in critical condition with congestive heart failure. Classically, prominent pulses are felt in the neck and upper limbs and the femoral pulses are weak, since they are supplied by the pulmonary flow from the ductus arteriosus and the small flow which passes through the coarctation. The use of prostaglandins may result in re-opening of the ductus and improved femoral pulses. Seventy five per cent of patients have associated anomalies such as bicuspid aortic valve, VSD and mitral valve anomalies, and these will make the corrective surgery more complicated.

In the critically ill neonate, the surgical correction will usually be performed as an emergency procedure. The surgery is done through a left thoracotomy at the 4th intercostal space without the use of cardiopulmonary bypass. The narrow portion of the aorta is removed and the ends are joined obliquely to reduce the risk of re-coarctation. In the presence of a significant VSD, pulmonary artery banding may be performed at the same time. The main complication of coarctation repair in infants is re-coarctation but, very rarely, paraplegia has been reported.

The older child with coarctation of the aorta may be asymptomatic but persistent cardiomegaly and hypertension will be indications for surgery.

AORTIC STENOSIS

Obstruction to left ventricular outflow may be found at valvular, subvalvular, supravalvular or combined levels. It can also be combined with other defects. Neonates and infants with critical aortic stenosis present with severe congestive cardiac failure, and reduced peripheral pulses, and therefore the need for urgent treatment.

Relief of aortic stenosis may be obtained with aortic valvotomy, aortic valve replacement in the older child, or aortic valve homograft insertion. The balloon dilation technique is growing in popularity.

INTERRUPTED AORTIC ARCH

This is a rare condition in which the aortic arch is not continuous and which will result in death within the first month if untreated. There are three types of interrupted aortic arch. These are:

- Type A, i.e. distal to the left subclavian artery.
- Type B, i.e. distal to the left carotid artery.
- Type C, i.e. distal to the right innominate artery.

Type B is the commonest while type C is very rare. A VSD is virtually always present, as is a PDA through which blood flows to the descending aorta. Truncus arteriosus and aorto-pulmonary windows are associated with this. Soon after birth, as the ductus arteriosus begins to close and the PVR decreases, excess blood flow to the lungs results in severe congestive heart failure. Primary surgical repair is the treatment of choice, but the operation is technically difficult and the post-operative course may be prolonged.

Long-term survival depends on early successful repair and adequate management of subsequent complications.

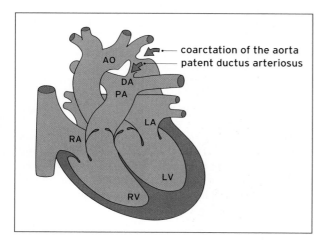

Figure 19.2 Coarctation of the aorta.

HYPOPLASTIC LEFT HEART SYNDROME

This defect is defined by aortic valve atresia or stenosis with associated hypoplasia of the left ventricle. The systemic blood flow derives almost entirely from the right ventricle through the ductus arteriosus. Depending on the degree of patency of the ductus arteriosus, the peripheral pulses may be normal, reduced or absent. Immediate management involves keeping the ductus patent with prostaglandins and avoiding large differences between systemic resistance and PVR. Sometimes, addition of carbon dioxide to the inspired gas mixture will assist by increasing PVR and improving systemic flow.

The surgical goal is to turn the single ventricle into the systemic circulation pump and allow the venous return from the body passively to enter the pulmonary circulation. Examples of this type of surgery are Fontan, total cavopulmonary connection and bidirectional Glenn shunt. Sometimes staged procedures are recommended to protect the lungs from developing pulmonary vascular disease.

Physiotherapy

It should be noted that different partial pressures of oxygen and carbon dioxide relative to each other in the blood will have a direct effect on how much blood flows to the lungs, such that:

- High carbon dioxide and low oxygen leads to an increased PVR and decreased pulmonary blood flow.
- High oxygen and low carbon dioxide leads to a decreased PVR and increased pulmonary blood flow.

Physiotherapy treatment. e.g. due to secretion retention, therefore may both create a detrimental imbalance in the flow ratio as well as correct an imbalance! Careful assessment of need for treatment is essential.

VASCULAR RINGS

A malformation of the aorta or pulmonary artery in which the trachea, the oesophagus or both are compressed is called a vascular ring. It may be asymptomatic and discovered incidentally at chest X-ray but when symptoms are present they usually occur early in infancy and are caused by compression of the trachea or oesophagus or both. Stridor, respiratory difficulties, repeated chest infections and feeding difficulties are commonly encountered. Head flexion may make the respiratory symptoms worse, and eating solids may also be difficult.

Diagnosis of tracheal stenosis may be made clinically, on chest X-ray and by rigid bronchoscopy.

Surgical repair involves relieving the vascular compression. Tracheal stenosis or tracheal malacia are frequently associated with vascular rings but many patients improve following surgical decompression.

Tracheal stenosis caused by complete tracheal rings ('stove-pipe trachea') complicates about 50% of the cases, and if respiratory symptoms persist then tracheal surgery may be indicated. Repair of tracheal stenosis is usually done on cardiopulmonary bypass. Tracheal resection and re-anastomosis is successful if the stenotic segment is short. In more complicated cases, tracheoplasty, or a more recent procedure, tracheal transplant, may be attempted.

Physiotherapy

The post-operative management of patients who have had tracheal surgery may involve long periods of ventilation, with or without tracheostomy. In the acute post-operative period, care should be taken with bagging as the tracheal anastomosis is not airtight and there is a risk of pneumothorax. In addition, the tracheal anastomosis will usually be distal to the end of the endotracheal tube, so care should be taken when suctioning, not to traumatise the site.

PALLIATIVE OPERATIONS

PULMONARY ARTERY BAND

The Pulmonary artery band (PAB) is designed to restrict excessive blood flow to the lungs by reducing the diameter of the pulmonary artery with a constricting tape. Infants that might benefit from this procedure are those with VSD, AVSD and truncus arteriosus. Excessive pulmonary blood flow is associated with heart failure, tachypnoea and, in the long term, development of pulmonary vascular disease and pulmonary hypertension. It is used when primary repair of the defect is not possible, to protect the lungs from the progression of pulmonary vascular disease.

MODIFIED BLALOCK-TAUSSIG SHUNT

Modified Blalock–Taussig shunt (MBTS) is the most commonly encountered palliative shunt procedure at present. The operation improves pulmonary blood flow by connecting the subclavian artery and the pulmonary artery. Used for cyanosed patients with poor blood flow to the lungs, e.g. caused by pulmonary and tricuspid atresia or tetralogy of Fallot, MBTS gives temporary improvement in lung perfusion. Phrenic nerve damage has been described following MBTS.

PHYSIOTHERAPY MANAGEMENT FOR CONGENITAL SURGICAL CONDITIONS

The general principles of physiotherapy assessment and treatment techniques are covered in previous chapters (see Chapters 16 and 18). Aspects specific to managing paediatric surgical patients will be discussed below.

After surgery, paediatric patients are at risk of respiratory morbidity from:

- Anaesthesia: this produces respiratory insufficiency which is characterised by reduced lung volumes and reduced lung and chest wall compliance. In addition, anaesthesia interferes with mucociliary clearance and phagocytosis and may impair the mechanism of hypoxic pulmonary vasoconstriction (HPV), which refers to the physiological event in which the lungs can selectively shut down perfusion to areas which are not being ventilated, thus improving the ventilation/perfusion match and maintaining good arterial oxygen tensions.

- Inspired oxygen: above 40% concentration, inspired oxygen is associated with a decreased rate of mucociliary clearance, diminished alveolar macrophage function and parenchymal damage.
- Mechanical compression of lung tissue: this takes place during surgery to optimise visualisation of the heart, and partial deflation of lungs on bypass means that considerable reversal of atelectasis is necessary post-operatively.
- Cessation of surfactant production: during cardiopulmonary bypass, the lungs are not perfused and surfactant production ceases, creating poor lung compliance post-operatively.
- Incision and chest drains: pain and guarded respiratory excursion may be caused by incision and chest drains.
- Paralysis during delayed sternal closure: this terminates normal lung clearance and prevents sighs, which will lead to atelectasis and reduced lung volumes.

PRE-OPERATIVE ASSESSMENT

There are several advantages to seeing children and their families before theatre.

A quick assessment of developmental milestones and quality of motor function will indicate any pre-operative neurological problems, which should be documented and managed post-operatively. Congenital defects may form part of a global mal-development that will have broader consequences.

Assessment of respiratory status will reveal problems that may prolong the post-operative course. Sometimes pre-operative chest clearance is indicated.

Parents and children will tend to feel less anxious if they know what to expect post-operatively, so a careful explanation of procedures and treatments will go a long way towards relieving fear of the unknown.

POST-OPERATIVE TREATMENT

Assessment

History

The age at which the defect was diagnosed, its type and the nature and severity of the symptoms will usually indicate how the child will progress post-operatively. Additional details such as lung dysfunction following prematurity or previous phrenic nerve injury may herald a problematic post-operative course.

Physical examination

Most children will return from theatre intubated and ventilated, with peripheral arterial and venous lines, central venous lines for drug delivery and measurement of central venous pressures (CVP), chest drains, pacing wires, electrocardiogram (ECG) leads, core and peripheral temperature and saturation probes, and urinary catheter for careful regulation of urine output and fluid balance. Lines measuring PAPs are sometimes present. Left atrial pressures are sometimes monitored if specific cardiac lesions make it useful to know both right and left atrial pressures.

The post-operative chest X-ray should be checked for pulmonary pathology and position of tubes, lines and drains.

Treatment

The child should not, in general, be subjected to physiotherapy treatment in the first few hours following surgery, the early aims of management being to achieve haemodynamic stability. There will rarely be exceptions to the rule, but if the post-operative chest X-ray shows lobar or segmental collapse with a loss of lung volume, if auscultation suggests retention of secretions, or if the blood gases are poor and ventilatory requirements exceed expectations, then the physiotherapist will be justified in attempting treatment. This treatment should be undertaken with extreme caution and constant vigilance for any deleterious haemodynamic effects.

Children having undergone closed heart procedures, e.g. ASD repair and palliative surgery, are generally ambulant on the first post-operative day and do not require any physiotherapy intervention. If the procedure has been performed via a thoracotomy then posture and shoulder movements may need attention.

Physiotherapy treatment is indicated for the prevention or treatment of atelectasis, the removal of pulmonary secretions, and for re-inflation and oxygenation of collapsed areas of lung, and to reduce the work of breathing.

Vibrations are usually well tolerated by intubated babies and children following cardiac surgery, but not by premature neonates. Vibrations performed intermittently with manual hyperinflations are very effective in moving secretions to the upper airways where they can be suctioned. Chest percussion should not cause pain, and therefore must not be performed over broken ribs, wound sites, chest drains or when there is active pulmonary haemorrhage. Percussion can be effective and comfortable to small babies by using a paediatric facemask.

After cardiac surgery, strict fluid restrictions can contribute to thick and tenacious secretions so saline instillation or mini-bronchoalveolar lavage (BAL) may be required to facilitate the removal of mucous plugs.

Postural drainage positions require to be modified in the paediatric cardiac unit because cardiac output and diaphragmatic function may be compromised in the head down position.

Prone positioning is an unsuitable position in the presence of abdominal distension, open sternum or anteriorly positioned chest drains.

Rehabilitation

Rehabilitation in terms of formal cardiovascular fitness programmes is usually not appropriate or necessary. Post-operative mobilisation will begin as soon as patients are free of inotropic support and most lines and drains have been removed. It is important to assess closely the neurodevelopmental needs of the child. If a pre-operative problem has been picked up this will need follow-up and if some new problem has developed as a complication of surgery or a long intensive care stay, advice and appropriate treatment should be implemented.

When Not To Treat

Confidence and accuracy in deciding when treatment is inappropriate or unnecessary is a difficult skill to acquire. Experience cannot be taught, but careful assessment will reveal the needs of the child in the ICU. In general, treatment should be avoided if the child is haemodynamically unstable, is very tachy- or bradycardic, or very hyper- or hypotensive. A child at risk of pulmonary hypertensive crisis and free of secretions should be left alone, and copious drainage of fresh blood from chest drains or endotracheal tubing may suggest an active bleeding point or deranged clotting. Physiotherapy should be postponed until these problems have resolved.

SPECIAL POST-OPERATIVE CONSIDERATIONS FOR PHYSIOTHERAPISTS

HIGH FREQUENCY VENILATION

High frequency ventilation (HFV) is rarely used after cardiac surgery but may be indicated to stabilise patients with intractable hypoxaemia, such as those with diaphragmatic hernias. The principle of HFV is to achieve ventilation by employing high respiratory rates (60–3000 cycles) and very small tidal volumes at moderate airway pressures. Increased gas mixing is facilitated by Brownian motion, which enhances gas exchange. The principal effect with this form of therapy is to decrease the movement of large volumes of gas through the chest and reduce barotrauma. Early thinking that chest physiotherapy is detrimental to these patients (because of the exchange of large volumes of gas during treatment) has begun to change and it appears that intermittent treatment (interrupting HFV) may be extremely beneficial in the presence of retained secretions.

EXTRACORPOREAL MEMBRANE OXYGENATION (ECMO)

ECMO is described in Chapter 20. If after technically successful corrective cardiac surgery a child is unable to come off bypass, then ECMO may be indicated to support the infant until the reversible cardiac dysfunction recovers.

PULMONARY HYPERTENSIVE CRISIS

Pulmonary hypertensive crisis can be a severe complication in paediatric cardiac patients post-operatively.

Children at risk of pulmonary hypertension are those who have had excessive shunting of blood flow from the left side of the heart to the pulmonary circulation on the right, e.g. VSD, AVSD and truncus arteriosus. Excessive blood flow to the lungs causes distension and damage to the pulmonary arteriolar walls, which become muscularised, unable to dilate normally and vulnerable to reactive vasoconstriction. Hypoxaemia, hypercapnia, metabolic acidosis, restlessness, handling (including physiotherapy)

and tracheal suctioning are all factors which may precipitate a pulmonary hypertensive crisis. During a major event, pulmonary vasoconstriction causes the PAP to rise above the systemic pressure with an increase in CVP. The systemic pressure may drop suddenly leading to cardiac arrest. This event will cause further hypoxaemia, acidosis and hypercapnia, which will worsen the pulmonary vasoconstriction, and the cycle may be very difficult to break. Manual ventilation with 100% oxygen, heavy sedation or paralysis, and nitric oxide or other pulmonary vasodilators, may help. Right ventricular damage may occur and the child may die during a crisis.

Appropriate treatment in certain infants can present a pulmonary hypertensive crisis; inattentive physiotherapy treatment, on the other hand, can precipitate this event. Pulmonary pathology related to secretion retention or lobar or segmental collapse following cardiac surgery will cause ventilation/perfusion mismatch, deterioration of blood gases and potential worsening of pulmonary hypertension. Treatment in a critically unstable patient should always be done *in situ*, and be short and effective under the protection of good sedation or paralysis with additional oxygen before, during and after treatment. Continual monitoring of the blood pressure, PAP and oxygen saturations will give an indication as to how well the treatment is being tolerated. A child receiving nitric oxide through the ventilator circuit, is often extremely dependent on the gas and it should be incorporated into the bagging circuit for physiotherapy treatment.

Nitric oxide is a therapeutic gas, delivered through the ventilator circuit, that acts as a potent pulmonary vasodilator. It is absorbed through the alveoli and terminal bronchiolar membranes, and has a local vasodilatory effect on the pulmonary vessels. It is, however, quite toxic except in extremely small doses (5–30 parts per million) and should be used with caution.

DELAYED STERNAL CLOSURE

Sternal closure following long and complicated cardiac surgery is sometimes not possible because of pulmonary, myocardial and chest wall oedema. Attempted chest closure may result in significant haemodynamic instability or respiratory compromise. Sternal closure may be delayed from 24 hours to 3 or more weeks, and during this time the patient is usually paralysed and sedated, and nursed in the supine or quarter turned position with a stent *in situ* to keep the edges of the sternum separate. Clearly, these patients are at enormous risk of pulmonary morbidity because of the prolonged anaesthesia, limited postural changes and their complete inability to maintain airway clearance. Competent physiotherapy is absolutely crucial in maintaining good pulmonary function, and although percussion is of little value, posterior and posterolateral vibrations (when the sternum is stented) and manual hyperinflations are usually well tolerated. The paralysed child will not cough and suction will retrieve only secretions at the end of the suction catheter. It may therefore be helpful to simulate cough by performing one or two vibrations during suction to optimise secretion yield per suction pass. This will reduce residual lung volumes, which will be poorly tolerated unless careful attention is given to pre-oxygenation and manual hyperinflation breaths after each suction. These breaths will help to recruit any lung areas that may have been compressed during the suction and vibration technique.

PHRENIC NERVE DAMAGE

Phrenic nerve damage during cardiothoracic surgery is well described and is the result of the close relation of the nerve to the mediastinal vessels and pericardium. Morbidity of this condition is worse in children under 2 years old, and may include inability to wean from ventilation and severe respiratory compromise. Paradoxical (upward) movement of a hemidiaphragm during inspiration may compress the ipsilateral lung and contribute towards mediastinal shift towards the contralateral side causing persistent loss of lung volume. Physiotherapy management will be indicated according to clinical symptoms, but head up positioning will relieve the thoracic cavity of the weight of the abdominal organs and reduce work of breathing. Surgical plication of the diaphragm will transform the flaccid paralysed hemidiaphragm into an immobile platform which will not move paradoxically.

CONCLUSION

Congenital conditions of the chest and heart are surgically managed in specialist paediatric units, but affected patients may be encountered in neonatal units or after surgery in district general hospitals, and are therefore included here. It has been possible only to provide a brief overview of the conditions, but further reading of relevant texts and articles will provide detailed understanding of any specific outstanding questions.

TRANSPLANTATION SURGERY IN CHILDREN

Adult cardiac and lung transplantation is discussed in Chapter 11, and although some principles of management in paediatric care may overlap, the paediatric population presents different challenges to the physiotherapist.

Transplantation may be offered to any patient with end stage cardiac or pulmonary disease that cannot be managed by further surgery or medical treatment. Paediatric patients waiting for transplantation encompass the entire age range from the neonate, e.g. with a hypoplastic left heart, to the young adult, perhaps awaiting heart–lung transplantation for cystic fibrosis (CF). The first neonatal heart transplant was performed in 1968, but before the introduction of effective immunosuppression (by cyclosporin) in 1980, most paediatric transplants were unsuccessful.

In the mid-1980s, heart–lung transplantation was introduced as an option for managing end stage disease in patients with CF.

ASSESSMENT FOR TRANSPLANTATION

The transplant assessment involves the evaluation of alternative forms of treatment, and suitability for transplantation, and the measurement of physical and physiological parameters. It is also a forum for providing parents and children with information. Unrealistic expectations are dispelled and the painful realities of transplantation are clarified (the long waiting list, infection and rejection, side effects of drugs, operative and late mortality). Many will have higher expectations of transplantation than are reasonable. Transplantation is not a cure; it is a hope for a better quality of life for a longer period of time than would have been possible with diseased organs. The children and their families are given time to weigh up the negative consequences of transplantation against the hope for a better quality of life.

Immunological evaluation for donor–recipient match includes blood type and cross-match, organ size and cytomegaloviral status. The physical assessment includes chest X-ray, lung function and thoracic volumes, a basic exercise test to assess distance covered in a set time, changes in oxygen saturations, oxygen dependency and nutritional status, and frequency of hospital admissions.

Cardiac catheterisation may be performed to assess PVR. Children with irreversible pulmonary vascular disease may be candidates for heart–lung transplantation.

Suitable children are placed on an active waiting list for transplantation as soon as donor organs become available. About half of the children waiting for transplantation will die before organs become available.

'Bridging to transplant' describes the process by which patients are kept alive by extraordinary means (ventilation, ECMO) in the hope that organs will become available. It becomes difficult to justify this practice in some paediatric age groups, when organs are difficult to come by and the wait can be very distressing for parents without guarantee of success in obtaining an organ.

TRANSPLANTATION SURGERY

The donor is assessed for irreversible brain damage, infection, ABO compatibility, normal gas exchange, good pulmonary compliance and a clear chest X-ray. A brief ventilation period and size match for the recipient are important.

Following transplantation, children return from surgery intubated and ventilated, with arterial and venous lines *in situ* for delivery of drugs and monitoring of CVP. Mediastinal and chest drains and atrial and ventricular pacing wires are standard post-operatively. A urinary catheter facilitates accurate assessment of fluid balance.

The surgery may take up to 8 hours. Extubation is hoped for within 48 hours and most patients are mobile within the first week of surgery.

Children who have undergone transplantation may spend about a month in hospital followed by a tapering routine of follow-up appointments so that maintenance levels of immunosuppressive drugs can be established and evidence of rejection can be closely monitored. Episodes of rejection are very common during the first 4–6 months post-operatively. Investigations for rejection include regular blood samples to monitor cyclosporin levels, myocardial and transbronchial biopsy and watching for signs of malaise.

LONG-TERM COMPLICATIONS

Major concerns in paediatric transplant are chronic rejection and the long-term side effects of immunosuppression. The tissue of the donor organ is immunologically different from the tissue of the recipient, and the recipient will mount an immune response (rejection) against the donor organ. This immune response can lead to destruction of the transplant graft. Because the body never develops a natural tolerance to the transplanted organ, life-long immunosuppression is required. Immunosuppressive therapy includes cyclosporin, corticosteroids, azathioprine and antithymocyte globulin. The side effects of these drugs are significant and include kidney and liver damage, diabetes, hypertension, tremors, seizures, hirsuitism, increased risk of infection, diabetes, osteoporosis, gastrointestinal ulceration, peripheral muscle wasting, cushingoid features, retarded growth and anaemia. Adolescent patients may find the altered body image from immunosuppressive therapy very difficult to accept and this may lead to poor compliance with medication.

There is an increased risk of malignancy, most commonly lymphomas associated with chronic immuno-suppression.

EXERCISE TOLERANCE AFTER TRANSPLANTATION

The ability to exercise aerobically depends on the ability to make energy (ATP) in skeletal muscle using oxygen. The supply of oxygen to skeletal muscle depends on the lungs' ability to exchange gas, the cardiac output and the muscles' ability to utilise oxygen. When the supply of oxygen is less than the demand, energy demands are supplemented by anaerobic metabolism. Anaerobic metabolism produces lactic acid, which increases fatigue and causes termination of exercise.

Transplant group members (heart, heart–lung and single- and double-lung transplants) have all exhibited lower maximal workloads when compared with normal subjects. They also all exhibit a peak oxygen uptake ($VO_{2\,max}$) of only 45–65% normal values. Resting heart rates are in general higher than in normal subjects, and peak exercise heart rates are in general lower than in normal subjects

The suboptimal ability to exercise following transplant is related to either the lungs' ability to exchange gas, cardiac output or the muscles' ability to utilise oxygen.

Gas exchange in the lungs following transplant is essentially normal, as are spirometry, lung function and the oxygen saturation of arterial blood (SaO_2). At maximal exercise there is still a reserve of about 30% voluntary ventilation, so gas exchange does not appear to limit exercise capacity. During exercise there appears to be no difference in oxygen consumption or carbon dioxide production between transplant group members and normal subjects.

Cardiac output depends on heart rate and stroke volume. Heart rate is regulated to a limited extent by vagal innervation. The transplanted heart is permanently denervated, and in the absence of vagal tone it was thought that heart rate is unable to increase appropriately in resonse to sudden increases in workload. During early exercise, compensation for increased cardiac output requirements comes from increased stroke volume. Heart rate is thus a poor measure of effort during exercise after transplant. In mid- and late exercise, increased cardiac performance is a result of increased heart rate from circulating catecholamines released by the adrenal gland. Training improves cardiac sensitivity to circulating catecholamines. It is, however, interesting to note that patients who have undergone single- or double-lung transplants (with intact cardiac vagal supply) exhibit the same limitations to maximal exercise capacity as patients with cardiac denervation. Cardiac denervation cannot thus be entirely responsible for limited exercise capacity.

It is proposed that the effects of chronic deconditioning pre-operatively may persist long after surgery, and that the ability of the muscles to utilise oxygen is primarily at fault in producing suboptimal exercise capacity. Muscle wasting before transplant will persist post-operatively, and studies have shown a significant correlation between muscle volume, maximal oxygen uptake, maximal heart rate and maximal workload. In addition, chronic anaemia and osteoporosis are frequently present after transplant, and this has been shown to reduce exercise capacity and maximal oxygen uptake directly.

If muscle atrophy is a significant contributor, then exercise performance can potentially be reversed by a formal rehabilitation programme. Further research into the feasibility of this option is required.

HEART TRANSPLANTATION

INDICATIONS FOR TRANSPLANTATION

The principal reasons for paediatric cardiac transplantation are acquired or viral cardiomyopathy, failed cardiac surgery for congenital cardiac defects, hypoplastic left heart syndrome and, rarely, restrictive coronary artery disease or ischaemic cardiomyopathy.

Contraindications to cardiac transplantation include irreversible pulmonary vascular disease (these patients may be candidates for heart–lung transplantation), renal failure and hepatic disease, active infection and malignancy.

METHOD OF HEART TRANSPLANTATION

The majority of paediatric heart transplantations are orthotopic transplants, in which the diseased heart is removed through a midline sternotomy, the donor heart then being substituted for it in the correct anatomical position.

COMPLICATIONS

The 5 year survival for all groups of paediatric cardiac transplant patients exceeds 70%, but by then coronary artery disease may have occurred in up to half the patients as a result of chronic immunosuppression. The concentric narrowing along the length of the coronary artery cannot be relieved by coronary artery bypass grafting. Sudden death may occur due to myocardial ischaemia, without the warning of angina-like symptoms because the heart is denervated. Re-transplantation is the only option for patients suffering from this complication.

PHYSIOTHERAPY MANAGEMENT

Pre-operative Assessment

The age at presentation varies widely in the paediatric heart transplant candidate, and the physiotherapist will need to assess the individual needs as the range of disability will be extensive. In general, the shorter the illness, the easier it is to recover function post-operatively. Sometimes the child will only be a few months old and, because of the fatigue and malaise associated with cardiac failure, will have failed to develop within normal parameters. Vigorous neuro-developmental rehabilitation before transplant is inappropriate and dangerous, but suggestions regarding positioning and gentle visual and tactile stimulation may help towards making the post-operative rehabilitation less difficult. Many children who are assessed for cardiac transplantation are free of respiratory symptoms, but if not, treatment should not be overly stressful.

Early Post-operative Management

Early post-operative management of the transplant patient is little different from that of other paediatric cardiac surgery patients, except that immunosuppression leaves these children at risk of infection and requires careful handling (Figure 19.3). Further infection risk comes from chronic deconditioning and potentially immature immune systems in the young recipients. Early post-operative goals are to keep the lungs free of secretions and facilitate good thoracic expansion while preventing circulatory complications. In addition, early mobility is encouraged within the limits of the individual's ability.

As soon as they are extubated and weaned from inotropic support (about the third post-operative day), patients should mobilise around the transplant cubicle and begin to use the exercise bike. Chest drains, pacing wires and intravenous lines are not contraindications to exercise.

The exercise bike is a valuable tool in the early rehabilitation of the transplant patient (Figure 19.4) because it can be moved into the transplant isolation cubicle and used on a daily basis until the patient is more immunocompetent. The exercise bike can also be taken to the physiotherapy gym.

The use of a pedal stand may be useful if the child is too weak to get on the exercise bike, and it may help to build confidence for trying out the exercise bike when most lines and drains have been removed. An exercise chart is helpful because it provides a tangible objective measure of improvement in function for the child, so maintaining motivation, and, further, is a good method of monitoring post-operative rehabilitation.

Most patients are given antithymocyte globulin in the perioperative period to maximise immunosuppression. Side effects may include muscle and joint pain, which may be worsened by exercise. Mobilisation should be

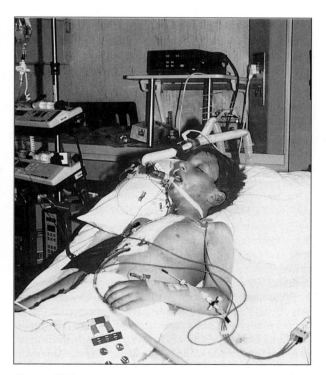

Figure 19.3 Day 1 post-operatively.

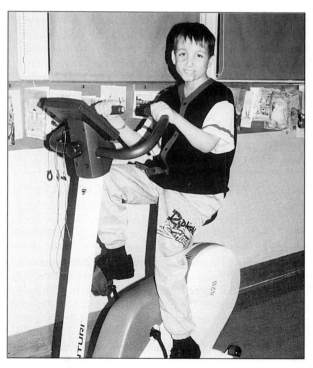

Figure 19.4 Early rehabilitation.

postponed for a short while if there is a suspicion of this side effect.

Late Post-operative Management

Prescriptive post-operative physiotherapy programmes are of limited value. All patients are different, and some may have been moribund before surgery while others may have been in relatively good physical condition. Some will suffer complications in theatre while others will have a smooth surgical course. In general, therapeutic aims will include improvement of exercise tolerance, power and range of movement to achieve early independence.

After surgery, the children (and some parents), having become used to a lengthy period of debilitation, may have lost confidence in their physical abilities. The rehabilitation programme after surgery aims not so much to achieve and maintain a high level of physical fitness, but to restore the confidence of the child (and parents) lost during the illness.

Individual physiotherapy rehabilitation programmes are designed to fit each patient depending on age, pre-operative condition and post-operative progress.

Policies regarding formal rehabilitation programmes will vary between transplant centres, and although there is little doubt from the literature that a comprehensive and sustained exercise programme will enhance the quality of life and possibly prolong it following transplant, there are logistical and ethical difficulties about enforcing such a programme. Most transplant centres will serve a large catchment area and will not be able to offer a supervised rehabilitation programme that a reasonable proportion of the population will be able to attend. In addition, the same variety of attitudes towards exercise will be encountered in the transplant population as in the general population, and it is impossible to enforce an exercise programme once the child has left hospital. It can only be hoped that any benefits experienced by the child or family from the exercise programme in hospital will be carried over to home life. The annual Transplant Games in the UK offer an excellent opportunity for children and adults to train for an event of their choice and enjoy the sense of achievement from participating.

LUNG AND HEART–LUNG TRANSPLANTATION

INDICATIONS FOR TRANSPLANTATION

More children require heart–lung transplantation than heart transplantation only, but fewer than 20% of donors whose hearts are suitable for transplantation have lungs that are also suitable for heart–lung transplantation.

Approximately two-thirds of paediatric patients requiring heart–lung transplantation have CF. For children with CF the options for transplantation include heart–lung transplantation or single- or double-lung transplantation. The procedure choice may be dictated by the availability of donor organs. Early mortality is the same for all groups but critical narrowing of the bronchial anastomosis accounts for much of the late mortality, especially in small children. For this reason, heart–lung *en bloc* with tracheal anastomosis is often

preferable. Single-lung transplant recipients are at risk of significant post-operative ventilation/perfusion mismatch. CF does not affect the transplanted lung and does not constitute additional risk in terms of survival and morbidity after transplant. Some children require both heart and lungs because of their primary pathology, and cannot accept single- or double-lung transplants. Some children with CF suffer terminal liver failure before developing significant pulmonary disease, and may need liver transplantation as a therapeutic priority.

Heart–lung transplantation for congenital heart disease may be required at all ages through to adult life. Most recipients will have Eisenmenger's complex (where PAP exceeds systemic blood pressure, causing poor pulmonary blood flow and cyanosis) as a result of longstanding left to right shunt. Other indications include absent connections between heart and lung, fibrosing alveolitis, interstitial pneumonitis and severe bronchopulmonary dysplasia. Rarely, congenital bronchial and tracheal abnormalities such as stove-pipe trachea require heart–lung transplantation.

Contraindications for transplantation include severe liver failure (although these patients may then theoretically be eligible for triple organ transplantation, there is currently only one centre in the UK which has performed this surgery, and only on adult patients to date), multiresistant organisms or *Aspergillus* infection, high steroid dependency (steroids are associated with poor healing of the tracheal anastomosis) and very poor nutritional status.

LUNG AND HEART–LUNG TRANSPLANTATION SURGERY

A median sternotomy or 'clam shell' surgical approach may be used.

Many children with CF who accept heart–lung *en bloc* organs donate their own relatively healthy heart to a child waiting for a heart transplant ('domino' transplant).

An early post-operative aim is to maintain a negative crystalloid balance to decrease pulmonary oedema. The transplanted lung may require high ventilation pressures post-operatively to assist reversal of distal airway closure.

After transplantation, children measure their own forced expiratory volume (FEV) twice daily with microspirometers, and a fall in these values of more than 10–15% may be an indication of rejection, which will be followed up by an urgent biopsy and drug treatment if indicated.

LONG-TERM COMPLICATIONS

The 5 year survival for heart–lung and single- and double-lung transplants is well below 50%. The long-term complications encountered in this patient group are obliterative bronchiolitis and narrowing of the tracheal or bronchial anastomosis.

Obliterative bronchiolitis continues to be the most stubborn obstacle to success in pulmonary transplantation. Most patients seem inevitably to develop this fibrosing inflammatory disease of the terminal airways, eventually leading to small airway obstruction and terminal lung disease. Although the mechanism of this process is not clearly understood, it is presumed to be a result of chronic subclinical rejection.

PHYSIOTHERAPY MANAGEMENT
Pre-operative Assessment and Treatment
Lung clearance techniques for children with CF must be optimised. The waiting list for transplantation is often long and unpredictable, and optimal chest physiotherapy may make the difference in extending survival until organs become available. Sometimes the child with end stage disease will perform less effective physiotherapy techniques, being unable to manage postural drainage. Alternatives, such as the active cycle of breathing techniques (ACBT), positive expiratory pressure (PEP), flutter or autogenic drainage, should be offered to optimise treatment.

Exercise tolerance and motivation should be determined during the assessment. Some children will have little interest in exercise, and so the loss of exercise tolerance becomes less of a factor in determining quality of life.

The reasons for pre-operative assessment mirror those for any pre-operative thoracic procedure: to assess current needs if any and to discuss the details of post-operative physiotherapy. Most people cope better under stressful situations when they know what to expect. If appropriate, some post-operative breathing techniques may be practised.

The degree and type of any specific neurological deficits or developmental delay should be noted but treatment should not be commenced pre-operatively if it compromises the child with end stage disease.

Early Post-operative Management
In the early post-operative period, fluid restriction may result in tenacious secretions which are difficult to clear. Early extubation is aimed at, but it is always useful to have at least one physiotherapy treatment before extubation to suction any residual debris from the anastomosis site.

An important factor to remember when treating the intubated patient is that the tracheal anastamosis in the transplanted lung is distal to the end of the endotracheal tube and may be traumatised during suction procedures. Great care should be taken with suctioning technique. In addition, the anastomosis site is not airtight for a few days after surgery, so bagging pressures should be equal to or slightly greater than pressures delivered safely by the ventilator, with a well functioning chest drain *in situ* to avoid the risk of pneumothorax.

Loss of ciliated epithelium around the tracheal anastomosis site may hinder the natural removal of secretions, and vagal nerve interruption causes permanent loss of sensation below the level of the anastamosis. The 'tickle' in the airways that usually indicates the presence of secretions and stimulates cough will not be present below the level of the anastomosis. Huff and cough should therefore be encouraged as a regular habit so that secretions audible below the anastomosis can be cleared.

Late Post-operative Management
Some transplant centres advocate that the pre-operative respiratory physiotherapy regimen performed by patients with CF be continued post-operatively. The argument is based on the theory that the airways above the anastomosis will continue to produce thick or infected secretions which may drip down into the transplanted lungs and cause infection. The denervated lungs are insensitive to the presence of secretions in the airways and will be vulnerable to infection.

However, most lung transplant patients have an unproductive cough after surgery, and there is no research evidence to date to support the argument that infected secretions drip down and infect the transplanted lungs, or that intensive respiratory physiotherapy will prolong survival after transplant. Physiotherapy is considered one of the most significant impediments to good quality of life pre-operatively. To continue it post-operatively in the absence of suppurative lung disease seems contrary to the objective of improved quality of life, and it would be difficult to expect compliance with a regimen that appears to carry no tangible benefit. It seems axiomatic to advise huff and cough on a regular basis to clear any secretions that are not 'felt' in the airways because of pulmonary denervation. In addition, patients should be advised to resume physiotherapy modalities to clear secretions during any intercurrent infections which result from immunosuppressive therapy. This is a relatively new and contentious area of physiotherapy, and more research will yield better understanding.

HOPE FOR THE FUTURE

LIVE DONORS
The potential for live donors (usually related family members) to donate a lobe or single lung is being utilised more commonly in the USA, but it has been attempted only once in the UK. The controversy surrounding this surgical option obviously centres on the justification for subjecting two human lives to risk instead of only one.

XENOTRANSPLANTATION
With an increasing shortage of donor organs there has been a renewed interest in xenotransplantation. Work is being done to produce 'transgenic' pigs, i.e. pigs which have organs genetically compatible with human tissue, which will create a potentially inexhaustible organ resource. Human trials will possibly commence within the next couple of years from the time of writing.

NEW DRUGS
In recent years an enormous amount of work has been done to produce immunosuppressive drugs that are more effective and less toxic over the long term, and may reduce the incidence of coronary artery disease and bronchiolitis obliterans. Since the late 1980s, seven promising new agents have been under investigation as potential replacements for the current regimens.

MECHANICAL ORGANS
Although mechanical pumps have been useful as bridges to transplantation or as long-term assist devices in adults who are ineligible for transplant, they have not yet been developed to serve patients of under 40 kg body weight.

GENERAL READING

Andrews M. Respiratory management of children following heart-lung transplant. *J Assoc Chart Physiother Respir Care* 1993, **22:**12-13.

Banner NR, *et al.* Cardiopulmonary response to dynamic exercise after heart and combined heart-lung transplantation. *Br Heart J* 1989, **61:**215-223.

Brown SE, Stansbury DW, Merrill EJ, Linden GS, Light RW. Prevention of suctioning-related arterial oxygen desaturation. Comparison of off-ventilator and on-ventilator suctioning. *Chest* 1983, **83(4):**621-627.

Crabtree, Goodnough SK. The effects of oxygen and hyperinflation on arterial oxygen tension after endotracheal suctioning. *Heart Lung* 1985, **14(1):**11-17.

De Leval MR, *et al.* Heart and lung transplantation for terminal cystic fibrosis. *J Thorac Cardiovasc Surg* 1991, **101:**633-642.

Dunn JM, *et al.*, ed. *Heart transplantation in children.* New York: Futura Publishing; 1990.

Durand M, Sangha B, Cabal LA, Hoppenbrouwers T, Hodgman JE. Cardiopulmonary and intracranial pressure changes related to endotracheal suctioning in preterm infants. *Crit Care Med* 1989, **17(6):**506-510.

Gunderson LP, Stone KS, Hamlin RL. Endotracheal suctioning-induced heart rate alterations. *Nurs Res* 1991, **40(3):**139-143.

Jordon SC, Scott O. *Heart disease in paediatrics.* London: Butterworth; 1989.

Jung RC, Gottlieb LS. Comparison of tracheobronchial suction catheters in humans. Visualisation by fiberoptic bronchoscopy. *Chest* 1976, **69(2):**179-182.

Jung RC, Newman J. Minimising hypoxia during endotracheal airway care. *Heart Lung* 1982, **11(3):**208-212.

Kavanagh T, *et al.* Cardiorespiratory responses to exercise training after orthotopic cardiac transplantation. *Circulation* 1987, **77(1):**162-171.

Landa JF, Kwoka MA, Chapman GA, Brito, M, Sackner MA. Effects of suctioning on mucociliary transport. *Chest* 1980, **77(2):**202-207.

Levick JR. *An introduction to cardiovascular physiology.* London: Butterworth; 1991.

Levy RD, *et al.* Exercise performance after lung transplantation. *J Heart Lung Transplant* 1993, **12:**27-33.

Perlman JM, Volpe JJ. Suctioning in the preterm infant: effects on cerebral blood flow velocity, intracranial pressure and arterial blood pressure. *Pediatrics* 1983, **72(3):**329-334.

Prasad SA, Hussey J. *Paediatric respiratory care–guide for physiotherapists and health professionals.* London: Chapman & Hall; 1995.

Riegel B, Forshee T. A review and critique of the literature on preoxygenation for endotracheal suctioning. *Heart Lung* 1985, **14(5):**507-518.

Sackner MA, Landa JF, Greenelich N, Robinson MJ. Pathogenesis and prevention of tracheobronchial damage with suction procedures. *Chest* 1973, **64(3):**285-290.

Savin WM, *et al.* Cardiorespiratory responses of cardiac transplant patients to graded, symptom limited exercise. *Circulation* 1980, **62(1):**55-60.

Shorten DR, Byrne PJ, Jones RL. Infant responses to saline instillations and endotracheal suctioning. *J Obstet Gynecol Neonatal Nurs* 1991, **20(6):**464-469.

Simbruner G, Coradello H, Fodor M, Havelec L, Lubec G, Pollak A. Effect of tracheal suction on oxygenation, circulation, and lung mechanics in newborn infants. *Arch Dis Child* 1981, **56:**326-330.

Stark J, de Leval M. *Surgery for congenital heart defects.* Philadelphia: WB Saunders; 1994.

Stone KS, Preusser BA, Groch KF, Karl JI, Gonyon DS. The effect of lung hyperinflation and endotracheal suctioning on cardiopulmonary hemodynamics. *Nurs Res* 1991, **40(2):**76-79.

Theodore J, *et al.* Cardiopulmonary function at maximum tolerable constant work rate exercise following human heart-lung transplantation. *Chest* 1987, **92(3):**433-439.

Wallwork J, ed. *Heart and heart-lung transplantation.* Philadelphia: WB Saunders; 1989.

Walsh JM, Vanderwarf C, Hoschett D, Fahey PJ. Unsuspected hemodynamic alterations during endotracheal suctioning. *Chest* 1989, **95(1):**162-165.

Whitehead B. Heart-lung transplantation in cystic fibrosis. *J Assoc Chart Physio Respir Care* 1993, **22:**10-12.

Williams TJ, *et al.* Maximal exercise testing in single and double lung transplant recipients. *Am Rev Respir Dis* 1992, **145:**101-105.

Young CS. A review of the adverse effects of airway suction. *Physiotherapy* 1984, **70(3):**104-108.

Young CS. A study of paediatric physiotherapy practice. *Physiotherapy* 1988, **74(1):**13-15.

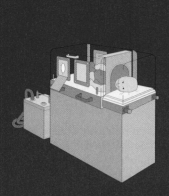

20 J Chapman, A Parker, L Yeo

THE NEONATAL UNIT AND SPECIALIST SUPPORT

CHAPTER OUTLINE

Neonatal unit:
- **Admission**
- **General problems**
- **Physiotherapy**

Specialised respiratory support:
- **Extracorporeal membrane oxygenation**
- **Negative pressure ventilation**

INTRODUCTION

The Neonatal Unit (NNU) is a distinctly different environment from both adult and paediatric Intensive Care Units (ICUs). The infants in a NNU have problems which vary considerably from those experienced by older children and adults. This is due to the differences in anatomy and physiology (see Chapter 15). The care and management of these problems are also very different.

Although physiotherapy has a major role to play in the respiratory, postural, orthopaedic and neuro-developmental care of the newborn, it is rare, in the UK, that an NNU has a full time physiotherapist. Most NNUs have physiotherapists who cover the unit as part of another role, e.g. paediatrics or obstetrics. Some NNUs do not have any input from a physiotherapist (Parker and Downs, 1991). On these units, physiotherapy techniques are carried out by neonatal nurses who may or may not have previously been taught by a physiotherapist.

Neonatal nurses are highly skilled, specialist nurses who are very aware of the problems of the sick neonate, and the physiotherapy techniques required are basic. Properly taught nurses can, therefore, easily give basic physiotherapy for the common problems they will encounter in these infants.

In order to be able to teach nurses how to handle infants safely, the physiotherapist must fully understand the problems of sick neonates, their management and the equipment used in their care. The NNU is not the place for an inexperienced physiotherapist so if an 'on-call' service is required, then it should be covered by physiotherapists who work in neonatal care, or only the nursing staff should treat overnight and at weekends.

REASONS FOR ADMISSION TO AN NNU

Reasons for admission to an NNU are:
- Low birthweight and pre-term birth.
- Perinatal problems.
- Congenital abnormalities.

LOW BIRTH WEIGHT AND PRE-TERM BIRTH

Each year about 7% of babies are born pre-term, i.e. before 37 weeks' gestation. Full-term is considered to be between 38 and 42 weeks of gestation. Some infants are born after a pregnancy lasting only 23 weeks.

About a third of pre-term infants will be small for gestational age (SGA), i.e. their birthweight will be less than the 10th centile for gestational age. This may be due to intra-uterine growth retardation (IUGR) caused by infection or placental insufficiency, for example.

Pre-term babies are often classified according to their birthweight, that is:
- Low birthweight (LBW), <2500 g.
- Very low birthweight (VLBW), <1500 g.
- Extremely low birthweight (ELBW), <1000 g.
- Ultra-low birthweight (ULBW), i.e. <750 g.

Problems Related to Pre-term Birth

The problems of pre-term infants are mainly due to the immaturity of the body systems, and those infants who are also SGA will have problems due to reduced reserves. The major problem for pre-term infants, and the main cause of death, is respiratory insufficiency.

Respiratory problems

The main cause of respiratory problems is respiratory distress syndrome (RDS). This is due to a lack of surfactant in the immature lung. Surfactant is a phospholipid material which reduces surface tension at the alveolar air/fluid interface and therefore reduces the work of breathing. The lack of a normal amount of surfactant causes atelectasis resulting in hypoxia. Surfactant is produced in the lung from about 24 weeks' gestation. The amount present gradually increases as gestational age increases, with a surge in production at about 34 weeks. The earlier infants are born, the more likely they are to develop RDS. Surfactant production is hindered by hypoxia and hypothermia.

RDS presents within a few hours of birth with sternal and costal recession, tachypnoea (respiratory rate >60 breaths/min) and grunting. Grunting is the sound made by the infant breathing out against a partially closed glottis to self-generate a positive pressure. The chest X-ray has a uniform 'ground glass' appearance with air bronchograms against unaerated alveoli.

Whatever the gestational age of the infant, surfactant will start to be produced at about 48 hours provided that the infant is not hypoxic or hypothermic.

Treatment of RDS is mainly supportive, with the infant being kept warm and any hypoxia being treated by some form of respiratory support, e.g. increased inspired oxygen (FiO_2), continuous positive airways pressure (CPAP) or mechanical ventilation. Antibiotics are given as it is not possible to distinguish clinical signs and chest X-rays of RDS from Group B streptoccocal septicaemia, which can be rapidly fatal. Antibiotics are given for at least 48 hours until cultures are known to be negative.

If pre-term labour can be stopped or slowed down, obstetricians can give the mother injections of steroids to try and stimulate surfactant production in the fetus. Steroids have been shown to give a 50% reduction in mortality and 70% reduction in incidence of RDS if given between 24 hours and 7 days before birth (Crowley et al., 1990).

RDS may also be prevented by the instillation of surfactant into the infant's lungs. Many studies have shown that surfactant therapy can reduce mortality by 50% (Morley, 1991). Surfactant may be natural, obtained from animal lungs or human amniotic fluid, or artificial, and it is very expensive. Several millilitres at a time are instilled directly into the infant's lungs via an endotracheal tube soon after birth. More research is needed to determine the best type of preparation, dosage regimens and which infants will benefit most.

Periventricular haemorrhage (PVH)

Periventricular haemorrhage (PVH) is a major cause of cerebral damage and death in the pre-term infant. It occurs in about 40% of VLBW infants but particularly in infants who have suffered hypoxia, hypercarbia and hypo- or hypertension. It is most common and tends to be most severe in the smallest and least mature infants. PVH most commonly occurs in the first week of life, particularly around the fourth day.

The haemorrhages arise from fragile capillaries in the floor of the lateral ventricles. Fluctuation of arterial oxygen (PaO_2) and blood pressure leading to variations in cerebral blood flow (CBF) will cause capillaries to rupture and bleeding to occur into and around the ventricles.

There are four grades of severity. Infants with:
- Grades I to II haemorrhages may be asymptomatic, require no specific treatment and have a good prognosis.
- Grades III to IV are very unwell and may not survive. Those that do may have hydrocephalus, and most will have varying degrees of neurological impairment.

PVH is regularly monitored by cerebral ultrasonography in infants who have had bleeds and those who are at risk.

Prevention of PVH is directed towards minimal handling of infants with avoidance of changes in PaO_2, arterial carbon dioxide ($PaCO_2$) and blood pressure. Drugs may also be used to minimise surges in CBF.

Periventricular leucomalacia

Periventricular leucomalacia (PVL) is a form of hypoxic ischaemic encephalopathy and may occur in utero or, most commonly, post-natally after cerebral hypoperfusion and ischaemia. Early detection and correction of hypotension to maintain blood pressure is extremely important in the early care of pre-term infants. PVL is associated with neurological impairment.

Persistent fetal circulation

Persistent fetal circulation (PFC) is a clinical syndrome consisting of pulmonary hypertension and right-to-left shunting through a patent ductus arteriosus (PDA) or foramen ovale. Infants present with tachypnoea and tricuspid or mitral regurgitation. Infants with PFC are extremely unwell and the slightest disturbance can precipitate severe hypoxaemia, so minimal handling is essential.

Treatment is supportive and vasodilator drugs may be used to dilate the pulmonary vasculature.

Temperature regulation

Pre-term infants have great problems maintaining their body temperature. They have a large surface area to bodyweight ratio and easily lose heat by evaporation and radiation through their very thin skin. Their central heat-controlling system is immature and they also have a smaller proportion of brown fat than do term infants. Thus they can rapidly become hypothermic. Hypothermia can cause acidosis, hypoglycaemia, increased oxygen consumption and decreased surfactant production. It is vital to maintain body temperature in the pre-term infant.

Infants should be nursed in the neutral temperature range, i.e. the temperature at which oxygen consumption is minimal in the presence of a normal body temperature. This will vary according to the infant's gestation and weight.

To maintain a neutral temperature range, infants are nursed in incubators or radiant warmers, and the ambient room temperature is kept high at 26–28°C.

Incubators are enclosed units of transparent material with portholes in the side for access. Carers must ensure not to leave portholes open, even briefly, as severe draughts will be caused. Radiant warmers are open-topped units with an overhead radiant heating device. This allows easy access to the infant but has the disadvantages of convective heat loss and insensible fluid loss. Infants may be nursed on radiant warmers when first admitted to the NNU, and then transferred to an incubator.

To reduce radiant heat loss, infants may be covered with plastic heat shields and/or an insulating material, e.g. bubblewrap, clingfilm, silver swaddlers. When an infant requires less intensive care monitoring, dressing is possible.

Infection

The pre-term infant is particularly vulnerable to infection. The skin is very thin and easily damaged. Only one type of immunoglobulin can cross the placenta, and the pre-term infant's white cells are functionally immature.

The most important means of preventing cross-infection is by scrupulous handwashing by all staff and visitors. Visitors to the NNU are usually kept to a minimum, e.g. parents, siblings and grandparents, and anyone with an infectious disease such as gastroenteritis should be excluded.

Prompt treatment of any infection with appropriate antibiotics is usual to prevent infection becoming severe and life threatening.

Jaundice

Physiological jaundice is common in the normal full-term infant, appearing after 2 days and usually disappearing by 7–10 days of life. The jaundice is due to a raised blood level of unconjugated bilirubin from the breakdown of fetal haemoglobin. Pre-term infants have impaired hepatic clearance of bilirubin and are at greater risk of the effects of hyperbilirubinaemia. Unconjugated bilirubin is fat soluble and easily diffuses through the blood–brain barrier, particularly into the basal ganglia. This can lead to a condition called kernicterus, which is characterised by athetoid cerebral palsy, deafness and mental retardation, and may occasionally be fatal.

Daily serum bilirubin levels are measured in blood taken by heel prick from jaundiced infants. Treatment consists of phototherapy where the infant is exposed to lightwaves of 400–500 nm which convert the bilirubin into a water-soluble non-neurotoxic product.

In severe cases, exchange transfusion may be required. In this procedure, blood is withdrawn from the infant in small amounts (5 or 10 ml) and is replaced by donor blood until twice the infant's blood volume has been exchanged. This procedure is not without complications.

Feeding

All neonates lose weight in the first few days of life, especially those born pre-term. Adequate nutrition and weight gain are important to avoid hypoglycaemia, persistent jaundice and delayed recovery from RDS. Feeding should be commenced early either enterally (oral or nasogastric feeds) or parenterally (intravenously).

Pre-term infants are initially unable to suck, and have impaired swallowing, cough and gag reflexes. Most will, therefore, need to be fed nasogastrically. Respiratory problems may be aggravated by the nasogastric tube obstructing one half of the upper airway. Food in the stomach may increase the work of breathing, lower the PaO_2 and cause apnoea. Pooling of milk in the stomach may also lead to gastro-oesophageal reflux and subsequent aspiration of milk into the lungs. Therefore, initially only small amounts (0.5 to 1 ml every hour) are given, preferably the mother's milk. Orogastric tubes may be used if the infant is struggling to breathe with a nasogastric tube *in situ*.

Feeds are more likely to be tolerated if the infant is positioned prone after feeding. If the infant is unable to tolerate enteral feeding, then intravenous feeding should be started and attempts made at enteral feeding every 2–3 days.

Hypoglycaemia

Hypoglycaemia in the pre-term infant causes symptoms of bradycardia and heart failure. Regular monitoring of blood sugar is essential and prompt treatment needed.

Apnoea

Apnoea may be due to immaturity of the respiratory centre or inco-ordination of the upper airway. It can also be a sign of other problems such as infection, hyperthermia, PVH and anaemia. Treatment depends on cause and severity.

Necrotising enterocolitis

Necrotising enterocolitis (NEC) is a serious bowel disorder precipitated by various factors, e.g. hypoxia, infection and severe IUGR. The infant becomes pale and unwell with abdominal distension. Treatment initially consists of gastric aspiration, intravenous nutrition and antibiotics. In severe cases a laparotomy may be required for resection of necrotic bowel.

Handling

No sick neonate will tolerate bad handling but pre-term infants are particularly at risk. Handling of any sort can cause hypoxia, which may result in severe sequelae.

A pre-term infant should not be handled unless absolutely necessary.

PERINATAL PROBLEMS

Perinatal problems occur at or around the time of birth.

Birth Asphyxia

This is defined as a delay in establishing respiration after birth. It occurs in about 10% of deliveries, and infants who are severely asphyxiated will require admission to an NNU.

Asphyxia may be due to:

- Occlusion or prolapse of the umbilical cord.
- Unco-ordinated hypertonic uterine contractions.
- Placental separation leading to antepartum haemorrhage.
- Malpresentation, e.g. breech delivery.

Asphyxia is more common in the pre-term infant and those suffering from IUGR.

The usual way of assessing severity of asphyxia is to use the Apgar score (Apgar, 1953). This grades five clinical features—heart rate, respiration, colour of trunk, muscle tone and response to oral suction—with scores from 0 to 2. Scoring is done at 1, 5, 10 and 15 minutes after delivery to indicate the degree of asphyxia and the success of resuscitation.

Severe asphyxia can lead to heart failure, cerebral damage and renal failure. The severity of cerebral damage may range from cerebral oedema to subdural or subarachnoid haemorrhage. Long-term neurological sequelae are difficult to predict in the early days and even severely asphyxiated infants occasionally make a reasonable neurological recovery.

Meconium Aspiration

Meconium is the thick green substance present in the fetal bowel which forms the first stool. Meconium aspiration occurs mainly in full-term infants who pass meconium *in utero* in response to acute or chronic hypoxia. If the hypoxia continues, the infant gasps and inhales meconium during delivery. Once meconium is inhaled it causes a chemical pneumonitis resulting in atelectasis, surfactant inhibition and mechanical obstruction with air trapping, and predisposes the infant to infection.

The incidence of meconium aspiration is very low in the UK (<0.2%) due to good preventive measures. A paediatrician is called to all deliveries when the mother's liquor is stained with meconium and there is fetal distress. At delivery, the infant's airway is suctioned immediately to prevent aspiration of meconium into the lungs when the first breath is taken. If meconium is aspirated then physiotherapy and suction are required urgently to remove plugs of meconium from the airways.

CONGENITAL ABNORMALITIES

Only infants with severe congenital abnormalities will need to be admitted to an NNU (see Chapter 19).

GENERAL PROBLEMS OF INFANTS IN AN NNU

PARENTAL-INFANT BONDING

It is usual that newly delivered infants are left with their parents. Unfortunately, this is not possible for infants who require resuscitation and subsequent transfer to the NNU.

The effect of early separation on parent–child relationships is controversial but it is generally accepted that any possible sequelae should be minimised as far as possible. Parents should be encouraged to visit the NNU and touch or stroke their baby. Cuddles are encouraged as soon as the infant's condition allows.

STRESS

Infants in an NNU experience many stressful stimuli; for example, they lay in a brightly lit room on a hard surface and undergo painful procedures. The average noise intensity in an NNU is 65 decibels (dB)—the same as in a busy street—while a bang on top of the incubator is 89 dB and closing one of the portholes 96 dB. Sudden loud noises cause a drop in the infant's PaO_2 and an increase in intracranial pressure and heart and respiratory rate.

To minimise stress, infants are nursed whenever possible on sheepskins or soft bean bags. Incubators are shielded from bright lights and lights are turned off or dimmed at night when possible. Painful stimuli are kept to a minimum and, when appropriate, analgesics are used. Staff should always close incubator portholes quietly and gently, and equipment should not be placed on top of the incubator.

VENTILATION OF THE NEONATE

In infants weighing <1000 g, ventilation will often be commenced from birth. Other indications are:

- Deteriorating blood gases.
- Recurrent or major apnoea.
- Pre- and post-operative major surgery.

Conventional Positive Pressure Ventilation

Full-term infants weighing >2500 g can be ventilated at rates of 30–40 breaths/min using time-cycled, pressure-limited ventilation. These ventilators inflate the lung for a preset length of time, e.g. 1 second, at a predetermined pressure, e.g. 20 mmHg.

In pre-term infants, the same ventilators are used but at much faster rates. In the first 48 hours of life, respiratory rate seems to be inversely proportional to gestational age. Infants born at 32 weeks' gestation have a respiratory rate of 70 breaths/min whereas those of 26–28 weeks' gestation have a respiratory rate of 100 breaths/min. Using fast ventilator rates fits more closely with natural rates, and infants often breathe in synchrony with the ventilator, enhancing oxygenation (Greenough et al.,1987). Some infants do not synchronise with the ventilator and the inspiratory phase of the ventilator cycle. This can cause a pneumothorax, so these infants are then paralysed and ventilated at a rate of <60 breaths/min. Ventilation settings are adjusted to maintain satisfactory blood gases, and infants are weaned from ventilation as soon as possible to reduce risks of infection, barotrauma and tracheal damage.

Patient Triggered Ventilation

During patient triggered ventilation (PTV), a ventilator breath is given every time the infant's breath is sensed by the triggering device. The triggering device needs to be very sensitive in order to respond to the very small changes in air flow made by these infants. This method of ventilation is less useful in pre-term infants whose respiratory efforts are inadequate and inconsistent.

Extracorporeal Membrane Oxygenation

Extacorporeal membrane oxygenation (ECMO) may be used in the full-term infant, e.g. after repair of a diaphragmatic hernia. However, it cannot be used in the pre-term infant as the anticoagulant therapy used in ECMO can precipate PVH. ECMO is discussed on page 313–315.

Negative Extrathoracic Pressure Ventilation

Negative extrathoracic pressure ventilation (VNEP) was originally used in the treatment of polio in children. It has now been adapted and is occasionally used in a NNU to wean infants with chronic lung disease from positive pressure ventilation. It is described in detail on page 316–318.

COMPLICATIONS OF RESPIRATORY SUPPORT IN THE NEWBORN

Pneumothorax

Occasionally pneumothoraces present spontaneously at birth but they are most commonly seen in pre-term infants having positive pressure ventilation. Infants with conditions such as RDS and meconium aspiration, where alveoli become hyperinflated, are particularly at risk. Other causative factors are high peak inspiratory pressure (PIP), positive end expiratory pressure (PEEP), long inflation times and active expiration against the ventilator's inspiration.

Small, asymptomatic pneumothoraces require no treatment. A large tension pneumothorax presents dramatically with pallor and shock, and needs urgent drainage with a chest drain. There is an association with PVH.

Pulmonary Interstitial Emphysema

Pulmonary interstitial emphysema (PIE) occurs when gas leaks out of an alveolus, tracks along the vascular bundles and remains trapped forming interstitial gas pockets. PIE is most common in pre-term infants, the incidence being inversely proportional to gestational age.

Treatment consists of fast rate, low pressure ventilation, and infants with unilateral lung PIE should be positioned with the affected lung lowermost. Severe PIE may require surgical resection of affected lung.

Chronic Lung Disease

About 20% of infants who have been ventilated remain oxygen dependent at 1 month of age; such infants are defined as having chronic lung disease (CLD). A small proportion of these infants have specific cystic abnormalities on their chest X-ray and are described as having bronchopulmonary dysplasia (BPD), which is the most severe form of CLD. The majority of infants with CLD will be oxygen dependent only for a few weeks, but infants with BPD often remain oxygen dependent for many months and may be discharged to continue oxygen therapy at home. BPD has a high mortality and, following discharge, infants have a higher incidence of sudden infant death syndrome (Greenough, 1995).

CLD occurs most commonly in infants who have had respiratory failure requiring high FiO_2 and high ventilator pressures. There is also an association with fluid overload, PDA and viral infection.

The infant with BPD has carbon dioxide retention and an increased oxygen requirement. Lung compliance is reduced and airway resistance is increased. The infant is tachypnoeic and has wheeze and persistent recession. The condition may be progressive, eventually leading to respiratory and cardiac failure and death.

Treatment of CLD consists of trying to reduce mechanical ventilation to a minimum and to wean from respiratory support as soon as possible. Pre-term infants are responsive to bronchodilators (Greenough and Milner, 1991) so wheeze can be treated successfully. Nebulised bronchodilators, however, can cause an initial drop in oxygen saturation so must be administered under observation.

Good nutrition is essential to encourage weight gain and lung growth. The infant may require diuretics, and antibiotics are frequently necessary as these infants are prone to chest infections.

Infants who survive are often small and underweight. They have recurrent upper and lower respiratory tract infections, wheezing and gastric reflux, particularly up to the age of 2 years. The long-term prognosis for those who survive to 2 years of age is good.

Subglottic Stenosis

This may occur in some infants following prolonged intubation, and can cause airway obstruction. Stridor is often present and severely affected infants will need a tracheostomy to maintain an airway. The tracheostomy will be required until the infant has grown and the size of the airway has increased sufficiently to allow adequate ventilation. This may take years. In order to prevent subglottic stenosis, endotracheal tubes are uncuffed and a small air leak should always be present during ventilation.

Retinopathy of Prematurity (ROP)

In this condition, the delicate capillaries in the retina proliferate leading to haemorrhage, fibrosis and scarring of the retina. This may cause permanent visual impairment. The exact cause is unknown, but periods of hyperoxia, i.e. PaO_2 above 12 kPa, are considered to be a major contributing factor. Continuous blood gas monitoring is essential to identify and prevent swings into hyperoxia for even brief periods.

PHYSIOTHERAPY

As many of the infants on an NNU have respiratory problems, chest physiotherapy, including suction, has a major role in maintaining clear lungs. However, physiotherapy, as with any form of handling, may cause detrimental effects such as hypoxia and bradycardia, so it is essential that a thorough assessment is made before each treatment. Physiotherapy and suction should never be carried out as a 'routine' procedure but given only when there is a definite indication and no contraindications.

RESPIRATORY ASSESSMENT OF THE NEONATE

Respiratory assessment is similar to that for children (see page 259) with some additional points.

History

It is important to ascertain from the medical notes the history of pregnancy, labour and delivery, Apgar scores, gestational age and weight, and course of illness from birth to present time.

Information from the Nurse

It is essential to discuss the infant's current condition with attending nurse or medical staff. Questions should include:

- How stable has the infant's condition been over the past few hours?
- What is the current respiratory status?
- How well is handling tolerated, e.g. does the infant become rapidly hypoxic or bradycardic?
- Does the FiO_2 or ventilation need to be increased before treatment for the infant to tolerate handling?
- Is the infant properly rested since the last handling episode?
- Is the infant being fed? If so, by which route? It is important to delay physiotherapy for at least 1 hour following a bolus enteral feed to avoid reflux and aspiration.

Vital Signs

Assessment of vital signs should include:

- Temperature—if this is <36.5°C in pre-term infants, non-essential handling should be left until the infant has warmed up.
- The trend of heart rate—tachycardia may be an indication of septicaemia or inadequate sedation in a ventilated infant. Pre-term infants may have self-limiting bradycardia (SLB), a temporary slowing of the heart rate which spontaneously resolves without intervention. More serious are persistent bradycardias which require some form of intervention from the attending nurse, e.g. tickling the infant's foot. These are known as bradycardias requiring stimulation (BRS). An increase in SLBs or BRSs may mean that an infant has become infected, has a progressing PVH or has retention of secretions requiring suction. Careful assessment is necessary to determine the cause.
- Apnoeic spells—in the infant these may indicate respiratory distress, sepsis or secretions in the upper and lower respiratory tract.
- The trend of arterial gases and the relationship to oxygen saturation—these should be noted together with the type of ventilation and inspired oxygen.

- Drug therapy, blood pressure, urine output and results of investigations.

Examination of the Infant

The examination should include noting the presence of lines, incisions and drains.

Signs of respiratory distress

In addition to the signs of tachypnoea, grunting, nasal flaring and pallor (see Table 16.1, page 260) the following may indicate that the infant is in respiratory distress:

- Recession—this is a pulling in of the sternum and ribs on inspiration. It occurs when the infant has to make a strong inspiratory effort to get air into very stiff non-compliant lungs, e.g. in RDS. The negative pressure generated on inspiration pulls in the very soft, compliant chest wall. In pre-term infants the chest wall is so soft that a certain amount of recession is always seen. However, if sternum and ribs are severely pulled in this is a sign that the infant is making increased respiratory effort.
- Stridor is the harsh sound made when there is partial obstruction of the larynx or upper trachea due to inflammation or collapse of the floppy tracheal wall. It can also occur following over-vigorous pharyngeal suction.
- Extension of the neck is often seen in the infant with respiratory distress making the airway straight in an attempt to lessen airway resistance. Overextension of an infant's neck will collapse the trachea.
- Head bobbing is seen in pre-term infants when they are using the sternomastoid and scalene muscles as accessory muscles of respiration. The neck extensors are weak and unable to stabilise the head, so the head moves rather than the chest wall.
- Infants who are having difficulty in breathing will be reluctant to feed, as they need to make frequent pauses from sucking.
- Cyanosis is an unreliable sign of respiratory insufficiency in infants as it depends on the relative amount and type of haemoglobin and the adequacy of peripheral circulation. For the first 3–4 weeks of life the neonate has an increased amount of fetal haemoglobin in the blood. This has a higher affinity for oxygen than adult haemoglobin so the oxygen dissociation curve is shifted to the left.
- Abdominal distension in a pre-term infant may indicate necrotising enterocolitis and may cause or increase respiratory distress. This is because the diaphragm, which is the main muscle of respiration in infants, is unable to work effectively against a distended abdomen.

Auscultation

The small size of an infant's chest means that localising findings in the chest is extremely difficult. Auscultation is really only useful for assessing air entry or listening for added sounds. In a ventilated pre-term infant, referred sounds, such as water in the ventilator tubing, can mask breath sounds or mimic crackles. In a non-ventilated pre-term infant, breaths are so small it can be impossible to hear anything at all.

Palpation

Crackles, including referred crackles, can easily be felt through the chest wall in infants.

PHYSIOTHERAPY TECHNIQUES

The physiotherapy techniques used in the treatment of neonates are similar to those used in adults and children. With the minimum of handling, these techniques should only be used if suctioning alone has not been effective.

Positioning and Postural Drainage (PD)

Body position affects ventilation and perfusion (V/Q) matching and PaO_2. Any position changes should be carried out extremely gently and carefully in order to minimise detrimental effects such as swings in blood pressure, PaO_2 and $PaCO_2$.

In the neonate, the prone position has been found to increase PaO_2 levels; supine is the least beneficial position (Dean, 1985). Neonates preferentially ventilate the upper lung in side lying (Davies et al., 1985). In the NNU, infants are usually nursed tilted head up as this position has been shown to increase PaO_2 in spontaneously breathing infants (Thoresen et al., 1988). However, pooling of secretions and atelectasis of dependent lung areas will occur if infants are left in one position for long periods. In infants, the right upper lobe is the area most commonly affected by collapse, particularly following extubation. Regular position changes, as tolerated by the sick infant, ensure that uppermost areas of lung are periodically drained and preferentially ventilated.

Specific postural drainage may not be appropriate in sick neonates, particularly the very pre-term. Infants who have unilateral lung disease may not tolerate the affected lung being uppermost for drainage of secretions. In this case, treatment is best given in the prone position, and these infants may need to be nursed with the unaffected lung uppermost in order to optimise gas exchange.

The head down position may be tolerated in full-term infants with lower lobe problems. However, this position should never be used for pre-term infants. It can cause hypoxia in spontaneously breathing infants and can increase the risk of PVH and gastro-oesophageal reflux (GOR). It is not well tolerated in infants with abdominal distension.

It is generally not practical to drain the apical segments of the upper lobes in the sitting position when infants are ventilated; the risk of dislodging the endotracheal tube is too great.

As pre-term infants are hypotonic and have soft, easily moulded bones, it is important to position them with a view to preventing or minimising postural deformities. Pre-term infants should be positioned with a flexed posture to avoid perpetuating the extended 'frog' posture they tend to adopt (Downs et al., 1991).

Manual Hyperinflation

The same precautious and contraindications apply for manual hyperinflation as in adults and children. This technique is less useful as a physiotherapy technique in infants, as the collateral ventilation channels, e.g. pores of Kohn, which allow diffusion of gas between alveoli and bronchioles, have not been identified in infants (Prasad, 1995).

Gas under positive pressure takes the line of least resistance so collapsed areas of lung will remain collapsed while being surrounded by areas of hyperinflation. Manual hyperinflation should not be used as a physiotherapy technique in pre-term infants as it increases the risks of barotrauma leading to PIE or pneumothorax. It can be used with caution in full-term infants provided the PIP used is limited to 20% above the PIP on the ventilator. Pressure should be monitored throughout by a manometer in the circuit. Detrimental effects can be reduced by giving one large hyperinflation interspersed with 3–4 tidal volume breaths (Hussey, 1992).

Percussion

In full-term infants weighing more than 3.0 kg, percussion can be given with the cupped hand. In pre-term infants, the middle fingers ('tenting') or padded cup-shaped objects, e.g. face masks, can be used.

Percussion seems to be better tolerated and more useful than vibrations in pre-term infants.

Vibrations

Vibrations can be effective in mobilising secretions in neonates because the chest wall is very compliant. However, this can also mean that the technique is less well tolerated, particularly in the pre-term infant, as vibrations increase intrathoracic pressure, reducing venous return to the heart, lowering cardiac output and increasing intracranial pressure. Vibrations to the left side of the chest have a similar effect to cardiac massage.

Vibrations are less useful in infants who are breathing or being ventilated at very fast rates because of the short expiratory time.

Precautions for percussion and vibrations

The use of percussion and vibrations should be avoided in very pre-term infants because they have thin fragile skin and are liable to bruise easily. These techniques should not be used in infants with osteoporosis as they may be implicated as the cause of rib fractures (Geggel et al., 1978). Fractures occurred in two infants with severe rickets, one of whom also had femoral and fibular fractures.

Suction

Suctioning should only be performed when secretions are present. It should never be carried out as a routine procedure. Suction may be necessary to maintain a clear airway but it is a potentially hazardous procedure, particularly in pre-term infants. The recognised side effects of suction are less common in paralysed and sedated infants (Fanconi and Duc, 1987).

Suctioning time should be kept to a minimum, e.g. 10 seconds in pre-term infants, to reduce the potential for hypoxia. Pre-oxygenation can prevent hypoxia but must be done with great caution in the pre-term infant to avoid a swing into hyperoxia and the risk of retinopathy of prematurity. Pre-term infants who are well oxygenated should only have their FiO_2 increased by 10%, e.g. by 40% immediately before passing the suction cathether. Following suction, the FiO_2 can again be increased if the infant continues to be hypoxic. Once recovery begins, the FiO_2 should slowly be reduced to the pretreatment level to avoid hyperoxia.

Pneumothorax has been reported due to perforation of a segmental bronchus by a suction catheter in pre-term infants with severe lung disease (Alpan *et al.*, 1984). The risk of perforation and mucosal trauma is reduced by only passing the suction catheter to only 1 cm past the end of the endotracheal tube. Suction catheters with centimetre markings are available to enable staff to know how far they are passing the catheter.

It is essential that good quality catheters are used, to reduce the amount of trauma. The optimum catheter should be smooth and well finished with a rounded tip. There should be an end hole with two small side holes to act as pressure relief outlets.

Ideally, the diameter of the catheter used should be less than 70% of the diameter of the endotracheal tube. In practice, the smallest catheter that is effective is a size 6 French gauge.

The amount of applied negative pressure used is important. If the pressure is too high more trauma will be caused, but if the pressure is too low thick secretions will not be aspirated up small bore catheters. Pressures should be set between 100 mmHg and 200 mmHg, depending on circumstances.

A gentle suctioning technique is essential, and the catheter should be withdrawn without a rotating motion or intermittently removing the thumb from the suction control port as such action can increase trauma and be less effective (Hough, 1991).

For infants not in an incubator, nasopharyngeal suction is important for clearing the upper airway but it can cause bradycardia and apnoea in the newborn. Suctioning must also be done with care in recently extubated infants in order to avoid aggravating laryngeal oedema.

Lavage

In many NNUs, suctioning is preceded by instillation of a diluent such as normal saline. The diluent may be instilled directly down the endotracheal tube or via a suction catheter (Downs, 1989).

The use of a diluent is thought to facilitate removal of secretions, and has been shown to reduce the risk of blockage of the endotracheal tube in one study (Drew *et al.*, 1986). In unparalysed infants, instillation of the diluent stimulates a cough, which may move secretions up the bronchial tree.

Humidification

Inadequate humidification of inspired gases in an intubated infant causes tracheobronchial secretions to become more viscous, and reduces mucociliary clearance. This may lead to blockage of the endotracheal tube.

In NNUs, heated humidifiers are usually used in ventilator circuits to adequately humidify inspired air. The humidifier temperature should be more than 36.5°C to reduce the risk of pneumothorax and CLD in VLBW infants (Tarnow–Mordi *et al.*, 1981).

CLINICAL INDICATIONS FOR PHYSIOTHERAPY

Physiotherapy is indicated when there is an increase or retention of secretions, or lobar collapse. Percussion and vibrations are only necessary if secretions have not been cleared by suction alone.

Lobar Collapse

If lobar collapse is caused by mucous plugging, the latter can be cleared with appropriate positioning and percussion, as tolerated by the infant.

When lobar collapse is caused by other problems, e.g. pulmonary interstitial emphysema in adjacent lung tissue, then physiotherapy techniques are of no benefit.

Meconium Aspiration

If an infant has inhaled meconium and initial attempts to remove it have been unsuccessful, then physiotherapy is essential. Positioning and vigorous percussion should be undertaken, preferably within 1 hour of aspiration, and continued regularly until meconium has been cleared. Treatment is usually well tolerated as these are mostly mature infants. If the meconium is not cleared, then a chemical pneumonitis develops. Physiotherapy is unhelpful at this stage as the lung becomes acutely inflamed and the infant is usually very unwell. Resolution of the pneumonitis may cause an increase in secretions, which may be cleared with positioning and percussion if suction alone is unsuccessful.

Aspiration of Feed/Vomit

Pre-term infants are prone to GOR and subsequent aspiration. Infants who have aspirated should be suctioned immediately to clear the airway. If this does not completely clear the lungs, then positioning and percussion, as tolerated, should be carried out as soon as possible.

In patients with recurrent aspiration due to GOR, physiotherapy may be unhelpful. Postural drainage, percussion and vibrations may aggravate GOR. Treatment should not be given in the horizontal or head down positions (Demont *et al.*, 1991). Physiotherapy should always be given before feeds and not before 1 hour afterwards.

In some cases the benefits of physiotherapy are outweighed by increased reflux and aspiration.

Chronic Lung Disease (CLD)

Infants with CLD may have persistent problems with increased secretions, so positioning and percussion may be helpful. If necessary, before discharge of the infant, parents should be taught the appropriate techniques.

In some infants wheeze and airway collapse are the main problems of CLD and these are aggravated by percussion and vibrations.

Careful assessment is needed in infants with CLD to ascertain whether physiotherapy is beneficial.

CONTRAINDICATIONS TO PHYSIOTHERAPY

Unstable Infant

Although there are rarely absolute contraindications to physiotherapy, the very unstable acutely ill infant should not be treated unless absolutely necessary.

Respiratory Distress Syndrome (RDS)

Physiotherapy is not indicated in early RDS as the main problem is lack of surfactant. Suction 12-hourly is sufficient to maintain a clear airway in early RDS (Wilson *et al.*, 1991). Routine chest physiotherapy in the first 24 hours of life in infants with RDS was associated with increased incidence of grade III–IV PVH when compared with suction alone (Raval *et al.*, 1987).

Pulmonary Haemorrhage

Severe acute bleeding from the lungs can occur spontaneously in pre-term infants and has also been associated with surfactant therapy.

Percussion and vibrations will aggravate bleeding, so are contraindicated. Careful suctioning to maintain a clear airway should be carried out as infrequently as possible.

When fresh blood is no longer being aspirated and secretions are brown and thick, then percussion and vibrations may assist clearance. If bleeding recurs treatment should be discontinued.

CONCLUSION

The NNU is not an area for the novice physiotherapist. The theoretical basis of management of neonates is complex. The treatment of acutely ill pre-term and term babies requires assessment skills beyond those developed in pregraduate training.

The role of the experienced physiotherapist in an NNU is to teach physiotherapy techniques to nursing staff, and to educate medical and nursing staff on the role physiotherapy has to play in the management of sick infants. The physiotherapist is also there to assess and treat infants with more complicated problems and to teach parents how to handle infants before discharge.

SPECIALISED VENTILATORY SUPPORT

This section covers two methods of unconventional ventilation (ECMO and VNEP) used successfully in the management of infants in a few specialist centres, and therefore not normally seen by physiotherapists. It should be noted that neither of these techniques is used exclusively with neonates. ECMO is also used in the treatment of adult ventilatory failure. Negative pressure ventilation (VNEP) in the form of 'iron lungs' was the only form of artificial ventilation before intermittent positive pressure ventilation (IPPV) was introduced in the 1960s. Both ECMO and VNEP are included here to assist the novice phyiotherapist in the management of infants and children who have undergone these forms of ventilation.

EXTRACORPOREAL MEMBRANE OXYGENATION (ECMO)

The origins of ECMO are related to the development of cardiopulmonary bypass techniques used to support patients undergoing cardiac surgery. The first patient to be successfully supported with ECMO was an adult with adult respiratory distress syndrome (ARDS). The patient was treated in 1972 by Hill in California (Hill *et al.*, 1972). In Michigan in 1975, Bartlett successfully supported a neonate with ECMO (Barlett, 1985). The use of ECMO in adults was abandoned in 1979, following poor results from a trial of ECMO versus conventional treatment for adults with ARDS, sponsored by the National Institute of Health of America (Zapol *et al.*, 1979). However, there has been a renewed interest in supporting adults with ECMO following the results of Gattinoni and co-workers (1986). Since then, the use of ECMO in all age groups has continued to develop. Commonly, the patients referred for ECMO have become unmanageable despite maximal conventional therapies. ECMO is practised within specialised centres and its use has spread world-wide.

ECMO enables prolonged extracorporeal life support of critically ill patients with reversible pulmonary and cardiac conditions for days or weeks, by using a modified heart–lung machine through extrathoracic cannulation. Access is achived either via a veno-arterial (VA) or venovenous (VV) route depending on whether the patient requires cardiorespiratory or respiratory support, respectively. Once the patient has been established on ECMO, the ventilator settings are reduced (Torosian *et al.*, 1995) to 'rest' settings: FiO_2, 30%; PIP, 20–25 cmH_2O; PEEP, 10 cmH_2O; respiratory rate 10 breaths/min. These 'rest' settings apply to neonates, children and adults. The reduced ventilator settings enable lung tissue to rest and recover from pathological or further ventilator-induced lung injury, i.e. barotrauma, volutrauma and oxygen toxicity, caused by high positive pressure ventilation with high oxygen supplementation.

A VA ECMO circuit is used if cardiac support is required. In addition, VA ECMO provides pulmonary support. Here blood is drained from the central venous circulation, commonly through the right internal jugular vein, and returned to the arterial circulation, commonly through the right carotid artery. This method offers circulatory support in the form of a partial to complete cardiopulmonary bypass. Associated with this is a reduction in the systolic diastolic gradient and a reduction of blood flow through the lungs, i.e. pulmonary hypoperfusion. VA ECMO supports cardiac function by capturing a proportion of the blood returning to the heart and therefore bypassing the heart. This enables the myocardium to 'rest' by reducing the preload on the right ventricle. As the blood is returned through an artery, the afterload on the left ventricle is increased. The disadvantages associated with VA ECMO include the possibility of microemboli being directly infused into the arterial circulation, and the carotid artery used for cannulation is likely to be ligated.

A VV ECMO circuit is used if pulmonary support is required. Here blood is drained from and returned to the venous circulation, e.g. draining from the right jugular vein and returning through the right femoral vein, or draining from the right femoral vein and re-infusing through the left femoral vein, or draining and re-infusing through the right atrium using a double lumen cannula. In VV ECMO, central venous pressures, pulmonary perfusion and cardiac output are unchanged, therefore VV ECMO does not provide any direct circulatory support. Because blood is drained from and re-infused into a venous system, some oxygenated blood will be re-circulated around the ECMO circuit. Despite this, the patient will still be adequately oxygenated so long as the circuit is managed at its optimum setting. Hypoxia, hypercarbia and acidosis cause pulmonary vasoconstriction that then leads to a further rise in pulmonary artery pressure, i.e. pulmonary hypertension.

Improved oxygenation counteracts these effects. ECMO ensures the patient is well oxygenated and carbon dioxide is adequately removed. As long as the underlying pulmonary condition is reversible, the pulmonary hypertension will resolve (Sosnowski et al., 1990). Often, the critically ill patient with worsening pulmonary function will also present with cardiovascular insufficiencies that require inotropic support. 'Hypoxic myocardial depression might be reversed by improvement in the ratio of myocardial oxygen delivery to consumption' (Cornish et al., 1993). Therefore as VV ECMO improves myocardial oxygenation the need for inotropic support decreases. 'Another advantage of VV perfusion is that, unlike VA ECMO, it preserves physiologic pulsatility. When compared to non-pulsatile flow, pulsatile flow decreases vascular resistance, decreases afterload and improves organ perfusion' (Cornish and Clark, 1995). The VV route also spares the ligation of the vessels used for cannulation (Peek et al., 1996).

All patients on ECMO are heparinised systemically with a continuous heparin infusion. Hence there is an increased risk of uncontrollable bleeding arising from heel sticks, venepunctures and intramuscular injections; they are therefore omitted. All drug infusions, parenteral

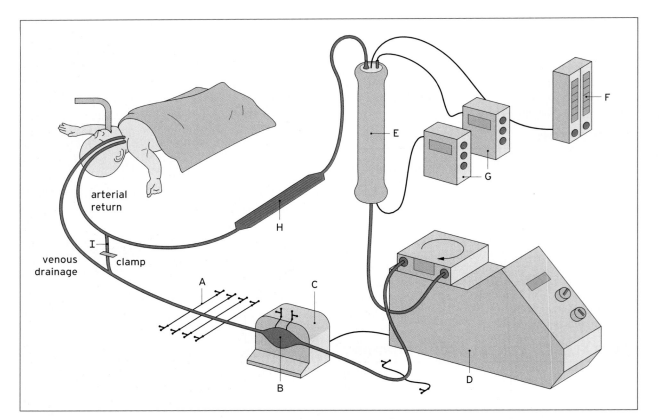

Figure 20.1 Diagram of a standard extracorporeal membrane oxygenation (ECMO) circuit.
(A) Series of 'pigtails' (3-way taps), (B) bladder, (C) bladder box, (D) semi-occlusive roller pump, (E) membrane oxygenator, (F) sweep gas control and supply, (G) membrane oxygenator pressure monitoring devices, (H) integral heater, and (I) bridge.

nutrition and haemofiltration (if required) are attached to the circuit. Activated clotting time (ACT) tests are performed at the bedside to determine the amount the heparin infused.

The Circuit

The integrity of the circuit (Figure 20.1) is constantly being reviewed by the ECMO specialist, who works closely with the nurse caring for the patient.

Blood is drained from the patient through the cannula by a gravity siphon (Bartlett, 1989). The blood then flows though polyvinylchloride (PVC) tubing past a series of 'pigtails'. These pigtails are access routes for the administration of intravenous medication and parenteral nutrition. If the patient goes into acute renal failure, the pigtails also offer access for the attachment of a haemofiltration circuit. The blood then flows into a small distendable bladder that is fitted to the bladder box, which is a pressure sensitive device that is linked to the roller pump. The bladder box servoregulates the circuit. The bladder collapses when venous drainage is impaired, triggering a microswitch that cuts off the pump, thus preventing the roller pump from generating a negative pressure. Inadequate venous drainage may be due to hypovolaemia, mediastinal shift caused by a pneumothorax or the occlusion of the drainage cannula. The tubing is fitted into a semi-occlusive roller pump that serves to generate the forward flow of the blood through the circuit. From the roller pump, the blood passes through the membrane oxygenator where it is oxygenated and carbon dioxide is removed. The membrane oxygenator is made of a spiral wound silicon envelope. Blood flows around the outside surface of the membrane envelope and oxygen is fed through the inside surface thereof, thereby allowing gaseous exchange to occur by diffusion across the membrane. The blood flows counter-current to the gas supply to allow the most efficient diffusion gradient. The gas flow rate through the oxygenator is known as the 'sweep rate', which determines the amount of carbon dioxide that will be blown off. The oxygen uptake capacity is determined by the 'flow rate' of the blood through the membrane oxygenator. From the oxygenator, the blood flows through a heat exchanger to ensure that any heat that may have been lost while the blood passed through the extracorporeal circuit is normothermic before it is returned to the patient. Maintaining normothermia is important to enable enzymes and clotting factors to function optimally.

The section of the circuit that precedes the pump is regarded as the venous side of the circuit and the section of the circuit after the pump, as the arterial side of the circuit. There is a connection between the venous side of the circuit and the arterial side of the circuit near the patient. This is known as the 'bridge'. The bridge serves to isolate the patient from the circuit while still enabling the circuit to operate. This serves as a safety feature in the event of any circuit problems and it is also used in VA ECMO trial off. Normally, this bridge is occluded by a clamp to prevent mixing of the arterial and venous sides of the circuit. To prevent the bridge from being occluded by a clot, the clamp is released regularly to allow blood to flush through the tubing.

Trial off ECMO

As the patient's clinical condition improves, ECMO support may be weaned. Once the patient reaches the minimum ECMO support, a procedure called a 'trial off' is carried out. With VA ECMO patients, complete isolation from the circuit is required. The venous drainage tube and arterial return tube are both clamped above the bridge. The bridge then enables the circuit to operate while 'trialling' the patient off ECMO support. With VV ECMO patients, a trial off the circuit simply involves the removal of the gas supply to the oxygenator. Regular arterial blood gas samples are taken during the trial off to assess the exchange capabilities of the lungs. Decannulation is carried out once adequate gas exchange on reasonable ventilator settings has been demonstrated and the patient is cardiovascularly stable. VA ECMO decannulation requires surgical removal of the cannulae.

PHYSIOTHERAPY CARE

The management of the ECMO patient requires a co-ordinated multidisciplinary team effort. It is essential that the physiotherapist is aware of the current patient care plan by communicating effectively with ECMO specialists, nurses and medics. This information is then incorporated into the physiotherapist's assessment to optimise any physiotherapy intervention.

When the patient is established onto ECMO, good pulmonary care is essential to assist the recovery of the lungs. When assessing the patient, additional information to consider includes the clotting status and the amount of ECMO support the patient is requiring. If the clotting status is greatly deranged, manual techniques and suctioning may trigger intrabronchial bleeding. Some of the patients may demonstrate severe ventilator-induced injury, presenting as pneumothoraces, PIE and/or a pneumomediastinum. In such situations, since ECMO supports the patient, the use of manual techniques should be delayed until the clotting status is within an acceptable range and the air leaks slow down or stop. In the presence of severe barotrauma, ventilation could be completely stopped and the patient kept on CPAP of 5–10 cmH$_2$O for 1–2 days to allow the air leaks to resolve. Commonly, the chest X-ray often worsens in the first 24 hours on ECMO. On auscultation, breath sounds may be very quiet or non-existent. The breath sounds tend to improve before radiological changes are evident.

The patient may be turned side to side to facilitate the drainage of pulmonary secretions (Cornish and Pettignano, 1995). If necessary, a head down tip to drain basal segments of the lung may also be carried out on adult and paediatric patients. When positioning the patient, great care should be taken to ensure the ECMO cannulae are unaffected. Therefore any movement of the patient should be carried out in the presence of the ECMO specialist to ensure the cannulae are still intact, secure and unoccluded during and after the manoeuvre.

ECMO patients often need to undergo aggressive diuresis. Subsequently, pulmonary secretions tend to become more tenacious. Bagging, after discussion with the consultant, and manual techniques such as percussion and vibrations may be employed to help mobilise secretions. Endotracheal suctioning should be performed at a frequency dependent on the amount of secretions produced. The instillation of saline may precede suctioning procedures to assist the removal of secretions (Bostic and Wendelglass, 1987). The amount of saline instilled is variable and dependent on assessment. Typically, larger amounts of saline can be used, with good effect, without any adverse reactions when compared with conventionally ventilated patients.

The careful positioning of the patient's limbs is important to prevent joint strains and contractures. Passive movements are carried out on adults. However, hip flexion movements that may affect groin cannulation sites should be avoided. With neonates, supporting their hips and shoulder girdles in a more physiological range using a rolls or padding reduces the need for handling.

It is important that the physiotherapist informs the nurse and ECMO specialist of preferred patient positions to assist with the continuity of pulmonary and joint care. These positions may then be incorporated into nursing careplans.

NEGATIVE PRESSURE VENTILATION (VNEP) OF NEONATES AND CHILDREN

There are reports of the use of VNEP as early as 1832. The early devices used hand-operated bellows or pumps to create negative pressure, which limited their application. However, the development of electrically powered bellows and the epidemics of poliomyelitis between 1910 and 1960,

led to a much wider use of VNEP. The ventilator was commonly known as the 'iron lung'. But the growing use of IPPV in the 1960s and 1970s led to a decline in the use of the iron lung. However, since the late 1980s, due to some technical improvements in design, there has been a renewed interest in the use of VNEP, especially in the management of neonates and young children (Figure 20.2).

The ventilator consists of a perspex tank, an electrical pump and some rigid hosing which connects the two. The tank rests on a bed or cot. Negative extrathoracic pressure ventilation is available in two modes, continuous negative pressure ventilation (CNEP) and intermittent negative pressure ventilation (INEP).

In both forms of VNEP, the child's body is sealed, at the neck, into the perspex chamber. A small opening in the lower third of a flat sheet of latex is cut and passed over the infant's head (like a tight fitting poncho). The latex is then secured to the outside of the tank to provide an airtight fit. The pump draws air out and creates a sub-atmospheric pressure around the chest wall. It is this pressure difference, between the inside and the outside of the chamber, that causes the airways to open and, if sufficiently high, draws air into the child's lungs via the nose or mouth.

APPLICATION
VNEP can be applied in one of two ways—as a continuous low negative pressure to support the child's own respiration or as an intermittent high negative pressure to provide artificial ventilation.

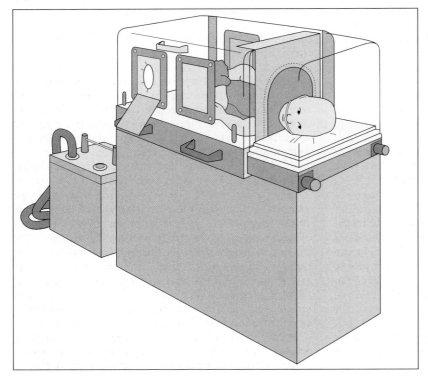

Figure 20.2 The negative pressure ventilation (VNEP) tank.

Continuous Negative Pressure Ventilation (CNEP)

A constant negative pressure of −4 to −8 cmH$_2$O is applied to the chest wall throughout the respiratory cycle to assist ventilation. The negative pressure applied to the thorax increases the transpleural pressure, which expands the lungs, opening up the small airways, and then acts like a splint to prevent collapse. CNEP is used to reduce the work of breathing in infants who are self-ventilating or to reduce the inflation pressure necessary to expand the lungs of infants receiving positive pressure ventilation.

Intermittent Negative Pressure Ventilation (INEP)

Alternate pressures of between −4 and −8 cmH$_2$O and between −20 and −30 cmH$_2$O are applied to the chest wall. While the low negative pressure acts to open up small airways, the high negative pressures cause air to be drawn into the lungs. As the negative pressure falls back towards atmospheric pressure, air is expelled from the lungs due to elastic recoil. INEP provides complete artificial ventilation without requiring intubation.

Supplemental Oxygen

Low flows of oxygen can be given via nasal cannulae while higher concentrations are best given via a headbox. The headbox is also the most effective way to provide humidification.

ADVANTAGES OF VNEP
Intubation

Unlike positive pressure ventilation, VNEP does not require the child to be intubated. Intubation is a difficult procedure, especially in neonates, and requires highly skilled staff both to carry out the procedure and to manage the intubated infant.

Sputum Retention

The presence of an endotracheal tube stimulates the production of secretions, which can lead to sputum retention. As intubation is not necessary for VNEP, secretions are less of a problem. Therefore suction is less likely to be required to maintain a clear airway than for a child on IPPV with an endotracheal tube *in situ*.

Oxygen Transfer and Cardiac Output

Studies have demonstrated that infants who are managed with VNEP compared with IPPV experience a decreased oxygen requirement. It is thought that VNEP leads to a reduced pulmonary vascular resistance, which improves oxygen transfer. It is also believed that VNEP does not reduce cardiac output to the same degree as IPPV.

Sedation and Weaning

As VNEP is well tolerated, the need for sedation is reduced. This is particularly important when trying to wean infants from ventilation.

Equipment

The equipment required to provide VNEP is simple to operate and maintain. It is also cheaper than a positive pressure ventilator. This has led to its use on general paediatric wards, and for a limited number of children in the home. Parents can learn to care for their child using the VNEP tank, and often manage their child with very little professional help.

DISADVANTAGES OF VNEP
Airway Obstruction

The main disadvantage of VNEP is that it may not be suitable for the management of infants with pre-existing upper airway obstruction. Negative pressure generated in the upper airways leads to further airway collapse. This may be overcome by the use of CPAP using either a face mask or a short nasopharyngeal tube.

INDICATIONS FOR THE USE OF VNEP
Short-term Respiratory Support

VNEP can be used to treat respiratory failure of any origin except in the presence of upper airway instability. However, there are some conditions where its use has significant advantages over positive pressure ventilation, e.g. RDS and CLD.

Long-term Respiratory Support

In conditions where respiratory support is likely to be required for many months or even years, VNEP is the ideal choice of ventilation as it provides the infant with the most realistic chance of going home. Conditions that have been treated include congenital myopathy, phrenic nerve palsy and central hypoventilation syndrome.

PHYSIOTHERAPY FOR INFANTS IN VNEP TANKS
Respiratory Care

Physiotherapy may be performed with the infant in the tank while it is receiving ventilatory support or, if the condition permits, during a short period out of the tank. As with all physiotherapy, liaison with the nursing and other medical staff is essential when planning the child's treatment programme.

If physiotherapy is to be carried out while the child is out of the tank, close monitoring of the child's respiratory status must be maintained. A fall in oxygen saturation or a rise in the level of carbon dioxide may indicate that the child is tiring and needs to be returned to the tank.

If physiotherapy is to be carried out in the tank, access is gained through the portholes. For an infant receiving INEP, the portholes should be opened during the expiratory phase, as this causes least disruption to ventilation. The physiotherapist should quickly insert his or her arms as far as possible into the tank, then draw them back to a comfortable position. This action allows the elasticated cuffs to make a good seal. A full assessment and treatment can be completed with the child in the tank, although there are some additional considerations when treating an infant on VNEP.

Treatment notes

Auscultation is possible although the noise of the pump can make this more difficult to interpret. Positioning the infant is limited as the mattress inside the tank is maintained in a headup tip of 10–20 degrees. However, the infant can be nursed in side lying, supine or prone positions. Changing the infant's position requires two people: one person to release and turn the infant's head, by inserting his or her fingers inside the latex around the infant's neck, and one person to turn the infant's body, by inserting his or her arms into the tank.

Percussion, especially in neonates, is best applied using a soft cup-shaped object such as the Bennett face mask. It can be difficult to percuss the apical lobes as the latex seal may be drawn into the tank covering the upper chest.

Manual hyperinflation is rarely indicated, and when it is used, the VNEP pump must be switched off to reduce the risk of pneumothorax. If manual hyperinflation is indicated in an emergency, the portholes should be opened.

After any procedure where the portholes have been opened, it is necessary to check that the pump is able to achieve the required pressure. Failure to reach sufficient negative pressures will occur if there is a leak in the system or a porthole is not properly closed.

Normal development

All infants nursed in a tank will need encouragement to develop normally. Special attention must be given to those infants who are likely to require negative pressure support for long periods. The physiotherapist has an important role to play in assessing the infant's development and the planning regimens that are geared towards achieving developmental milestones. However, it is the parents, play therapists and nurses who are most likely to actualise these plans so they must be involved in assessment and goal setting.

Infants should be encouraged to look around, so toys and mobiles must be within focus. In addition, parents, nurses and therapists must get close enough to make eye contact. Own-body recognition and eye–hand co-ordination also must be learned by the infant. If the infant is nursed in the tank, large mirrors may be useful to achieve this. If the infant is able to come out of the tank for short periods, play should be directed to gaining head control and later sitting balance.

REFERENCES

Alpan G, *et al*. Pneumothorax due to endotracheal tube suction. *Am J Perinatol* 1984, **1:**345-348.

Apgar V. A proposal for a new method of evaluation of the newborn infant. *Curr Res Anaes Analgesia* 1953, **32:**260-267.

Bartlett RH. Esperanza (ASAIO Presidential address) *Trans ASAIO* 1985, **30:**723-725.

Bartlett RH. Extracorporeal life support in neonatal respiratory failure. *Surg Rounds* August 1989:41-50.

Bostic J, Wendelgass ST. Normal saline instillation as part of suctioning procedure. *Heart Lung* 1987, **16:**532-536.

Cornish JD, Clark RH. Principles and practice of venovenous extracorporeal membrane oxygenation. In: Zwischenberger JB, Bartlett RH, eds. *Extracorporeal cardiopulmonary support in critical care*. Ann Arbor: Extracorporeal Life Support Organisation; 1995.

Cornish JD, Heiss KF, Clarke RH, Strieper MJ, Boecler B, Kesser K. Efficacy of venovenous extracorporeal membrane oxygenation for neonates with respiratory and circulatory compromise. *J Paed* 1993, **122(1):**105-109.

Cornish JD, Pettignano R. Clinical management of neonates on VA ECMO. In: Zwischenberger JB, Bartlett RH, eds. *Extracorporeal cardiopulmonary support in critical care*. Ann Arbor: Extracorporeal Life Support Organisation; 1995.

Crowley P, Chalmers I, Keirse M. The effects of corticosteroid administered before pre-term delivery: an overview of evidence from controlled trials. *Br J Obstet Gynaecol* 1990, **97:**11-25.

Davies H, *et al*. Regional ventilation in infancy. *New Engl J Med* 1985, **313:**1626-1628.

Dean E. Effect of body position on pulmonary function. *Phys Ther* 1985, **65:**613-618.

Demont B *et al*. Effects of respiratory physical therapy and nasopharyngeal suction on gastro oesophageal reflux in infants less than a year of age with or without reflux. *Arch Fr Pediatr* 1991, **48:**621-625.

Downs J. Endotracheal suction: a method of tracheal washout. *Physiotherapy* 1989, **75:**54.

Downs J, *et al*. Effect of intervention on development of hip posture in very pre-term babies. *Arch Dis Child* 1991, **66:**797-801.

Drew J, Padoms K, Clabburn SL. Endotracheal management in newborn babies with hyaline membrane disease. *Aust J Physio* 1986, **36:**3-5.

Fanconi S, Duc G. Intratracheal suctioning in sick pre-term infants: prevention of intracranial hypertension and cerebral hypoperfusion by muscle paralysis. *Pediatrics* 1987, **79:**538-543.

Gattinoni L, Pesenti A, Mascheroni D, *et al*. Low frequency positive pressure ventilation with extracorporeal CO_2 removal in severe acute respiratory failure. *JAMA* 1986, **256:**881-885.

Geggel R, Pereio G, Spackman T. Fractured ribs: unusual presentation of rickets in premature infants. *J Pediatrics* 1978, **93:**680-682.

Greenough A. Common neonatal disorders. In: Prasad S, Hussey J, eds. *Paediatric respiratory care*. London: Chapman & Hall; 1995.

Greenough A, Milner AD. Prematurity and asthma–is there a link? *Curr Med Lit Paediatr* 1991, **4:**87-91.

Greenough A, Poole J, Greenall F, *et al*. Comparison of different rates of artificial ventilation in pre-term neonates with respiratory distress syndrome. *Acta Paediatr Scand* 1987, **76:**706-712.

Hill D, O'Brien TG, Murray JJ, *et al*. Extracorporeal oxygenation for acute post traumatic respiratory failure (Shock-lung syndrome); use of the Bramson membrane lung. *N Engl J Med* 1972, **286:**629-634.

Hough A. Methods to clear secretions. In: Hough A, ed. *Physiotherapy in respiratory care*. London: Chapman & Hall; 1991.

Hussey J. Effects of chest physiotherapy for children in intensive care after surgery. *Physiotherapy* 1992, **78:**109-113.

Morley C. Surfactant treatment for premature babies: a review of clinical trials. *Arch Dis Child* 1991, **66:**445-450.

Parker A, Downs J. Chest physiotherapy in neonatal ITU. *Paed Nurs* 1991, **3:**319-321.

Peek GJ, Firmin RK, Moore HM, Sosnowski AW. Cannulation of neonates for venovenous extracorporeal life support. *Ann Thorac Surg* 1996, **61:** 1851-1852

Prasad SA. Growth and development of the cardiorespiratory system. In: Prasad SA, Hussey J, eds. *Paediatric repiratory care*. London: Chapman & Hall; 1995.

Raval D, *et al*. Chest physiotherapy in pre-term infants with respiratory distress syndrome in the first 24 hours of life. *J Perinatol* 1987, **7:**301-304.

Sosnowski A, Bonser SJ, Field DJ, Graham TR, Firmin RK. Extracorporeal membrane oxygenation. *BMJ* 1990, **301:**303-304.

Tarnow-Mordi W, *et al*. Low inspired gas temperature and respiratory complications in very low birth weight infants. *J Pediatr* 1981, **114:**438-442.

Thoresen M, Cavan F, Whitelaw A. Effect of tilting on oxygenation in newborn infants. *Arch Dis Child* 1988, **63:**315-317.

Torosian MB, Bastwrous A, Statter MB, Arensman RM. Management of children with ECLS. In: Zwischenberger JB, Bartlett RH, eds. *Extracorporeal cardiopulmonary support in critical care*. Ann Arbor: Extracorporeal Life Support Organisation; 1995.

Wilson G, *et al*. Evaluation of two endotracheal suction regimes in babies ventilated for respiratory distress syndrome. *Early Hum Dev* 1991, **25:**87-90.

Zapol WM, Snider MT, Hill JD, *et al*. Extracorporeal membrane oxygenation in severe acute respiratory failure. *JAMA* 1979, **242:**2193-2196.

SECTION 5

RESEARCH AND AUDIT

RESEARCH AND CLINICAL AUDIT

CHAPTER OUTLINE

- Reliable data
- Valid data
- Evaluating a research paper
- Performing research

- Standards
- Outcome measures
- The audit cycle

INTRODUCTION

Research and clinical audit both require the systematic collection and objective analysis of validated and reliable data. Physiotherapists should understand the principles, even if not actively involved in the design and implementation of these projects. The two topics have the same ultimate aim: to improve the quality of care of patients. The two disciplines have fundamental differences, which are summarised below (Table 21.1). Research is a process which intends to further our knowledge. It is achieved by the collection of complex data in a precise and highly controlled manner. Clinical audit is the monitoring of standards in current practice based on our present knowledge. This involves the accumulation of simple and uncontrolled information, and comparing it with the expected results.

Using reliable and valid measuring tools is an essential part of both research and audit, therefore these two terms require defining.

RELIABLE DATA

A reliable measurement tool is one that will produce the same results when the study is repeated by a different person or using different equipment.

Example

Arterial blood gas analysis is highly reliable provided the analyser is calibrated and procedures are correctly followed.

Pulse oximetry is much less reliable and there can be a discrepancy of up to about 4% in saturations recorded above 80%. Reliability falls with poor peripheral perfusion, and, below 80%, decreases greatly. Reliability is also dependent on the manufacturer of the apparatus (Yelderman and New, 1983).

VALID DATA

Validity compares the results against those of another method of measuring changes; the greater the correlation between the two methods of testing, the higher the validity.

Example

The visual analogue for dyspnoea correlates well with changes in peak expiratory flow rate (PEFR) in asthmatics and patients with chronic obstructive pulmonary disease (COPD) (Gift, 1989).

To summarise, research and clinical audit tools are methods that respiratory physiotherapists can use to evaluate their treatments. Research takes a detailed look at a topic and audit will assess its effect on current practice and treatment. The rest of this chapter will introduce the principles of research and clinical audit in the context of physiotherapy respiratory care.

RESEARCH

Respiratory physiotherapy had its beginnings in an era before clinical trials routinely investigated the main effect, indication and side effects of a new technique. Experienced practitioners may know a technique will be effective on a particular patient, but lack the research evidence to back up their hypothesis. Currently the medical field demands such evidence and physiotherapists must address this problem.

EVALUATING A RESEARCH PAPER

Historically, very few respiratory physiotherapists have had the knowledge, self confidence, time or financial support to perform evaluative research. This is not restricted to respiratory care, but as a profession physiotherapists have been slow to realise the need to perform and publish the results of research (Parry, 1994), leaving a gap which has been filled by others. The greater part of published research in the medical journals evaluating the effects of respiratory physiotherapy has been performed by individuals with little understanding of our practice. Prescriptive physiotherapy has been replaced by assessment-based treatment over the past 20 years, but research is still being published and reference is often based on outdated clinical practice. These papers appear to evaluate the effects of physiotherapy, but all too often contain one or more flaws in their design. These include:

- Controlling the physiotherapeutic techniques, thus making them ineffective for the patients in the study.
- Not standardising the physiotherapy and/or not describing it.
- Applying prolonged and/or multiple physiotherapy techniques in a manner that would inevitably have detrimental effects on the patient.
- Applying the results from normal people to those with pulmonary pathology.
- Applying techniques to mobilise chest secretions to a group of patients without secretions.
- Not controlling non-physiotherapeutic sources of haemodynamic stress.

The results and conclusions of any studies containing these design errors should be treated with appropriate caution. Unfortunately does not occur, and sweeping generalisations are made about the effects of respiratory physiotherapy. In the case of percussion, these range from the technique being considered ineffective to it being considered so detrimental as to contraindicate its use.

Example

The use of manual hyperinflation and percussion on all intubated and ventilated patients was common practice in the 1970s, but as a result of published research (Gormezano and Braithwaite, 1972; Connors et al., 1980; Klein et al., 1988; Hammon et al., 1992) the use of both these techniques fell into disrepute. Accurate assessment should mean that the intubation and ventilation of a patient do not automatically infer that respiratory physiotherapy is necessary (Webber, 1991), while not meaning that manual hyperinflation or percussion are never indicated.

It is easy to dismiss most published research on the basis of its flaws. The research designs used are often described as experimental but as they are not performed under laboratory conditions discrepancies will occur. As all individual patients are inherently unique even if their diagnosis, age, sex and socioeconomic groupings are identical, clinical trials using patients can never be perfect. The skill of evaluating research papers lies in being able to distinguish between reasonable allowances and the unacceptable.

When reading a research paper, do not take what is written at face value. Is the paper written in a clear empirical manner without jargon? Highly complex papers give the impression of being very learned, but this may just be a smoke screen for indifferent research. Has the paper been printed in a reputable journal in which items have been peer reviewed? Then, the following questions about the paper have to be considered:

Title and Abstract

Is there a clear summary of the purpose, methodology, results and conclusions of the research?

Introduction and Literature Review

Is the hypothesis clearly stated, and is the literature review thorough, up to date and relevant?

Differences between research and clinical audit	
Research	**Audit**
One-off activity	Cyclical activity
Highly controlled variables	Uncontrolled variables
Looks to the future	Examines current practice
Extends current knowledge	Incorporates knowledge into current practice

Table 21.1 **Differences between research and clinical audit.**

Methodology

When looking at the methodology:

- Is the design described appropriate for testing the hypothesis?
- Is there only one variable tested?
- Is the control of other variables adequate?
- Is the subject sample unlikely to introduce bias?
- Is the data sensitive enough to measure changes?
- Is any apparatus used reliable and valid?

Results

Has the appropriate statistical analysis been used, and are tables and graphs clear, relevant and not open to misinterpretation?

Discussion

When reading the discussion:

- Are the results interpreted in an unbiased fashion?
- Are clinical and statistical significance clearly differentiated?
- Are any limitations of the research acknowledged?
- Are any practical implications presented?
- Are any generalisations from a small sample to the population appropriate?

If the answer is yes to all these questions, then the contents of the research paper should be viewed with respect. The paper may present results which contradict the current basis of treatment but this does not mean the paper should be dismissed. The purpose of research is to increase knowledge, and if we ignore good quality research it will be to our peril!

PERFORMING RESEARCH

The number of respiratory physiotherapists in full time research posts is small, and until this is rectified the gap needs to be filled by practising clinicians. This is daunting to the many physiotherapists educated by diploma. The graduates of BSc (Physiotherapy) courses containing an element of research as part of the final grade, are bringing the ethos of research to the practical field.

Embarking on a research project needs careful consideration. Are there enough suitable subjects to test your hypothesis on? The project may take many months to finish, therefore you need to be very interested in the area you are researching. Enthusiasm tends to wane if you encounter problems, so set yourself short-term target dates for completing the literature search, protocol and data collection to reduce the chances of getting bogged down in one section.

The basic steps to be taken to perform research are outlined below:

Identify the Topic

The idea for a topic can arise for many reasons, for example, the initial thought of why? what? how? when? may be a puzzle that has just occurred to you as a result of treating a patient, reading someone else's research, seeing a new piece of apparatus, or observing an old technique being applied in a different environment.

Perform a Literature Search

This should look into the subject in depth and breadth. Examine papers published within the past 5 years. If there are few available, extend the search to 10 years. Searches have been made quicker by computer but choose your key words carefully to avoid wasting time.

Form a Hypothesis

This is a statement of what the research expects to prove. It is usually stated in the null form (H°), i.e. there is no difference between the results from the treatment group and those from the control group; this is to encourage greater objectivity.

Design the Study

Deciding what and how data are to be collected is dependent on the nature of the H°. If the research requires quantitative results (e.g. Does stair climbing affect the restrictive lung defect after coronary artery surgery?) the number of stairs climbed and the pulmonary function test results are numeric data which produce objective and reliable results. When the question is qualitative (e.g. Has breathing re-education had an effect on the quality of life of a chronic hyperventilation patient?) the data required will be subjective, and therefore the answers then have to be given a numeric score for statistical analysis. For any design, use of a previously validated and reliable testing method will enhance the credibility of the study.

A clinical trial, single case study and questionnaire are the commonest research designs used in physiotherapy. No design is ideal for all circumstances; each has its advantages and faults (Table 21.2) and in a particular situation the researcher must choose the most appropriate to test the hypothesis.

Produce a Research Protocol

A research project involving patients will require permission from their consultant and from the health authority's ethics committee. A written protocol, outlining the aims and means of the project, will have to be submitted to this committee. This short description of the study should include the title, researcher, hypothesis, a brief literature review, the research methodology, any personnel involved and how ethical issues will be dealt with. This should be addressed to the ethics committee, giving them plenty of time to consider the proposal before you intend to commence. A similar protocol including a breakdown of the costs can also be used to obtain funding in the form of money or equipment from a relevant company or charity, or a research grant. If the project has been funded it must be acknowledged when the results are published.

Perform a Pilot Study

This tries out the research methodology on a small sample to spot any problems with the design. The data from the pilot group should not be included in the main samples results.

Advantages and disadvantages of research designs		
	For	**Against**
Clinical trial	Rigorous	Control difficult
	Able to generalise	Physiotherapy rarely standard Unethical to withhold treatment
Single case study	Good for generating a hypothesis	Not able to generalise No statistical analysis
	Patient acts as own control	May be confused with descriptive case studies
Questionnaire	Easy to collect data from a scattered population	Bias introduced by having results from a self-selecting group of responders
	How the patient feels	Depth limited by number of questions

Table 21.2 Advantages and disadvantages of research designs.

Collect the Data

Data should be collected by a person who does not know the hypothesis, to prevent the researcher introducing bias to the results. This is not always possible and in those cases this should be acknowledged in the results.

Analyse the Data

Simple data can be analysed by taking averages or plotting graphs but complex data requires statistical analysis to determine its significance. Statistical analysis has been made much easier by the introduction of specific computer software available at postgraduate centres or local universities. There may be some facilities available to help you in this task.

Make Conclusions

Has the H° been proven? Decide what the implications of the results are, and if further research is needed.

Publish

The results can be disseminated by oral or poster presentations at seminars, conferences etc., but to reach the widest audience the research needs to be written in a clear concise manner, and sent to a reputable refereed journal.

CLINICAL AUDIT

The Department of Health define clinical audit as 'the systematic and critical analysis of the quality of medical care, including the procedures used for diagnosis and treatment, the use of resources and the resulting outcome and quality of life for the patient' (Department of Health, 1989). Data comparing the functioning of each health authority to the national standards of practice have to be collected by all departments. The increasing demand for evidence-based practice throughout the acute sector encourages physiotherapists to evaluate their skills. This can be done through clinical audit. Also, if a change in practice is required due to external forces, physiotherapists can use the audit to monitor its effects on patients, by looking at objective outcomes or subjective measures, e.g. patient satisfaction.

CLINICAL AUDIT AND THE PHYSIOTHERAPIST

The Department of Health has demanded that clinical audit forms part of the normal routine of health-professional practice. Physiotherapists may perform the audit themselves or employ their health authority audit department to perform the data collection and analysis for them. As audit projects are dependent on the analysis of available data, keeping accurate written clinical notes is the responsibility of all physiotherapists.

Physiotherapists contemplating a clinical audit are not limited to evaluating their professional practice in isolation; as we are part of the multidiciplinary team, the patient outcome is not normally purely as a result of only our intervention.

Example

Following routine cardiac surgery, early mobilisation combined with instruction in supported coughing is effective in the prevention of post-operative chest infection. If all routine patients are to be mobilised, the nursing staff need to be involved in the continuation and encouragement of this practice outside normal working hours. In addition, the medical staff have to be aware of the need to prescribe appropriate and adequate analgesia for the patients to be able to cough effectively.

STANDARDS

Setting standards is an integral part of clinical audit, providing a baseline from which to compare. The Association of Chartered Physiotherapists in Respiratory Care (ACPRC) has set 15 standards in respiratory care (ACPRC, 1994). These cover patient referral, assessment and treatment. There are also standards for emergency work and professional development. In addition to national standards, each health authority will have locally agreed guidelines for some treatments, e.g. the use of respiratory equipment, continuous positive airway pressure, biphasic positive airway pressure, and negative intermittent positive pressure. Both standards and guidelines can be audited by a variety of means including examining documentation, comparing outcomes, peer review, or patient satisfaction survey, whichever is the most applicable.

OUTCOME MEASURES

Research and evaluation of respiratory care have been hampered by the shortage of reliable and valid outcome measures. The effectiveness of a treatment for sputum retention could be evaluated by measuring the amount of sputum production, but is volume or weight the more reliable test? The clearance of sputum does not affect pulmonary function tests or radio-isotope clearance, and therefore is not a valid measure. A valid outcome for the treatment of this problem would give an indication that the patient was less distressed or had a reduced work of breathing on re-assessment.

A few measures have been identified as either reliable or valid and are listed below (Table 21.3). Choose your outcome measure carefully to be sure you can identify changes in the patient's status.

THE AUDIT CYCLE

Audit looks at how research has affected practice. As identified at the beginning of this chapter, clinical audit is a cyclical activity, involving studying current practice, changing as appropriate and then reviewing the effects of the change. This is commonly called the audit cycle (Figure 21.1), and is the recognised plan for producing a clinical audit. The procedure is described in more detail below.

Identify Area for Review

This could be a problem, new technique, change in work practice or a new standard.

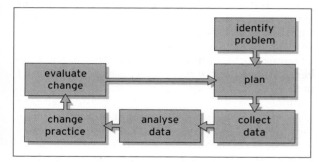

Figure 21.1 Audit cycle.

Plan

The condition

The causes and the normal progression of the medical condition need to be identified, so that the effect any physiotherapy has can be measured. Examples are:
- The natural progression of cystic fibrosis is prolonged deterioration in pulmonary function. The effect of physiotherapy can be measured taking this progression into account.
- Post-operative lobar atelectasis after upper abdominal surgery without concurrent infection will resolve when the patient becomes mobile. Routine physiotherapy for these patients cannot be justified if the patient is mobile.

The treatment

Perform a literature search looking for evidence of the effectiveness of the physiotherapy treatment.

The standard

Based on the research, decide on the standard or locally agreed guideline that is to be tested.

The analysis

Select an appropriately sensitive outcome measure (Table 21.3).

Collect the Data

Devise a system of data collection, and select the personnel responsible for gathering them. The data need to be collected from a large sample of patients, at least 10% of the annual patient load (a higher percentage if the total number of patients per annum is less than 100), so that the results are not influenced by patients on the extremes of the sample.

Analyse the Data

This can be in the form of averages or frequencies, comparing the results with the expected outcome from the literature.

Present the Results

Present the results to the relevant managers, with recommendations for changes in practice, service or funding.

Change Practice

The audit results may mean implementing a change in practice. To ensure this change is working, the cycle is then repeated. To ensure standards are maintained a periodic review is recommended.

Three different examples of clinical audit are briefly outlined below:

Example 1

Problem: A large number of patients with COPD in exacerbation have been admitted to the unit. On assessment it has been noted that many have been unable to use their bronchodilator inhaler effectively.

Audit: Does the patient have any reversible airway obstruction? If yes, can the patient effectively use the inhaler?

Outcome measures		
Measure	**Reliability**	**Validity**
Auscultation	50%	
Chronic Respiratory Disease questionnaire	Stable patients 90%	More sensitive to clinical change than 6 minute walk or Visual Analogue Scale
Peak expiratory flow rate	Diurnal variation up to 20% in normal subjects	
Percussion (diagnostic)	55%	Poor—improves if lesion <5 cm below surface or >3 cm size
Pulmonary function tests	FVC highly reliable but poor sensitivity to slight or moderate abnormalities	
Pulse oximetry	Dependent on machine used When perfusion is poor, SO_2 very unreliable	SO_2 80–100% with a range of +/- 4%. Increasingly invalid with hypoxia compared with arterial blood gas analysis

Table 21.3 **Outcome measures.**

- Use PEFR before and after to confirm visual assessment.
- Who prescribed the inhaler?
- Who taught its use?
- Produce data and present to medical staff.
- Change practice: In-service training for those involved in patient management, i.e. doctors, practice nurses and community physiotherapists.
- Re-audit: Is there a change in results?

Example 2

A pulmonary rehabilitation programme has been set up and its effect needs to be evaluated. Research shows that patients participating in the programme will show no benefits in pulmonary function tests but the chronic respiratory disease questionnaire is sensitive to changes. This audit can be extended into the multidisciplinary setting by monitoring the number of visits these patients make to their doctor, and their admission rate to hospital before and after entry on the programme.

Example 3

Research shows that 20.5% of patients who have upper abdominal surgery will succumb to a chest infection (Dilworth and White, 1992). The local guideline states that all patients will be given an incentive spirometer and be encouraged to use this hourly. The number of proved chest infections can be used to evaluate this practice based on temperature, purulent sputum, positive sputum culture, raised white cell count, evidence of retained secretions, or consolidation on auscultation. The natural disease process shows that oxygenation will improve spontaneously after the first post-operative day, therefore this can not be used as an outcome measure.

CONCLUSION

Examining current research and performing clinical audit are now part of the respiratory physiotherapist's daily practice. The two areas are inextricably linked, with clinical audit looking at how research has affected our practice, for the benefit of our patients. Physiotherapists not actively researching need to remain up to date with current practice, e.g. attending courses, reading professional journals, participating in local and national respiratory interest groups. Finally, it must be remembered that the purpose of all this activity is to improve the quality of care of our patients.

REFERENCES

Association of Chartered Physiotherapists in Respiratory Care. *Standards for respiratory care*. London: Chartered Society of Physiotherapy; 1994.

Connors AF, Hammon WE, Martin RJ, Rogers RM. Chest physical therapy: the immediate effect on oxygenation in acutely ill patients. *Chest* 1980, **78:**559-564.

Department of Health. *Medical audit working paper 6*. London: HMSO; 1989.

Dilworth JP, White RJ. Postoperative chest infection after abdominal surgery: an important problem for smokers. *Respir Med* 1992, **86:**205-210.

Gormezano J, Braithwaite MA. Effects of physiotherapy during intermittent positive pressure ventilation. *Anesthesia* 1972, **27:**258-264.

Hammon WE, Connors AF, McCaffree DR. Cardiac arrhythmias during postural drainage and chest percussion of critically ill patients. *Chest* 1992, **102:**1837-1841.

Klein P, Kemper M, Weissman C, Rosenbaum SH, Askanazi J, Hyman AI. Attenuation of the hemodynamic responses to chest physical therapy. *Chest* 1988. **93:**38-42.

Parry A. Physiotherapy journals—why bother? *Physiotherapy* 1994, **80:**22-27.

Webber BA. Evaluation and inflation in respiratory care. *Physiotherapy* 1991, **77:**801-804.

Yelderman M, New W. Evaluation of pulse oximetry. *Anesthesiology* 1983, **59:**349-352.